AUDITORY DISORDERS IN SCHOOL CHILDREN

THIRD EDITION

AUDITORY DISORDERS IN SCHOOL CHILDREN

The Law • Identification • Remediation

THIRD EDITION

Ross J. Roeser, Ph.D.
Director, Callier Center for Communication Disorders
Professor, Program in Communication Disorders
University of Texas at Dallas
Dallas, Texas

Marion P. Downs, M.A., D.H.S.
Professor Emeritus, Department of Otolaryngology
Division of Audiology
University of Colorado
Health Sciences Center
Denver, Colorado

1995

Thieme Medical Publishers, Inc.
Georg Thieme Verlag • Stuttgart • New York

Thieme Medical Publishers, Inc.
381 Park Avenue South
New York, New York 10016

AUDITORY DISORDERS IN SCHOOL CHILDREN
Third Edition
Ross J. Roeser and Marion P. Downs

Library of Congress Cataloging in Publication Data
Auditory disorders in school children/edited by Ross J. Roeser and Marion P. Downs. — 3rd ed.
   p.   cm.
   Includes bibliographical references and index.
   ISBN 0-86577-550-8 (Thieme Medical Publishers). — ISBN 3-13-599803-7 (Georg Thieme Verlag)
   1. Hearing disorders in children.   2. School children—Diseases.   3. Hearing impaired children—
Rehabilitation.   I. Roeser, Ross J.   II. Downs, Marion P.
   [DNLM: 1. Hearing Disorders—in infancy & childhood.   2. Hearing Disorders—rehabilitation.
3. Remedial Teaching.   4. Education, Special—United States.   WV 271 A912 1994]
RF291.5.C45A85   1994
618.92 '0978—dc20
DNLM/DLC
for Library of Congress   94-23587
                                                                                                                  CIP

Important note: Medicine is an ever-changing science. Research and clinical experience are continually broadening
our knowledge, in particular our knowledge of proper treatment and drug therapy. Insofar as this book mentions
any dosage or applications, readers may rest assured that the authors, editors, and publishers have made every
effort to ensure that such references are strictly in accordance with the state of knowledge at the time of production of the book. Nevertheless, every user is requested to carefully examine the manufacturers' leaflets accompanying each drug to check on his own responsibility whether the dosage schedules recommended therein or the
contraindications stated by the manufacturers differ from the statements made in the present book. Such examination is particularly important with drugs that are either rarely used or have been newly released on the market.

Some of the product names, patents, and registered designs referred to in this book are in fact registered trademarks
or proprietary names even though specific reference to this fact is not always made in the text. Therefore, the
appearance of a name without designation as proprietary is not to be construed as a representation by the publisher
that it is in the public domain.

Printed in the United States of America.

5 4 3 2 1

TMP ISBN 0-86577-550-8
GTV ISBN 3-13-59980 3-7

CONTENTS

Part I. The Law

Part II. Identification

Part III. Remediation

PREFACE
TO THE
THIRD EDITION

In this third edition of *Auditory Disorders in School Children*, we have made significant modifications and provide innovative and new challenging concepts for those working with children having auditory disorders. You will note that throughout the text we pay particular attention to the use of person-first reference, that is, "hearing-impaired children" are "children with hearing loss," "deaf children" are "children with deafness," and so on. We are committed to making the individual with handicap first a person and then address the handicap. The *individual* child with an auditory disorder is a paramount concept we have promoted throughout this text.

Most educators and school administrators are now familiar with the laws that govern handicapped children; these laws change more quickly than the typical life expectancy of a textbook. However, in Part I of our text we present an update of issues dealing with the law.

In the second and third sections of our book, the materials cover unique material related to:

- New concepts in medical management
- Advances in screening techniques for auditory disorders and middle ear function
- New strategies in identifying and providing remediation for central auditory disorders
- Assistive listening devices as they relate to school-aged children
- Providing assistance to students with deafness with cochlear implants and tactile instruments
- Presenting a comprehensive listing of resource materials for use with students having hearing impairments
- Enhancing the self-image of children with hearing loss

This text brings together experts from all disciplines who present innovative ideas on how to provide help for the individual child with auditory disorders in the best possible way. Knowledge of material presented in this text is mandatory for students who are planning careers in the schools. All practicing clinicians working with school children having hearing impairment must also be aware of the contents of this book so that children with auditory disorders will be served appropriately and reach their maximum educational potential.

Ross J. Roeser
Marion P. Downs

ACKNOWLEDGMENTS

This volume was prepared in part as a result of the 1994 Bruton Conference on Advances In Educating Children Hearing Loss, held at the University of Texas at Dallas, Callier Center for Communication Disorders. The conference was underwritten by the David Bruton, Jr., Endowment Fund. We are very grateful to the David Bruton family for supporting the conference and enabling the scientific and clinical insights that developed from it. Over the past 11 years, the Bruton Endowment has promoted the exchange of innovative research and clinical knowledge at the Callier Center For Communication Disorders/UTDallas. We are pleased to acknowledge the contribution of the Bruton Endowment to the conference and this volume, recognizing that the exchange of knowledge that occurred will lead to improved clinical service delivery for young children with hearing impairments and will enhance research efforts and the delivery of services in the area.

We are also indebted to the help of Linda Sensibaugh, Jennifer Deming, M.S., and Georgeanne Self, M.S.; and to our contributors. Without their assistance and adherence to our short deadlines, we would never have met our demanding publication schedule.

Finally, thanks are extended to Miss Nelle Johnston and Mrs. Paula Dennard of the Foundation for the Callier Center. Their meaningful efforts in helping children with deafness have had a profound and lasting impact. We thank, admire, and respectfully salute them.

Ross J. Roeser
Marion P. Downs

CONTRIBUTORS

CAROL AMON, M.A.
Supervisor, Colorado Department of Education, Special Education Services, Denver, Colorado
Legislative Impact on the Education of Children with Auditory Disorders

R. RAY BATTIN, Ph.D.
Clinical Neuropsychologist-Audiologist, The Battin Clinic, Houston, Texas
Psycho-Educational Assessment of Children with Auditory Language Learning Problems

VIRGINIA BERRY, M.S.
Assistant Professor, Department of Speech and Hearing Sciences, University of Southern Mississippi, Hattiesburg, Mississippi
Classroom Intervention Strategies and Resource Materials for Children with Hearing Loss

KAREN A. CLARK, M.A.
Head, Education Division, Callier Center for Communication Disorders, University of Texas, Dallas, Texas
A Collaborative Framework for Intervention

CARL C. CRANDELL, Ph.D.
Assistant Professor, Callier Center for Communication Disorders, University of Texas at Dallas, Dallas, Texas (Currently–Assistant Professor, University of Florida, Gainesville, Florida)
Classroom Acoustics

MARION P. DOWNS, M.A., D.H.S.
Professor Emeritus, Department of Otolaryngology, Division of Audiology, University of Colorado, Health Sciences Center, Denver, Colorado
Contribution of Mild Hearing Loss to Auditory Language Learning Problems

CAROL FLEXER, Ph.D.
Professor, Audiology, School of Communicative Disorders, University of Akron, Akron, Ohio
Classroom Amplification Systems

M. SUZANNE HASENSTAB, Ph.D.
Professor, Assistant Director, Division of Audiology, Department of Otolaryngology, Medical College of Virginia, Richmond, Virginia
Remediation of Children with Auditory Language Learning Disorders

ROBERT W. KEITH, Ph.D.
Professor and Director, Division of Audiology and Vestibular Testing, Department of Otolaryngology, University of Cincinnati Medical Center, Cincinnati, Ohio
Tests of Central Auditory Processing

ROBERT E. KRETSCHMER, Ph.D.
Associate Professor, Special Education, Teachers College, Columbia University, New York, New York
The Psycho-Educational Assessment of Children with Hearing Impairment

JOAN LAUGHTON, Ph.D.
  Associate Professor, Department of Communicative Sciences and Disorders, University of Georgia, Athens, Georgia
  Remediation of Children with Auditory Language Learning Disorders

DAVID LUTERMAN, D.Ed.
  Professor, Communication Disorders, Emerson College, Boston, Massachusetts
  Counseling for Parents of Children with Auditory Disorders

HELEN McCAFFREY, Ph.D.
  Audiologist, Faculty Associate, Callier Center for Communication Disorders, University of Texas at Dallas, Dallas, Texas (Currently–Private Practice, Austin, Texas)
  Techniques and Concepts in Auditory Training and Speechreading

CAROLYN H. MUSKET, M.A.
  Clinical Lecturer, Communication Disorders; Coordinator, Assistive Devices Center, Callier Center for Communication Disorders, University of Texas at Dallas, Dallas, Texas
  Maintenance of Personal Hearing Aids
  Assistive Devices for Students with Hearing Impairments

ROSS J. ROESER, Ph.D.
  Director and Professor, Callier Center for Communication Disorders, University of Texas at Dallas, Dallas, Texas
  Audiometric and Immittance Measures: Principles and Interpretation
  Screening for Hearing Loss and Middle Ear Disorders In The School
  Cochlear Implants and Tactile Aids for the Students with Profound Deafness

PETER S. ROLAND, M.D.
  Associate Professor, Otolaryngology, University of Texas, Southwestern Medical Center at Dallas, Dallas, Texas
  Medical Aspects of Disorders of the Auditory System

SUSAN P. RUSSELL, M.A.
  Auditory Services Specialist, Auditory Programs, Montgomery County Public Schools, Rockville, Maryland
  Enhancing the Self Image of the Mainstreamed Child with Auditory Disorders

JOSEPH J. SMALDINO, Ph.D.
  Department Head and Professor, Communicative Disorders, University of Northern Iowa, Cedar Falls, Iowa
  Classroom Acoustics

DIANA L. TERRY, M.S.
  Communication Specialist, Dallas Regional Day School for the Deaf, Callier Center for Communication Disorders, University of Texas at Dallas, Dallas, Texas
  A Collaborative Framework for Intervention

The Law   I

INTRODUCTION

Federal legislation governing children with disabilities in the schools has a long and varied history, but the struggle for the landmark legislation currently affecting the schools began about two decades ago. At that time, children with disabilities were excluded overtly from public schools, and little was done to provide educational programs for them. With the enactment of milestone statutes, the plight of the child in the schools with disabilities has changed dramatically.

The Rehabilitation Act of 1974 (PL 93-112, Section 504) helped awaken public interest in the millions of children, youths, and adults with disabilities who suffered the indignity and despair of isolation, discrimination, and maltreatment as a result of their disabilities. This act provided qualified individuals with disabilities in the United States with the legal means to prevent exclusion from or participation in any program or activity receiving federal financial assistance solely by reason of their disabilities. Although Section 504 was landmark legislation in providing services for children with disabilities, there was still a problem. The most important legislation for school-aged children came when the Education for All Handicapped Children Act (PL 94-142) was enacted into law in November 1975. This act was originally introduced into the Senate as S.3614 on May 16, 1974. Through numerous and hard-fought debates, the law was adopted primarily based on the fact that only one half of the approximately 8 million children with disabilities requiring special education and related services were receiving an appropriate education. PL 94-142 became effective October 1, 1977, with a staggered timetable for full implementation. This law stated that by 1980 all children with disabilities aged 3 to 21 years must be provided with an appropriate education through the public school systems.

PL 94-142 has been labeled a "civil rights act for the disabled." This civil rights concept is based on seven guarantees to all children with disabilities and their parents specifically outlined in the law.

RIGHT TO AN EDUCATION

Until PL 94-142 was enacted, many children with disabilities were denied educational opportunities because of the philosophies that some children were uneducable and/or simply more trouble than their education was worth. In addition, education was denied simply because appropriate educational support was lacking in terms of personnel and programs. PL 94-142 guarantees the right of all children, disabled or not, to an education. This law assumes the basic premise that all children are capable of benefiting from an education and should not be excluded from educational opportunities.

RIGHT TO A FREE EDUCATION

PL 94-142 recognizes that states are obligated to finance education for all of its children, whether they are normal or disabled. This provision specifies that the educational services provided to a child with a disability should be "free." Free indicates that education, and the services necessary for an appropriate education, should be provided without charge to the parents. Costs covered under 94-142 include, for example, special tutoring or therapy, tuition, transportation, room and board in private settings, and so on. Financing of education by school systems is mandated so there will be no financial barriers to educational opportunities.

RIGHT TO AN APPROPRIATE EDUCATION

Because PL 94-142 operates on the premise that all children are educable given an appropriate program, the law mandates that an Individualized Educational Program (IEP) be developed for and provided to each and every child with a disability. The IEP is the heart of the law.

The IEP was mandated because of the apparent gross negligence reported in developing programs for children with disabilities. The IEP serves two basic purposes. First, it is a "blueprint" for the child's educational program; all of the special services for the child are included in the IEP. Second, the IEP helps determine the proper educational placement for the child. The proper educational placement means the setting most conducive to the accomplishment of the child's goals.

Under the concept of "appropriate" education comes the issue of comparability and access. Can or should appropriate education for a child with a disability be comparable to that of a child without disability? Limited program time, adequate personnel, and other such factors affect comparability. Access problems have to do with factors such as the availability of physical education and extracurricular activities, as well as a full range of services necessary for an appropriate education for the child.

PL 94-142 makes it clear that access to a full range of services is mandatory, and 13 related services are specified. For example, for the child with hearing impairment this requirement means that provisions must be made for the following audiological services:

(1) Identification of children with hearing loss.
(2) Determination of the range, nature, and degree of hearing loss, including referral for medical or other professional attention for the habilitation of hearing.
(3) Provision of habilitative activities, such as language habilitation, auditory training, speech reading (lipreading), hearing evaluation, and speech conservation.
(4) Creation and administration of programs for prevention of hearing loss.
(5) Counseling and guidance of pupils, parents, and teachers regarding hearing loss.
(6) Determination of the child's need for group and individual amplification, selecting and fitting an appropriate aid, and evaluating the effectiveness of amplification.

RIGHT TO A LEAST RESTRICTIVE ENVIRONMENT (LRE)

The LRE, as stated in PL 94-142, affords the child with a disability equal accessibility opportunity to an environment that would be the most appropriate and conducive to his or her specific academic, social, and emotional maturity. Explicit in the LRE concept is the statement that education with nondisabled children, in a neighborhood school, and in life with the family is the most normal environment.

With LRE comes the term "mainstreaming"—integrating the child into the normal classroom. The idea behind mainstreaming is that segregation is harmful; integration is beneficial. As stated in the law, the range of settings in which mainstreaming can occur includes:

(1) *The regular classroom.* Placement in the regular classroom must legitimately be considered for each child.

(2) *The regular classroom with itinerant instruction.* "Supplemental aids and services" in the regular classroom should be attempted before a more restrictive setting can be justified.

(3) *The regular classroom for all academic and nonacademic programs possible and the resource room for the remainder of the activities.*

(4) *Full time in a special class in a neighborhood school that has nondisabled children.*

(5) *Assignment to a special school as close to the child's home as possible.*

(6) *Educational services provided in a nonschool setting such as home, hospital, or institution.*

RIGHT TO DUE PROCESS

PL 94-142 states that parents have the right to be heard, informed, and involved. In addition, parents have the right to question and challenge decisions, be informed in writing of proposed actions and reasons for them, examine records, and evaluate results and have them explained. Moreover, parents have the right to agree or disagree, and if disagreement occurs they have the right to a hearing conducted by an impartial hearing officer. During this hearing, parents have the right to use their own witnesses, experts, and evaluators. If the parents speak in a foreign language, all communication must be in their native language or the assistance of an interpreter must be available.

The right to due process has given parents a powerful tool to be assertive when they feel it necessary. The overwhelming barrier that the schoolhouse door has often symbolized is now gone. No longer can children be changed in their placement, or dismissed or discharged from schools without the explicit knowledge and participation of the parents.

RIGHT TO CONFIDENTIALITY

PL 94-142 explicitly states that all records must be kept confidential. No identifiable data can be shared inappropriately or without the written consent of the parents or guardians. This safeguard is extended to all information, including results of evaluations, due process outcomes, LEA reports, and other such documents.

RIGHT TO NONDISCRIMINATORY EVALUATION

PL 94-142 mandates that diagnostic and educational evaluations cannot discriminate on the basis of race, culture, language, or communication methods. This ruling is based on the previous lack of recognition given to children with disability of "minority" cultures on test performance. The implications of this ruling are that tests must be appropriate and have been validated for each target population in question. In addition to being certified and qualified to do the testing, evaluators must be articulate in the child's native language or the provision for an interpreter must be made during testing.

In 1986, PL 94-142 was amended through PL 99-457 to lower the age of eligibility to 3 years. The Handicapped Infants and Toddlers Program was also established by PL 99-457 and lowered the age further to birth through age two for those who require early intervention services because they: (1) are experiencing educational delays; (2) have a diagnosed physical or mental condition that has a high probability of developmental delay; and (3) risk having substantial developmental delays if early intervention services are not provided.

In October 1990, PL 94-142 was further amended through 99-457. A significant change in 99-457 was that the name of the legislation was changed from *Education of the Handicapped Act to Individuals with Disabilities Education Act* (IDEA). PL 99-457 embraces the concept of parent–child intervention as the best way to serve infants and toddlers and establishes the Individualized Family Services Plan (IFSP). The IFSP is the cornerstone of current educational planning and must state precisely the types of early intervention services each infant or toddler will receive. These services must be determined with full participation of the parents. What effect has federal legislation had on children with auditory disorders in the schools? This section of our text deals with this topic.—*RJR, MPD*

LEGISLATIVE IMPACT ON THE EDUCATION OF CHILDREN WITH AUDITORY DISORDERS

1

Carol Amon

One of the greatest delusions in the world is the hope that the evils of this world can be cured by legislation.

—Thomas B. Reed, 1839–1902

All children with disabilities, including those with auditory disorders, must have available to them a free, appropriate public education in the least restrictive environment, which includes special education and related services designed to meet their unique needs.

Through enactment in 1975 of the Education of All Handicapped Act (Public Law 94-142), which has now become the Individuals with Disabilities Education Act (IDEA), the federal government appears to have guaranteed that all school children with auditory disorders will receive adequate education.[1-3] Section 504 of the Rehabilitation Act of 1973 also guaranteed that discrimination on the basis of disability would not occur in any program or activity that received federal financial assistance. Both IDEA and Section 504 were based on the concept of "protected class" status. They were conceived of as a response to national concern during the 1960s that many members of our society, including those with disabilities, had been prevented from enjoying their full civil rights due to discrimination.

Persons with auditory disorders, as part of the protected class, were ensured individual rights by having guaranteed access to all societal institutions, including schools, and by having additional support necessary to achieve that access. We were in the golden age of special education. Specialists in hearing assumed the responsibility for designing specific methodologies, curricula, classes, and supports for students with auditory disorders, and emphasis was placed on the need for a continuum of placement options ranging from regular classrooms to residential placement.

As a result of that legislation, however, advocates for persons with disabilities began to place heavy emphasis on the least restrictive environment (LRE) provisions, insisting that classes,

buildings, and transportation be accessible to all and that separate programs or accommodations for the disabled were not a satisfactory substitute. A great emphasis was placed on educating children with auditory disorders in regular schools and classrooms by some of these advocates, theorizing that placements in or closer to the regular classroom were somehow inherently less restrictive for all children with disabilities.

Some deaf consumers, parents, and professional personnel took great issue with this interpretation and application of the LRE provisions and suggested that regular settings may be completely isolating linguistically, psychologically, and socially for students with auditory disorders. In February 1988, the Commission on Education of the Deaf issued to the President and Congress of the United States its *Toward Equality: Education of the Deaf.* The Commission stated that it received more input regarding LRE than on any other issue, citing LRE as the issue that most thwarts attempts to provide an appropriate education to children who are deaf. It was the contention of many that a critical mass of deaf students is necessary for providing the intensive language-rich environment and social environment required for an appropriate education.

More recently, we have been bombarded with federal and state proposals for education reform in general. The kind of far-reaching education goals and standards envisioned in the "Goals 2000: Educate America Act," for example, are termed an economic imperative and a social imperative for a vital society. It is often suggested that such words as reform, inclusion, outcomes, diversity, and standards replace such words as compliance, LRE, mandates, access, and special education.

Much of the deaf community, on the other hand, does not see the integration of deaf people into hearing society as beneficial and has begun to insist that deafness is not a disability, but rather a linguistic minority or subculture. They are especially concerned about the integration of deaf students into regular public schools where they may become isolated and made to fit into a hearing world as opposed to embracing their own deaf "culture." They do not see as positive the medical and technological advances that may minimize the effects of hearing loss.

THE CHALLENGE

We have before us today federal and state legislation that "protects" students with auditory disorders, ensuring that they be identified and then provided with special education. This protected class status assumes that: (1) some populations have need for protection and to guarantee access, therefore, they must be identified objectively; (2) there is a need for unique instruction, curriculum, and support; (3) designated resources are needed to ensure that unique instruction occurs; and (4) funding should be tied directly to resources that are tied directly to identified students. We also have before us today general educational reform that suggests that we eliminate special education, moving to a unified system that embraces diversity and inclusion. This unified system assumes that: (1) no protected status is necessary and therefore identification is not necessary or desired and access is assumed for all; (2) all students need unique instruction for some things; (3) resources will be combined to provide a wide variety of instruction for all; and (4) funding should be combined to one source to allow maximum flexibility. Diametrically opposed to both of these positions is the voice of the deaf community who want neither designation as disabled nor inclusion, but rather recognition of deafness as a culture, allowing deaf persons to be educated within their culture.

Programming for students with auditory disorders is obviously a complex task. We know that these students can attain the same performance levels as those that are seen as desirable for all students, but that outcomes for these students often fall short of what most professionals and parents would consider acceptable. The major obstacle to resolving this problem appears to be the quest for a homogenous solution to the problems of a heterogeneous set of students. Whether we believe in the "protected class" status that current legislation addresses, a unified system which embraces societal and general educational inclusion, the recognition of deafness as a separate culture, all of the above or none of the above, the challenge before us is to provide each student with auditory disorders with an appropriate education. An appropriate education for each child is one that is designed by parents and educators in partnership and one that is instructionally differentiated to respond to the child's unique needs and goals. Each child must have the opportunity to develop language, communication skills, and a strong, secure identity at a rate commensurate with hearing children. This can only occur if programming is individualized, if a variety of placement options are available, and if an effective monitoring system is in place to assure growth commensurate with chronological age. Legislation, alone, neither ensures nor prohibits this from occurring.

Administrators, service providers, parents, and consumers need to concentrate on *what* each child with an auditory disorder needs and *how* this can best be learned by this specific child and spend less time debating *where* services to students with auditory disorders should be provided and *who* should provide them. When the emphasis in on *where* instruction occurs, students are made to fit into the existing systems of regular or special education based on the assumption that once the proper location has been determined, appropriate instruction is guaranteed. *What* a student needs and *how* he or she learns should drive *where* the service is provided and by *whom*.

IDENTIFICATION, LOCATION, AND EVALUATION OF CHILDREN WITH DISABILITIES

IDEA Regulation: 34 C.F.R. 300.128(a) Each State. . .must. . .ensure that (1) All children with disabilities, regardless of the severity of their disability, and who are in need of special education and related services are identified, located, and evaluated. . .

Federal legislation mandates that all children with disabilities who are in need of special education and related services are identified, located, and evaluated. Local unified systems would suggest that identification is not necessary but that the unique instructional needs would automatically be identified. Education within the deaf culture assumes that needs would be automatically known. Regardless of where these unique needs are identified or by whom, it is critical that we understand the physical, cognitive, linguistic, and emotional functioning of each child with auditory disorders and how this relates to his or her educational achievement and life skills performance.

The public must be made aware of the effects of hearing loss on a child's development, hearing screening opportunities must be available to all children on a year around basis, procedures must be in place for referring a child for audiological assessment, and follow-up procedures for medical treatment and educational evaluation and possible intervention must exist.

303.531 Before any action is taken with respect to the initial placement of a child with a disability in a program providing special education and related services, a full and individual evaluation of the child's educational needs must be conducted. . . .

303.532(3) The evaluation is made by a multidisciplinary team or group of persons, including at least one teacher or other specialist with knowledge in the area of suspected disability. (f) The child is assessed in all areas related to the suspected disability, if appropriate, health, vision, hearing, social and emotional status, general intelligence, academic performance, communicative status, and motor abilities.

The process of interpreting and sharing information about a student's current level of functioning, achievement, and performance provides the basis for individualization. Unlike diagnosis, which is focused on confirming the existence of a particular problem or deficit, evaluation refers to the process of putting together all information to construct a whole picture of the child.

The intended result of the evaluation process is the most complete understanding possible of the child. This can only be done by a collaborative team effort of parents and professionals integrating the unique information that each contributes. By sharing ideas and perspectives, the team enhances the quality of planning necessary to ensure an appropriate education.

Interpreting and reporting assessment results is often seen by professionals as a logical, effortless task for which most have been trained.

Parents, however, often view this process as frustrating, meaningless, and a waste of time. "Professionals spend several hours testing our children, but never share what it all means." "They take our kids apart by disciplines and never put them back together as whole children." "It feels like each professional must prove his or her worth by giving lengthy assessment reports that are meaningless to us and others." "They usually have already discussed and made decisions about our child and are there simply to tell us parents their conclusions." Interestingly, some professionals agree with these parental perceptions. "We've got to look good to these parents. If we don't meet ahead of time, we might say something that we don't all agree on and we can't disagree in front of the parents.

Parents should have an integral part in the evaluation process from the beginning. Just as each professional assesses functioning and prepares an assessment report, so should the parents. Proving them with a worksheet that asks them to note their child's strengths and areas of difficulty at home and in the community can facilitate this. The letter in Table 1–1, sent to parents at least 2 weeks prior to the meeting where assessment results are discussed, is suggested.

Table 1–1 Letter to Parents

Dear Parents:

For us to get a better understanding of your child's strengths and areas of difficulty, it would be helpful if you and your family would provide the information listed on the attached questionnaire. Your child may function differently at home than he or she does in school, and it is important that we know and understand these differences.

Please complete the questionnaire and bring it with you to the meeting, so that your information is used when we discuss your child's current level of functioning and needs. We look forward to working with you.

It is important that parents have the opportunity to think through and record their thoughts on their own and not through an interview process by a professional. It then becomes even more critical that the meeting in which these thoughts and observations are shared be structured in such a way as to allow parents to contribute their own information. Parents report that there is nothing more degrading and humiliating than to have a professional report for them. Statements such as "Mrs. Jones reported. . ." or "The child's father said. . ." or "During my interview with the family it was learned that. . ." serve no purpose other than to confirm the parents' feelings of insecurity and inadequacy.

An example of questions for parents is provided in Table 1–2 and may be useful; however, it is important to structure the questions to the language and socioeducational level of the parents.

Table 1–2 Sample Questions for Parents

1. What does your child hear at home?
2. How well does your child learn and remember things? How quickly does your child understand something new?
3. How does your child communicate at home with you, with his or her siblings?
4. How do you think your child views himself or herself? What does your family see as desirable and undesirable behaviors?
5. How well does your child follow directions? Does he or she have responsibilities at home?
6. What do you think your child needs to continue to learn and grow?
7. What would you like to see your child accomplish in the next year, in the next 3 years?

Providing parents with such a structure accomplishes several things. First, facilitating the recording of their specific observations may help with the denial of reality. It is far easier and healthier for parents to recognize the child's weaknesses than for a professional to tell them. Second, it facilitates communication among family members, which often breaks down in families of children with disabilities due to different coping styles. Third, it gives credibility to parent perceptions during the meeting in which assessment and observations are discussed. Often, if a parent disagrees with a professional observation, that disagreement is viewed by the professionals as parent denial of reality or emotional reaction to information difficult to hear. When parents have noted this information previously and bring it to the meeting, it is viewed by the professionals as more credible. If a professional's assessment report is filed with the student's records, it is important to include the parents' reports.

Regular education teachers also need to be encouraged to be strong partners in the evaluation. It is important to let them know that their information is just as important as that of the specialists. Their knowledge of what and how the child learns, daily performance, learning style, group participation, and patterns of behavior is unique and critical.

INDIVIDUAL EDUCATIONAL PLANNING

300.343(a) Each public agency is responsible for initiating and conducting meetings for the purpose of developing, reviewing, and revising the IEP of a child with a disability.

300.345(a) Each public agency shall take steps to ensure that one or both of the parents of the child with a disability are present at each meeting or are afforded the opportunity to participate.

300.346(a) The IEP for each child must include (1) A statement of the child's present levels of educational performance; (2) A statement of annual goals, including short-term instructional objectives; (3) A statement of the specific special education and related services to be provided to the child and the extent that the child will be able to participate in regular educational programs; (4) The projected dates for initiation of services and the anticipated duration of the services; and (5) Appropriate objective criteria and evaluation procedures and schedules for determining, on at least an annual basis, whether the short term instructional objectives are being achieved; (b)(1) The IEP for each student, beginning no later than age 16, must include a statement of the needed transition services including, if appropriate, a statement of each public agency's and each participating agency's responsibilities or linkages, or both, before the student leaves the school setting.

IDEA 34 C.F.R. Appendix C to Part 300—Notice of Interpretation Question #26. What is the role of the parents at an IEP meeting? The parents of a child with a disability are expected to be equal participants along with school personnel, in developing, reviewing, and revising the child's IEP. This is an active role in which the parents (1) participate in the discussion about the child's needs for special education and related services, and (2) join with the other participants in deciding what services the agency will provide to the child.

The individual educational planning (IEP) process, whether a federally mandated process or a local informal process, should be a systematic process of sharing and interpreting information about a child, through group discussion, so as to understand him or her completely and then to design a plan for the provision of appropriate education. When developing, reviewing, or revising an IEP, participants in the planning meeting should draw on and consider information from a variety of sources, including information from the family, ensure that information obtained from all of these sources is documented and carefully considered, and reach decisions through group discussion and consensus.

It is the responsibility of every participant in the IEP meeting to: (1) come to the meeting prepared; (2) be present physically and emotionally; (3) share his or her information and point of view, giving the best descriptions possible; (4) listen to others do the same; and (5) be open to reaching decisions about appropriate education through group discussion and consensus. Participants should not (1) read assessment reports, (2) be committed to an outcome, or (3) determine services based on availability.

Current Levels of Functioning, Achievement, and Performance, and Needs

If we are truly going to individualize for each child, then it is important that we understand that child from a global point of view, not just from one perspective, assessment, or observation. It is not just the speech and language specialist, for example, who has information about a child's communicative functioning. The child communicates at home, in the community, and at school. Therefore, it is important to understand his or her communication ability from several perspectives.

The traditional "round robin" reporting that is often done at IEP meetings does not allow for true discussion and consensus for many reasons. First, there is the issue of "pecking order." Many parents and professionals feel that if an expert gives an assessment report, it is not wise to offer a different opinion, since this would appear as a challenge to that expert. Second, when lengthy reports are given, it is difficult to listen to and integrate all the information. Third, it is human nature, when "in the spotlight," to perform in such a way as to impress professional peers with the breadth and length of information known. Much of the information reported is not viewed as critical to the understanding of the child.

A preferred way of structuring this meeting is to facilitate a child-centered discussion. "Let's talk about the child's communication. Mom and Dad, how does he communicate at home? Is that what you see in the classroom? What did formal testing reveal? Why might we see that discrepancy? Who else has information on this? What I'm hearing

then is . . . but in some situations we might see . . ., is that correct?" It is the synthesis of information that is recorded on the child's IEP. Often, it is helpful to ask the parents to share their information first, when beginning each area of discussion, before they get caught up in the jargon of others and before they react emotionally to difficult-to-hear information. This also allows them to feel like equal partners in the discussion and decision-making process.

Goals and Short-Term Instructional Objectives

After using information about the child's functioning and needs, the team should decides what the child can reasonably be expected to accomplish within a 12-month period. Again, it is important to use a child-centered structure for discussion and decision-making and important to understand parental desires. It is often helpful to ask about dreams for the child, and also about fears, which can easily lead into a discussion of goals. Short-term instructional objectives are measurable, intermediate steps between the present levels of performance and the annual goals that are established for the child. The objectives are developed based on a logical breakdown of the major components of the annual goals and can serve as milestones for measuring progress toward meeting the goals.

Determination of Specific Special Education and Related Services

300.17(a)(1) The term "special education" means specially designed instruction, at no cost to the parents, to meet the unique needs of a child with a disability.

300.16(a) The term "related services" means transportation and such developmental, corrective, and other supportive services as are required to assist a child with a disability to benefit from special education, and includes speech pathology and audiology, psychological services, physical and occupational therapy, recreation, including therapeutic recreation, early identification and assessment of disabilities in children, counseling services, including rehabilitation counseling, and medical services for diagnostic or evaluation purposes. The term also includes school health services, social work services in schools, and parent counseling and training.

If we accept the premise that regular education curricula and methods are designed to meet the needs of the majority of students, then we must consider this also to be appropriate for students with auditory disorders, making only those modifications and adaptations needed as a result of their unique needs. Assuming that students with auditory disorders need a totally special program, with special curricula, methodologies, and instructional techniques, is counterproductive. It is important, however, to take into consideration their unique needs, so that these students have the same opportunity to learn as any other student. To individualize for each student, the team should respond to the following questions in order.

1. What are the subjects and activities in regular education in which this student can participate with no modifications or adaptations and from which he or she can benefit? Some students may be able to benefit from many subjects or activities; others may only be able to benefit from lunch and recess activities. The real world into which the student with auditory disorders may want to integrate does not automatically provide modifications for his or her auditory deficits. For this reason, it is important to expose the student to that world, if that is a goal for him or her, throughout his or her educational experience. This should only be done, however, to the extent that benefit can be gained and feelings of isolation do not occur.

2. What are the subjects and activities in regular education from which the student can benefit so long as specific modifications or adaptations are made? What are those modifications and adaptations? The team can refer back to the list of needs for much of this information. The following is an example of modifications or adaptations that might be considered.

   Techniques
   Directions and instruction given individually or in writing
   Key words and concepts of verbal instruction reinforced in writing
   Extra time allowed for processing
   Short-phrase answers allowed
   All verbal instruction interpreted into signs
   New vocabulary and concepts introduced in advance
   Content, Materials
   High-interest, low-vocabulary materials utilized

Written materials utilized to be at no greater than ____th grade reading level
Scripts or notes of lecture presentations provided
Vocabulary lists provided
Environment
Preferential seating
Direct student-to-teacher amplification
Classroom accommodations relating to acoustics, reverberation, lighting, seating
Classroom safety accommodations, such as flashing fire alarm
Assistive listening and communication devices, such as: personal FM systems, auditory trainers, telecommunication devices, and telecaption devices
Evaluation
Tests given orally, individually, or with reading assistance
Verbal/signed responses allowed rather than written responses
Extra time to complete tests
Daily work and participation evaluated in lieu of tests

After determining what specific modification and adaptations the child needs, the team may decide who is responsible for them—the regular education teacher, a specialist, both, one in consultation with the other, etc.

3. What alternative curriculum or instruction does the student need that is not offered as part of regular education? Specific instruction in language or reading, functional mathematics, independent living skills, or affective education are examples of alternative instruction.

4. What supportive training does the student (or family) need in relation to deficit areas and how much? This may include receptive or expressive language training, speech intelligibility training, auditory training, or counseling. It may include parental skill development training in expansion of language, sign language, hearing aid maintenance, etc. The amount of individualized training in each area needs to be determined with no regard to availability of services. Once that is identified, based on student need, the team may assign any service provider or a combination of service providers. Speech intelligibility training, for example, can be facilitated by many types of service providers. Speech therapists may only need to serve as consultants. An example of this concept was well-illustrated in a junior high school where a student with severe auditory disorders was having difficulty expressing

anger appropriately. When angry, he would often resort to kicking in lockers or putting his fist through classroom windows. The IEP team determined that a goal for this student would be to express anger appropriately, specifically through verbalizing rather than through physical actions. A psychologist was available in that building only once a week, which, of course, did not usually coincide with when the student became angry. Creatively, the team decided that "one person whom the student liked and trusted should be available at all times to whom he could go at will and express feelings of anger." A counselor was not available and he did not trust his teacher or principal. It was determined that the ideal service provider would be the custodian. The custodian was approached, happily accepted this challenge, and received some consultation from the psychologist. It worked.

5. What behaviors need to be carried out consistently by all service providers, including the parents? If, for example, a goal for a child is to gain attention by vocalizing rather than gesturing, it is important that all service providers, including the parents, ignore gesturing and respond only to vocalization. Such consistency is also usually necessary in behavior management strategies. These types of needs should be addressed by the team so that everyone has ownership in them and will thus be working toward them. Speech therapists alone cannot cause language or speech development; psychologist alone cannot change a child's behavior.

300.18(a) "Transition services" means a coordinated set of activities for a student, designed within an outcome-oriented process, that promotes movement from school to post-school activities, including post secondary education, vocational training, integrated employment, continuing and adult education, adult services, independent living, or community participation. (b) The coordinated set of activities...must (1) Be based on the individual student's needs, taking into account the student's preferences and interests; and (2) Include needed activities in the areas of (i) Instruction; (ii) Community experiences; (iii) The development of employment and other post-school adult living objectives; and (iv) If appropriate, acquisition of daily living skills and functional vocational evaluation.

---

6. (If applicable.) What specific services or community experiences does the student need to assist with transition from school to post-secondary education, vocational training, employment and independent living? What will agencies' responsibilities be and what are the linkages?

Most students go through the process of transition naturally, weighing and sorting out their knowledge of themselves and their values in relation to the world around them. This conceptual process, of which most students may not even be aware, may be different for students with auditory disorders. They often have not heard family, peers or members of the community discussing the multitude of issues relating to independent living and the adult world. In addition, many students with auditory disorders may have been deprived of opportunities to become self-directed, self-controlled individuals, due to the overzealous support and assistance often given by teachers, parents, and specialists.

It is critically important that we provide services that build functional bridges spanning the gulf between the security and structure offered by the school and the home, and the opportunities and risks of adult life. Too often, students with auditory disorders leave the educational system without meaningful occupations, skills for independent living, and knowledge of services available from other agencies.

Specific transition plans should be developed no later than the 10th grade, as part of the IEP process, and the student must take part in the development of that plan. Such a plan will facilitate decision-making. High school courses can be selected accordingly. Vocational education or work study programs can be used. Specific training in searching, applying for, and interviewing for a job can be provided. Specific guidance can be given on job retention skills and adjusting to competitive standards. Specific opportunities for using recreational facilities and for participation in a wide variety of leisure time activities can be provided. Specific instruction in daily living skills, such as managing personal finances, selecting and managing a household, buying, preparing, and consuming foods, and exhibiting responsible citizenship, can be provided. Personal and social skills can be discussed and developed in relation to socially responsible behavior, interpersonal communication, problem-solving, independence, self-awareness, and self-confidence. Career interests can be refined to match aptitudes. For example, a person interested in becoming a lawyer, but without the ability to do so, can be guided toward becoming a courtroom clerk or paralegal.

We may need to deemphasize our traditional remedial academic instruction and focus on the development of competencies to facilitate the student's living as independently and happily as possible in today's society. Students with auditory disorders need specific instruction in obtaining and utilizing interpreters, rights as a disabled citizen, support systems and their use such as TDDs and Relay Systems.

LEAST RESTRICTIVE ENVIRONMENT

> 300.305 Each public agency shall take steps to ensure that its children with disabilities have available to them the variety of educational programs and services available to non disabled children in the area served by the agency, including art, music, industrial arts, consumer and homemaking education, and vocational education.
>
> 300.306(a) Each public agency shall take steps to provide nonacademic and extracurricular services and activities in such manner as is necessary to afford children with disabilities an equal opportunity for participation in those services and activities.
>
> 300.550(b) Each public agency shall ensure (1) That to the maximum extent appropriate, children with disabilities, including children in public or private institutions or other care facilities, are educated with children who are non disabled; and (2) That special classes, separate schooling or other removal of children with disabilities from the regular educational environment occurs only when the nature or severity of the disability is such that education in regular classes with the use of supplementary aids and services cannot be achieved satisfactorily.
>
> 300.552(d) In selecting the LRE, consideration is given to any potential harmful effect on the child or on the quality of services that he or she needs.

The education of students with auditory disorders has historically been an area of conflicting values and opinions among professionals, parents, and consumers. The concept of a LRE and the process for determination of LRE will undoubtedly continue to be areas of discussion and disagreement. It is imperative, therefore, that decisions for each child be made by a team of parents and professionals who are open to designing an appropriate education for this particular child, regardless of their individual beliefs. Focus should be on what environment will be most productive for the child, given the goals that have been determined for him or her and the services he or she needs. LRE is currently guaranteed by federal legislation; however, the process by which to determine LRE is with the school and family. Every child with auditory disorders has a right to an appropriate education. This right cannot be taken away by the schools or by the parents. The decisions must be made together through discussion and consensus building.

ADMINISTRATIVE LEADERSHIP

Whether our emphasis is on compliance with federal and state special education mandates or moving toward a unified system, administrative leadership appears to be a key element in the provision of appropriate education to students with auditory disorders in our schools.

Regular education administrators must demonstrate ownership of all students in their buildings, including those with auditory disorders, and show support for all staff, including those with specific skills in the area of hearing. They must support the needs of students with auditory disorders and encourage regular education staff to make the necessary modifications. They must assign service providers with the characteristics that will enhance learning, such as enthusiasm, flexibility, teaching style, patience, ability to communicate, willingness to rephrase and repeat, willingness to provide individual instruction, willingness to adapt and modify curriculum, and ability to work as an effective team member. They must develop a budget sufficient to carry out effective identification and services to students with auditory disorders, and they must provide time to specialists in hearing for on-going communication and consultation.

Sufficient personnel must be employed to provide for identification, assessment, and planning and for instructional and related services, including audiologists, speech language specialists, teachers, and educational interpreters when needed. Case loads and student teacher ratios must be reasonable, and trained and qualified substitute teachers and support personnel must be provided when needed.

Facilities must be adequate and appropriate for instructional and related services to students with auditory disorders, considering noise, lighting, and seating. Sufficient funds and resources must be allocated to support the unique needs of students with auditory disorders, including materials, equipment, and assistive technology devices.

> 300.303 Each public agency shall ensure that the hearing aids worn by children with hearing impairments including deafness in school are functioning properly.
>
> 300.308 Each public agency shall ensure that assistive technology devices or assistive technology services, or both, are made available to a child with a disability if required as a part of the child's (a) Special education, (b) Related services, or (c) Supplementary aids and services.

Staff who provide services to students with auditory disorders must be appropriately qualified, certified, licensed or registered, and well trained. Teachers must be skilled in the use of the communication modes of the student being served. Educational interpreters must have skills commensurate with the students' language level and communication mode.

A comprehensive system of personnel development must be implemented. Promising practices in the area of hearing must be known and utilized. Staff development programs in hearing must reflect current research on effective instructional practices. Needs assessment must be conducted. Opportunities for in-service training and personal growth must be provided.

A FREE APPROPRIATE PUBLIC EDUCATION

> 300.8 Free appropriate public education means special education and related services that (a) Are provided at public expense, under public supervision and direction, and without charge; (b) Meet the standards of the State Educational Agency, (c) Include preschool, elementary school, or secondary school education in the State involved; and (d) Are provided in conformity with an IEP.

There is no dispute over the fact that children with auditory disorders have a right to a free appropriate public education. Disputes begin to arise over the definition of "appropriate." Legally, services are appropriate when they are in conformity with an IEP. Emotionally, each of us often considers them to be appropriate when they are commensurate with our beliefs and opinions. Objectively, they are appropriate when the child is provided the opportunity to attain the same performance levels as those attained by students without auditory disorders. This can be done and is being done by understanding each child, completely individualizing services for that child, and then monitoring progress weekly, not allowing the student to progress slower than that commensurate with chronological age.

As caring individuals, we often deprive students with auditory disorders of the only experience that can really promote their growth and development—the experience of using their own strengths. In our zealous attempt to support, modify, and accept these students, we may assume responsibility for their success. It is important constantly to remember our end product—a student who thinks for himself or herself as a self-directed, self-controlled individual. He or she needs to become personally accountable and able to act without guidance, assistance, or supervision and to be answerable for his or her behavior. Students with auditory disorders need to find a sense of responsibility for themselves and their actions.

An important component of the system of services for students with auditory disorders, then, is personalized instruction. This does not happen automatically. This would include assistance in personalizing, internalizing, and applying information; in developing a realistic view of self; and in planning, implementing and evaluating personal goals. This is accomplished by providing formal and informal counseling to the student and is performed by monitoring and providing training to professionals and parents. This must be pervasive throughout the student's program and not a separate entity providing mostly for "here-and-now" situations. We must allow students with auditory disorders "to do" rather than being "done to."

SUMMARY

With an appropriate education, children with auditory disorders can learn, achieve, and grow commensurate with their chronological age;

however; this often does not happen. The major obstacle to this occurring appears to be the quest for a homogenous solution to the needs of a heterogeneous set of students. Legislation, alone, neither ensures nor prohibits the provision of an appropriate education. We as parents, consumers, service providers, and administrators must work in partnership to identify the needs of and goals for each of these students, to design an individualized education plan in response to these needs and goals, and to monitor growth constantly, changing our plan as needed.

REFERENCES

1. Department of Education, Final Regulations for the Assistance to States for the Education of Children with Disabilities Program under part B of the *Individuals with Disabilities Education Act. Fed Reg*, 57 (no. 289; September 29, 1992), 44794–44852.
2. Commision on the Education of the Deaf (COED): *Toward Equality: Education of the Deaf*, Report to the President and Congress of the United States (1988).
3. United States Congress, *Goals 2000: Educate America Act.*

Identification | II

INTRODUCTION

The quest for the most appropriate test to identifying hearing loss in school children began as early as 1927, at which time the Western Electric 4-C Group Speech Test was introduced as a screening technique. Following this early effort, procedures for hearing screening in the schools emphasized group tests and for 30 to 35 years such tests were in vogue. However, this trend changed with the discovery of the many pitfalls that exist in group tests, and at present individual tests are performed in school hearing screening.

With sophistication of equipment and advancement of audiological techniques comes the requirement that the personnel involved in auditory screening programs have greater skills. Also is the requirement that they have concern for the total program, so that the individual needs of each child are met. No longer should school personnel be content with simply identifying the child with hearing loss. School personnel must be concerned about: identifying those children with all types of auditory disorders, including minimal hearing loss and middle ear disorders; referring those children failing the screening for appropriate medical follow-up; and providing remedial educational programs for those children who have sustained hearing loss. All facets of the process must be established and carried out on each child for the program to be effective.

The emphasis on individual testing and the gradual collection of data on hearing loss in school children has given a new direction to school hearing conservation programs. It is now well established that middle ear disorders, even those that are transient, can have a significant impact on speech and language development. This fact, coupled with the introduction of immittance measures, makes it possible to detect middle ear disorders, even when they do not significantly impair hearing threshold sensitivity.

There has been controversy regarding the place of screening for middle ear disorders with immittance tests. This controversy has resulted in endorsements from several national organizations against the use of immittance measures for mass screening. While there may be pragmatic reasons why immittance measures can be questioned, the decision against mass screening does not appear to be in the best interest of the individual child; if the program is designed in the best possible interest of the individual child, there would be little question that auditory screening programs must include appropriate screening of middle ear function along with audiometric screening for hearing loss.

This part of our text covers information on the identification process. It is imperative that those involved in audiometric and immittance screening have a thorough understanding of the principles underlying the measurements obtained and be able to interpret the data collected from the screening tests and from additional diagnostic testing. This information is covered in Chapter 2. The physician plays a key role in the diagnosis and management of auditory disorders in school children. Chapter 3 covers medical aspects of hearing loss that must be known by the school personnel involved in the identification program.

Too often, school personnel involved in the screening do not have a general overview of the purpose of screening and the philosophies underlying the screening process. Moreover, there are numerous sets of guidelines that have been published on screening for hearing loss and middle ear disorders. In Chapter 4, the screening process is reviewed and guidelines are presented that summarize an effective program. Chapter 5 covers the difficult area of central auditory testing; practical guidelines are given on how to identify and assess this most perplexing population of children. In Chapters 6 and 7, psychoeducational assessment of children with hearing impairment and language learning problems are covered, respectively.

In this part of our book, we bring together all of the knowledge and expertise one should have in developing and carrying out an effective hearing conservation program and in assessing the child with auditory impairment in the schools.—*RJR, MPD*

2

AUDIOMETRIC AND IMMITTANCE MEASURES: PRINCIPLES AND INTERPRETATION

Ross J. Roeser

There are in fact two things, science and opinion; the former begets knowledge, the latter ignorance.

—Hippocrates, 460–377 B.C.

THE PHYSICAL BASES OF HEARING

Sound

Most people are aware that the human ear responds to sound, but few are familiar with the technical aspects of sound and the terms used to describe its physical characteristics. To have a working knowledge of hearing loss, and the possible difficulty that an individual loss of hearing may present, an understanding of both the technical aspects and physical characteristics of sound is needed.

Two elementary concepts are necessary to understand sound. First, sound is created by vibration or the movement of molecules in the air. Vibration refers to the back-and-forth movement, or oscillation, of molecular particles. To give rise to a sound wave, an object, or vibrator, must be set into motion by a force causing molecular displacement or disruption of air particles.

The second elementary concept is that vibrations are propagated in an elastic medium. The elastic medium propagating sound in our environment is typically air. This implies that if a vibrator was set into motion in a vacuum, the sensation of hearing would not occur because no medium exists to transmit the vibrations.

With the three factors of vibrator, force, and medium, sound can be created. However, simply causing the physical conditions needed for sound may not be enough. Some also believe that to create sound, it is required to have an ear. Thus, if a vibrator were set into motion and air particles were carried by a medium but no one perceived the vibrations, with the requirement that an ear also be present, sound did not occur.

Figure 2–1 is a summary of the concepts just presented. In this figure the four elements

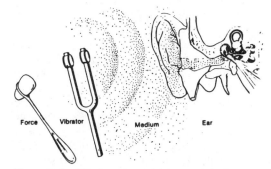

Figure 2–1. The four elements necessary for the production of sound.

necessary for sound are presented: a force, a vibrator, a medium, and an ear.

Frequency and Intensity

Two parameters of sound that define its basic characteristics are frequency and intensity.

Frequency. The physical measurement of what is psychologically perceived as pitch is frequency. Frequency specifies the number of back-and-forth oscillations, or cycles, produced by a vibrator in a given time as a sound is created. The term used to describe frequency is "Hertz," abbreviated Hz, and this term specifies the number of cycles that occur in 1 second. For example, if a vibrator (tuning fork) were set into motion and completed 1000 back-and-forth cycles in 1 second, it would have a frequency of 1000 Hz. Frequency and pitch are related in that as the frequency of a sound increases, the listener perceives a tone of a higher and higher pitch.

A sound can be made up of only one frequency or, as in most instances, of many different frequencies. The simplest acoustic signal is created when only one frequency is present; this form of sound is called a pure tone. In the example just given, the 1000 Hz vibrator was generating a pure tone because only one frequency occurred.

Pure tones do not exist in our everyday environment; they must be created electronically. However, pure tones are the basic acoustic signal used in auditory testing, primarily because they are the simplest form of sound to generate, the easiest to control, and, most important, they test the auditory system for frequency-specific problems.

The sounds we encounter in our everyday environment are complex and contain many different frequencies. The human ear responds to frequencies between 20 and 20,000 Hz. Frequencies that are below this range are *infrasonic* and those above this range, *ultrasonic*. For example, a sound with a frequency of 10 Hz is infrasonic and would not be perceived by the normal ear, and a sound with a frequency of 30,000 Hz is ultrasonic and would also not be perceived. Even though the ear responds to frequencies ranging from 20 to 20,000 Hz, only those frequencies between 300 and 3000 Hz are actually critical for the perception of speech. This means that it would be possible for an individual to have essentially no hearing above 3000 Hz and have only marginal difficulty in hearing speech in a quiet environment. This observation explains why pure tones are important in assessing the auditory system.

In audiometric testing the standard frequencies evaluated range from 125 or 250 Hz through 8000 Hz. This frequency range is generally the most audible to the human ear and provides guidelines on how well the individual is able to perceive speech because the speech frequencies fall within this range.

As part of a standard audiometric evaluation, pure-tone thresholds are typically assessed at *octave intervals* and sometimes at *half-octave intervals*. Thus, the frequencies 250, 500, 1000, 2000, 4000, and 8000 Hz are routinely tested and 750, 1500, 3000, and 6000 Hz are sometimes tested when additional information is warranted. However, more and more it is becoming the custom to include 3000 and 6000 Hz in the standard audiometric evaluation, especially when hearing loss is present.

Intensity. The physical measurement of what is psychologically perceived as loudness is intensity. The intensity of a sound is determined by the amount of movement or displacement of air particles that occurs as a sound is created. The greater the amount of displacement, the more intense, or louder, the sound. Intensity is measured in units called *decibels*, abbreviated dB, a term that literally means one tenth of a bell (named after Alexander Graham Bell). The decibel is technically defined as the logarithmic ratio between two magnitudes of pressure, or power.

As indicated by the technical definition, intensity is far more complicated than frequency, and to understand the decibel fully requires knowledge of advanced mathematical functions. The decibel is based on logarithmic function because the ear responds to a very large range of pressure changes and logarithms allow these changes to be expressed by smaller numbers than would be required for a linear function. There are excellent references that the interested reader may consult for additional information on how to compute decibels using logarithms (eg, Berlin[1]).

Although the concepts underlying the decibel are somewhat complicated and will not be covered in this chapter, a less difficult concept is that the decibel is a relative unit of measurement. This means that simply saying, for example, 10 dB or 20 dB has no specific meaning without specifying the reference for the measure. There are two decibel reference levels most often used in audiometric testing: *sound pressure level (SPL)* and *hearing level (HL)*.

These two reference levels are described as follows:

dB SPL. Sound pressure level refers to the absolute pressure reference level for the decibel. The pressure reference used to determine dB SPL is 0.000204 dynes/cm^2, so 0 dB SPL is equal to a pressure force of 0.000204 dynes/cm^2 and 10 dB or 20 dB SPL equals 10 or 20 dB above the 0.000204 dynes/cm^2 force. Because dB SPL is a physical measure, it is not affected by the frequencies present in sound.

dB HL. The reference for the decibel used to express deviation from normal hearing sensitivity is dB HL. As will be pointed out later, the ear is not sensitive to all frequencies at the same intensity. That is, hearing sensitivity changes as a function of the frequency of the sound. Therefore, 0 dB HL represents an intensity equal to the threshold sensitivity of the normal ear at each frequency. Audiometers are calibrated in dB HL, so that any decibel value above 0 dB HL represents a deviation from normal hearing levels. For example, 25 dB HL is 25 decibels above the normal hearing threshold for that frequency.

Over the past 44 years, four standards have been used to define the absolute SPL levels at which the normal ear responds as a function of frequency. The standards are: the American Standards Association (ASA),[2] adopted in 1951; the International Standards Organization (ISO),[3] adopted in 1961; and the American National Standards Institute (ANSI), first adopted in 1969[4] and revised in 1989.[5] At present, all audiometers should conform to the 1989 ANSI standard.

In some instances, decibel hearing threshold level (HTL) will also be used. When dB HTL is used, it implies that the decibel value given was a measured threshold from a patient, that is, the value was an actual level obtained during threshold assessment.

Frequency and Intensity Function of the Human Ear Figure

As already pointed out, the ear responds to different absolute intensities, or different SPLs, as a function of frequency. Stated in another way, it takes a different SPL to reach the level at which the normal ear will perceive the sound (threshold level) at different frequencies. Figure 2–2 illustrates the threshold sensitivity function of the normal ear and gives the 1989 ANSI levels required to reach threshold at each frequency for normal ears (0 dB HL). As shown in Figure 2–2, the ear is most sensitive in the midfrequencies, around 1000 to 1500 Hz. Since audiometers are calibrated in dB HL, it is not necessary to know the absolute dB SPL/HL difference at each frequency. The audiometer automatically corrects for the dB SPL/HL difference as the frequency is changed.

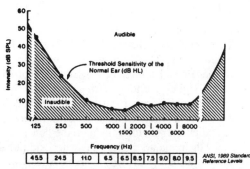

Figure 2–2. The threshold sensitivity of the normal ear as a function of frequency. The numbers at the bottom are the 1989 ANSI dB SPL values required to reach normal threshold sensitivity at each frequency.

THE AUDIOMETER AND AUDIOMETRY

The Audiometer

An audiometer is technically defined as an electronic device that generates signals used to assess hearing. There are various types of audiometers presently available from numerous manufacturers. The types of audiometers commercially available vary from simple screening models to very complex clinical instruments, and the signals generated range from simple pure tones to more complex stimuli, which are used in comprehensive testing.

Basic Functions. Audiometers were first designed to generate the same frequencies as those produced by tuning forks, for example, 256, 512, and 1024. However, audiometer manufacturers have now standardized their instruments on a scale based on even thousands of Hertz. Therefore, audiometers today generate at least all the following test frequencies: 250, 500, 750, 1000, 1500, 2000, 2500, 3000, 4000, 6000, and 8000 Hz.

Several models of audiometers with limited versatility have been recommended for screening. Screening audiometers generally provide a choice of several discrete frequency pure tones as well as a method of precisely controlling the intensity of the tones. These audiometers range in price from about $600 to $800.

Diagnostic audiometers provide, in addition to pure tones, a speech circuit and are designed so that many special diagnostic (site of lesion) auditory tests may be performed. The cost of this type of instrument ranges from $10,000 to $20,000, and more, and its use requires a commercially built, sound-treated room. Diagnostic audiometers are generally found in clinical or medical settings and are not usually available in the school setting.

Regardless of the make or model, pure-tone audiometers have certain basic controls and switches in common. These components may vary in appearance and location according to different designs; however, they perform the same basic functions. To show the diversity that can be found in audiometers, Figure 2–3 illustrates two different commercially available audiometers with the external controls and parts of the instruments appropriately labeled. The correct way that the audiometer should be placed and examiner should be seated in relation to the child when screening is shown in Figure 2–3B. As shown in Figure

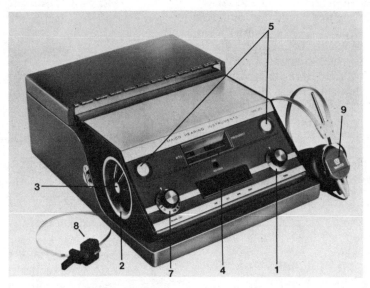

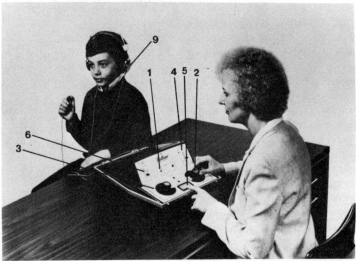

Figure 2–3. Components of two commercially available audiometers (see text for description). *(Top, courtesy of Maico Hearing Instruments. Bottom, courtesy of Beltone Electronics.)*

2–3B, the child should be readily observable by the tester. However, to prevent false responses, the examiner should be out of the child's peripheral vision.

The following describes the function of each major control shown in Figure 2–3.

Power Supply (not shown). Audiometers are equipped with standard three-pronged plugs for 120 volt power. However, some portable screening audiometers are battery powered. Battery-powered instruments are desirable because they can be used when power outlets are unavailable. However, the use of battery-powered audiometers is discouraged because the battery current may vary with usage, resulting in large variability in the output of the test stimuli.

On-Off or Power Switch (1 in Fig. 2–3). After the audiometer has been plugged in, it should be turned on and allowed to warm up for approximately 10 minutes prior to testing. This procedure assures that the proper current has reached all parts of the instrument for optimal functioning. The audiometer should remain in the "on" position for the remainder of the day when additional testing is to be performed, as there is less wear on the electrical components to leave it on all day than to turn it on and off several times during the day.

Attenuator or Hearing Level Dial (2 in Fig. 2–3). The intensity of the stimuli is controlled by the attenuator, or HL dial. The attenuator is actually a group of resistors built into the output circuit to control the intensity in small steps. Most attenuators are designed to operate in 5 dB steps, although some operate in steps of 1 or 2 dB. The attenuator dial has a range of 0 to 110 dB HL for air conduction testing, with 0 dB HL at each frequency being the threshold sensitivity for normal listeners. Not all of the test stimuli are capable of being presented at intensities of 110 dB HL. Specifically, 250 and 8000 Hz have limited outputs, and the maximum output for each frequency is specified on the frequency selector dial. Bone conduction testing is limited to 0 to 40 or 0 to 60 or 70 dB HL, depending on the frequency.

Frequency Selector Dial (3 in Fig. 2–3B). The frequency selector dial allows stimuli to be varied in discrete steps from 125 to 8000 Hz in octave and half-octave intervals. As already mentioned, the frequency selector dial also shows, by use of smaller numerals on the dial, the maximum output (dB HL or dB HTL) that the audiometer is capable of producing at each test frequency.

Output Selector Switch (4 in Fig. 2–3). Test signals may be delivered to the right earphone, left earphone, bone conduction oscillator, or, in the case of diagnostic audiometers, through loudspeakers. The output selector switch determines which of these devices is activated. Some audiometers may also have a "group" position on the output selector switch. This position is used when the audiometer activates multiple earphones for group testing. Because group tests are seldom used in school screening, the group output selector position is rarely, if ever, used.

Tone Interrupter (5 in Fig. 2–3) and Tone Reverse Switch (6 in Fig. 2–3B). The tone interrupter is a button, bar, or lever used either to present or interrupt the test stimuli, depending on the position of the tone reverse switch. The tone reverse switch allows the tone to be "normally on" or "normally off." In the "normally on" position, the tone is turned off by depressing the tone interrupter. In the "normally off" position, the tone is presented by depressing the tone interrupter.

In audiometric testing the tone reverse switch should always be in the "normally off" position. Serious errors can result if the tone reverse switch is in the "normally on" position. The "normally on" position is used only during calibration and for special audiometric tests not performed as part of screening.

Masking Dial (7 in Fig. 2–3A). In some instances, a masking sound must be applied to the nontest ear to ensure that crossover of the test signal is not occurring. The masking dial controls the level of the masking signal noise. Masking is a complicated procedure to understand and is not used in screening programs.

Bone Conduction Oscillator (8 in Fig. 2–3A). The bone conduction oscillator is used to obtain threshold measures of bone conduction sensitivity. Bone conduction testing is a diagnostic procedure and should not be performed as part of routine screening unless specifically designed and supervised by an audiologist. The capability to perform bone conduction tests is not necessary in audiometers used in screening programs.

Earphones (9 in Fig. 2–3A, B). The earphones are secured in a standard headband and transmit test tones to each ear individually according to a standardized color code: red for the right ear and blue for the left ear. Important points regarding earphones are: (1) earphones are calibrated to one specific audiometer and should always be considered an integral part of that particular instrument; (2) earphones should never be interchanged between audiometers unless the equipment is recalibrated; and (3) the tension of the headband and resiliency of the earphone cushions are important factors for reliable test results.

The standard audiometer earphone is made up of a driver mounted in a supra-aural (MX-41/AR) cushion (see example in Fig. 2–4). Although supra-aural cushions are standard equipment on audiometers, noise-excluding earphone cushions have been suggested for use in screening because they reduce (attenuate) ambient noise more effectively than the standard MX-41/AR cushion. This feature implies that accurate tests may be performed in the presence of higher background noise levels.

Figure 2–4 shows a diagram of the supra-aural cushion, and two types of noise-excluding cushions, the circumaural cushion, and the combined (circumaural/supra-aural) cushion. Although noise-excluding cushions do attenuate ambient noise more effectively than the standard cushion, research has shown that there is no advantage for using the circumaural cushion in audiometry, due to the excessive volume created by incomplete coupling of the driver to the pinna.[6,7] The use of the combination-type cushion does provide both proper coupling and superior attenuation of ambient noise, which allows for accurate testing to

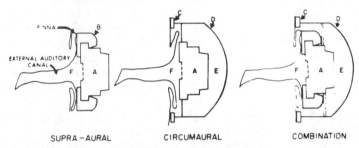

A = Electro-Acoustic Driver
B = Supra-Aural Cushion (MX-41/AR)
C = Resilient Cushion
D = Circumaural Dome
E = Foam Filled Cavity
F = Enclosed Volume of Air

SUPRA-AURAL   CIRCUMAURAL   COMBINATION

Figure 2–4. Schematic showing the components of a supra-aural earphone cushion, a circumaural cushion, and a combination-type (circumaural/supra-aural) cushion. *(Reprinted with permission from Musket and Roeser.[8]).*

be conducted with children and adults in test environments having excessive noise.[8] A commercially available combination-type (noise excluding) earphone is shown in Figure 2–5. Due to their size and complexity

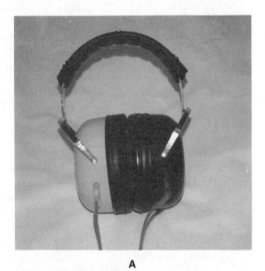

A

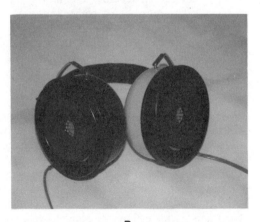

B

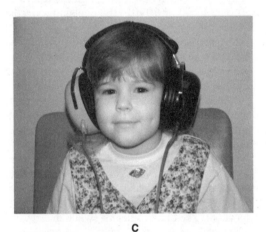

C

Figure 2–5. A combination-type noise-excluding earphone system. Note in figure 2–5B that a standard cushion is contained within the plastic enclosure that surrounds the pinna. Figure 2–5C shows show they are placed on the child.

noise-excluding earphones are more difficult to use and they have not been endorsed for general use in hearing screening in the schools. However, when used properly by the seasoned tester, they are beneficial.

A new type of earphone, which inserts directly into the ear canal, has been developed. Figure 2–6 shows the Etymotic Research tubephone. As shown, these insert earphones consist of two rectangular plastic cases, that contain the transducers (to change the electrical signal into an acoustic signal). Plastic tubing is attached to each case and at the end of the tubing is a foam plug that is inserted into each ear canal during testing. The use of insert-type earphones has distinct advantages: (1) they attenuation external noise in the environment better, which means that more accurate testing can be performed outside sound treated

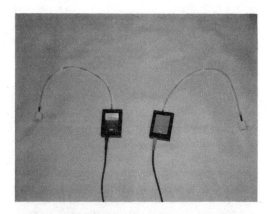

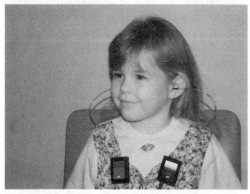

Figure 2–6. Etymotic, model ER3A, insert earphones. The top photograph shows the components of the system (see text for description), and the bottom photograph shows how they are placed on a child.

rooms; (2) interaural attenuation is increased, which means that crossover to the nontest ear is less of a problem when unilateral hearing loss is present; (3) ear canal collapse is eliminated; and (4) they are more comfortable.

Insert earphones are especially helpful in performing the threshold screening test for children who fail the pure tone sweep-check screening. Those using this type of earphone must learn to insert the form tip into the ear canal properly to achieve the maximum attenuation of background noise.[9] False-positive identifications will be reduced with proper use of insert earphones.

Calibration of Audiometers. All audiometers, whether they are used for screening or diagnostic purposes, must meet minimum requirements set by ANSI. The standard currently in effect for audiometers is ANSI S3.6-1989 and can be obtained for a fee by writing to the American National Standards Institute at 1430 Broadway, New York, NY 10018, or the Acoustical Society of America at 335 East 45th St., New York, NY 10017. Although it is not mandatory

to have the standard, it will be helpful to have it if the school system has the basic equipment necessary for electronic calibration.

Studies have documented the unfortunate finding that audiometers used for school hearing screening tend to go out of calibration frequently. For example, Walton and Wilson[10] found that 82% of the 50 audiometers used in a school hearing conservation program that were routinely serviced had one or more calibration problems that could have interfered with test results. Problems with mechanical conditions, internal noise, intensity, use time, attenuator linearity, and frequency accounted for the major errors. Some manufacturers have updated their equipment and are using more modern electronic components, such as digital electronics and integrated circuits, which should increase the reliability and durability of screening audiometers. However, field studies have not yet been reported.

The user of the audiometer is responsible for checking the equipment and providing for the regular calibration. Calibration is necessary to ensure that the audiometer is producing a pure tone at the specific frequency and intensity, that the stimulus is present only in the earphone to which it is directed, and that the stimulus is free from unwanted noise, interference, and distortion.

There are four types of calibration schedules. These include a daily listening check, a monthly biologic check, a periodic check (yearly), and an exhaustive check (every 5 years).

Daily Listening Check. Each morning following an appropriate warm-up time (10 minutes), the tester should listen to the signal emitted from the audiometer at various intensities and at all frequencies for transient clicks or distortions of the signal. The tester should also determine that the signal is in the correct earphone. It is far better to discover a malfunction in the equipment at the beginning of testing than to face inappropriate referrals.

Biologic Calibration. Each month that the audiometer is in use, a biologic calibration check is required on at least one subject whose hearing threshold is known. The procedure involves obtaining baseline threshold measurements on three to five individuals with normal hearing who will be available for comparison testing throughout the year. If on the monthly check, a threshold difference greater than 5 dB HL is found for one of the individuals for any test frequency between 500 and 6000 Hz, then the other subjects should be checked. If a shift greater than 5 dB in the same direction is confirmed by the additional biologic checks, an electronic calibration of the audiometer is required. The results from each monthly biologic calibration check should be recorded on a form that is kept in a calibration file maintained for each audiometer.

Periodic Electronic Calibration.   At least once a year, every audiometer should have an electronic calibration to ensure that it meets the minimum standards defined by ANSI. This service is provided by electronic or acoustic firms using specialized equipment. If it is necessary to ship the audiometer to another location for calibration, it should be packed carefully so that the instrument will be protected from damage in transit. As soon as the audiometer is returned from calibration or repair, the user should perform a biologic check to reestablish new baseline threshold records on subjects, as just described.

Exhaustive Electronic Calibration.   Every 5 years, each audiometer must have an exhaustive electronic calibration. This calibration is more comprehensive than the periodic electronic calibration and includes the testing of all settings on the frequency and intensity (HL/HTL) dials, as well as replacing switches, cords, and earphone drivers and cushions.

BASIC AUDIOMETRIC TESTS

Pure tone and speech stimuli are used in routine audiometry. Pure-tone stimuli are used to obtain air conduction and bone conduction thresholds and results are displayed on a pure-tone audiogram. The term "threshold" is used to define the lowest or least intense level at which the individual being tested responds to the signal presented in a given number of trials; usually defined as two of four or three of six (50%). Standard psychophysical procedures have been developed for use in threshold assessment.[11] Speech stimuli are used in obtaining speech reception thresholds, also referred to as spondee thresholds, and speech or word discrimination scores. Results from speech testing are typically recorded in a table next to the pure-tone audiogram.

Pure-Tone Audiometry

Pure Tone Air Conduction Audiometry.   This type of testing involves the measurement of auditory sensitivity using specific pure tones presented to the listener through earphones mounted in a headset and placed over the ears.

Pure tones provide information regarding the differential effects of lesions in the auditory system.

Pure Tone Bone Conduction Audiometry.   Bone conduction testing is part of diagnostic audiometric testing. In bone conduction testing, thresholds are established in much the same manner as air conduction thresholds. However, instead of using earphones, a single bone conduction oscillator, secured in a standard headband (see 8 in Fig. 2–3A), is placed behind the ear on the mastoid bone. The signal from the bone conduction oscillator sets the bones of the entire skull into motion, thus stimulating both inner ears (cochlea). Because both cochleas are stimulated, the response obtained may reflect the auditory sensitivity of the better cochlea. Thus, in bone conduction testing it may become necessary to mask the ear not being tested when a hearing loss is present.

Speech Audiometry

Many individuals first become aware that they have a hearing loss when their ability to understand speech becomes impaired. Pure tone measurements only give limited information concerning communication difficulties. To quantify communication difficulty, it is necessary to assess the individual's ability to detect and understand speech material.

In standard speech audiometry, words are spoken into a microphone (live voice presentation) or delivered using a tape or compact disc (recorded presentation) with the output signal regulated by the audiometer. The listener wears earphones, is instructed to repeat the test words, and one ear is tested at a time. With children, several standardized tests have also been developed using picture-pointing responses rather than written or spoken responses. Using these basic procedures, the threshold for speech and the ability to understand speech sounds is measured.

Speech Recognition Threshold.   The original term used for the threshold for speech was the "speech reception threshold" and many clinics still use this term. However, the preferred term is "speech recognition threshold," because it more accurately describes the procedures used in the test.[12] The SRT is a measure of auditory threshold sensitivity for speech. The standard procedure in obtaining the SRT uses spondee words, which are compound or bisyllabic words, such as "railroad," "toothbrush" and "outside," presented with equal stress on both syllables. The main function of the SRT is to confirm the pure tone thresholds; in addition, it serves as a reference for the level at which word recognition or identification testing is performed.

The primary frequencies used to discriminate speech sounds are between 300 and 3000 Hz. Thus, the SRT should be in agreement with the thresholds that fall within this region. The three octave frequencies tested within the 300 to 3000 Hz range are 500, 1000, and 2000 Hz. Together these three frequencies are used to calculate the pure-tone average (PTA). For example, if thresholds are 60, 75, and 80 dB HL at 500, 1000, and 2000 Hz, the PTA would be 72 dB HL. The SRT and PTA should agree to within −8 to 6 dB[13]; in the above example, the SRT should be 64 to 78 dB HL.

In some cases, when there is a large difference in one of the three frequencies, only two frequencies are used to calculate the PTA.[14] If the PTA and SRT are not in close agreement, it suggests that the listener may not understand the task or may not be fully cooperating with the testing (pseudohypoacusis).

When hearing loss is in the severe to profound range, and word recognition or identification is very poor, a reception threshold to spondee words may not be obtainable. In such cases a speech detection threshold (SDT), sometimes referred to as a speech awareness threshold, is obtained. Rather than a measure of speech reception, the SDT simply quantifies the lowest level at which speech is detected. The SDT will agree with the pure-tone audiogram in that it will be within 5 to 10 dB of the best (lowest) threshold on the audiogram. The SDT may also be influenced by the threshold at 125 Hz and, although this frequency is not routinely tested, it should be when the SDT does not agree with the pure-tone audiogram.

Speech Discrimination/Word Recognition. This test was first referred to as a "speech discrimination test." However, a suggestion has been made that the terminology be changed to "word recognition test" or "speech recognition test" to reflect the procedures used in the testing.[15] In this chapter the terms "speech discrimination" and "word recognition" will be used synonymously. The traditional tests use standardized, phonetically balanced lists of single syllable (monosyllabic) words. Phonetically balanced indicates that the distribution of phonetic elements in the lists approximates the distribution found in everyday conversation. Some advanced tests use sentences. When sentences are used, the terminology "speech recognition" more accurately describes the procedure.

Word recognition scores are calculated in percentage correct; a score of 100% means that all speech stimuli were discriminated correctly. The following is a general guide for interpreting most standard word discrimination test scores:[16]

90 to 100%—within the range of normal
75 to 90%—slight difficulty
60 to 75%—moderate difficulty
50 to 60%—poor discrimination
50% or less—very poor discrimination

The Audiogram

The audiogram is a graph or grid on which audiometric data are displayed. Many clinics use audiograms to record their data, but some prefer to use a tabular form to record audiometric results. Figure 2–7 compares the same pure tone

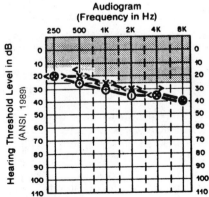

	RIGHT EAR				LEFT EAR				
Freq.	AC	Mask	BC	Mask	AC	Mask	BC	Mask	Sound Field
250	20		20		20		20		
500	25		15		20		20		
750									
1000	30		25		25		25		
1500									
2000	35		30		30		30		
3000									
4000	35		35		35		30		
6000									
8000	40				40				

Figure 2–7. Comparison of audiometric findings on a standard graphic audiogram form (left) and a grid-type form (right).

findings on a standard graphic audiogram and a tabular form.

A wide variety of symbols and symbol systems have been used by different clinics to record results on audiograms. In this diversity is the potential for confusion and misinterpretation, especially when records are exchanged between clinics.[17] Because of the potential for misinterpretation, the American Speech and Hearing Association (ASHA) has developed a standard audiogram format and symbol system for audiograms.[18] In constructing an audiogram, it is recommended that one octave on the frequency scale be equivalent in span to 20 dB on the HL scale. In addition, grid lines of equal darkness and thickness should appear at octave intervals on the frequency scale and at 10 dB intervals on the intensity scale.

The symbol system recommended by ASHA is illustrated in Figure 2–8. An important criterion used in developing the recommended symbol system was that it not be necessary to use different colors to differentiate between ears, as some symbol systems do. The ASHA guidelines also recommend that when no response is obtained at the maximum output of the audiometer, an arrow be attached to the lower outside corner of the appropriate symbol about 45° outward from the frequency axis, pointing to the right for left ear symbols and to the left for right ear symbols.

Sound field tests are noted on the audiogram by placing the symbol "S" on the audiogram form. Sound field tests utilize one or two loudspeakers rather than earphones, and when unilateral hearing loss is present, thresholds represent only the sensitivity of the better ear. When the presence of unilateral hearing loss is unknown, one must assume that the thresholds reflect only the sensitivity of the better ear and thresholds under earphones must be obtained to complete the evaluation.

Because of the potential confusion that can occur as a result of using different symbol systems, audiograms should follow the ASHA guidelines. It is also important that the symbol system used, and an explanation of any the notations used, appear in a legend on the audiogram form.

Audiometric Interpretation

Types of Hearing Loss. The type of hearing loss determined through audiometric testing identifies that part of the auditory mechanism with

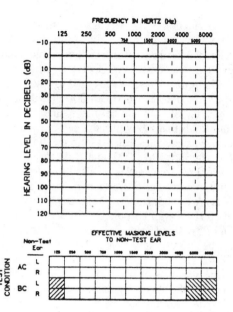

Figure 2–8. Example audiogram form (top), showing approriate dimensions, and audiometric symbols (bottom) recommended by ASHA.[18] Note that on the audiogram form 20 dB on the ordinate equals 1 octave on the abcissa.

impairment. Through audiometric tests, three types of hearing loss can be identified: *conductive, sensorineural,* and *mixed.* Figure 2–9 illustrates the difference between these types of hearing loss on the basis of the anatomic site involved. In addition, *pseudohypoacusis* (also referred to as functional, nonorganic, or psychogenic hearing loss) may be found (see later).

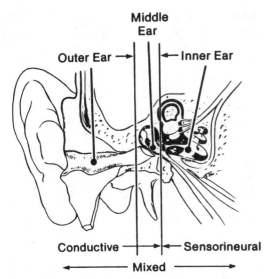

Figure 2-9. The three types of hearing loss classified according to anatomic site involved.

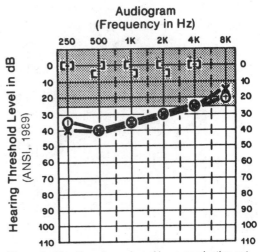

Figure 2-10. Pure-tone air and bone conduction pattern for conductive hearing loss.

Conductive Hearing Loss. Conductive hearing loss is by far the most common type of hearing loss found in school children. Conductive hearing loss literally means that part or all of the mechanical conducting components of the auditory mechanism are inefficient. The mechanical components of the auditory mechanism include the pinna, external ear canal, eardrum, middle ear ossicles and muscles, and the middle ear cavity (see Fig. 2-9). A purely conductive hearing impairment assumes no disorder of the inner ear or cochlea or of the auditory nerve.

Congenital anomalies of the outer ear may cause conductive hearing loss, but most conductive loss is acquired. The most common cause of an acquired conductive impairment in children is serous otitis media, an inflammation of the middle ear cavity accompanied by fluid.[19] Impacted ear wax (cerumen), perforated eardrum, and otosclerosis, a spongylike growth originating on the footplate of the stapes, are some of the other common factors causing conductive hearing loss.

Figure 2-10 presents the audiometric pattern for conductive loss. As shown, the pure tone audiometric pattern for conductive hearing loss is normal bone conduction thresholds and abnormal air conduction thresholds. In addition, with conductive loss, immittance measures (described later) are most likely abnormal. Two behavioral symptoms separate those persons with conductive hearing loss from those with sensorineural hearing loss.

Individuals with conductive hearing loss will demonstrate normal word recognition ability when the signal is made sufficiently loud. Moreover, the individuals's speech may be softly spoken, because he hears his own voice louder than normally, due to an "occlusion effect" resulting from the conductive hearing loss. Fortunately, with a conductive hearing loss, spontaneous recovery is frequent, or the loss can be reversed through medical and/or surgical treatment.

Sensorineural Hearing Loss. A hearing loss due to pathologic changes in the inner ear, or along the nerve pathway from the inner ear to the brainstem, is referred to as a sensorineural hearing impairment. The inner ear contains the cochlea and sensory receptors or hair cells located on the basilar membrane, a structure within the cochlea.

The hair cells transmit information to nerve fibers and the information is then fed to the temporal lobe of the brain via the VIIIth cranial nerve and auditory pathway. A pure sensorineural impairment exists when the sound conducting mechanism (outer and middle ear) is normal in every respect, but a disorder is present in the cochlea or auditory nerve, or both.

The pure-tone audiometric pattern for sensorineural hearing loss is shown in Figure 2-11. With sensorineural hearing loss, air and bone conduction thresholds are both elevated and within 10 dB of each other. The immittance measures of the tympanogram and static admittance (compliance), described later, are normal, and acoustic reflexes may be present, elevated, or absent, depending on the degree of hearing loss.

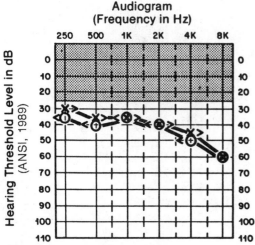

Figure 2–11. Pure-tone air and bone conduction pattern for sensorineural hearing loss.

Causes of sensorineural hearing impairment can be congenital (prior to or at birth) or acquired after birth. Congenital sensorineural hearing loss may result from hereditary factors, which can cause underdevelopment or early degeneration of the auditory nerve, in utero viral infections, or birth trauma. Acquired sensorineural loss may be caused by factors such as noise exposure, acoustic tumor, head injury, or the toxic effect of certain drugs. In virtually all cases, sensorineural hearing loss is not amenable to medical or surgical treatment.

Several symptoms characteristic of sensorineural hearing loss are shouting or talking in a loud voice, poor word recognition ability, and recruitment. Shouting or speaking in a loud voice may occur with sensorineural loss because the impaired person does not have normal hearing by bone conduction. Hence those with sensorineural hearing loss do not hear their own voice or other voices normally and may have difficulty regulating the intensity level of the voice. Not all persons with sensorineural hearing loss speak loudly and not all with conductive loss speak softly; many learn to regulate their voice levels appropriately.

The frequent decrease in word recognition associated with sensorineural hearing loss is due to distortion of the speech signal caused by nerve fiber loss. The typical sensorineural hearing loss is characterized by better hearing in the low frequencies than in the high frequencies. Consonants contain high-frequency information and vowels are predominantly low in frequency. Therefore, consonant sounds may be easily con-

fused or not heard at all. Shouting at the individual with sensorineural loss may result only in agitation rather than improved comprehension because the person may hear voices, but not be able to understand them.

The third symptom of sensorineural hearing impairment, recruitment, refers to an abnormal, rapid growth in loudness once the threshold of hearing has been crossed. After the signal is intense enough to be perceived, any further increase in intensity may cause a disproportionate increase in the sensation of loudness. Because of recruitment and word recognition difficulty, individuals with sensorineural hearing loss experience greater difficulty in noisy surroundings than those with normal hearing or conductive hearing loss.

Mixed Hearing Loss. With a mixed hearing loss, a significant conductive impairment is superimposed on a sensorineural hearing loss. Causes of mixed hearing loss may be any combination of the causes described previously for conductive and sensorineural hearing loss. The conductive component of the mixed hearing loss may be amenable to medical treatment, but the sensorineural component is not reversible. Figure 2–12 shows audiometric data depicting a mixed hearing loss. With mixed hearing loss, air conduction and bone conduction thresholds are elevated, but bone conduction thresholds are better than air conduction thresholds by 10 dB or more.

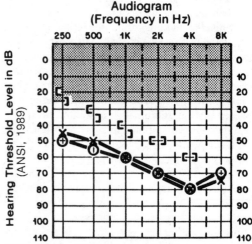

Figure 2–12. Pure-tone air and bone conduction pattern for mixed hearing loss.

Pseudohypoacusis. As stated before, pseudohypoacusis is also referred to as functional hearing loss, nonorganic hearing loss, or psychogenic hearing loss. Pseudohypoacusis literally means false (pseudo), abnormally low (hypo), hearing (acusis). The diagnosis of pseudohypoacusis is made when an individual claims to have a hearing loss, but discrepancies in audiometric test findings and behavior suggest that the loss does not exist or does not exist to the degree that is indicated by voluntary test results.

Several factors may explain causes for pseudohypoacusis. Some believe that emotional stress may lead an individual to unconsciously develop a "hearing loss" as a protective device or an escape from what seems to be an intolerable situation. Another motive for pseudohypoacusis may be pecuniary, and the individual may be well aware of the true status of auditory sensitivity. Whenever pseudohypoacusis is found in children, referral to a professional family counselor should be made to investigate the motives behind the need for feigning the loss of hearing.

Degree of Hearing Loss

Once a hearing loss has been identified, it becomes necessary to classify it according to the degree of difficulty it presents to the individual. The term "deaf" is sometimes used by nonprofessionals to refer to all persons who have a hearing impairment. However, the term "deaf" is technically reserved for the individual with hearing loss whose auditory mechanism is so severely impaired that only a few or none of the prosodic and phonetic elements of speech can be recognized. The individual who is deaf must rely mainly or entirely on speech reading or other forms of visual receptive communication for the perception of language.[20] Few individuals with hearing loss would be classified as being deaf under this definition.

On the other hand, the term "hard-of-hearing" refers to an individual with hearing loss who can identify enough of the distinguishing features of speech through hearing alone to permit at least partial recognition of spoken language. With the addition of the visual system, individuals with hearing loss may understand even more language, provided the vocabulary and syntax are within the linguistic code.

Although it is difficult to draw firm boundaries between individuals who are deaf and those who are hard-of-hearing on the basis of the loss demonstrated by pure tone findings alone, the following classification, based on the PTA (500, 1000, and 2000 Hz) is a general guide to the degree of hearing loss as it relates to children[21]:

15 to 30 dB HL—mild
31 to 50 dB HL—moderate
51 to 80 dB HL—severe
81 to 100 dB HL—profound
100 dB HL+—anacusis or total hearing loss

The classification used with adult populations is as follows:[22]

−10 to 26 dB HL—within normal limits
27 to 40 dB HL—mild loss
41 to 55 dB HL—moderate loss
56 to 70 dB HL—moderate-to-severe loss
71 to 90 dB HL—severe loss
91+—profound loss

The relationship between the degree of hearing loss (PTA) and the amount of handicap it presents is provided in Table 2–1.

In addition to the degree of loss, a complete description of an individual's hearing impairment should include whether one ear (unilateral) or both ears (bilateral) are involved and a statement regarding the type of loss. Besides the degree of loss through the speech frequencies, the overall effect of the hearing loss will depend on whether it involves one ear, both ears equally, or one ear to a lesser degree. For example, the child with significant hearing loss in one ear and normal hearing in the other will appear to hear normally, especially in a quiet listening environment. However, when noise is present, the child with unilateral hearing loss will have significant difficulty in discriminating speech.

Table 2–2 lists common terms used to describe pure-tone audiograms and provides the general contour for each.[23] These terms will give those interpreting audiograms a general feeling for the configuration of the loss.

AUDIOMETRIC TESTS IN CHILDREN

When standard methods cannot be applied to young children successfully, or for children with special problems, procedures using behavioral methods are available. This section describes advanced tests used with these children. The tests described would not be used in school screening programs but are presented to explain the types of tests that are available in the audiology clinic. Table 2–3 lists four procedures that are used by audiologists with young and difficult-to-test-children. Included are: Behavioral observation audiometry (BOA), conditioned orientation reflex

Table 2–1   Degree of Communication Difficuly as a Function of Hearing Loss

Communication Difficulty	Level of Hearing Loss (Pure-Tone Average 500, 1000, and 2000 Hz)	Degree of Hearing Loss
Demonstrates difficulty understanding soft-spoken speech; needs preferential seating and may benefit from speech reading training; good candidate for a hearing aid	25–40	Mild
Demonstrates an understanding of speech at 3–5 feet; requires amplification, preferential seating, speech reading training, and speech therapy	40–55	Moderate
Speech must be loud for auditory reception; difficulty in group and classroom discussion; may require special classes for hearing-impaired; plus all of the above needs	55–70	Moderate to severe
Loud speech may be understood at 1 ft from ear; may distinguish vowels but no consonants; requires classroom for hearing-impaired and mainstreaming at a later date	70–90	Severe
Does not rely on audition as primary modality for communication; may work well with a total communication approach; may eventually be mainstreamed at higher grade levels	90	Profound

Adapted from Goodman.[22]

(COR) audiometry/visual reinforcement audiometry (VRA), tangible reinforcement operant conditioning audiometry (TROCA), and play conditioning audiometry (PCA).

The use of these specialized techniques requires a calibrated sound field system, diagnostic audiometer, and sound-treated room. The procedure with BOA and COR/VRA involves placing the child in the sound-treated room, presenting stimuli in the sound field through calibrated speakers, and observing the child's behavior for expected reactions. Depending on the technique used, the child can be reinforced for responding to the sound. Although these are gross tests of hearing, valuable information can be obtained through BOA, COR, or VRA with children who are young and difficult to test.

Tests using speech stimuli are sometimes more successfully used with children who are young and difficult to test because speech is more meaningful than pure tones, and the child will respond more readily. A common procedure for the audiologist is to present the stimulus either through earphones or, in sound field and to observe the child, or, when possible, to have the child respond by pointing to pictures. However, even if responses to speech are within normal limits, pure-tone testing is required because speech stimuli do not test the high frequencies and significant hearing loss could still be present.

Roeser and Yellin[25] present a detailed description of the four procedures; they are described below briefly.

Behavioral Observation Audiometry. BOA provides only minimal information about hearing sensitivity, but often it is the only successful behavioral test that can be applied to children who are difficult to test. Testing usually takes place in sound field, although if the child will accept earphones they are placed on the ears.

Stimuli are presented to the child and behavioral responses are observed. Ideally, two evaluators should observe the child and a comparison of their observations made.

Testing must proceed quickly, as the child may fatigue, lose interest, or become restless. Stimuli are initially presented at low to moderate intensities and if no response is noted an intense stimulus is presented to cause a startle response. Expected responses and levels have been developed for infants and by 2 years of age the developmentally normal child should respond at near threshold levels.

BOA has many limitations but is useful as a gross test of hearing sensitivity. Significant hearing loss can be ruled out, and conditioning levels for other behavioral test procedures can be determined. Results from BOA must be viewed cautiously, as responses tend to be elevated and only represent sensitivity in the better ear when sound field testing is used.

Conditioned Orientation Reflex/Visual Reinforcement Audiometry. COR/VRA rely on conditioning. That is, when a child orients to a sound, reinforcement is provide by presentation of a visual reinforcer. This procedure is based

Table 2–2   Common Terms Used to Describe Pure-Tone Audiograms

Term	Description	Audiometric Configuration
Flat	There is little or no change in thresholds ($\pm$ 20 dB) across frequencies	
Sloping	As Frequency increases, the degree of loss increases	
Rising	As frequency increases, the degree of loss decreases	
Precipitious	There is a very sharp increase in the loss between 1 and 2 octaves	
Scoop or through shape	The greatest hearing loss is present in the mid frequencies, and hearing sensitivity is better in the low and high frequencies	
Inverted scoop or trough shape	The greatest hearing loss is in the low and high frequencies, and hearing sensitivity is better in the mid frequencies	
High frequency	The hearing loss is limited to the frequencies above the speech range (2000–3000 Hz)	
Fragmentary	Thresholds are recorded only for low frequencies, and they are in the severe to profound range	
4000–6000 Hz notch	Hearing is within normal limits through 3000 Hz and there is a sharp drop in the 4000–6000 Hz range, with improved thresholds at 8000 Hz	
Carhart's notch	There is a mixed hearing loss, and bone conduction thresholds have a characteristic configuration, with a maximum loss at 2000 Hz	

Reprinted with permission from Roeser.[23]

on the visual orientation reflex; when a light stimulus is presented, a young child will turn reflexively toward the light source. By pairing an auditory stimulus with the light stimulus, the child can be conditioned to orient to the light when the sound stimuli alone are perceived.

COR/VRA is a quick and efficient procedure. The main advantage is that the child need not perform a voluntary motor task, which makes it especially helpful when evaluating children younger than 3 years of age.

Tangible Reinforcement Operant Conditioning Audiometry. TROCA is a procedure that uses an object to reinforce a child's response to an auditory stimulus. The technique requires use of specially designed equipment that will dispense a tangible reinforcer to the child on activating a switch. The reinforcer may be food, such as candy or cereal; a drink, such as juice or soda; a small trinket or toy; or another tangible reinforcer that the child is accustomed to using. The tangible reinforcer is paired with the auditory stimulus until the auditory stimulus is conditioned to elicit a response. Children who are difficult to test will require several training sessions that last no longer than about 15 minutes to obtain reliable responses. Parents, teachers, or speech-language pathologists may include test training in their daily activities to expedite the testing.

Table 2–3 Summary of Audiological Evaluation Procedures for Infants and Children*

Name of Test	Explanation of Technique	Indicates for Use	Advantages/Disadvantages
Behavioral observation audiometry (BOA)	*Conditioning:* None A variety of test signals are presented through loudspeakers. Minimal intensity is determined where behavioral changes are observed (eg, alerting, scanning, cessation or activity, or change in sucking during testing) *Reinforcement:* None	Infants under 6 months and older youngsters with severe developmental delays *Alternative:* Auditory evoked responses (particularly if test findings suggest a signficant hearing loss)	*Advantages:* Can be used with unconditionable children *Disadvtanges:* 1. Rapid habituation of unconditioned behavior 2. Unilateral losses may be missed 3. Can only rule out severe and profound losses because relatively high intensities are required to elicit unconditioned responses even in infants with normal hearing
Conditioned orientation reflex audiometry (COR) Visual reinforcement audiometry (VRA)	*Conditioning:* Establish bond between auditory signal and flashing lighted toy *Reinforcement:* Lighted toy as well as social praise during test phase	Toddlers from 6 to 24 months and many older children with developmental delays *Alternative:* Auditory evoked responses	*Advantages:* 1. Stimuli can be presented by earphones, bone conduction, or loudspeaker 2. Does not require voluntary response 3. Capitalizes on heightened visual alertness of children with hearing impairments *Disadvantages:* 1. Approximately 35% of infants under 12 months of age cannot be conditioned 2. Many toddlers will not accept earphones initially 3. If stimuli are presented in the sound field, a unilateral hearing loss may be missed
Tangible reinforcement operant conditioning audiometry (TROCA)	*Conditioning:* Connection is established between auditory stimuli and "button-pressing" *Reinforcement:* A tangible reinforcement (such as cereal) that is automatically dispensed following a correct response	Preschoolers, especially those with short attention spans and those who work best with structure. Also many older mentally retarded children *Alternative:* VRA (auditory evoked responses)	*Advantages:* 1. Stimuli can be presented by earphones, bone conduction, or loudspeakers 2. Can be used in conjunction with frequency-specific measures *Disadvantages:* 1. Time-consuming and requires repeated sessions to establish conditioning 2. Children will often insist upon eating the reinforcer between trials, thus increasing the length of the test session substantially
Play conditioning audiometry (PCA)	*Conditioning:* Connection is established between auditory stimuli and play activity *Reinforcement:* Play activity and social reinforcement during conditioning and testing. May also use visual reinforcement	Preschoolers, 30 months to 4 years, and older children with mild developmental delays *Alternatives:* TROCA or VRA (auditory evoked responses)	*Advantages:* Can be used in conjunction with any frequency-specific measures *Disadvantages:* A variety of activities are needed to maintain interest in the activity; otherwise, response behavior habituates

*Adapted from Matkin.[24] Reprinted by permission.

Play Conditioning Audiometry. PCA is the most reliable method for children who are difficult to test when it can be applied. PCA makes testing a game. The child is trained to perform a simple motor task, such as dropping a block into a box, stacking rings, or snapping beads together. The activity is accompanied by verbal praise, which becomes reinforcing.

PCA is carried out by conditioning the child to perform the response before proceeding to threshold testing. Conditioning is carried out by presenting suprathreshold stimuli and guiding the child through the response mode. This can be accomplished by laying the headphones on a table in front of the child and presenting the stimuli at high intensities (100 to 110 dB at 1000 Hz). When responses occur without the evaluator's urging or guidance, the headphones are placed on the child, the intensity is lowered to 50 to 60 dB, responses are reestablished, and the intensity is gradually lowered in 5 to 10 dB steps until threshold is obtained. Thresholds obtained with PCA are considered very accurate.

A technique that is most helpful in PCA is play audiometry reinforcement using a flashlight (PARF). PARF is an effective procedure with very young children, as young as 2 to 2 1/2 years of age, as well as older children who are difficult to test. PARF is used to initiate the test by teaching the child the correct task to be performed in response to light and then replacing the visual stimulus with the pure-tone auditory stimulus.

The steps used in the procedure using ring stacking are illustrated in Figure 2–13 and are as follows. With the flashlight in the examiner's hand, the child holds a ring to the light (Fig. 2–13A). Once the light is flashed on and off briefly (1 to 2 seconds), the examiner takes the child's hand and moves it to the stack and helps the child to place the ring on the stack (Fig. 2–13B). Usually, after two or three trials, the child knows the response and the flashlight is put completely out of sight.

Earphones are then placed on the child's ears and the examiner takes the child's hand, which has a ring in it, and places it to the child's cheek (Fig. 2–13C). A tone is presented at 1000 Hz at 50 dB HL, and the examiner guides the child's hand to the stack and helps him to place the ring on the stack. If the child does not appear to respond at 50 dB HL, the tone is increased in intensity in 10 dB steps until a response is obtained. After the child learns the correct response, usually after three or four trials, the intensity is

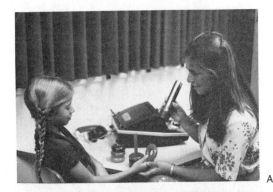

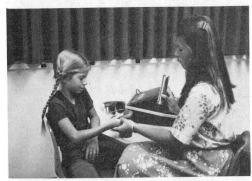

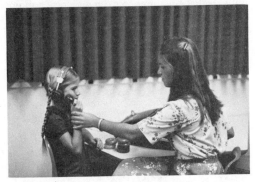

Figure 2–13. Play audiometry reinforcement using a flashlight (PARF). A. Conditioning the child to respond to the light. B. Teaching the correct response. C. Transferring to the auditory-only stimulus.

lowered in 20 dB steps until the stimuli are presented at 20 dB or higher if necessary. After 1000 Hz is tested, the procedure is continued at 2000 and 4000 Hz and then the other ear is screened.

Play conditioning can be used successfully with younger children. Generally, the procedure is limited when children are less than 30 months of age.[24]

Test Training. Test training is used with PCA when children cannot be conditioned in one or two sessions with play techniques. The procedure involves teaching the child over a series of sessions to respond by block dropping, inserting pegs into a board, or performing some other overt behavior to the presentation of an auditory stimulus. The purpose of the training is to establish a behavior that can be used in screening or testing.

The procedures used in test training are essentially the same as those described for play conditioning, but the training occurs over several, sometimes numerous, sessions. The number of sessions required to train a child will vary with each child; sometimes only five to six sessions are required and sometimes many more. It is important to keep sessions brief (10 to 15 minutes) and frequent (once or twice per school day).

The speech pathologist, whose schedule permits frequent, short contacts, often is the most likely person to do the actual training. It is advisable to set up the test training program under the direction of the audiologist because children who are in this difficult-to-test category should be tested by an audiologist after the child's behavior has been shaped.

PARF can also be used in test training. In fact, a rule to follow is that if a child will not condition to the visual stimulus with PARF, it is highly unlikely that conditioning to an auditory stimulus will be possible. Auditory stimuli are more abstract than the visual stimuli used with PARF.

Children Who Are Impossible to Test

When behavioral tests are unreliable or cannot be used, valid information on hearing sensitivity can be obtained through the use of auditory brainstem response (ABR) audiometry and otoacoustic emissions.

Auditory Brainstem Response Audiometry. ABR has also been called brainstem evoked response audiometry, but ABR is the widely accepted term. ABR has proven to be highly successful in evaluating those children who are impossible to test with behavioral procedures, including infants only a few hours old.

The procedure used to obtain ABR results involves placing small electrodes on the head and the mastoids of the individual being tested. Auditory stimuli, usually a rapid secession of clicks presented at a rate of about 10/s, are delivered to the relaxed, preferably sleeping patient. The electrodes pick up the minute electrical activity emanating from the brain and this activity is fed into a computer averager. The computer extracts the auditory signal from the ongoing electroencephalographic (EEG) activity of the brain.

The electrical signal extracted from the EEG activity reflects the sound-induced neuronal activity of the auditory nerve and brainstem pathways. The resulting response has three distinct peaks (total of seven) and the amplitude of the peaks and the time required for these peaks to appear is measured. The threshold of the ABR is used along with the time (latency) and amplitude of the peaks to determine whether hearing loss is present and the functional status of the auditory system.

The primary advantages of the ABR technique are that it is an objective procedure used for evaluating auditory sensitivity that does not require voluntary participation on the part of the patient, and it is noninvasive. As long as the patient can be maintained in a relaxed state, it is possible to obtain information on auditory sensitivity. Many clinics sedate their patients for testing.

The ABR technique is highly valuable for the patient who is impossible to test. However, a major limitation is that the test only evaluates high frequencies in the 1000 to 4000 Hz range. Thus, only partial information is obtained regarding hearing sensitivity. In addition, ABR tests auditory sensitivity only and not "hearing" (ie, cognitive interpretation of sound such as in speech audiometry). As such, ABR provides no clue as to how the patient interprets sounds even if results are normal. These two limitations make long-term monitoring of the child necessary until behavioral tests can be performed and more complete audiometric information obtained. Although these limitations do affect the predictive value of the ABR test, the technique has proven useful for those children who are impossible to test with behavioral methods. Hall[26] provides a comprehensive overview of the auditory evoked response procedures, including ABR.

Otoacoustic Emissions. Otoacoustic emissions (OAEs) are obtained by coupling a small microphone to the external ear canal, similar to the system used in immittance measures, and using averaging procedures similar to those used with ABR testing. The equipment, procedures, and interpretation used in OAE testing are quite sophisticated, but the procedure is becoming more and more clinically useful in assessing auditory sensitivity in difficult-to-test populations. In fact, OAEs have recently been endorsed as the primary test for infant hearing screening (see chapter 4).

There are two basic categories of OAEs: spontaneous otoacoustic emissions (SOAEs) and evoked (or stimulated) otoacoustic emissions (EOAEs). SOAEs, as indicated by the name, occur in the absence of stimulation to the ear. SOAEs are low intensity sounds that usually are inaudible to the individual and the meaning of their presence is still not fully understood. EOAEs are recorded by introducing different types of stimuli to the ear. The type of stimulus determines which of three types of EOAEs that are recorded: transiently evoked otoacoustic emissions (TEOAE), stimulus-frequency otoacoustic emissions (SFOAE), or distortion product otoacoustic emissions (DPOAE).

TEOAEs appear after delivering a brief stimulus (click) to the ear. SFOAEs appear during the presentation of a tonal stimulus and occur at the frequency of the stimulus. DPOAEs appear during stimulation of the ear by introducing two tonal stimuli simultaneously. DPOEAs occur at frequencies that are different from the stimulus frequencies and the observed response has a mathematical relationship to the frequencies of the primary stimuli.

Glattke and Kujawa[27] present an excellent summary of OAEs for those interested in more material on this promising clinical procedure.

THE IMMITTANCE INSTRUMENT AND MEASURES

The terminology used for measures of middle ear function has changed over the past several years and can be confusing. The following definitions should help clarify this confusion.

Impedance: opposition to the flow of energy (in the outer and middle ear) expressed in ohms. The impedance of a system is influenced by the mass, stiffness, and frictional resistance that is present. The term "impedance measures" was first used to describe the clinical procedures involved in testing middle ear function.

Admittance: the ease with which acoustic energy is transmitted (in the outer and middle ear) expressed in mhos (mho is ohm spelled backward). Admittance and compliance are terms that are used synonymously.

Immittance: Because middle ear measures are electronically or electroacoustically based on the measurement of *impedance* or *admittance*, the term "immittance" was created to encompass both techniques.[28]

Compliance: The inverse of stiffness, which relates to the ease of acoustic energy transmission (see admittance above). The terms "compliance" and "admittance" have been used synonymously; however, admittance is the suggested terminology.[29,30] Compliance and admittance are measured in equivalent volumes of air using cubic centimeters or milliliters (1 cm³ is the same volume as 1 ml; or $1.0 \text{ cm}^3 = 1.0 \text{ ml}$). Because not all have adopted the use of the term "admittance," in this chapter "admittance (compliance)" will be used.

Routine immittance measures do not assess hearing but provide objective information on the mechanical transfer function of sound in the outer and middle ear. That is, routine immittance measures assess the functional state of the conductive mechanism of the ear. Through such assessment, it is possible to detect and define disorders in the outer and middle ear system objectively.

One distinct advantage of immittance measurement is that successful testing does not rely on a behavioral response. The measures can be obtained on a child who is semicooperative, usually in less than 1 minute per ear with little difficulty. With the child who is uncooperative, more time is usually required; there are also some children who cannot be tested without major variations in the testing protocol.

Because little cooperation is required, immittance tests can be performed on younger children, as well as children who are difficult or impossible to test. The advantage of being able to apply immittance to previously untestable populations successfully has tempted many to use routine immittance measures in an effort to assess hearing sensitivity. Although there is a relationship between measures, the use of immittance measures does not eliminate the need for audiometric testing. A child can have perfectly normal findings on routine immittance tests and still manifest a significant bilateral sensorineural hearing loss.

Although the procedures used to administer immittance tests are relatively simple and can be learned in a matter of hours, the difficulty with the immittance testing lies in interpretation. To interpret the diagnostic value of the results from the immittance test battery, a thorough understanding of the auditory system and the principles of immittance are required. Such understanding includes a comprehensive knowledge of the acoustic and physiological principles underlying the immittance technique and auditory system, as well as the various pathologic conditions that may affect the auditory system. This section presents the basics of the immittance technique as they apply to immittance screening and interpretation of results. Chapter 4 describes screening principles, pure tone and immittance screening criteria and their application.

Principles of Immittance Measurement

The total or complex immittance of the ear is based on a number of physical characteristics, including mass, stiffness, and friction. For the serious student of immittance measurement, these factors and the relationship between them must be known. However, because the ear is a stiffness-dominated system, immittance can be explained simplistically by considering stiffness only.

The clinical measurement of immittance is based on the principle that when a known quantity of sound (acoustic energy) is applied to the ear, a certain amount of measured energy is reflected; the amount of reflected energy will vary depending on the stiffness (immobility) or flaccidity (mobility) of the system. The stiffer or less flaccid or less compliant (mobile) the system, the greater the amount of energy that will be reflected (which means that less energy will be admitted). Conversely, the less stiff, more flaccid, or more compliant (mobile) the system, the smaller the amount of energy that will be reflected (which means that more energy will be admitted). Note that stiffness and admittance (compliance) are reciprocally related. As one increases, the other decreases.

Various disorders in the outer and middle ear affect the stiffness of the system, which concomitantly affects mobility or admittance (compliance). When the reflected energy varies from a known normal range, many disorders affecting the outer and middle ear can be detected. This principle can be understood better by reviewing the mechanics of the immittance instrument itself.

The Immittance Instrument

The immittance instrument is sometimes called an "immittance audiometer" or an "immittance bridge," but neither of these terms is technically appropriate. An audiometer is a device used to assess hearing. Since immittance measures do not assess hearing, it is misleading to refer to an immittance instrument as an audiometer. The term "immittance bridge" was adopted because the instrument circuit contains an electronic component called a Wheatstone bridge. Because this is only one component of a more complex system, the terminology is also not accurate.

The ANSI standard for immittance instruments is ANSI S3.39-1987 (ASA 71).[31] As with audiometers, the standard can be obtained for a fee by writing to American National Standards Institute at 1430 Broadway, New York, NY 10018 or to the Acoustical Society of America at 335 East 45th St., New York, NY 10017. All current immittance equipment should meet the 1987 ANSI standards.

Basic Functions. The manner in which immittance testing is performed has changed significantly in recent years. Initially, immittance instruments were operated manually, but with computer technology we now have microprocessor-based instruments that operate automatically. Figure 2–14 shows a microprocessor-based diagnostic immittance instrument. This instrument allows the user to perform simple screening testing as well as advanced diagnostic procedures (such as reflex decay and reflex latency) and can be used in an automatic mode or manually.

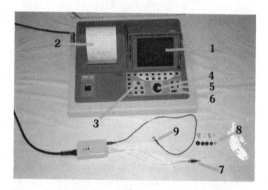

Figure 2–14. A diagnostic immittance instrument (see text for description).

The function of each major component will be described.

CRT Screen (1 in fig. 2–14). This screen displays the data that are collected during immittance measurements.

Print out (2 in Fig. 2–14). A hard copy of the data shown on the CRT screen can be printed (see example in Fig. 2–22).

Manual control (3 in Fig. 2–14). Allows the user to run each applicable test procedure manually.

Pressure control (4 in Fig. 2–14). The pressure control operates an air pump that is used to increase and decrease the air pressure in the external auditory canal during manual tympanometry. A manometer measures the pressure change as it occurs. The range of pressures available in most immittance instruments is from 200 to −400 or −600 daPa. Originally, immittance units measured pressure in millimeters of water pressure, and older equipment will express pressure in this terminology. Because decaPascals and millimeters of water are virtually the same in the pressure ranges used to perform immittance measures on the ear (97.8 daPa = 100 mm/H^2O), the two measures can be considered equivalent.

Reflex Eliciting Stimulus (5 in Fig. 2–14). Allows the examiner to choose either from puretone stimuli at octave frequencies from 250 to 4000 Hz, or broad band noise, low pass filtered noise, or high pass filtered noise.

Intensity Control (6 in Fig. 2–14). Allows the examiner to choose the intensity of the reflex eliciting stimuli from 35 to 110 dB HL for ipsilateral presentation and 35 to 120 dB HL for contralateral stimulation. Exposure to intensity levels above 110 dB HL can be harmful and extreme care should be taken when presenting acoustic reflex stimuli at high intensities.

Probe (7 in Fig 2–14). The probe is inserted into the external auditory canal; the ear into which the probe is inserted is the ear from which the immittance measures are being recorded.

Probe Tips (8 in Fig. 2–14). Various sized plastic or rubber tips are placed at the end of the probe. These tips allow the probe to be inserted into the external auditory canal so that the necessary hermetic (airtight) seal can be obtained during immittance measures.

Contralateral Reflex-Eliciting Earphone (9 in Fig. 2–14). For this instrument, an insert-type earphone is used; other instruments use a standard supra-aural earphone. The contralateral acoustic reflex-eliciting earphone is placed into the ear opposite (contralateral to) the probe ear. The reflex-eliciting earphone is used to present a signal to the ear opposite the probe ear to determine the presence or absence of acoustic reflexes.

Figure 2–15 shows how the probe is placed in the ear canal (top) and how the headset of the immittance instrument is placed for testing (bottom). With the headset in one position, immittance findings are obtained for one ear (the probe ear); the ipsilateral acoustic reflex stimulus is delivered to the probe ear, and the contralateral acoustic stimulus is delivered to the ear opposite the probe ear (contralateral reflex-eliciting ear).

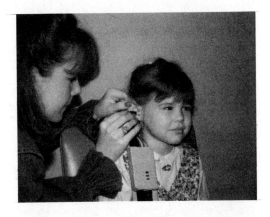

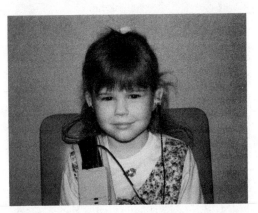

Figure 2–15. Placement of the probe into the external auditory canal (top). The bottom photograph shows how the instrument would be placed for obtaining the immittance values in the probe right ear; the left ear canal has an insert earphone placed into it for stimulation of the contralateral acoustic reflex.

The headset is then reversed and the procedure is repeated.

In Figure 2–15, the immittance and ipsilateral reflex of the right ear are being measured. The contralateral acoustic reflex-eliciting signal is being delivered to the left ear; the acoustic reflex from the left ear stimulation is being recorded in the (contralateral) right ear. When describing immittance results, it is helpful to describe them in reference to the probe ear. In this way, no confusion will exist about the ear being described.

Figure 2–16 is a schematic representation of the principles used to determine the immittance in the probe ear. The diagram illustrates the closed cavity between the probe tip of the immittance instrument and the external ear canal: the area from the end of the probe tip to the tympanic membrane. As shown in Figure 2–16, the probe tip is connected to three components in the immittance instrument: a loudspeaker (2a), an air

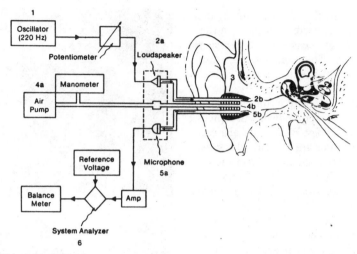

Figure 2-16. Principles of immittance measurement in the probe ear (see text for description).

pump and manometer (4a), and a microphone (5a). The immittance probe apparatus measures the stiffness or admittance (compliance) of the middle ear system in the following way: a 220 Hz or 226 Hz (other probe frequencies are used when advanced tests are performed) probe tone emitted from the loudspeaker (2a) is introduced into the external ear canal through a port in the probe tip (2b). Depending on the state of the ear canal and middle ear, some energy is absorbed and transmitted to the inner ear and some energy is reflected. The reflected energy is picked up through a second port in the probe tip (5b) and delivered to the microphone (5a), and the system analyzer (6) compares the input signal to the reflected energy.

As already described, the immittance instrument acts like a small sound pressure measuring device in determining the state of the middle ear. The amount of reflected energy picked up by the microphone from the probe tone determines the functional state of the ear. A high amount of reflected energy means that the system is more stiff or less compliant than normal, and vice versa. Conditions such as otitis media and ossicular chain fixation result in high stiffness or low admittance (compliance); in such cases the reflected energy would be higher than normal. Conversely, low stiffness or high admittance (compliance) would be caused by conditions such as disarticulation of the ossicular chain or a scarred, flaccid tympanic membrane. Under these conditions, more energy would pass through than normally, so the amount reflected would be less than normal.

The third port in the probe tip (4b) is connected to an air pump and manometer (4a). The air pump and manometer act together to increase, decrease, and measure the air pressure in the outer ear canal. This system is used in obtaining the tympanogram (described later).

Microprocessor (automatic) immittance units are being used more frequently in audiology clinics and in screening programs. This type of equipment is designed to be used in situations in which rapid assessment of middle ear function is required, such as in large-scale screening programs and with the pediatric population, where the child typically will not remain quiet for more than few seconds. Figure 2-17 shows an automatic immittance unit in use during screening. The primary advantages of using this type of equipment is that obtaining an airtight seal requires only that it be held over the entrance of the ear canal, simplifying the procedure; and only about 5 to 10 seconds is required to perform tympanometry, static admittance, and ipsilateral acoustic reflex measures for each ear. Following the data collection, the information is displayed on a light-emitting diode screen or a hard copy can be printed. An example is provided in Figure 2-18.

Immittance Measures

Table 2-4 lists the four basic immittance procedures used to assess middle ear function: tympanogram, tympanogram height, physical volume, and acoustic reflex. In addition, a comparison is

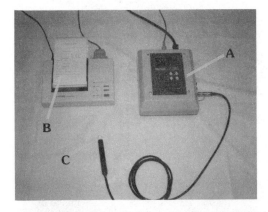

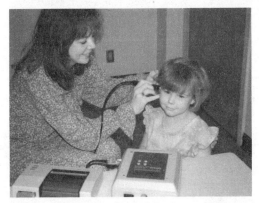

Figure 2–17. Example of a microprocessor-based screening immittance unit (top): A is the processor, B is the printer, and C is the probe tip. Data are obtained by holding the probe against the external auditory canal for about 5 seconds (bottom).

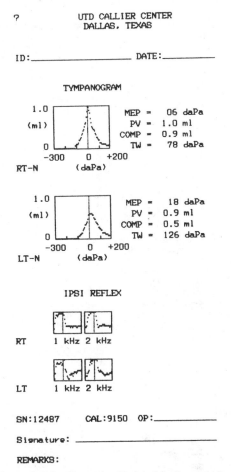

Figure 2–18. Example of printed findings obtained from a microprocessor-based screening immittance unit. Results shown would indicate normal middle ear function (see text for description).

made between the classic (descriptive) immittance method and the absolute (microprocessor-based) method. As shown, the two procedures use essentially the same information, but classify results differently for the tympanogram. The classic method describes the tympanogram shape (type A, B, and C).[32] However, the absolute method provides objective measures of the tympanogram: Tympanometric peak pressure (TPP), tympanometric width/gradient (TW or GR), and tympanogram height (static admittance-peak Y).[29,30] Table 2–5 lists the mean norms for each of the basic immittance procedures and gives the 90% ranges for children and adults separately. Although each test provides significant information by itself, immittance tests are not performed or interpreted in isolation. Diagnostic capabilities are strengthened when the results of all test procedures are interpreted together.

Tympanogram. The tympanogram measures eardrum admittance (compliance) or mobility as a function of mechanically varying the air pressure in an hermetically sealed external ear canal. The admittance (compliance) or mobility of the eardrum at an air pressure ranging from +200 to −400 daPa is recorded on a graph referred to as a tympanogram. The tympanogram is plotted by introducing the positive and negative air pressure into the probe ear, and recording the admittance (compliance) of the ear, based on the amount of reflected energy.

To comprehend how varying the air pressure in the external auditory canal affects the amount of reflected energy from the tympanic membrane, one must understand the pressure/admittance (compliance) principle. Figure 2–19 illustrates this principle in a normal ear. Recall that stiffness and admittance (compliance) are reciprocally related and that by measuring one of these characteristics, the other can be derived.

In Figure 2–19, the amount of reflected energy is at its lowest point when the pressure in the

Table 2–4   Summary of Immittance Tests and Comparison of Classic and Absolute (Microprocessor-Based) Procedures

Procedure	Purpose	Classic Description	Units of Measurement	Absolute Description	Unit of Measurement
Tympanogram	Assess the pressure/ compliance function of the eardrum	Type A, B, C	Relative units	Tympano-metric peak pressure (TPP)	daPa
				Tympano-metric width (TW) gradient (GR)	daPa
Tympanogram height	Classification of tympanogram	Static compliance	cm³/ml*	Static admittance (peak Y)	mmho or cm³/ml*
Physical volume	Measures the equivalent volume of the space be-tween the probe tip and the eardrum	Physical volume test	cm³/ml*	Equivalent ear canal volume (V$_{ec}$)	cm³/ml*
Acoustic reflex	Indirect measure of stapedial muscle contrac-tion to intense sound	Acoustic reflex	Relative change in eardrum admittance (compliance)	Acoustic reflex (AR)	Relative change in eardrum admittance (compliance)

*Cubic centimeters and milliliters are identical volumes (1 cm³ = 1 ml).

Table 2–5   Mean Norms and 90% Ranges for Immittance Measures*

Tympanometric Peak Pressure (TPP)	Tympanometric Width/Gradient (TW/GR)	Static Admittance/ Compliance (Peak Y)	Ear Canal Volume (V^{ec})
Borderline – 100 to – 200 daPa	Children mean = 100 daPa	Children mean = 0.5 mmho/cm³/ml†	Children mean = 0.7 cm³/ml†
	90% range = 60–150 daPa	90% range = 0.2–0.9, mmho/cm³/ml†	90% range = 0.4–1.0, cm³/ml†
Abnormal More negative than – 200 daPa	Adult mean = 80 daPa	Adult mean = 0.8, mmho/cm³/ml†	Adult mean = 1.1 cm³/ml†
	90% range = 50–110 daPa	90% range = 0.3–1.4, mmho/cm³/ml†	90% range = 0.6–1.5 cm³/ml†

*Adapted from American Speech and Hearing Association Committee on Audiometric Evaluation[28] and from Margolis and Heller.[29]
†Cubic centimeters (cm³) and milliliters (ml) are identical volumes (1 cm³ = 1 ml).

external auditory canal is at atmospheric pressure (0 daPa). Under this condition, in the normal ear: (1) there is equal pressure between the external and middle ear cavities; (2) the amount of energy absorbed by the tympanic membrane and middle ear structures from the probe tone is at the great-est level; and (3) the amount of reflected energy from the probe tone is at its lowest level, which means that the admittance (compliance) is at its highest point. However, when either a positive or negative pressure is introduced into the ex-

ternal ear canal, the force exerted on the normal tympanic membrane stretches and stiffens it and other middle ear structures. The increase in stiff-ness, with a concomitant decrease in admittance (compliance), increases the amount of reflected energy. In Figure 2–19, the amount of reflected energy is highest at 200 and −300 daPa, which indicates that admittance (compliance) is at its lowest point at these two pressures for this ear.

Modern, microprocessor-based immittance in-struments are quick and efficient; the immittance

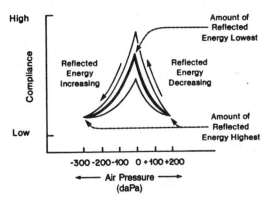

Figure 2–19. Schematic representation of how varying air pressure in the external ear canal affects the stiffness of the eardrum and the reflected energy of the probe tone (see text for description).

data are recorded automatically in just a few seconds by simply placing the probe into the ear canal. However, by using these automatic instruments, the examiner may not fully understand how the data are being collected. The procedure for manually plotting the data is more helpful in explaining the principles of immittance measurement.

Figure 2–20 shows a manually plotted tympanogram. Air pressure is introduced into the ear canal at 200 daPa. The 200 daPa pressure establishes a stiff system with low admittance (compliance), and the amount of reflected energy is greater than at atmospheric pressure. At this point, the first reading (1 in Fig. 2–20) is obtained; in the example in Fig. 2–20 the reading is 1.4 ml. This reading also represents the equivalent physical volume of the system (see Physical/Ear Canal Volume later).

In the normal ear the admittance (compliance) obtained at 200 daPa will be low. The air pressure is then gradually reduced from 200 daPa until it reaches the point where the amount of reflected energy is the lowest, and the admittance (compliance) is the highest. This point is termed the point of maximum admittance (compliance) and indicates that the air pressure is equal between the external ear canal and middle ear cavity. At this point, the second reading (2 in Fig. 2–20) is noted on the tympanogram. In the normal ear, the point of maximum admittance (compliance) is at or near atmospheric pressure (0 to −50 daPa). Finally, a third reading (3 in Fig. 2–20) is made at a more negative pressure, about −200 daPa less pressure than the point of maximum admittance (compliance), to complete the tympanometric configuration. When the three points are connected, a pattern results that can be classified according to normal or various abnormal middle ear conditions.

Tympanograms can be plotted using a relative or absolute scale. Examples of the two methods are shown in Figures 2–18 and 2–20. Note that for relative measures the 200 daPa reading is always at 0 ml. With absolute measurements, the 200 daPa reading also provides information on ear canal volume (see Physical/Ear Canal Volume later).

Classical (Descriptive) Method. Several systems have been proposed to classify tympanograms. Due to its simplicity, the classic (descriptive) method shown in Figure 2–21 has been the most popular. The three type A classifications represent normal middle ear pressure; the sub-

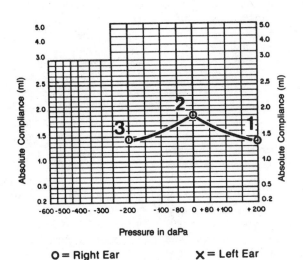

O = Right Ear   X = Left Ear

Figure 2–20. Example of a manually plotted tympanogram (see text for description).

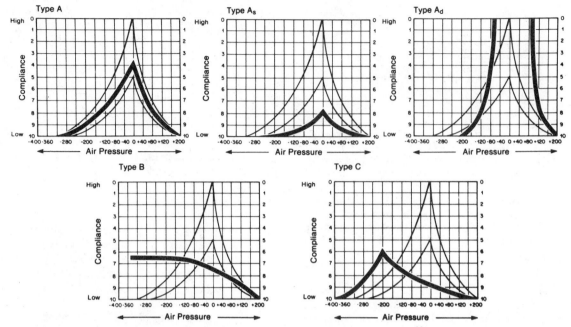

Figure 2–21. The classic (A, B, C) classification of tympanograms (after Jerger[32]).

classifications of types Ad and As represent abnormally high and low admittance (compliance), respectively. The type B classification represents little or no admittance (compliance) in the conductive system, regardless of the air pressure in the external ear. This is the most abnormal tympanogram that can be found. The type C classification represents abnormal negative pressure in the middle ear.

Absolute Method. Although the classic method for describing tympanograms is simple, it is subjective and not all tympanograms fall into the A, B, and C classifications. The absolute method quantifies tympanogram classification using TPP and (TW or GR).

TPP is a direct measure of the air pressure in the middle ear. Negative pressure occurs when the gas (air) is absorbed in the middle ear due to eustachian tube closure. Negative TPP is indicative of the early stages of otitis media; positive TPP is found in early stages of acute otitis media. Table 2–5 provides mean norms for TPP, as well as three other basic immittance measures. Normal middle ear pressure ranges between +50 and −100 daPa. As shown in Table 2–5, between −100 and −200 daPa middle ear function borderlines on abnormal, and beyond −200 daPa middle ear function is abnormal. Research has shown that large fluctuations can be found in TPP; abnormal TPP in the absence of other middle ear anomalies does not reflect significant changes in other middle ear function,

and abnormal TPP cannot be observed reliably with an otoscope. Due to these observations, TPP is not used as a unitary criterion for referral (see Chapter 4).

(TW or GR) describes the shape of the tympanogram surrounding the peak. TW/GR is calculated by measuring the pressure range corresponding to a percentage of reduction in static admittance from the maximum peak admittance. The procedure is: (1) the peak (maximum) admittance is determined (for example, 1.0 cm³/ml); (2) the peak admittance is reduced by a percentage (for example, 50%); (3) the values on the positive and negative pressure tails of the tympanogram are noted (at 0.5 cm³/ml); and (4) the distance between the positive tympanogram tail and negative tympanogram tail is measured in decaPascal. The current norms provided in Table 2–5 are based on a 50% criterion.[30]

TW/GR measures appear to be sensitive to middle ear diseases that are not detected by other immittance measures or otoscopy. However, this is a relatively new measure and more data are needed to establish efficiency. It should be noted that when tympanograms are flat (type B) the TW/GR cannot be measured properly (see Fig. 2–26).

Tympanogram Height: Static Admittance (Compliance)

In addition to peak pressure and width, proper interpretation of the tympanogram depends on

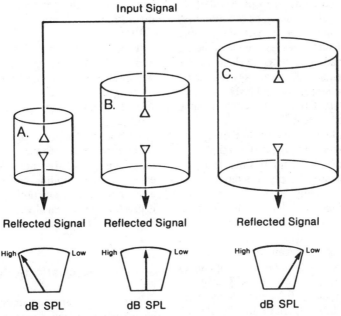

Figure 2–22. The effects of volume change on the input/output function of an acoustic signal for a small cavity (A), a medium cavity (B), and a large cavity (C).

specifying its height. Static admittance (compliance) provides objective information on tympanogram height by quantifying its peak relative to the tail value (obtained at 200 daPa).

Static admittance (compliance) measurement can be explained using the volume principle, which states that the absolute size of a cavity of known physical characteristics (a hard wall cavity) can be determined by knowing the amount of reflected energy from an input signal of known intensity. Figure 2–22 illustrates this concept. Figure 2–22A shows a fixed volume cavity with an input acoustic signal and a reflected SPL value, which is high compared with Figure 2–22B and C. In Figure 2–22B, the same input acoustic signal is used, but the output SPL is reduced due to the increased volume in the larger cavity. With a larger cavity, there is more absorption, which causes less resistance and, as a result, there is less reflection of energy. In Figure 2–22C, the same input acoustic signal is also used, but once again output SPL is reduced due to an even larger cavity. Based on this simple principle, the absolute volume of a cavity can be determined as long as the physical characteristics of the cavity are specified.

Static admittance is measured by introducing a positive pressure into the external auditory canal. In a normal ear the increased stiffness of the tympanic membrane sets up an artificial

acoustical "wall." Under this condition, the volume of the cavity from the probe tip of the immittance instrument to the ear drum is measured in volume units (cubic centimeters or milliliters) equivalent to a cavity of known physical characteristics. Note that the term "equivalent" is used because the physical characteristics of each ear canal will vary, and the reflected energy must be used in comparison to a standard cavity (a hard-wall cavity) of known physical characteristics. The pressure is then removed, the tympanic membrane returns to its natural resting place, and the artificial acoustical wall will no longer be present. Under this condition, the cavity from the probe tip, including the external canal and middle ear space, is measured in equivalent units.

The procedure used to obtain static admittance is to place the probe tip into the external ear canal, which directs the probe tone into the ear canal, and introduce a pressure of 200 daPa. The positive air pressure serves to stretch and stiffen the tympanic membrane, resulting in a large amount of reflected energy. An admittance (compliance) reading is obtained, which gives an equivalent volume (cubic centimeters or milliliters) at this positive air pressure setting. When the ear drum is intact, this reading is the equivalent volume of the external ear canal (sometimes referred to as the C1 reading). The air pressure is then adjusted from 200 daPa to the point of maximum admittance (compliance) (at or near 0 daPa in the normal ear) and a second reading is made (sometimes referred to at the C2 reading). This reading is the equivalent volume of the total outer and middle ear system. Static admittance (compliance) is calculated by subtracting the first reading (C1) from the second reading (C2). This derived value represents the equivalent volume of the middle ear system. In Figure 2–20 the static admittance (compliance) is 0.5 ml (1.9 ml minus 1.4 ml). With microprocessing immittance units, the user simply sees the resulting admittance value. In Figure 2–18 the static admittance (compliance) is 0.9 ml for the right ear (0.9 ml minus 0 ml) and 0.5 for the left (0.5 minus 0 ml).

Table 2–5 provides the mean normal values and 90% ranges for static admittance (compliance) for children and adults separately. As shown, for children the mean value is 0.5 mmho/cm³/ml with a range of 0.2 to 0.9 mmho/cm³/ml. For adults, the mean value is 0.8 mmho/cm³/ml, with a range of 0.3 to 1.4 mmho/cm³/ml.

Physical/Ear Canal Volume

In the presence of a flat tympanogram, static admittance (compliance) measures help to detect ear drum perforation and determine whether a pressure equalization (PE) tube (surgically placed in an ear drum) is patent (open). This additional information is available when the first reading (at +200 daPa; the C1 reading) is obtained. The measure is sometimes called the physical volume test (PVT) but the ASHA standard[30] refers to this measure as "ear canal volume."

The PVT is accomplished by introducing positive air pressure into the external auditory canal and obtaining a reading at +200 daPa (a C1 reading). Mean ear canal volume norms and 90% ranges are provided in Table 2–5 for children and adults separately. For children, the mean is 0.7 cm³/ml with a 90% range of 0.4 to 1.0 cm³/ml. For adults, the mean is 1.1 cm3/ml with a 90% range of 0.6 to 1.5 cm³/ml. If a reading is unusually high, often exceeding 4.0 to 5.0 cm³/ml in adults, and a flat (type B) tympanogram is obtained, a perforation is present or if a PE tube was previously placed it is patent (open). In Figure 2–18 ear canal volume (PV) is given in digital form (1.0 ml for the right ear and 0.9 ml for the left). In Figure 2–20 the ear canal volume is provided on the tympanogram

in absolute equivalent volume [1.4 ml, which is the admittance (compliance) reading at +200 daPa].

It should be recognized that the size and shape of the probe tip and its placement in the ear canal will influence the ear canal volume reading. This may result in some test/retest variability, but should not change the interpretation of the test significantly.

When testing an ear with a perforation or open PE tube, the pressure may suddenly release when introducing a positive pressure into the external ear canal. This finding would indicate that the eustachian tube is functioning. When a PE tube is present and ear canal volume is normal or below normal, the ventilating tube may be blocked.

Acoustic Reflexes

The acoustic reflex occurs when a small muscle in the middle ear, the stapedius, contracts due to high intensity stimulation; this reflex should occur in both ears (bilaterally). The fact that the acoustic reflex is bilateral means that a signal directed to one ear can elicit a recordable reflex in the opposite (contralateral) ear.

When the stapedius muscle contracts in the normal ear, there is a resulting stiffening of the tympanic membrane. This stiffening of the tympanic membrane during contraction is detected by the immittance instrument as a change in the reflected energy from the probe tone. The change is monitored by the system analyzer and projected to the immittance instrument. It is important to realize that the immittance procedure does not measure middle ear muscle contraction directly, but *measures the effect of middle ear muscle contraction on tympanic membrane stiffening.* This has an important implication in interpreting the clinical value of acoustic reflex results, because mechanical changes in the middle ear can obliterate recording the acoustic reflex when it occurs. That is, the middle ear muscles may contract, but the presence of middle ear pathologic changes will obliterate the affect of the contraction on the stiffness change necessary to record the contraction with the immittance instrument.

Contralateral measurement of the acoustic reflex is achieved by presenting different acoustic signals through the reflex-eliciting earphone to one ear and measuring the change in stiffness that results due to the muscle contraction in the probe ear. This test should be performed with the middle ear system at the point of maximum admittance (compliance). If the reflex is not measured at the point of maximum admittance (compliance), it may be obliterated due to the pressure imbalance between the ear canal and the middle ear cavity.

Ipsilateral reflex measurement is achieved by stimulating and measuring the reflex in the same (probe) ear. The advantages of ipsilateral reflex measurement in diagnostic testing are reviewed by Jerger.[33]

Acoustic reflexes can be assessed by obtaining the threshold at which the reflex occurs, or screened by presenting the reflex-eliciting tone at a fixed intensity (100 or 105 dB HL). In the normal ear, acoustic reflexes are elicited between 85 and 95 dB HL. Once threshold is established at one frequency, the level is recorded and other frequencies can be tested. However, in immittance screening only one frequency is typically screened at a fixed intensity of about 100 dB (see Chapter 4).

Figure 2–23 A and B provide graphic displays of acoustic reflex threshold measurement from two different ears; for both measures only ipsilateral reflexes were obtained. In Figure 2–23A the test frequencies were 1000 and 2000 Hz, and the thresholds were 85 dB HL at 1000 Hz and 95 dB HL at 2000 Hz. In Figure 2–23B the test frequencies also were 1000 and 2000 Hz; the thresholds were 85 dB HL for both frequencies. Note how the amplitude changes in the recordings by varying the intensity of the eliciting signal.

The presence of reflexes within normal limits at all frequencies is consistent with normal middle ear function; there is also a high probability that auditory sensitivity is within normal limits. However, acoustic reflexes may occur at expected intensities at all frequencies when mild or moderate to severe sensorineural hearing loss is present. For this reason, acoustic reflexes cannot be used to predict hearing threshold sensitivity with absolute assurance. Hearing threshold sensitivity must be assessed behaviorally if there are questions regarding hearing loss.

If reflexes are absent, some form of middle ear disease may be indicated. Absent reflexes may also indicate a moderate to severe sensorineural hearing loss without recruitment, or a paralysis of the VIIth cranial nerve in the central auditory pathways. Absent reflexes have also occasionally been observed in individuals with normal or near-normal hearing, which may indicate middle ear disease or neurological involvement of the VIIIth or VIIth nerve.

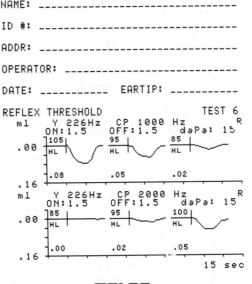

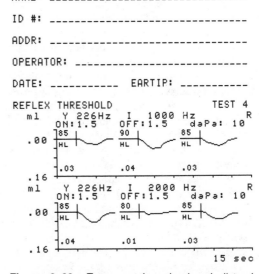

Figure 2–23. Two · examples showing ipsilateral acoustic reflex recordings. The presence of a reflex is indicated by a downward deflection of the tracing (see text for additional discription).

Partial or elevated reflexes may also be recorded. "Partial" means that a reflex is present at some frequencies tested and absent at others, and "elevated" refers to reflexes that are present at a hearing level exceeding 100 dB HL. Partial or elevated reflexes may indicate the presence of a hearing loss at those frequencies in which they are absent.

Acoustic reflex measures provide a powerful diagnostic assessment of middle ear function and neurological functioning of the auditory system, as well as an index of auditory sensitivity. However, as pointed out in Chapter 4, because of their high level of sensitivity, acoustic reflexes are not used as a referral criterion for screening.

CLASSIFYING IMMITTANCE FINDINGS

Table 2–6 classifies the common findings that are obtained from the standard immittance test battery (see Table 2–4) into 11 different categories. This classification system compares the classic (descriptive) method of describing the tympanograms with the absolute method and allows for a direct comparison of the different measures that are obtained. Table 2–7 provides the clinical implications for each of the 11 categories. These categories should help to develop appropriate referral strategies.

Category I findings represent normal middle ear function.

Category II findings represent normal peak pressure, tympanometric width, and admittance (compliance), but the acoustic reflex is absent. Middle ear disorder or hearing loss is suggested.

Categories III through VI represent normal peak pressure, but tympanometric width and admittance (compliance) values fall outside the range of normal limits. The presence of the acoustic reflex for categories III and V would suggest that the abnormal tympanometric width and admittance (compliance) is not significant. However, in the presence of abnormal tympanometric width and admittance (compliance), an absent acoustic reflex (categories IV and VI) would suggest middle ear disorder.

Categories VII and VIII represent little or no admittance (compliance); TPP and TW are either absent or higher than normal, and static admittance (compliance) is lower than normal. For these two categories, when physical/ear canal volume is normal or low (category VII) the physical/ear canal volume predicts effusion; when physical/ear canal volume values are high (category VIII), a perforated eardrum or open PE tube is indicated.

Category IX represents abnormal negative pressure in the middle ear cavity. Abnormal middle ear pressure is a precursor to or possible resolution of middle ear effusion. Although middle ear disorder is predicted, large middle ear pressure variations are common (see Chapter 4). Abnormal middle ear pressure in isolation does not warrant follow-up or treatment.

Category X represents abnormal middle ear pressure, higher tympanometric width, and reduced admittance (compliance). This category suggests effusion in the middle ear.

Category XI includes all other possible outcomes.

Application of Audiometric and Immittance Principles

The following four cases will be used to integrate and clarify the audiometric and immittance principles discussed in this chapter. Figure 2–24 shows findings for normal hearing and normal middle ear function bilaterally. On the audiogram, thresholds are no poorer than 5 dB HL at any test frequency. As expected, speech audiometry reveals normal SRTs, agreeing with PTAs, and word recognition (Discrim) scores within the normal range (90 to 100%). Tympanograms are type A bilaterally, with tympanometric peak pressure (Figs. 2–24 through 2–27 shown tympanometric peak pressure as MEP), static admittance/compliance (COMP), and tympanometric width (TW) within the normal range for the left ear; static admittance/compliance (COMP) is at the lower range of normal for the right ear, which explains why tympanometric peak pressure (MEP) and tympanometric width (TW) were not recordable. Ipsilateral acoustic reflexes are present bilaterally at 1000 and 2000 Hz. Immittance results are classified as category I bilaterally (normal middle ear function).

Figure 2–25 shows findings for a mild to severe bilateral sloping sensorineural hearing loss. Thresholds are within the range of normal limits at 250 and 500 Hz and drop into the moderate to severe range at higher frequencies. SRTs are within normal limits and agree with the two frequency PTA (500 and 1000 Hz). In this case, because of the large difference between thresholds at 1000 and 2000 Hz, only 500 and 1000 Hz are used to calculate the PTA. Word recognition (Discrim) scores are reduced bilaterally, with a poorer score in the left ear (70%) than in the right (82%).

Normal tympanograms (type A) with tympanometric peak pressure (MEP), static admittance/compliance (COMP), and tympanometric width

Table 2–6   Categories of Common Immittance Findings by Classic (Descriptive) Method (Type A, B, C) and Absolute Measures

Category (Designator)	Classic (Descriptive) Method (Type)	Tympan-ometric Peak Pressure (TTP)	Typan-ometric Width/ Gradient (TW/GR)	Static Admittance/ Compliance (Peak Y)	Ear Canal/ Physical Volume Test (PV/V$_{ec}$)	Ipsilateral Acoustic Reflex (AR)
I	A	Normal	Normal	Normal	Normal	Present
II	A	Normal	Normal	Normal	Normal	Absent
III	Ad	Normal	Higher than normal	Higher than normal	Normal	Present
IV	Ad	Normal	Higher than normal	Higher than normal	Normal	Absent
V	As	Normal	Lower than normal	Lower than normal	Normal	Present
VI	As	Normal	Lower than normal	Lower than normal	Normal	Absent
VII	B flat	Absent or lower than normal	Absent or higher than normal*	Lower than normal	Normal or low	Absent
VIII	B flat	Absent or lower than normal	Absent or higher than normal	Lower than normal	Higher than normal	Absent
IX	C	More nega-tive than normal	Normal	Normal	Normal	Present or absent
X	"Rounded" C	More nega-tive than normal	Higher than normal	Lower than normal	Normal	Absent
XI Other						

*See Table 2–7 for interpretation of categories. See text for abbreviations.

Table 2–7   Clinical Implictions of Categories Listed in Table 2–6 for Middle Ear Disorders

Category	Clinical Implications for Middle Ear Disorder
I	Normal middle ear function
II	When other immittance results are within normal limits, but the acoustic reflex is absent, if significant sensorineural hearing loss is not present and neurological function is normal, middle ear disorder is predicted
III	Increased admittance (compliance) (mobility) in the eardrum or middle ear system; when acoustic reflexes are present, in the absence of conductive hearing loss, middle ear disorder is not predicted
IV	Increased admittance (compliance) (moblity) in the eardrum or middle ear system; when acoustic reflexes are absent, in the presence of conductive hearing loss, middle ear disorder (disarticulation of ossicular chain) is predicted
V	Decreased admittance (compliance) (mobility) in the eardrum or middle ear system; when acoustic reflexes are present, in the absence of conductive hearing loss, middle ear disorder is not predicted
VI	Decreased admittance (compliance) (mobility) in the eardrum or middle ear system; when acoustic reflexes are absent, in the presence of conductive hearing loss, middle ear disorder (fixation of the ossicular chain) is predicted
VII	Little or no admittance (compliance) (mobility) of the eardrum or middle ear system; when the physical volume (V$_{ec}$) is within normal limits, possible effusion (fluid) in middle ear or other significant middle ear disorder is predicted
VIII	Little or no admittance (compliance) in the system; when the physical volume test (V$_{ec}$) is high, the equivalent volume of the ear canal and middle ear are being measured. Perforation of the eardrum is predicted, or if PE (tympanostomy) tube is in eardrum it is patent (open)
IX	Abnormal negative pressure in the middle ear cavity. Possibly precursory to or resolution of middle ear effusion
X	Abnormal negative pressure in the middle ear cavity and reduced admittance (compliance) (mobility) of the eardrum and/or middle ear system. Middle ear effusion or other significant middle ear disorder is predicted
XI	Other. Classifications I through X describe the preponderance of immittance findings; however, other outcomes are possible

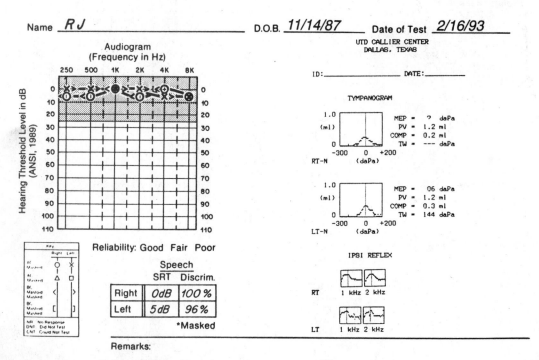

Figure 2–24. Audiometric and immittance findings within normal limits bilaterally (category I).

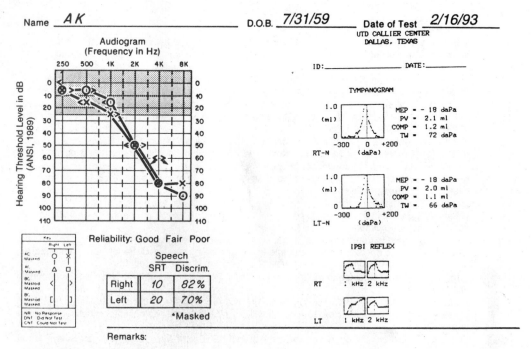

Figure 2–25. A mild to severe sloping high-frequency sensorineural hearing loss bilaterally. Immittance results are classified as category I bilaterally.

(TW) within normal limits are shown bilaterally. Note that acoustic reflexes are present bilaterally despite the presence of the high-frequency hearing loss. Immittance results are classified as category I bilaterally (normal middle ear function).

Individuals with audiometric findings like those shown in Figure 2–25 would be difficult to identify without pure-tone audiometric tests. Such individuals will usually respond to speech within normal limits, because of the normal thresholds in the 250 to 1000 Hz range. However, such individuals will have considerable difficulty in discriminating speech, especially in the presence of background noise; and this difficulty may not be readily apparent to others. In addition, abnormal speech production may be present, because high-frequency fricative and sibilant sounds would be distorted. Only through audiometric screening/ testing would individuals with audiometric results like those shown in Figure 2–25 be detected.

The results in Figure 2–26 show normal hearing in the right ear with a mild rising conductive hearing loss in the left ear. SRTs are in agreement with the PTA for both ears and support the degree of hearing loss in the left ear. Word recognition (Discrim) scores are within normal limits bilaterally.

Immittance findings support normal middle ear function for the right ear and the presence of a conductive hearing loss in the left ear. For the right ear, the tympanogram is normal (type A), with tympanometric peak pressure (MEP), static admittance/compliance (COMP) and tympanometric width (TW) within the normal range. The left ear shows a flat (type B) tympanogram with unmeasurable static admittance/compliance (COMP). Note that the physical volume (PV) for the left ear is within normal limits, suggesting that the ear drum is intact. Acoustic reflexes are present in the right ear and, due to the conductive pathologic condition, absent in the left ear. Contralateral acoustic reflexes were not measured but would be absent bilaterally. Immittance results are classified as category I for the right ear and category VII for the left.

Figure 2–27 shows audiometric results for a hearing loss in the severe to profound range bilaterally. Thresholds between 250 and 500 Hz range from 65 dB HL; no responses were recorded at 110 dB HL above 1000 Hz. SRTs and word recognition (Discrim) scores could not be obtained due to the severity of the loss. Note that even though the SRTs could not be measured, speech detection/awareness thresholds (SAT)

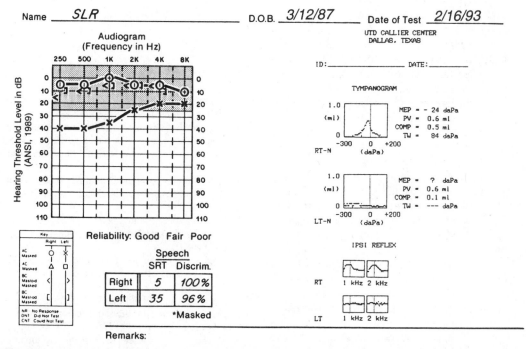

Figure 2–26. A mild left ear rising conductive hearing loss with normal hearing in the right ear. Immittance findings are classified as category I for the right ear and category VII for the left.

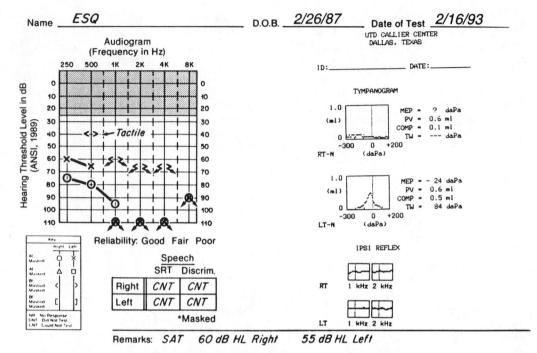

Figure 2–27. A severe to profound bilateral (primarily) sensorineural hearing loss with abnormal immittance findings for the right ear. Immittance findings are classified as category I for the right ear and category VII for the left.

were obtained and agreed with thresholds in the 250 Hz region. Response by bone conduction was obtained at 250 Hz at maximum limits of the audiometer (40 dB HL) for each ear, but no responses were obtained above this frequency. Because bone conduction threshold responses were present only at 250 Hz at equipment limits (40 dB HL), they are considered tactile stimulation rather than auditory; the child felt them rather than heard them.

The tympanogram was normal for the right ear, but abnormal (flat; type B) with low static admittance/compliance (COMP) for the left ear. The physical volume was within the normal range for the left ear, indicating that the eardrum was intact. As expected, due to the degree of hearing loss present, acoustic reflexes were absent bilaterally. Immittance data are classified as category I for the left ear and category VII for the right.

The data in Figure 2–27 point out the value of immittance measures when severe to profound hearing loss is present. Due to the output limitations of bone conduction testing, it is impossible to detect conductive hearing loss when air conduction thresholds exceed 70 dB HL. Therefore, the only means available to detect conductive disorders with a loss this severe is through the use of immittance testing. The results in Figure 2–27 suggest the presence of a significant conductive

disorder and the child should be referred for medical examination.

REFERENCES

1. Berlin CI: Programmed instruction in the decibel, in Northern JL, ed: *Hearing Disorders* (Boston: Little, Brown, & Co., 1967).
2. Specification of the council on physical medicine and rehabilitation of the American Medical Association. *JAMA*, 146 (1951), 255–257.
3. Standard Reference zero for calibration of pure-tone audiometers. ISD recommendation R389 (New York: American National Standards Institute, 1964).
4. Specifications for audiometers. ANSI S3.6-1969. (New York: American National Standards Institute, 1970).
5. Specifications for audiometers. ANSI S3.6-1989. (New York: American National Standards Institute, 1989).
6. Roeser RJ, Glorig A: Pure tone audiometry in noise with auraldomes. *Audiology*, 14 (1975), 144–151.
7. Roeser RJ, Seidel J, Glorig A: Performance of earphone enclosures for threshold audiometry. *Sound Vibration*, 10, No. 9 (1975), 22–25.
8. Musket CH, Roeser RJ: Using circumaural enclosures with children. *J Speech Hear Res*, 20 (1977), 325–333.

9. Clark JL, Roeser RJ: Three studies comparing performance of the ER-3A tubephone with TDH-50P earphone. *Ear Hearing*, 9 (1988), 268–274.

10. Walton WK, Wilson WR: Stability of routinely serviced portable audiometers. *Lang Speech Hear Serv Sch*, 3 (1972), 36–43.

11. Carhart R, Jerger J: Preferred method for clinical determination of pure tone thresholds. *J Speech Hear Disord*, 24 (1959), 330–345.

12. American Speech-Language-Hearing Association (ASHA). Guidelines for determining threshold level for speech. *ASHA*, 30 (March 1988) 85–88.

13. Hopkinson NT: Speech reception threshold, in Katz J, ed: *Handbook of Clinical Audiology*, ed 2 (Baltimore: Williams & Wilkins, 1978).

14. Fletcher H: A method of calculating hearing loss for speech from an audiogram. *J Acoust Soc Am*, 22 (1950), 1–5.

15. Konkle DF, Rintelmann WF: Introduction to speech audiometry, in D. F. Konkle, W. F. Rintelmann, eds: *Principles of Speech Audiometery* (Baltimore: University Park Press, 1983).

16. Goetzinger CP: Word discrimination testing, in Katz, J, ed: *Handbook of Clinical Audiology*, ed 2 (Baltimore: Williams & Wilkins, 1978).

17. Martin FN, Kopra LL: Symbols in pure tone audiometry. *ASHA* 12 (1970), 182–185.

18. American Speech and Hearing Association (ASHA), Guidelines for Audiometric Symbols. *ASHA*, 32 (suppl 2) (1990), 25–30.

19. Northern JL, Downs MP: *Hearing in Children*, ed 4 (Baltimore: Williams & Wilkins, 1991).

20. Boothroyd A: Hearing aids, cochlear implants, and profoundly deaf children, in Owens E, Kessler, DK, eds: *Cochlear Implants in Young Deaf Children* (Boston: College-Hill Press, 1989).

21. Green DS: Pure tone air conduction testing, in Katz J, ed: *Handbook of Clinical Audiology*, ed. 3 (Baltimore: Williams & Wilkins, 1985).

22. Goodman A: Reference zero levels for pure tone audiometers. *ASHA*, 7 (1965) 262-263.

23. Roeser RJ: *Diagnostic Audiology*, (Austin: Pro-Ed, 1986).

24. Matkin ND: The audiologic examination of young children at risk. *Ear, Nose, Throat*, 58 (1979) 297–302.

25. Roeser RJ, Yellin W: Pure-tone tests with pre-school children, in Martin FN, ed: *Hearing Disorders in Children* (Austin: Pro-Ed, 1987).

26. Hall J: *Handbook of Auditory Evoked Responses* (Boston: Allyn and Bacon, 1992).

27. Glattke TJ, Kujawa SW: Otoacoustic emissions. *Am J Audiol*, 1 (1991), 29–40.

28. American Speech and Hearing Association (ASHA) Committee on Audiometric Evaluation. Guidelines for acoustic immittance screening of middle ear function. *ASHA*, 21, No. 4 (1979), 282–288.

29. Margolis R, Heller JW: Screening tympanometry: Criteria for medical referral. *Audiology*, 26 (1987), 197–208.

30. American Speech-Language-Hearing Association (ASHA). Guidelines for screening hearing impairment and middle ear disorders. *ASHA*, 32 (Suppl 2) (1990), 17–24.

31. Specifications for instruments to measure aural acoustic impedance and admittance (aural acoustic immittance). ANSI S3.39-1987. (New York: American National Standards Institute, 1987).

32. Jerger J: Clinical experience with impedance audiometry, *Arch Otolaryngol*, 92 (1970), 311–324.

33. Jerger S: Diagnostic use of impedance measures, in Jerger J, ed: *Handbook of Clinical Impedance Audiometry* (Acton, MA: American Electromedics Co., 1975).

MEDICAL ASPECTS OF DISORDERS OF THE AUDITORY SYSTEM

Peter S. Roland

The desire to take medicine is perhaps the greatest feature which distinguishes man from animals.

—Sir William Osler, 1849–1919

HISTORY

Children present to the otologic physician with a limited number of complaints. Adequate evaluation of each child requires complete elucidation of their difficulties. The following information should be gathered for each presenting symptom:

1. When the symptom was first noted.
2. Whether the symptom is constantly present or intermittent.
3. If the symptom is intermittent, how often does the symptom occurs and how long does it lasts with each occurrence. Do the symptoms come in clusters?
4. How severe is the symptom?
5. Whether, in general, the symptom is improving or worsening.
6. Is the symptom bilateral or unilateral? If bilateral and intermittent, does it occur in each ear simultaneously or independently? If bilateral, did it begin simultaneously in both ears?
7. If more than one symptom is troubling the patient, one must establish if the symptoms occur independently or clustered together to form a symptom complex (syndrome).

Tinnitus

Millions of persons experience varying degrees of tinnitus, indeed; at some time or another almost everyone experiences brief episodes of tinnitus, usually in quiet environments. Most individuals are not bothered by such brief episodes, but when tinnitus remains sustained they may experience considerable discomfort. Some persons find the symptom annoying. Others are kept awake at night and may have difficulty concentrating. A few individuals find the tinnitus disabling and are prevented from pursuing their usual daily activities. An occasional individual may find the experience so tortuous that sui cide is contemplated to escape it.

The same general considerations that apply to adults apply to children. One must take into account, however, that children may have much greater difficulty in expressing and describing their subjective sensations. On the whole, tinnitus seems to be a less bothersome symptom in the pediatric age group than it is among adults. Nonetheless, some children have their hearing loss first identified as part of an evaluation for tinnitus.

Hearing Loss

Although formal audiometric testing is the most critical component in assessing hearing loss, it is often useful to gain some understanding of how much difficulty the child experiences due to hypoacusis. This can be somewhat difficult, especially in younger children. Consultation with family and teachers is critical. Parents are usually acute observers of their own child's hearing acuity and may be aware of fairly subtle changes. Although parents can be (and often are) manipulated by children, the parent's assessment should always be taken at face value. Subsequent information may sometimes demonstrate that the parent's assessment was inaccurate. One should establish how much difficulty the child experiences, in what circumstances he or she experiences difficulty, and how troublesome these difficulties are.

The time course of the hearing change is the most useful piece of historical information.

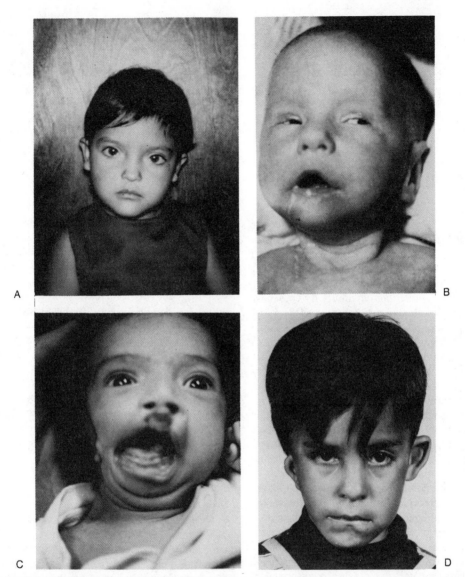

Figure 3-1. Examples of genetic birth defect syndromes with associated hearing loss. (A) Waardenburg syndrome. This patient does not have a white forelock; she has the increased medial intercanthal distance, severe hearing loss, and brilliant blue eyes. (B) Rubella syndrome. This infant had microcephaly, microphthalmia, carp-shaped mouth, large abnormal ears, a bulbous nasal tip, and a fixed stapes. (C) Treacher Collins syndrome with severe facial malformations, a very small mandible, which caused the tongue to obstruct the airway and caused his death. Temporal bone pathologic findings showed a malformed monopod stapes, and the facial nerve exited directly from the side of the skull. (D) Microtia-atresia. Both the malformed right ear and the normal-appearing left ear had conductive losses. The left ear hearing loss was due to stapes fixation. (Figure 3–1B reprinted with permission from Hemenway.[4] Figure 3–1C reprinted with permission from Sando et al.[5]; Figure 3–1D reprinted with permission from Bergstrom.[6]

Losses that have occurred many years prior to the current evaluation and are stable are not likely to require medical intervention. In making such determinations the availability of previous audiograms is extremely helpful and efforts should be made to obtain any previous audiograms. Inquiries should be made into the circumstances of long-standing losses, and any association with febrile illness, antibiotic therapy, noise exposure, trauma, or surgery must be noted.

If other family members have hearing loss, the nature of such losses should be explored and audiograms obtained. The time at which children first note the loss, how they noted it, and its rate of progression should always be determined if possible. Each child should be specifically evaluated to see if his hearing fluctuates and if so under what circumstances, how frequently, and with what severity. Any association of the hearing loss with vertigo or tinnitus, otalgia, otorrhea, upper respiratory infection, nasal stuffiness, headache, dysarthria, dysphagia, visual changes, numbness or tingling in the extremities, or focal motor weakness should all be established.

Otalgia

Otalgia (ear pain) precipitates many physician visits and has a myriad of causes. In a high percentage of adults, otalgia is not otogenic. It is estimated that in the primary care setting, only 50% of cases of ear pain in adults are caused by ear disease. Although nonotogenic otalgia is less common in children, the child may also experience ear pain as occurring within the structures of the ear when it is, in fact, referred from other embryologically related structures. The pain of otologic origin is usually dull, aching, and relatively constant. Pain that comes and goes frequently during the day is rarely otogenic. Otalgia is commonly due to disorders affecting the larynx, pharynx, and tonsils. Tonsillitis and pharyngitis are two common causes of referred otalgia in children. Disorders of the muscles of mastication and the temporomandibular joint are also often perceived as ear pain. Many important otologic conditions such as cholesteatoma, other forms of chronic otitis media, Meniere's disease, and acoustic tumor are not associated with pain at all.

Otogenic ear pain may be due to cerumen impaction, infection, and, quite rarely, neoplasms. The most common causes of otogenic ear pain are infection. Both external otitis and acute otitis media may cause excruciating pain that precipitates a physician visit, usually on an emergency basis. Since most such cases are treated in the primary care setting, the incidence of ear pain due to otologic disease is actually lower in a referral otologic practice than it is in a general practice.

Otorrhea

With the rare exception of cases in which spinal fluid drains through the ear, otorrhea (drainage from the ear) is related to infection. The child's history is especially important. Painless drainage is usually the result of chronic otitis media. This may be cholesteatoma, chronic mastoiditis due to irreversible mucosal disease, and tympanic membrane perforation or chronic reflux through the eustachian tube. Otorrhea may occur sporadically as the result of an otherwise asymptomatic tympanic membrane perforation, especially if water has inadvertently entered the middle ear space. Children with a history of painless drainage going back for months or years are highly suspect of harboring a temporal bone cholesteatoma. This is especially true if the drainage fails to resolve after vigorous treatment with systemic and topical antibiotics. Drainage associated with pain is more likely to be caused by an acute infectious process. Perforated otitis media may be preceded by very severe ear pain. Acute external otitis is frequently manifested by the simultaneous occurrence of aural drainage and acute ear pain. The prolonged use of antibiotic drops should alert the examiner to the possibility of fungal otitis, which occurs principally as a complication of broad spectrum topical antibiotic treatment.

Patients who routinely occlude the external auditory canal with hearing instruments or protective earplugs are much more difficult to treat because occlusion of the external auditory canal interferes with the normal cleansing mechanism of the ear.

Vertigo

Vertigo (dizziness) has myriad causes, many of which are entirely unrelated to the temporal bone and ear. A detailed history is the single most important piece of information in establishing a diagnosis. The following points should be clearly elucidated in every patient history. What exactly does the child mean by "dizziness"? What does he or she experience? The answers to these questions vary dramatically. Vertigo arising from the vestibular system generally has as its principal component "the illusion of motion." This may be a sense of rotation or the sense of falling to one side or the other. When the child uses such terms as "light-headed", "giddy", "confused", or "faint" the sensation is not likely to be labyrinthine in origin. When did the symptom first occur, how often does it occur, and how long does it last when it does occur? What is the shortest and longest time the dizziness has lasted? Is the dizziness associated with nausea, vomiting, or sweating? Is the child aware of any change in hearing before, during, or after the dizzy spell? Do any activities reliably bring on the dizzy spell? Is the dizzy spell associated with any difficulty in swallowing, speaking, or any change in vision? Is consciousness ever completely lost during a dizzy spell? Is there associated tinnitus or feeling of aural fullness? Can the child tell when a dizzy episode is about to occur? A special inquiry should be made into whether the child has headaches before, during, or after each episode of vertigo or disequilibrium. It should be established whether there is a familial history of migraine. Migraine is a much more common cause of episodic vertigo in childhood than in adulthood and accounts for a substantial number of children with intermittent dizzy spells. Careful evaluation of the history in light of basic audiometry will usually establish whether the vertigo is likely to be otogenic in etiology and will probably suggest a diagnosis. Further diagnostic tests can then be ordered to confirm or deny these initial conclusions.

PHYSICAL EXAMINATION OF THE EAR

Examination of the ear begins with examination of the auricle. The size and shape of the auricle and its position should be carefully noted. Some children will have no auricle due to congenital aural atresia, some will have one that is abnormally small or poorly formed, and other children may have an auricle placed either unusually low with respect to the remainder of the facial skeleton or unusually high.

The size and adequacy of the external auditory canal should be assessed. Some children have collapsing external auditory canals with a slitlike opening. This should be noted prior to audiometry so that insert earphones can be used to assess the tympanic membrane and middle ear conduction mechanism.

To assess the likelihood of collapse and the adequacy of the size of the external auditory canal, the auricle should be drawn backward and upward. This opens the lateral portion of the cartilaginous canal and permits assessment of the bony canal. The presence of flaking skin, which suggests chronic seborrheic dermatitis, should be noted at this time. An otoscope may then be used to examine the external auditory canal and tympanic membrane. Preliminary examination of the size of the canal will allow the appropriate size speculum to be selected. The largest speculum that can be comfortably inserted into the patient's external auditory canal should be chosen. Specula for use in the external auditory canal are designed in such a way that they rarely protrude further into the ear than the cartilaginous portion of the external auditory canal. This portion can be stretched and manipulated with minimal or no discomfort. Should the speculum reach the inner third of the ear canal, even the slightest pressure will be extraordinarily painful. The patient's head needs to be tilted toward the opposite shoulder to account for the normal upward direction of the ear canal.

It will often be necessary to remove cerumen from the external auditory canal to examine the tympanic membrane. This may be accomplished by using an ear syringe or Water-Pik for the instillation of water to "flush" the cerumen out of the external auditory canal (see Chapter 4). Alternatively, the cerumen may be removed using small curettes or a cerumen spoon with or without the adjunctive use of an operating microscope. Cerumen that has been impacted into the external auditory canal by the repeated use of Q-tips may be extraordinarily difficult to remove. Such children should be referred to an otolaryngologist who can remove the cerumen using the operating microscope if irrigation techniques have failed. Occasionally, a general anesthetic will be required for cerumen removal.

Every attempt should be made to visualize the entire tympanic membrane. Otoscopic or microscopic examination of the ear cannot be considered complete until the entire tympanic membrane, including the pars flaccida, has been visualized. Figure 3–2 shows the landmarks on the tympanic membrane. The anulus tympanicum should be followed anteriorly and posteriorly until it meets the anterior and posterior malleolar folds. The pars flaccida lies between these two folds. Perforation or deep retraction of the pars flaccida is virtually always diagnostic of a cholesteatoma. Both the long and short process of the malleus can be seen in the normal drum and their presence should be noted. The long process of the incus and chorda tympani can frequently, although not invariably, be seen through a normal tympanic membrane. However, if the head of the malleus or body of the incus is seen, there has been erosion of the superior external auditory canal and lateral wall of the middle ear space. This is seen almost exclusively in cholesteatoma (Figure 3–3). Occasionally, a retracted drum lies directly on the incudostapedial joint, forming a "myringostapediopexy." In such circumstances, long-term retraction probably due to eustachian

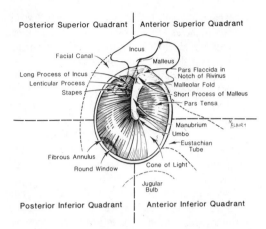

Figure 3-2. Diagram of the lateral surface of the tympanic membrane. Special note should be made of the pars flaccida. Failure to examine the pars flaccida is a common cause of missed cholesteatoma. The head of the malleus and incus are not normally seen. When the heads of these ossicles can be seen, this reliably indicates the presence of bony erosion almost always due to cholesteatoma. Reprinted with permission from Meyerhoff and Carter.[7]

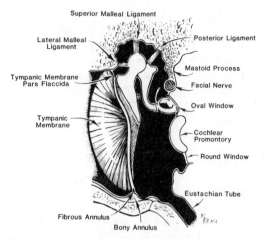

Figure 3-3. Diagram of the middle ear space seen in coronal cross-section. The funnel shape of the tympanic membrane can readily be appreciated. One can appreciate that the heads of the ossicles should not normally be seen. A very close relationship between the facial nerve and the footplate of the stapes is readily appraent in the diagram. The inferior position of the round window should also be noted. Reprinted with permission from Meyerhoff and Carter.[7]

tube insufficiency can be assumed. Surprisingly, hearing can often be near normal in such situations. The examiner should be wary of the "dimeric membrane." Frequently perforations of the tympanic membrane heal without the middle fibrous layer of the eardrum regenerating in normal fashion. The result is an extremely thin "secondary" membrane that is always translucent and often transparent. Such secondary membranes may be indistinguishable from perforations without the use of the operating microscope.

The pneumatic otoscope is used to create positive or negative pressure on the tympanic membrane. Such pressure changes normally cause visible movement of the tympanic membrane. Using the pneumatic otoscope, the examiner can assess the degree of mobility of the tympanic membrane. Chronic middle ear effusion, for example, usually promotes a sluggish or immobile tympanic membrane. In addition, brisk tympanic movements virtually excludes the possibility of tympanic membrane perforation. Pneumatic otoscopy using the handheld otoscope may occasionally induce movement in healed secondary membranes, which makes it apparent that the drum is indeed intact although quite thin.

Masses behind the tympanic membrane may be caused by a variety of different sorts of pathologic processes. Color is important and may be a clue to etiology. White masses suggest cholesteatoma, tympanosclerosis, or, very rarely, middle

ear osteoma. Dark blue masses suggest venous vascular structures, such as a high jugular bulb. Dark red masses suggest highly vascular tumors such as glomus tympanicum tumors or granulation tissue. The presence of pulsations within a mass strongly suggests that it is arterialized and vascular in etiology. This can sometimes be confirmed by applying positive pressure to the tympanic membrane using the pneumatic otoscope. Positive pressure reduces blood flow within the mass and causes blanching of the drum overlying the middle ear mass. Such blanching is referred to as a positive Brown's sign and strongly suggests a vascular neoplasm. Occasionally, a red blotch will be seen in the area of the oval window. This may not be a mass but may represent the hypervascular bone characteristic of an active focus of otosclerosis.

No otologic examination is complete without examination of the facial nerve. The patient should be asked to frown, smile, wrinkle his nose, whistle, show his teeth, and shut his eyes. Any asymmetry between sides or the inability to perform any of these motions should be clearly noted.

The earliest and most subtle sign of facial weakness is lagophthalmos. The eyelid closes a bit more slowly on the affected side than on the normal, contralateral side. This is clearly evident when the patient blinks spontaneously. The blink on the affected side appears to lag behind its normal contralateral partner.

DISEASES OF THE EXTERNAL AUDITORY CANAL

A variety of conditions affect the external auditory canal, most of which occur in children. Of special importance are the congenital aural atresias that are generally diagnosed in childhood and require staged management of both the auditory and cosmetic components.

Dermatitis

Two types of dermatitis affect the external auditory ear with some frequency. The seborrheic dermatitides are much the most common. Seborrheic dermatitis is usually manifested by chronic itching of the external auditory canals and frequently associated with dry, flaky skin over the conchal bowl and medial portions of the external auditory canal. Careful physical examination often reveals the complete or near absence of cerumen. The condition is important not only because the itching is subjectively very distressing, but because the chronic irritation of the skin of the external auditory canal reduces its effectiveness as a barrier to infection. Thus, children with chronic seborrheic dermatitis are much more susceptible to chronic bacterial external otitis (swimmer's ear) than are the unaffected, normal population. Indeed, after careful questioning, many children who have recurrent episodes of external otitis will be discovered to have chronic, dry, flaking and pruritic external auditory canals. In some children the same condition waxes and wanes on an irregular and unpredictable basis. Many children will have little or no difficulty for years, with sporadic "flare-ups" lasting weeks or months. Seborrheic dermatitis of the external auditory canal responds favorably to the use of very low dose steroid preparations at infrequent intervals. The use of 2% hydrocortisone cream applied to the conchal bowl and medial external auditory canal two or three times a week is frequently sufficient. In more difficult cases, the use of a steroid containing antibiotic drop that is placed into the external auditory canal may also be required. Some cases respond to the simple application of mineral oil or other emollient without the use of any medication whatsoever.

The other dermatitis that is seen with some frequency is allergic or atopic dermatis. The majority of these cases occur in response to exogenous materials placed in or around the external auditory canal. Many allergic reactions are seen in response to topical antibiotic drops. Neomycin is especially likely to produce topical sensitization and result in allergic reaction. Allergic reactions to neomycin (and other topical antibiotics) occur in two somewhat distinct forms. A fulminant form is occasionally encountered that results in massive swelling of the external auditory canal and a dramatic drug eruption involving the conchal bowl, lobule, and frequently the skin of the neck. The eruption is associated with cutaneous weeping of serosanguinous fluid and is accompanied by intense pain and tenderness. Such reactions, of course, require the immediate discontinuance of the offending agent and often the use of both topical and systemic steroid medications. A more indolent form of hypersensitivity is manifested simply by the failure of a typical external otitis to resolve in response to what appears to be appropriate antibiotic therapy. Long-term drainage, edema of the external auditory canal, pain, and tenderness persist in the presence of the use of both topical drops and mechanical cleansing. Such reactions can be adequately treated by discontinuing the offending agent and treating the external otitis with a nonantibiotic drop containing an antiseptic with or without a topical steroid.

Atopic reactions occur to the materials from which both ear molds and earplugs are made. Again, the reaction may be fulminant with clear-cut swelling, pain, and tenderness or may be more indolent with only minimal swelling and moderate tenderness. The mainstay of treatment is replacement of the offending agent with a more hypoallergenic material.

External Otitis

The most common cause of bacterial infections of the external auditory canal is bacterial external otitis or "swimmer's ear." In more than 90% of cases, the offending organism is *Pseudomonas aeruginosa*. This organism is relatively ubiquitous in the environment and in the appropriate circumstances may be pathogenic. It is, however, extremely sensitive to the local acidity (pH) of its environment. *Pseudomonas* is incapable of growing or reproducing in acid media. One of the functions of cerumen appears to be maintenance of a slightly acidic environment, which prevents the growth of *Pseudomonas*. Introduction of water into the external auditory canal by swimming (or other means) washes out the normal acidity of the canal and may substitute a nonacid environment. In such circumstances, the ubiquitous *Pseudomonas* may produce a purulent bacterial infection. The incidence of acute bacterial external otitis is significantly higher in June, July, and August because most swimming occurs during these months. As already mentioned, the presence of an impaired skin barrier, as can occur with seborrheic dermatitis, may significantly increase the chances of the development of bacterial external otitis.

The disorder is of relatively sudden onset and is characterized by very severe pain localized to the affected external auditory canal. An important diagnostic feature is extreme sensitivity to any movement of the auricle or tissues surrounding the external auditory canal. This is helpful in distinguishing external otitis from middle ear problems. Acute otitis media is unaffected by even fairly vigorous auricular movement. Examination will show mucopurulent exudate accumulating in the external auditory canal, marked swelling of the tissues of the external auditory canal, and frequently erythema, edema, and occasionally "weeping." In many cases it is not possible to examine the tympanic membrane fully because of the exquisite tenderness of the canal and a marked amount of canal swelling. The disorder is rarely, if ever, associated with fever, malaise, or other signs of systemic infection.

Treatment follows logically from the known etiology of the infection. Reacidification of the external auditory canal is almost always sufficient to cure the disorder, unless the external auditory canal is so swollen as to prevent the acidifying fluids from entering or there is so much accumulated mucopurulent debris that the drops do not come in contact with the infected tissues. An external canal that is swollen closed can be dealt with effectively by placing a small wick into the external auditory canal. The wick is made of an expandable material and draws the acidifying solution into the canal. When a large amount of mucopurulent debris has accumulated in the canal, mechanical removal of the debris using the operating microscope and suction is essential and often crucial to successful management. In severe cases, such cleansing may need to be done two or three times on an every other day basis. Antibiotic drops should be continued at least a week beyond remission of pain.

Antibiotic drops directed against *Pseudomonas* are also effective in eliminating infection but are generally unnecessary. The use of antibiotic drops carries with it the risk of producing a topical allergic reaction and the promotion of fungal external otitis. For that reason, I avoid their use for infections limited to the external auditory canal.

Fungal External Otitis

Most fungal growth that occurs within the external auditory canal is saprophytic. The fungi grow on desquamated epithelium, cerumen, or the inspissated mucopurulent debris from a previous bacterial infection. True fungal external otitis with tissue invasion of fungal elements is uncommon and almost completely limited to individuals who are significantly immunocompromised. Individuals taking high-dose steroids, using immunosuppressive agents, or with immunodeficiency disorders are candidates for such infections. An exception to this general rule may be healthy individuals who have had long-term treatment with systemic antimicrobials or topical antibiotics. In such individuals, fungi are frequently cultured from a chronic draining external auditory canal, and they may be etiologically important. Such fungal external otitis is best treated by withdrawal of the antibiotic therapy and the use of topical antiseptics like Mercurochrome or gentian violet. Antiseptics have the advantage of being fairly universal in their toxicity. Thus, they are much less likely to select out resistant organisms, which can then grow unrestrained by their usual bacterial competitors. Acidifying agents are also useful in the treatment of fungal external otitis as many of the fungi are sensitive to ambient pH. Occasionally, especially in immunocompromised individuals, the use of topical or even systemic antifungal agents may become necessary.

Congenital Aural Atresias

Congenital aural atresias can involve the pinna, external auditory canal, middle ear space, or ossicles. Such malformations may occur alone or in association with other regional or distant malformations. A variety of different syndromes have been identified associated with malformations of the ear and are listed in Table 3–1. When there is associated gross malformation of the auricle, the atresia is usually identified promptly, often on the day of birth. However, when the pinna is normal, identification of the stenotic or atretic external auditory canal may be delayed for a number of years. Identification may await the child's failure to meet developmental guidelines or failure of screening audiometric tests in school.

Table 3–1   Syndromes Associated with Congenital Aural Atresia

1. Alport's syndrome
2. Crouson's disease
3. Marfan syndrome
4. Osteogenesis imperfecta
5. Treacher Collins syndrome
6. Pierre Robin syndrome
7. Goldenhar's syndrome
8. Franceshetti syndrome
9. Nager's acrofacial dysostosis
10. Wildervanck's syndome
11. Sprengel's deformity
12. Pyle's syndrome
13. Paget's disease
14. Möbius' syndrome
15. Levy-Hollister's (LADD) syndrome
16. CHARGE syndrome
17. Alagille syndrome
18. Andersen's disease
19. Fraser's syndrome
20. Lenz's syndrome
21. Noonan's syndrome

Malformations of the external and middle ears occur approximately once in every 10,000 to 20,000 births. It appears that a significant percentage of cases of atresia are not due to genetic causes. Fortunately, the malformation occurs unilaterally four times more frequently than it does bilaterally. The etiology in unilateral cases often remains obscure, but many cases may be acquired as the result of vascular injury to the branchial arches, which can occur in utero. Since embryological development of the ear is finished by week 28 of gestation, injuries that occur in late pregnancy will not affect development of the ear. Portions of the external auditory canal and middle ear develop from the same underlying embryological structures, so middle ear malformations are frequently associated with malformations of the external auditory canal. Fortunately, however, the cochlea, semi-circular canals, and VIIIth cranial nerve are rarely affected. Most individuals with congenital aural atresia have normally functioning neurosensory auditory systems. The anatomic course of the facial nerve is frequently altered in malformations of the ear and temporal bone, which makes surgical correction somewhat more hazardous, but facial nerve function is rarely affected by the malformation. The tympanic membrane is frequently replaced by a bony plate and there are a large variety of identified malformations and deformities of the ossicles.

Management of the child with congenital aural atresia should begin with a complete evaluation so as to detect any associated abnormalities. If there is an external auditory canal present, it should be carefully evaluated. An attempt needs to be made to see whether the canal is complete or whether it becomes stenotic or atretic medially. This is often difficult to do in the small child and may occasionally require radiographic imaging.

· More important than radiographic assessment is accurate determination of hearing thresholds. Differentiation of conductive from neurosensory components is important but often difficult in the young child. The use of both air and bone conduction auditory brainstem response (ABR) for threshold assessment may be pivotal.

Since hearing rehabilitation must occur long before these children are surgical candidates, amplification needs to be considered even in those individuals who may later benefit from reconstructive operations. The need for hearing restoration is immediate and should not be delayed even a few weeks beyond birth. Educational and social development can be retarded by hearing loss and the restoration of hearing after the critical developmental period may not compensate for the handicapping effects of early hearing loss. The available options include the use of conventional amplification, externally applied bone conducting hearing aids, and implantable bone conducting hearing aids. As a general rule, when conventional amplification can be used, it is the treatment of choice. I prefer the use of the implantable bone conducting aid, when appropriate, in patients with bilateral maximal conductive hearing losses and normal bone levels if they cannot be successfully fitted with conventional hearing aids (Figure 3–5).

In patients with only conductive hearing losses, even if maximal, the continued use of amplification may provide perfectly adequate hearing restoration. Surgical repair of the external auditory canal, tympanic membrane, and middle ear space can be accomplished by a variety of different surgical techniques. Favorable outcomes are more likely in individuals with the least severe abnormalities. Whether surgical repair should be undertaken depends entirely on the patient and his parents. It is often useful to wait until the child is old enough to participate in the decision for surgical repair of the congenital atresia. Surgical intervention is not without risks and complications. Frequently, the air-bone gap can be closed to 30 dB or less but failure to close the air-bone gap is the most common problem associated with reconstructive surgery. Restenosis of the external auditory canal is relatively common. Finally, although the rate remains low, facial nerve injury occurs significantly more commonly after repair of congenital lesions than after repair of acquired lesions.

DISORDERS OF THE TYMPANIC MEMBRANE, MIDDLE EAR AND MASTOID

Tympanic Membrane Performances

Tympanic membrane perforations can arise either as a consequence of infection or trauma. Acute otitis media frequently results in perforation of the tympanic membrane. Generally speaking, such perforations heal spontaneously, but occasionally the perforation fails to heal and is left as a permanent feature of the tympanic membrane. Severe, acute, necrotizing otitis media has a much higher incidence of tympanic membrane perforation associated with it than the usual middle ear infections. Chronic infection with an unusual organism, such as tuberculosis, produces a much higher rate of permanent tympanic membrane perforation than occurs in the epidemic otitis media of schoolchildren.

A variety of different types of trauma can produce tympanic membrane perforation. For the most part, this is blast trauma, although penetrating trauma is occasionally involved. The results of a slap to the side of the head, which completely occludes the external auditory canal, forcing a column of air down onto the tympanic membrane and rupturing it, is one form of blast trauma. It is apparently this mechanism of injury that is most frequently responsible for the tympanic membrane perforations associated with water-skiing. Injuries involving water or traumatic tympanic membrane perforations contaminated with water shortly after their occurrence are less likely to heal.

When infection complicates an acute tympanic membrane perforation, the probability of spontaneous healing is significantly reduced. With those caveats in mind, most tympanic membrane perforations heal spontaneously and without significant or meaningful residue.

Perforations of the tympanic membrane diagnosed on physical examination should be first categorized as to their location. They may occur either in the pars tensa or the pars flaccida. Per-forations of the pars flaccida may be assumed to be cholesteatomas and should be managed as such. Perforations in the pars tensa can be divided into those that are central and those that are marginal. A central perforation has a small rim of intact tympanic membrane around it. Marginal perforations extend all the way to the bony anulus of the external auditory canal. It is often difficult and sometimes impossible to determine whether an anterior perforation is marginal because the anterior canal wall makes it difficult to see the most anterior portion of the tympanic membrane. The distinction between central and marginal perforations is important because marginal perforations have the potential to develop into cholesteatomas and, therefore, should be considered dangerous. Central perforations, on the other hand, are unlikely to develop into cholesteatomas and are sometimes referred to as "safe" perforations. The size of the tympanic membrane perforation should also be determined. Size can be recorded either in terms of an estimate of diameter in millimeters or estimate of the percentage of tympanic membrane involved in the perforation. The location should be identified. Both location and size are important factors in determining the amount of conductive hearing loss associated with the particular type of perforation.

Three sorts of difficulties arise from chronic perforations of the tympanic membrane: (1) formation of cholesteatoma, (2) significant conductive hearing loss, and (3) recurrent infection.

Hearing loss caused by tympanic membrane perforations is highly variable. Small pinpoint perforations may have no associated hearing loss and larger perforations may produce losses up to 50 dB. Perforations directly over the round window niche may produce significant hearing loss because of phase cancellation effects. Conductive hearing losses greater than 40 to 50 dB suggest associated ossicular discontinuity or fixation.

By permitting the ingress of bacteria from the external auditory canal into the middle ear space, perforations may lead to recurrent infections of the middle ear and mastoid. If water is allowed to enter the external auditory canal, it is particularly likely to carry bacteria into the middle ear space and further increase the likelihood of infection. Protection of the middle ear space from water-borne bacterial contamination is an essential part of management. Thus, ear protection should be used for swimming or bathing.

Obstruction of the external auditory canal also increases the likelihood of infections. Persons who utilize hearing aids or earplugs in an ear with a chronic perforation are much more likely to experience difficulty with recurrent mucopurulent infections and chronic otorrhea.

The treatment of tympanic membrane perforations is surgical repair. In individuals with marginal perforations, the propensity of these perforations to form cholesteatomas is sufficient to warrant surgical repair in most cases. Repair of central perforations, however, is entirely elective.

Otitis Media

Figures 3–3 and 3–4 show the middle ear space and associated mastoid air cell system and eustachian tube. Abnormal eustachian tube function appears to be a common pathologic feature in the development of most forms of otitis media. The normally functioning eustachian tube remains closed at rest but should open episodically to equalize middle ear pressure with ambient barometric pressure. The eustachian tubes are opened by active muscular contraction of small palatal muscles during swallowing or yawning. If the eustachian tube is always open (patulous), then bacterial laden secretions from the nasopharynx may enter the middle ear and produce infection. In fact, such secretions may be forced into the middle ear if the eustachian tube is open during active sneezing or nose blowing. If the tube remains chronically shut, negative pressure will develop in the middle ear. Negative middle ear pressure may result in the development of a retracted tympanic membrane and middle ear effusion. Over time, such fluid may thicken and become mucoid ("glue" ear). If bacteria find their way into such an effusion, acute purulent bacterial otitis media will rapidly develop. By producing swelling of the mucous membranes of the eustachian tube and inhibiting normal ciliary function, middle ear effusions (either infected or uninfected) may themselves produce dysfunction of the eustachian tube and perpetuate their own condition (Figures 3–4, 3–5).

Infants and children are predisposed to otitis media because their eustachian tubes are more horizontal, shorter, and wider than those of adults. Palatal muscle function, as with muscle function generally, is less efficient in infants and small children than it is in adults; therefore, the active tubal opening is less reliable and vigorous. Inflammation of the nasal end of the eustachian tube can produce sufficient swelling to obstruct

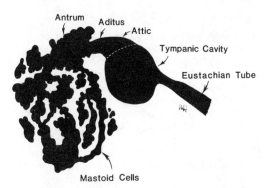

Figure 3–4. Diagram of the middle ear system and associated mastoid air cells. This schematically shows the relati o nship of the middle ear space, the mastoid air cell system and eustachian tube. (Reprinted with permission from Meyerhoff and Carter.)

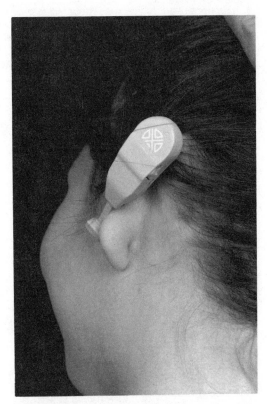

Figure 3–5. An Audiant™ Bone Conducting™ hearing aid as seen in position just above the deformed auricle of an individual with congenital aural atresia.

it mechanically. Such inflammation may result from viral (a cold) or bacterial infection, chemical irritation (tobacco smoke, chlorinated pool water), or inhalant allergy. The consequences of long-term eustachian tube dysfunction include not only persistent or recurrent middle ear effusions with or without infection, but also pathologic

Case study 3–1. J.M. is a 4-year-old child who had a 1- to 2-year history of multiple recurrent episodes of otitis media. Indeed, during the previous 18 months, he had been on antibiotics for almost 12 months. This included one 3-month period during which he received prophylactic antibiotics in an attempt to eliminate middle ear infections. However, even during this period of time he developed one episode of acute otitis media. Approximately 3 months ago, he was referred for an evaluation for speech and language delay and attention deficit disorder. He was deemed to be approximately 3 to 6 months behind in the acquisition of both expressive and receptive language skills. He had difficulty concentrating, could not attend well to tasks, and fell asleep easily and frequently during the day. He had chronic nasal congestion and was a chronic mouth breather, according to his parents. He snored loudly at night and gagged on his food during meals.

Examination showed that he had bilateral middle ear effusions with no evidence of infection. He had mucus coming from both nostrils and was breathing loudly and heavily through his mouth. Intraoral examination showed very large hypertrophic tonsils, that met at the midline ("kissing").

Audiometric evaluation showed that he had bilateral flat 40 decibel conductive hearing loss, tympanograms were flat bilaterally (see Audiogram 1). Soft tissue lateral x-ray of his neck showed that in addition to his large, obstructive tonsils he had large pads of adenoid tissue that completely prevented movement of air through his nose.

He underwent bilateral adenotonsillectomy with insertion of tympanostomy tubes. His snoring resolved immediately and many of the symptoms of his attention deficit disorder disappeared. He no longer fell asleep during the day and was able to concentrate much better because he was getting a good night's sleep. Approximately 6 months after the operative intervention he had "caught up" and had age-appropriate speech and language skills.

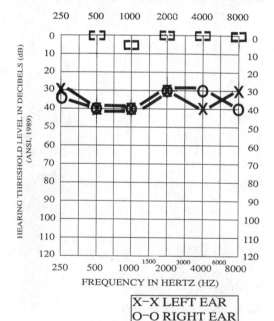

X–X LEFT EAR
O–O RIGHT EAR

Audiogram 1. Audiometric configuration showing binaural flat conductive hearing loss. See case histroy #1.

alterations of the tympanic membrane and complications associated with the inner ear, mastoid, or the central nervous system. Chronic or repeated retraction of the tympanic membrane will produce stretching and thinning. A chronically retracted tympanic membrane may rest on the long process of the incus and incudostapedial joint and produce ossicular erosion, ossicular discontinuity, and moderate to severe conductive hearing loss. Further atrophy will leave the tympanic membrane draped over the medial wall of the middle ear. This will produce functional elimination of the middle ear space. When the eardrum is left in this configuration for an extended period of time, fibrosis and scarring will occur, and the process will become irreversible (adhesive otitis media). Recurrent infection can deposit hyalin (a calcium-like substance) in the middle ear. These hyalin deposits, termed "tympanosclerosis," may be limited to the tympanic membrane or may involve the heads of the ossicles within the middle ear space. Tympanosclerotic plaques limited to the tympanic membrane are easily noticed but, although they may present a dramatic appearance, rarely produce hearing loss or other alteration of middle ear function. On the other hand, tympanosclerotic deposition around the heads of the ossicles will produce fixation and maximum conductive hearing loss. The process of the development of tympanosclerosis of the tympanic membrane and middle ear space appear to be independent. Although there is good evidence that development of tympanosclerosis of the tympanic membrane is associated with injury to the drum (tympanic membrane perforation), the apparent etiology of middle ear tympanosclerosis is entirely unknown. Fortunately, middle ear tympanosclerosis is uncommon.

If thinning and retraction of the tympanic membrane occurs in the posterior quadrant and

Case study 3–2.   B.Q. is an 8-year-old who had been treated for right-sided "external otitis" for the last year. He had virtually continuous, foul-smelling, mucopurulent drainage from the right ear. It was not associated with pain. He had multiple episodes of otitis media and middle ear effusion as a child and had two sets of tympanostomy tubes. Audiograms performed between the ages of 3 and 5 years showed mild conductive hearing loss that fluctuated 10 to 15 dB. However, after extrusion of his second set of tympanostomy tubes at the age of 5 years, he had two entirely normal audiograms.

Examination showed a normal left tympanic membrane except for the presence of some tympanosclerosis. The pars tensa of the right tympanic membrane also had some tympanosclerosis. However, in the area of the pars flaccida a perforation could be seen. A large amount of mucopus could be seen issuing from this perforation. After extensive cleansing and careful evaluation with the Zeiss operating microscope, a small amount of squamous epithelium could be removed from the perforation. It was apparent that the perforation represented the open neck of a large cholesteatoma.

Audiometric evaluation was normal, including tympanometry.

The nature of cholesteatoma was carefully explained to the parents and the necessity for surgical removal emphasized. The child's father, however, had recently taken a new position and wished to wait 9 months until the child's cholesteatoma would be covered by their insurance policy.

Six months after his initial presentation, the child's parents called because B.Q. had woken up acutely dizzy. He was seen immediately that day and audiometric evaluation showed a significant neurosensory hearing loss. He was, therefore, taken to the operating room immediately. A large cholesteatoma was found filling the mastoid. It has eroded into the horizontal semicircular canal. The cholesteatoma was carefully removed and a piece of tissue placed over the open semicircular canal. The vertigo remitted promptly, but he was left with a significant neurosensory hearing loss (see Audiogram 2).

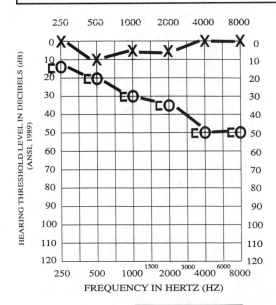

X–X LEFT EAR
O–O RIGHT EAR

Audiogram 2.   Audiometric evaluation showing significant neurosensory hearing loss in the right ear. See case history #2.

portions of the drum are sucked into the mastoid cavity, a cholesteatoma will develop. The lateral surface of the tympanic membrane consists of skin and, like skin in other portions of the body, it sheds epithelial cells ("desquamates").

Acute otitis media is one of the most common diseases of early childhood and effects at least 70% of children prior to the age of 6 years. It is the most common reason for the administration of antibiotics to children. Prior to the use of antibiotic medications, acute otitis media was the cause of significant mortality in infancy and childhood. Fortunately, current antimicrobials have significantly reduced (but not completely eliminated) the incidence of life-threatening complications. The peak incidence occurs between 6 and 24 months of age. It occurs more frequently during the winter months. Exposure to second-hand cigarette smoke and placement in day-care centers seems to increase the incidence of acute otitis media significantly. The disease is caused by infection with a number of different relatively common bacteria and generally responds to the institution of prompt antibiotic therapy. A worrisome new development is increasing resistance of these organisms to currently available antibiotics. Concern has recently developed that antibiotic resistance may increase the prevalence to the point where serious life-threatening complications are again common.

Acute otitis media is a purulent infection that begins with edema, hyperemia, and hemorrhage in the subepithelial space of the middle ear mucosa. This is then followed by the local infiltration of white blood cells and the accumulation of pus within the middle ear space. Typically, acute otitis media is of relatively sudden onset. Because it represents the accumulation of pus within a closed body cavity, it is associated with significant systemic signs of infection, such as elevated temperature, malaise, and elevated white blood cell count. The ear is exquisitely painful, although there is no tenderness in the area of the auricle or periauricular tissues, as is seen with external otitis. In untreated cases, the condition resolves with spontaneous rupture of the tympanic membrane. The opening in the tympanic membrane allows the pus to drain out of the external auditory canal. Rupture of the tympanic membrane is associated with very rapid relief of pain and prompt defervescence. In more than 90% of cases, the tympanic membrane heals spontaneously and there is no residua.

Prior to the development of antibiotic therapy, most cases of acute otitis media resolved after spontaneous perforation. However, a significant minority did not resolve and the affected child developed chronic mastoiditis, sigmoid sinus thrombosis, facial nerve paralysis, labyrinthitis with complete neurosensory hearing loss, meningitis, or brain abscess. Many children died as a consequence of one or another of these complications.

A single episode of otitis media treated with appropriate antibiotics will generally produce an effusion that clears within 1 month. In 90% of cases, an effusion due to an initial episode of acute otitis media clears within 3 months.

When the middle ear space continues to harbor fluid, for more than 3 months after an episode of acute otitis media, the condition has become chronic otitis media with chronic middle ear effusion. Although culture of such fluid shows that it does contain small numbers of viable bacteria, the condition is not an infection in the usual sense of the word. There is no associated pain, fever, or development of pus. Indeed, the condition is frequently asymptomatic and 50% of cases are "silent." Such cases can be diagnosed only on routine "well-baby" evaluations. The persistence of fluid behind the tympanic membrane presents difficulties if and only if it produces either significant conductive hearing loss or promotes frequently recurrent acute otitis media. The presence of this fluid in and of itself is of no great consequence. Therefore, an estimate of hearing threshold is crucial in the intelligent management of chronic middle ear effusion. A child with normal hearing thresholds who has relatively few middle ear infections need not be treated aggressively for the mere presence of middle ear fluid.

When persistent middle ear fluid causes significant conductive hearing loss (greater than 15 dB in a child) or is associated with more than four to six episodes of acute otitis media per year, then treatment should be implemented. The use of prophylactic antibiotics has been advocated for many years. However, the rapid development of antimicrobial resistance in the organisms commonly responsible for acute otitis media now make such protracted antibiotic treatment controversial. Since many of these conditions are caused by chronic eustachian tube dysfunction, the use of antihistamines or decongestants would seem to make sense. However, several good clinical studies have shown that antihistamines and decongestants are of essentially no use whatsoever in the treatment of persistent middle ear fluid in children. The use of steroids remains controversial but can be effective. If effusions persist greater than 12 weeks and are associated with significant hearing loss, consideration should be given to the insertion of tympanostomy tubes. However, the mere presence of fluid will not be a compelling reason for surgical intervention. This is especially true if the effusion is unilateral. In children with bilateral effusion who have conductive hearing losses greater than 15 or 20 decibels, justification for tympanostomy tube insertion is considerably reinforced. One must remember that the conductive hearing loss associated with middle ear effusions is variable and audiometric evaluation may occur when a child is hearing relatively well. The observations of parents or teachers should be given great credence. When there is a documented or even suspected problem with the acquisition of speech and language skills, or difficulty in school, then insertion of tympanostomy tubes should be considered to eliminate the possibility of mild conductive hearing loss as an etiologic or confounding variable.

Some children have special predisposing factors for otitis media with effusion. Children with cleft palate or Down's syndrome and patients with craniofacial syndromes such as Treacher Collins or Crouzon's syndrome are especially predisposed to otitis. These patients should be evaluated individually, bearing in mind their congenital anomalies. Almost all will benefit from tympanostomy tubes. In children with concurrent neurosensory hearing loss the use of tympanostomy tubes may be more urgent. If the sensorineural component is severe or profound, elimination of the conductive component may be the difference between aidable and unaidable hearing. Children with other medical problems that produce febrile conditions or with drug allergies may benefit from the early insertion of tympanostomy tubes to eliminate acute otitis media as a confounding variable. Children readily subject to febrile seizures may have little tolerance for the acute episodes of otitis media that most children deal with easily.

In patients over the age of 4 years, a number of studies have now shown that hypertrophied adenoid tissue plays a significant etiologic role in the persistence of middle ear effusion. In children more than 4 years old with persistent fluid consideration should be given to simultaneous adenoidectomy at the time of tympanostomy tube insertion.

The insertion of tympanostomy tubes is a relatively simple procedure. In many children over the age of 7 or 8 years it can be performed as an outpatient office procedure, as is generally done with adults. However, in younger children, a short general anesthetic is necessary. The tympanostomy tubes act as prosthetic eustachian tubes. At the time of tympanostomy tube insertion, the fluid is mechanically aspirated from the middle ear space. The tympanostomy tube then permits effective pressure regulation, equalizing the ambient pressure between the ear canal and the middle ear space and draining middle ear fluid through the tube into the ear canal. The tubes are spontaneously extruded from the tympanic membrane after about 1 year. Complications related to the insertion of tympanostomy tubes are relatively infrequent. Ten to 25% of patients will develop otorrhea drainage from the middle ear through the tympanostomy tube into the ear canal at some time.

Although the tympanic membrane heals completely after extrusion of tympanostomy tubes in 97 to 98% of cases, in 2 to 3% the tympanic membrane fails to heal after extrusion of the tube. This is somewhat more common with larger tubes and is more likely to occur when the tube is extruded in the presence of active infection. Even though the rate of permanent perforation related to tympanostomy tube placement is low, tympanostomy tube insertion has become sufficiently frequent so that this now accounts for a significant number of permanent tympanic membrane perforations in young children. In the vast majority of such cases, the infection can be effectively eliminated with a 5 to 7 day course of topical antibiotic drops placed into the external auditory canal. Persistent tympanic membrane perforation occurs in about 3% of patients and may require operative repair after tube extrusion. Tympanosclerosis of the tympanic membrane can occur but is generally of no consequence. Such complications need to be compared with the rather serious complications of persistent otitis media and the developmental and educational consequences of persistent conductive hearing loss.

Cholesteatoma

The lateral surface of the tympanic membrane consists of skin and, like skin in other portions of the body, it sheds epithelial cells (desquamates). The normally functioning external auditory canal removes these shed components as they are produced. If a sufficient portion of the tympanic membrane is retracted far enough into the mastoid, these shed epithelial cells can no longer escape out of the external auditory canal, and they accumulate as a mass of dead skin within the temporal bone. Such collections of desquamated skin cells will erode bone slowly through a combination of pressure necrosis and enzymatic activity. Such a collection of dead skin trapped within the middle space or temporal bone and increasing slowly in size is termed a "cholesteatoma." The condition may also be referred to as a "keratinoma" or "epidermoid inclusion cyst" or, in the older otologic literature, as a "pearly tumor." The dead skin components at the center of such skin-filled cysts are an excellent medium for bacterial growth and eventually infection will develop. Infection accelerates the process of bony destruction. Infections in such cysts are difficult to eradicate because blood-borne antibiotics are not delivered to these nonvascular areas and topical drops cannot penetrate to the core of the mass of dead skin. As cholesteatomas expand, they do so only at the expense of surrounding normal structures. Thus, cholesteatomas may result in any one of the following complications: (1) Destruction of one or all of the ossicles producing conductive hearing loss; (2) erosion of the bone of the labyrinthine capsule with penetration of the membranous labyrinth, causing a severe or profound neurosensory hearing loss (Figure 3–6) and overwhelming vertigo (labyrinthine fistula); (3) bacterial infection of the labyrinthine fluids producing bacterial labyrinthitis. Since the fluids within the labyrinth are in direct communication with the cerebrospinal fluid, bacterial

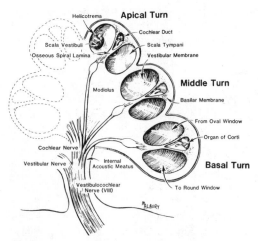

Figure 3-6. Diagram of the normal cochlea. The cochlea duct (scala media) is the site for a variety of inner ear fluid imbalances. Incomplete formation of the cochlea is responsible for a large variety of congenital neurosensory hearing losses. (We have reproduced with permission from Meyerhoff and Carter).

meningitis frequently develops as a consequence of bacterial labyrinthitis. Untreated bacterial meningitis may be fatal within a matter of only a few hours; (4) erosion into the cranial cavity producing either meningitis or brain abscess; (5) thrombosis or infection of the veins draining the brain, producing brain swelling, stroke, coma, and death; (6) thrombosis and infection of the major venous outflow tract (sigmoid sinus) may produce metastatic infection, brain abscess, and death; and (7) erosion into and paralysis of the facial nerve.

Surgical removal is the only reliable treatment and requires mastoidectomy in virtually all cases. Since the complications of cholesteatoma may be fatal, surgical therapy has as its goal complete removal of cholesteatoma and creation of a "safe" ear not subject to recurrent disease. Reconstruction of the disrupted middle ear transformer mechanism is of secondary importance. Even so, every effort is made to restore hearing when this is consistent with elimination of serious disease.

Otosclerosis

Otosclerosis is more properly termed "otospongiosis." However, the term "otosclerosis" is so enshrined in the literature that its continued widespread use is irresistible. Otosclerosis is a disease process in which vascular spongy bone replaces the normally hard bone of the labyrinthine capsule. It occurs most frequently in the area of the oval window. In about 10% of affected

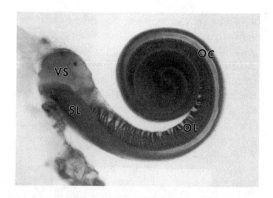

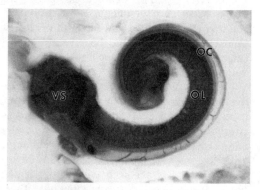

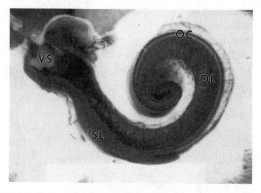

Figure 3-7. Microdissection: a) normal cochlear morphology in a specimen from a 16-year-old female, b) Mondini dysplasia in a 2-year-old female with trisomy 21, and c) Mondini dysplasia from an infant with CHARGE syndrome. Only one and a half turns of the cochlea have been developed. VS = Vestibule, OL = Osseus Spiral Lamina, OC = Organ of Corti. (Photographs and specimens courtesy of Gary C. Wright, Ph.D.)

individuals the otosclerotic process extends to involve the footplate and annular ligament. When this occurs, mobility of the footplate will be progressively reduced and a conductive hearing loss will develop slowly. Three quarters of all patients will develop disease in both ears.

There is evidence to support the notion that release of toxic enzymes into the perilymphatic

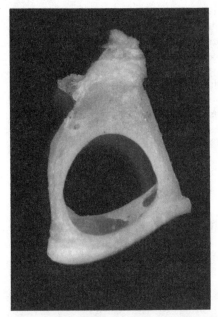
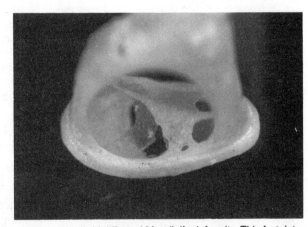

Figure 3–8. Multiple perforations in the footplate in this patient with bilateral Mondini's deformity. This footplate was removed from the patient described in case study 3–3.

spaces of the inner ear may cause progressive neurosensory hearing impairment and that this can be arrested by treatment of sodium fluoride. However, the diagnosis is difficult, especially in patients without concurrent stapes fixation, and the frequency with which "cochlear" otosclerosis occurs is not known. The disease is hereditary in many (but certainly not all) cases. Although the exact mechanism of inheritance is unknown, a dominant pattern with variable penetrance is favored by most researchers. Definitive diagnosis depends on middle ear exploration with visualization of the otosclerotic focus and mechanical verification of stapes fixation. Presurgical diagnosis is based on the presence of slowly progressive conductive hearing loss in the absence of concurrent or preceding chronic ear disease. Presurgical diagnosis is accurate in about 90% of cases. The cardinal audiometric finding in otosclerosis is a progressively increasing air-bone gap. Early in the course of the disease, when only the anterior portion of the stapes is fixed, a marked low-frequency gap is seen. As footplate fixation becomes complete, high frequencies become involved and the loss becomes a flat, conductive hearing loss. Sensorineural hearing loss may be depressed in some individuals but not all. Depression of bond conduction scores isolated to the 2000 Hz range is characteristic of otosclerosis and referred to as "Carhart's notch."

When surgical correction is desired, the fixed stapes is completely or partially removed and replaced with a prosthesis. The operation takes about 45 minutes and may be performed under local anesthesia. It is a day surgical procedure and does not require hospitalization. A wide variety of different sorts of prosthesis and techniques have been used and most have produced excellent results. Indeed 95% of patients undergoing surgery for otosclerosis will experience a closure of the air-bone gap to within 10 dB. Three to 5% of patients will experience no improvement and will therefore continue to be good candidates for amplification. The biggest risk associated with stapedectomy is the 1 to 2% chance of complete and profound neurosensory hearing loss associated with the operative procedure. The reason for such catastrophic loss has never been completely clarified, but it does not seem to be necessarily related to technical intraoperative difficulties.

Ossicular Discontinuity

Ossicular discontinuity may occur from a variety of causes. In children the most frequent cause is necrosis of the long process of the incus due to recurrent or persistent middle ear infection or effusion. In most such cases, the ossicular discontinuity is not complete, but rather the necrotic distal segment of the long process of the incus is replaced by a thin band of fibrous tissue. The connection between the long process of the incus and the capitulum of the stapes thus becomes fibrous rather than bony. As such, it transmits sound inefficiently and a significant conductive hearing loss is apparent. However, it is uncommon for the conductive hearing loss to be maximal in nature. A significant percentage of these children have a rather interesting audiometric finding. The air-bone gap becomes larger in the higher frequencies than in the lower. This high-frequency accentuated air-bone gap is thought to be characteristic of fibrous unions of the incudostapedial joint.

Previous surgical procedures can leave discontinuities in the ossicular chain. Oftentimes, surgery for cholesteatoma requires removal of part or all of one or more of the ossicles. Most frequently, the incus needs to be removed because of irremediable involvement with cholesteatoma. The head of the malleus may also have to be removed and, frequently, the capitulum of the stapes. In many cases, bony destruction of the ossicles by the cholesteatomatous process has occurred prior to surgical intervention.

Trauma can produce ossicular dislocation. In general, trauma produces inferior dislocation of the incus. The long process loses contact with the capitulum of the stapes. The incudomalleolar joint can be disrupted at the same time. Less frequently, trauma produces subluxation of the stapes into the oval window. When this occurs, there may be associated dizziness and neurosensory hearing loss as well as a conductive hearing loss. If such a situation is suspected, then immediate surgical intervention should be recommended to limit the amount of neurosensory hearing loss and to close the opening between the inner and middle ear space (perilymph fistula).

Treatment of ossicular discontinuity or dislocation is called "ossiculoplasty." Repair of the ossicular chain is possible in most cases. Unfortunately, results are not as good with repair of

defects involving the malleus and incus as stapes replacement is for repair of otosclerosis. Closure of the air-bone gap to 10 dB probably occurs in less than three quarters of all patients but depends somewhat on the nature of the hearing deficit. When the malleus and incus and stapes superstructure are gone and a total ossicular replacement prosthesis must be used, closure of the air-bone gap to within 30 dB is considered a good result. On the other hand, when the conductive hearing loss is caused by necrosis of the long process of the incus, complete closure can frequently be obtained.

INNER EAR AND INTERNAL AUDITORY CANAL

Sensorineural Hearing Loss

There are a large variety of causes for neurosensory hearing loss. These can roughly be divided into congenital and acquired etiologies. Congenital neurosensory hearing losses may be divided into genetic and nongenetic etiologies. As listed in Table 3-1, there are a large variety of known genetic inner ear hearing loss syndromes.

A variety of nongenetic neurosensory hearing losses that are congenital in nature have also been described. The most common is probably the maternal rubella syndrome in which deafness is associated with congenital cataracts and congenital heart disease (Figure 3-1). The availability of vaccines to prevent this disease have significantly reduced the incidence of hearing loss attributable to rubella. Toxoplasmosis and syphilis are other infections that can involve the developing embryo and produce postnatal hearing loss. Both of these processes can produce progressive neurosensory hearing losses of childhood.

Ototoxic drugs given to the mother during pregnancy may produce congenital hearing loss. Hypoxia during intrauterine development may produce significant injury to the auditory system. Injury to the vascular system of the branchial arches can produce either unilateral or bilateral hypoplasia of the membranous labyrinth.

Perinatal hypoxia due to birth trauma may also result in sensorineural hearing loss, as may intracranial hemorrhage complicating delivery.

Delayed sensorineural hearing loss can also be divided into genetic and nongenetic forms. The nongenetic etiologies are well-known and probably consist most frequently of those losses due to infection, neoplasm, the administration of ototoxic agents, or trauma. Noise-induced hearing

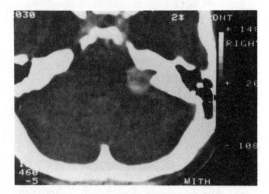

Figure 3–9. This is a computerized axial tomogram showing an acoustic neuroma in the cerebellopontine angle.

Case study 3-3. C.F. is an 8-year-old child who first presented to the otolaryngology department because of a cerebrospinal fluid leak in her left ear. She had two previous episodes of meningitis due to cerebrospinal fluid leak. The leak has been identified using special radiographic techniques. Audiometric evaluation at the time of this first visit showed that she had no hearing in her left ear and a 60 dB hearing loss in her right ear (see Audiogram 3a). However, her speech and language development was much better than one would expect with such a hearing loss, and it was assumed that she had the better hearing when younger and that it had progressively deteriorated. At that time, she was taken to the operating room where the left inner ear was completely filled with muscle and the ear closed off to prevent further spinal fluid leakage and meningitis. She did well for 2½ years, after which she had an additional episode of meningitis. She was, therefore, seen again in the otolaryngology department. Review of her computed tomography scans confirmed that she had bilateral Mondini's deformity. It was apparent that she now had developed cerebrospinal fluid leakage from her other ear. Audiometric evaluation at this time showed approximately a 90 dB "corner" audiogram (see Audiogram 3b). To prevent recurrent meningitis, it would be necessary to "pack" completely the cochlea with muscle or fat. This would eliminate C.F.'s residual hearing. It was, therefore, elected to place the electrode array of a Nucleus cochlear implant into the cochlea at the time of surgery. At operation, she was found to have a multiple congenital defect of her stapes footplate. Insertion of the implant was accomplished even though she had only a single "common" cavity. Because the electrode array was "coiled" within the common cavity, only the middle electrodes were stimulated. Postoperatively, she has done well. She has had no recurrent meningitis and her hearing is functionally better than it was preoperatively. She is doing well in a regular classroom situation.

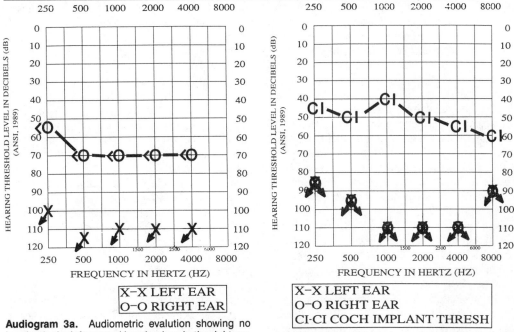

Audiogram 3a. Audiometric evaluation showing no hearing in the left ear and hearing loss in the right ear. See case history #3.

Audiogram 3b. Audiometric evaluation showing a 90 dB "corner" audiogram. See case history #3.

loss falls into this category. There are a large variety of genetic causes for delayed neurosensory hearing loss. Cochlear otosclerosis has already been mentioned as one such manifestation. Progressive neurosensory hearing loss can be attributed to a large variety of syndromes displaying musculoskeletal features. Among them are Paget's disease, van der Hoeve de Kleyn syndrome,

Alport's disease, and all of the mucopolysaccharidoses, such as Hunter's syndrome, Hurler's syndrome, Sanfilippo's syndrome and the syndromes of Morquio and Maroteaux-Lamy. Other well-document syndromes are associated with visual problems, such as Alstrm's syndrome, Refsum's syndrome, and Cockayne's syndrome. However, the largest variety of delayed, genetically mediated neurosensory hearing losses occur sporadically as a consequence of a recessive inheritance pattern and are fortunately not associated with specific syndromes.

Progressive Neurosensory Hearing Loss

A goodly number of children with hearing impairment develop progressive neurosensory hearing loss. Many of these children have well-identified syndromes such as Alport's, renal tubular acidosis, branchio-otorenal syndrome, Archer's syndrome, Refsum's syndrome, Norrie's syndrome, Wallenberg's syndrome, osteogenesis imperfecta, osteopetrosis, or mucopolysaccharide storage diseases. Some will have familial tumors.

However, a significant number of children with progressive neurosensory hearing loss have no obvious etiology.

Brookhauser et al[1,2] have reported on 114 children who showed progressive neurosensory hearing loss that appears to be noise induced. There was a striking male predominance. One quarter of these cases occurred prior to 10 years of age. Inquiry as to noise exposure must be made in children with high-frequency progressive types of losses.

Inner ear fluid imbalance is another apparent cause of progressive neurosensory hearing loss. It may involve perilymphatic fistula or Meniere's disease. The evaluation of children with progressive neurosensory hearing loss can identify an etiology in as many as 50 to 60% of cases. This should include complete history and computed tomography scan to identify labyrinthine anomalies or neurofibromatosis.

Perilymph fistula should be suspected if sensorineural hearing loss develops or progresses during or after a bout of otitis media. Vertigo or disequilibrium may accompany the hearing loss about half the time. Reilly and Kenna[3] have documented that up to 6% of all children with sensorineural hearing loss had perilymph fistula. Perilymph fistula can be difficult to diagnosis without surgical exploration. The likelihood of perilymph fistula is increased if there is a history of antecedent head trauma or barometric trauma. Abnormal electrocochleography certainly increases the possibility of perilymph fistula being the etiology of the progressive neurosensory loss. If perilymph fistula is the cause, then operative repair may prevent further deterioration and, although infrequently, in some patients may improve thresholds.

Meniere's Disease

Meniere's disease can occur in childhood, although it is unusual. Its diagnosis requires comprehensive evaluation. Meniere's disease or syndrome is a disorder with four principal clinical features: (1) episodes of whirling vertigo lasting several minutes to several hours; (2) low-pitched roaring tinnitus occurring or worsening during a vertiginous attack; (3) fluctuating low tone neurosensory hearing loss; and (4) a sense of fullness or pressure in the affected ear that can be very severe. Only about 3 to 4% of patients with Meniere's disease present in the pediatric age group. When endolymphatic hydrops or Meniere's disease is suspected, the use of electrocochleoraphy and other vestibular testing may be helpful. Electronystagmography (ENG) and sinusoidal harmonic acceleration can be useful in documenting unilateral labyrinthine dysfunction and confirming the diagnosis of Meniere's disease.

Most children are entirely asymptomatic between episodes, although some experience a chronic, mild disequilibrium, tinnitus, or aural fullness between vertiginous episodes. The disease is usually progressive. Early in the course of the disease, hearing often returns completely to normal between attacks, but over months or years a permanent hearing loss usually develops. The hearing loss may follow any pattern, but low-frequency losses are more common in the early course of the disease. Children with long-standing disease, on the other hand, are more likely to have flat losses.

It is not possible to predict the course of the disease in individual patients. Some children will experience a relatively indolent variety with attacks separated by years, others will loose all hearing and balance function over a period of several months. Most children follow a middle course, with attacks coming in clusters lasting several weeks and separated by months or even years of symptom-free periods. The development of anacusis is uncommon. The disease is bilateral in 15 to 20% of patients. Older children with Meniere's disease frequently complain of dysacusis and diplacusis, which are relatively unusual symptoms. Word discrimination scores are variably affected but often well preserved. The definitive diagnosis is difficult and depends on the documentation of a fluctuating low-tone neurosensory hearing loss associated with abnormal vestibular function. The presence of abnormal electrocochleography strongly reinforces the diagnosis. Primary therapy consists of vigorous salt restriction and the use of diuretic therapy. When such therapy fails, consideration can be given to the use of endolymphatic sac decompressive surgery. Endolymphatic sac decompressive surgery is helpful in 75% of patients in terms of relieving vertiginous symptoms. However, the evidence for hearing improvement is equivocal.

Tumors of the Internal Auditory Canal and Cerebellopontine Angle

Children may develop tumors of the temporal bone or cerebellopontine angle that can produce unilateral hearing loss and vestibular dysfunction (Figure 3–9). All children with unilateral otologic symptoms should be evaluated for such tumors. Such evaluation should include at least an evaluation of the word discrimination score and interpeak latencies on ABR. In many cases, radiographic imaging should be obtained. Symptoms of mass lesions involving the temporal bone or cerebellopontine angle may be subtle and slow to develop. Classically, the child experiences progressive high frequency neurosensory hearing loss over several months or years. Older children may complain of associated tinnitus. As the tumor enlarges, nerves in the surrounding area may become sufficiently distorted and stretched so as to produce numbness of the external auditory canal or face or weakness of facial muscles and facial paralysis. Continued growth results in compression of the brainstem with obstruction of the normal flow of cerebrospinal fluid, consequent hydrocephalus, and death. Early diagnosis of such tumors is critical if they are malignant. Early diagnosis in such a setting may permit life-saving intervention. Even when the tumor is benign, early diagnosis permits the tumor to be removed much more easily and safely with much lower surgical morbidity and mortality. The ability of the surgeon to preserve normal function of the facial nerve while achieving total tumor removal correlates directly with tumor size at the time of the diagnosis in benign tumors. The larger the tumor the more likely permanent facial weakness becomes. Diagnosis depends on a high incidence of suspicion and the frequent use of ABR examinations in children with unilateral complaints. More than 90% of children with cerebellopontine angle or temporal bone tumors affecting hearing will have abnormal ABRs. Stapedius reflex testing frequently shows stapedius reflex decay when there is compression of the VIIIth cranial nerve.

Acoustic neuroma or meningioma accounts for the large majority of tumors that affect hearing in children. Children with acoustic neuromas frequently have neurofibromatosis (von Recklinghausen's disease) and in such individuals there may well be a positive family history as the disease is inherited as an autosomal dominant. Other varieties of benign and malignant tumors occur sporadically.

REFERENCES

1. Brookhouser PE, Worthington DW, Kelly WS: Unilateral hearing loss in children. *Laryngoscope*, 101 (1991), 1264–1272.
2. Brookhouser PE, Worthington DW, Kelly WJ: Noise-induced hearing loss in children. *Laryngoscope*, 102 (1992), 645–655.
3. Reilly JS, Kenna MA: Congenital perilymphatic fistula: An overlooked diagnosis? *Am J Otol*, 10 No. 6 (1989), 496–498.
4. Hemenway WG, Sardo I, McChesney D: Temporal bone pathology following material rubella. *Arch Exp Ohren Nasen Kehlkopfheilkd*, 195 (1969), 287–300.
5. Sando I, Hemenway WG, Morgan RW: Histopathology of the temporal bones in mandibulofacial depostosis. *Trans Am Acad Opthalmol Otolaryngol*, 72 (1968), 913–924.
6. Bergstrom L: Congenital deafness, in English GM, ed: *Otolaryngology Loose Leaf Series*, Vol. 1 (Philadelphia: Harper and Row).
7. Meyerhoff WL, Carter JB: Scope of the problem and fundamentals, in Meyerhoff WL, ed: Diagnosis and management of hearing loss (Philadelphia: WB Saunders, 1984).

SCREENING FOR HEARING LOSS AND MIDDLE EAR DISORDERS IN THE SCHOOLS

| 4 |

Ross J. Roeser

A few honest men are better than numbers.

—Oliver Cromwell, 1599–1658

The foremost purpose of any hearing conservation program is to identify the children in the population who have hearing impairment that will interfere with their educational development.[1] Any significant loss in hearing sensitivity or auditory function will influence the overall educational process of the involved child.

A school system could implement a program of "identification audiometry" with the sole purpose of locating those children with hearing impairment. However, this limited program could not be considered adequate because the actual identification of children with hearing impairment is only the initial step in the development of a school hearing conservation program. More than identification of hearing loss is needed to meet the special educational needs of those children found to have significant hearing loss.

Experience suggests that the vast majority of hearing conservation programs are effective in identifying children with hearing impairment, but oftentimes are not effective for follow-up and providing comprehensive services to those who are identified. Once a child is found to have significant hearing impairment, it is imperative that provisions be made for proper medical diagnosis and treatment. For example, amplification may be indicated. In all cases, special educational intervention should be considered. Without provisions for these comprehensive follow-up services, children with significant hearing loss will continue to be sensorially deprived and will not attain their maximum educational potential.

Anderson[2] points out that hearing conservation programs lacking requisite comprehensive follow-up services actually are worse than programs not providing screening. Inadequate screening programs delude school administrators into assuming that an effective program exists when it does not. It cannot be stressed enough that all aspects—identification, audiological and medical referral or follow-up, and special educational considerations—must be included in any school hearing conservation program.

A major question in defining the overall purpose of a hearing conservation program in the schools is deciding whether to attempt to identify only those children with significant auditory impairment or to have the dual purpose of identifying children with auditory impairment and middle ear disorders.

Traditionally, hearing screening programs have used pure-tone air conduction hearing tests (the pure-tone sweep-check test) to identify children with peripheral hearing impairments. Such tests have proven to be effective in identifying significant hearing loss, but it is now well established that there are serious limitations in identifying middle ear pathologic conditions with air conduction tests. A number of studies have pointed out that audiometric screening alone will fail to detect about one half of the children with confirmed middle ear disease.[3-6]

Prior to 1970, there were no practical means for routine screening or middle ear disorders, especially in school children. The only valid procedure was to examine the ear with an otoscope; this procedure requires a trained observer and is not sensitive to many types of middle ear disease. However, with the emergence of immittance measures of the ear (described in Chapter 2), a feasible method of identifying middle ear disorders in school children is available. From a theoretic point of view, few audiologists and other health professionals would argue that immittance is a valuable part of school hearing conservation and belongs in every program. Such a statement is based on the validity and reliability of immittance tests and the relative ease with which immittance measurements are performed. However, several pragmatic factors should be considered before any school system implements an immittance screening program. These factors will be outlined later in this chapter.

When a school system elects to perform immittance screening, the one point that must be stressed emphatically is that immittance measures will not replace pure tone screening. That is, immittance measures screen for middle ear disorders; they do not provide direct information on hearing sensitivity. Even when a child has normal results on immittance measures, it is still necessary to perform tests to assess hearing sensitivity. By providing immittance screening, the school system is expanding its hearing conservation program to include detection of middle ear disorders; it is not replacing the procedures used in the hearing screening program. However, because of the high incidence of middle ear disorders in school children (especially in the primary grades; see Chapter 9) and its effects on educational achievement, immittance screening should be considered as an integral part of all elementary school hearing conservation programs, especially in the early grades.

This chapter reviews basic principles underlying screening. In addition, considerations and procedures for hearing and immittance screening programs for school children are presented. Guidelines are also presented that will allow for the implementation of an effective program to identify hearing loss and middle ear disorders in school children. Readers who are not completely familiar with audiometric and immittance principles should review them in Chapter 2 before reading this chapter.

PRINCIPLES OF SCREENING

The Concept of "Pass" and "Fail"

The purpose of screening is to identify those individuals having a defined disorder as early as possible, who would have otherwise not been identified, and to administer treatment at a time when it will either remediate the disorder or retard its rate of development.[7] Screening can be viewed as the general process by which groups of people are separated into those who manifest some defined trait, or those who do not. In this sense, it is a binary process—either passing the

individual who is considered a likely candidate not to have the disorder, or failing the individual who is considered a likely candidate to have the disorder.

Although screening is an "either/or" process, disorders may exist on a continuum from "not present at all" to "present in the most severe form." Based on this principle, it is incorrect to think that those individuals who pass the screening are completely free from the disorder for which the screening is being conducted. Instead, one should view those who pass the screening as individuals who do not manifest the disorder for which the screening is being conducted in a form severe enough to warrant consideration for additional testing.

This viewpoint is especially relevant for the screening of auditory disorders in school children because of the constraints that typically are put on such screening programs. As will be pointed out in later sections of this chapter, the procedures used for identifying auditory disorders in school children are limited, due to the nature of the tests themselves and the environment in which they are performed. Therefore, if a child successfully passes a school auditory screening test, it is not appropriate to think that the child's auditory system is completely normal, because the child may, in fact, have some auditory impairment. However, if the criteria are appropriate and the child passes the school screening, one can say that the child's auditory system is not impaired to the extent that it will interfere with educational achievement, and if hearing loss does exist, it is not significant enough to warrant additional audiological testing.

To illustrate, a child is screened at 500, 1000, 2000, and 4000 Hz at a level of 25 dB hearing level, and the pass-fail criterion is failure to respond to two frequencies in the same ear. Children who do not respond at 4000 Hz in either ear will pass the screening. Although it has been estimated by the school's screening criteria that the child's hearing loss will not cause significant educational problems, the child still does have hearing loss; hearing is not "normal." This concept of "pass" and "fail" must be maintained throughout the development and implementation of all hearing conservation programs, especially those in the schools.

Reliability and Validity

Four related terms are used to describe the general effectiveness of any type of screening test:

reliability and *validity*, and *sensitivity* and *specificity*. Reliability deals with the consistency of the test. That is, if the test is administered and then repeated by a different or the same tester at another time, will the test results be the same (test-retest or intraexaminer reliability). Without a high degree of reliability, the screening tool is ineffective, because the results of the test will vary from test session to test session and from tester to tester.

It is not difficult to envision how poor reliability will have serious consequences on screening tests; the reliability of a test must be high for the test to be effective. However, just because a screening test is reliable, it still may not be an effective test if it fails to identify the problem for which the screening is being conducted. To illustrate, one could use the color of children's hair as a screening test for deafness, and in all probability this measure would have a high degree of test-retest and intraexaminer reliability. However, hair color is a very poor index of deafness, because it is not a *valid* test for deafness. Another more realistic example would be the use of pure-tone screening tests to identify middle ear disorders. As has already been stressed, pure-tone testing fails to identify about one half of the children with middle ear disorders. Therefore, pure-tone testing is not a valid measure to assess the state of the middle ear and should not be used for identifying middle ear problems.

The validity of a screening test, then, is the degree to which results are consistent with the actual presence or absence of the disorder. In other words, validity determines whether the test is actually measuring the trait for which the screening is being conducted. It is important to realize that newly developed screening procedures must be validated in some way before they are put into widespread use. Such assessment would involve calculating the percentage of *false-positive* and *false-negative* identification, and the *sensitivity* and *specificity* of the test.

False-Positive and False-Negative Identifications

It would be ideal if a screening test was 100% accurate in its classification, if all those with and without the disorder were correctly identified. However, this situation is rarely if ever the case, and there are always an expected number of false-positive and false-negative identifications. These two conditions are illustrated in the tetrachordic table in Figure 4–1. As shown in Figure 4–1, diagnostic test results indicate whether the disorder is actually present or not present (this is considered "truth").

As an example, for hearing loss the diagnostic procedure would be pure-tone threshold tests performed in a sound-treated room. Results from the screening test, shown along the side of the figure, can either be positive, indicting failure on the screening, or negative, indicating that the screening was passed. These cells represent all possible outcomes once the results of both the screening and diagnostic tests are known. The results of this

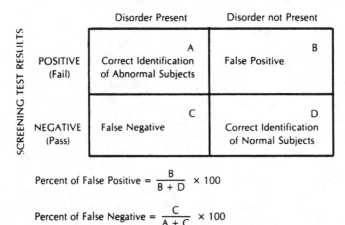

Figure 4–1. Tetrachordic table classifying results into correct identifications (cells A and D), false-positive identifications (cell B), and false-negative identifications (cell C).

analysis has three outcomes: correct identification of the abnormal and normal subjects (cells A and D), false-positive identifications (cell B) and false-negative (cell C) identifications. As illustrated, a false-positive identification occurs when an individual fails the screening test, but actually does not have the disorder. A false-negative identification occurs when an individual passes the screening test but has the disorder. The formulas in Figure 4–1 show how the percentage of false-positive and false-negative identifications can be calculated. Examples of how the formulas are used are presented later.

Neither false-positive nor false-negative identifications are desirable in screening programs and represent a liability or "cost" to the screening process. The cost can be the actual dollars that are spent as a result of the screening, or the needless expenditure of time, effort, or any other resource. Frankenberg[7] lists the following as costs of false-positive identifications: (1) the cost associated with retrieving the child for further evaluations; (2) the cost of additional screening or diagnostic tests that will fail to confirm the disorder; (3) mental anguish of the parents and the child; and (4) the cost and danger of unnecessary treatment, if the absence of the disease is not detected by diagnostic tests.

False-positive results are most likely to interfere with the overall acceptance of the screening program in the community it serves. This especially is true for hearing screening, because the cost of false-positive identifications may be high. An office visit to an otolaryngologist or audiologist can be expensive, and it is quite disconcerting for a parent to be told for such a fee that his child is "normal." Only a few parents voicing their dissatisfaction over this unnecessary visit would be needed before false-positive identifications would ultimately jeopardize acceptance of the program. Thus, from the perspective of the administrator of the screening program, false-positive identifications must be avoided.

The costs of false-negative identifications are: (1) the loss of the benefits associated with early identifications and diagnosis; and (2) false reassurance, which will delay correct identification of the child's problem, even when symptoms persist. In the case of hearing impairment, time lost in providing the necessary educational and possibly medical intervention is detrimental to the child; if this delay is too great, the child may be deprived of full educational potential.

Sensitivity and Specificity

Sensitivity and specificity are used to measure the validity of a screening test. The sensitivity of a test is its accuracy in correctly identifying

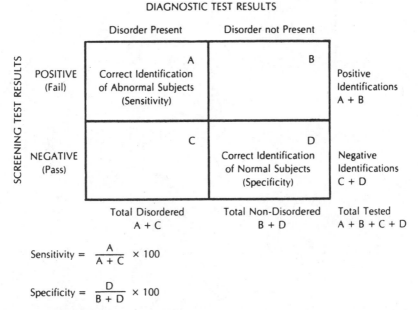

Figure 4–2. Correct identification of abnormal subjects—sensitivity (cell A)—and normal subjects—specificity (cell D)—for a screening test.

the disordered subjects. Specificity is the test's accuracy in correctly identifying the subjects without the disorder. Figure 4–2 is an extension of Figure 4–1, and illustrates how these two terms are applied. Cell A represents those subjects who failed the screening test and actually had the disorder. Data from cell A are used to calculate the sensitivity of the screening test. Cell D represents subjects who passed the screening and did not have the disorder. Data from this cell are used to calculate the specificity of the screening test. The sensitivity and specificity of a given test are computed using the formulas provided at the bottom of Figure 4–2.

Figure 4–3 presents data showing how the false-positive, false-negative, sensitivity, and specificity values of a screening test can be calculated using hypothetical data from a hearing screening test on 1000 children. Of these 1000 children, diagnostic test results showed that 92 actually had hearing loss (cells A + C), and 908 actually were free from hearing loss (cells B + D). The screening test identified 96 children with hearing loss (cells A + B), and 904 children

without hearing loss (cells C + D). Based on the data presented in Figure 4–3, the sensitivity of this test is calculated to be 95.7% and the specificity 99.1%. Stated differently, the screening test correctly identified 95.7% of those subjects who actually had hearing loss and 99.1% of the subjects who were free from hearing loss. The false-negative and false-positive rates were calculated to be 4.3% and 0.9%, respectively.

The hypothetical data in Figure 4–3 would strongly support the validity of the screening test being used to detect hearing loss, because both the sensitivity and specificity are high, and the false-positive and false-negative rates low. This is a desired result that one attempts to achieve in any screening program.

In designing a screening test, the sensitivity and specificity must be considered together because they are related, and they directly influence the false-positive and false-negative rates. The overall goal is to maintain a balance between the factors that determine the validity of the test, so that the sensitivity and specificity, as well as the related false-positive and false-negative rates, are within

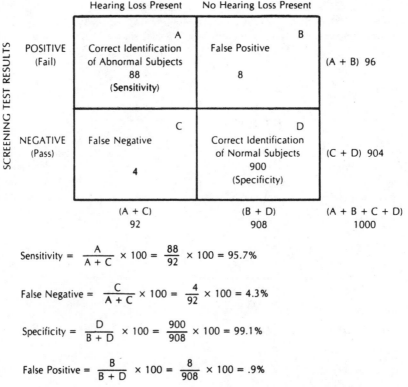

Figure 4–3. Calculating the sensitivity, false-negative rate, specificity, and false-positive rate for a screening test administered to 1000 subjects.

a predetermined acceptable range for the screening that is being conducted. An extreme example is the case in which the screening test fails all those screened (cells A or B). Such a test will produce 100% sensitivity. However, the false-positive rate would also be 100%, and the specificity and false-negative rates each 0%, making the test worthless. Conversely, redesigning the same test so that all those screened would pass the test, results in 100% specificity. However, in this case the false-negative rate would be 100% and the sensitivity and false-positive rates 0%, also providing a worthless test.

Co-Positivity and Co-Negativity

It is possible to compare two different types of screening tests that are screening for the same disorder and to evaluate the performance of a given tester by comparing the test results with those obtained by an expert. In either case, for the results obtained, the *co-positivity* and *co-negativity* can be determined. The co-positivity is the extent to which the two tests agree in identifying those with the disorder (the positive results), and the co-negativity is the agreement in identifying those without the disorder (the negative results). An example of two different audiometric tests would be the comparison of results from a test using speech signals to those using pure tones presented at a fixed intensity. To compare tester performance, results that are obtained by the tester would be compared directly to those obtained from the same subjects by a certified audiologist.

The co-positivity and co-negativity of a test are calculated using the same formulas for calculating sensitivity and specificity, respectively. However, unlike sensitivity and specificity, measures of co-positivity and co-negativity, while providing valuable information on the reliability of a screening test, do not measure the test's validity.

Program Evaluation

Program evaluation should be an integral part of any screening process and can occur at a number of levels, from evaluation of the equipment to evaluation of the procedures and personnel used in the program. Of course, routine calibration checks of the equipment are mandatory (see Chapter 2). With the information previously given, it is possible to conduct a methodological

evaluation of the screening procedures and personnel, provided one of two steps is added to the screening process—either the reliability of the procedures can be evaluated by comparing test results from those individuals who perform routine screening with those obtained by an audiologist (co-positive and co-negativity), or the validity of the procedures can be evaluated by comparing screening results with diagnostic findings (sensitivity and specificity).

Co-positivity and Co-negativity. An example of evaluating the reliability of the program by calculating its co-positivity and co-negativity follows: Two audiometric support personnel screen 868 children and the school's audiologist immediately rescreens the children. Figure 4–4 shows the data after they have been categorized into a tetrachordic table. The co-positivity and co-negativity for Support Person 1 were 76% and 94%, respectively, with commensurate false-negative and false-positive rates of 24% and 6%, respectively. However, for Support Person 2 the respective values were 97% and 99.3% for co-positivity and co-negativity and 3% and 0.7% for the false-negativity and false-positive rates.

The data in Figure 4–4 would indicate that for some reason the results of the screenings performed by Support Person 1 are inferior to those obtained by Support Person 2, when compared with the audiologist's results. In fact, these hypothetical data would be alarming if they were actually obtained through program evaluation, because of the high false-negative rates found for Support Person 1. To check Support Person 1, the equipment being used would be examined to ensure that it is in proper calibration and there are no malfunctions, and the actual test procedures used in the screening would be evaluated carefully. If findings similar to those in Figure 4–4 were revealed through program evaluation, careful scrutiny of the performance of Support Person 1 should be made until it is within limits similar to those for Support Person 2.

Sensitivity and Specificity. Whenever results from a screening test can be compared to results from a diagnostic test, the sensitivity and specificity of the screening test can be calculated to determine the validity of the results. Such an evaluation can be performed retrospectively, after the results have been obtained and reported, or it can be planned prospectively by including a diagnostic test with the screening test. An example of retrospective evaluation is as follows: Wilson and Walton[8] evaluated a fixed-intensity pure-tone screening technique with 1168 children.

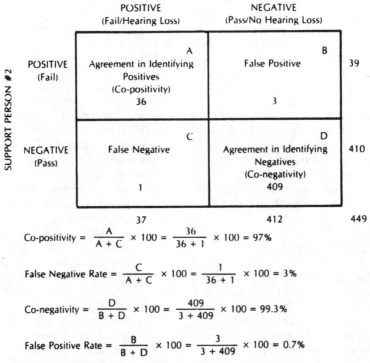

AUDIOLOGIST'S RESULTS

POSITIVE
(Fail/Hearing Loss)

NEGATIVE
(Pass/No Hearing Loss)

SUPPORT PERSON #1

POSITIVE
(Fail)

A
Agreement in Identifying
Positives
(Co-positivity)
16

B
False Positive

22

38

NEGATIVE
(Pass)

C
False Negative

5

D
Agreement in Identifying
Negatives
(Co-negativity)
376

381

21   398   419

Co-positivity = $\dfrac{A}{A+C} \times 100 = \dfrac{16}{16+5} = 76\%$

False Negative Rate = $\dfrac{C}{A+C} \times 100 = \dfrac{5}{16+5} \times 100 = 24\%$

Co-negativity = $\dfrac{D}{B+D} \times 100 = \dfrac{376}{22+376} \times 100 = 94\%$

False Positive Rate = $\dfrac{B}{B+D} \times 100 = \dfrac{22}{22+376} \times 100 = 6\%$

AUDIOLOGIST'S RESULTS

POSITIVE
(Fail/Hearing Loss)

NEGATIVE
(Pass/No Hearing Loss)

SUPPORT PERSON #2

POSITIVE
(Fail)

A
Agreement in Identifying
Positives
(Co-positivity)
36

B
False Positive

3

39

NEGATIVE
(Pass)

C
False Negative

1

D
Agreement in Identifying
Negatives
(Co-negativity)
409

410

37   412   449

Co-positivity = $\dfrac{A}{A+C} \times 100 = \dfrac{36}{36+1} \times 100 = 97\%$

False Negative Rate = $\dfrac{C}{A+C} \times 100 = \dfrac{1}{36+1} \times 100 = 3\%$

Co-negativity = $\dfrac{D}{B+D} \times 100 = \dfrac{409}{3+409} \times 100 = 99.3\%$

False Positive Rate = $\dfrac{B}{B+D} \times 100 = \dfrac{3}{3+409} \times 100 = 0.7\%$

Figure 4–4. Calculating co-positivity and co-negativity of a screening test for two support personnel.

Following the screening, threshold tests were performed on all children in a sound-treated room. Interestingly, they report that the overall accuracy of the screening test was 94.7%; the results from both screening and threshold tests would pass the subjects 91.4% of the time and fail the subjects 3.3% of the time. The false-positive and false-negative rates were stated to be 3.2% and 2.0%, respectively, producing an "inaccuracy" rate of 5.2%. From these data, they concluded that the screening procedures used were highly accurate in identifying hearing loss. However, they failed to recognize the importance of the sensitivity and specificity of the test, as previously described.

Figure 4–5 presents the data of Wilson and Walton's[8] calculated in the manner described in Figure 4–3. As shown in Figure 4–5, the respective sensitivity and specificity of the screening test were 63% and 97%, and the false-positive and false-negative rates were 3% and 37%. These data mean that 97% of the children with normal hearing were correctly identified, producing an overreferral rate of 3%. This rate is well within acceptable limits. However, a discouraging result was that only 63% of the children with hearing loss were correctly identified, leaving 37% im-

properly classified as having no significant loss. When viewed in these terms, the results from this screening survey do not support the use of the screening test that Wilson and Walton were evaluating under the conditions in which it was used, because of the low sensitivity and high false-negative rates. For a screening test for hearing loss to be acceptable, the sensitivity should be within the 90 to 95% range and the corresponding false-negative rate 5 to 10%. These ranges appear to be reasonable as goals, given the present state of knowledge in the area of hearing screening.

It is unfortunate that most school hearing conservation programs do not routinely evaluate the reliability and validity of their procedures. Program evaluation does require extra time on the part of the personnel in the program, which ultimately translates into added dollars. However, without appropriate evaluation, the basic issue of the program's reliability and validity will always be subject to questions. Although the examples given in this section have only used tests of hearing sensitivity, similar evaluations can and should be performed for other measures used in screening, such as immittance measures and otoacoustic emissions.

THRESHOLD TEST

		Disordered (Fail) (Hearing Loss)	Non-Disordered (Pass) (No Hearing Loss)	
SCREENING TEST RESULTS	POSITIVE (Fail)	A 3.3% (39)	B 3.2% (38)	Total (A + B) 77
	NEGATIVE (Pass)	C 2.0% (23)	D 91.4% (1068)	(C + D) 1091
		(A + C) 62	(B + D) 1106	(A + B + C + D) 1168

$$\text{Sensitivity} = \frac{A}{A + C} \times 100 = \frac{39}{39 + 23} \times 100 = 63\%$$

$$\text{False Negative} = \frac{C}{A + C} \times 100 = \frac{23}{39 + 23} \times 100 = 37\%$$

$$\text{Specificity} = \frac{D}{B + D} \times 100 = \frac{1068}{38 + 1068} \times 100 = 97\%$$

$$\text{False Positive} = \frac{B}{B + D} \times 100 = \frac{38}{38 \times 1068} \times 100 = 3\%$$

Figure 4–5. Retrospective analysis of hearing screening data reported by Wilson and Walton.[8]

THE PREVALENCE OF HEARING LOSS AND MIDDLE EAR DISORDERS IN CHILDREN

Frasier[9] and Stewart[10] estimate that congenital, profound hearing loss occurs in 1 in 1000 births worldwide. These reports only represent severe hearing loss, so the true incidence of all hearing loss in infants and children would be significantly greater. Northern and Downs[11] indicate that there were 42,000 children with severe hearing impairment attending special schools or classes for the hearing-impaired in the United States in 1991. Berg[12] estimates that there are another 950,000 hard-of-hearing children having losses in the 26 to 55 dB HL range, who will require assistance in the classroom.

Data from studies on screening for ear disease in school children suggest that the prevalence of ear disease is much greater than that of hearing loss. Based on a survey of 3197 children between the ages of 0 to 5 years, Klein[13] estimates that the occurrence of middle ear disease ranges between 8.3% and 25.3%. Jerger[14] states that estimates of the prevalence of otitis media with fluid, the primary middle ear disorder that causes hearing loss in children, range up to 30% and have seldom been less than 15%. By conservative estimates, this prevalence rate implies that there are some 2,500,000 children between the ages of 0 to 6 years in this country affected by middle ear disease. Furthermore, Jerger states that as many as 8,000,000 to 9,000,000 children in the 0- to 6-year-old age range have experienced at least one bout of otitis media with fluid. Brooks[15] points out that undetected (and therefore untreated) middle ear disease can lead to numerous possible serious complications that require surgery or cause permanent hearing loss.

The data just presented clearly document the need for hearing conservation programs and screening for middle ear disorders in the schools. However, these estimates do not address questions regarding the number of children expected to fail a given audiometric screening test or a screening test for middle ear disorders. Answers to these questions are important to school personnel in the overall planning of the program.

With respect to hearing loss, Anderson[2] contends that a referral rate of between 5 and 10% is reasonable. This estimate is the range typically quoted in virtually all of the literature. For example, Silverman, and David[16] conclude that, "Our best estimate. . . is that 5 percent of school-age children have hearing loss, in one ear at least." Results from the Pittsburgh study[17] also support the 5% incidence figure. However, is this range realistic? Should about 5% of the children screened in the program fail the test? Moreover, if the 5% figure is representative, by how much can the rate vary before there is concern about the false-positive and false-negative identifications?

Connor[18] reviewed three separate studies conducted between 1926 and 1960. Depending on the particular study, he found that the incidence of hearing loss ranged from 0.5 to 21%. Although this survey is almost 20 years old, more recent surveys on the incidence of hearing disorders demonstrate the same inconsistencies. Melnick et al[3] screened 860 children and failed 135 (15.7%) of the population. Fay et al,[19] on the other hand, failed 90 of 336 children, representing a failure rate of 26.8%. However, Robinson et al[20] reported a failure rate of only 3.5%.

The discrepancies in findings of these studies can be related to variables such as the types of tests used, the instruments used to perform the screening, the training of the testers, environmental noise present during the hearing screening, and the pass-fail criteria. However, even when these factors are controlled as closely as possible, variability still exists. For example, Table 4–1 presents results from audiometric screening of 54,370 children in the Dallas public schools using a pure-tone sweep-check test at 500, 1000, 2000, and 4000 Hz at a level of 25 dB HL. Six different testers were used in the program, but the procedures, equipment, and pass-fail criteria were identical, and all testers had the same training. Despite this uniformity in the program, the percentage of failures between testers ranged from 0.9 to 3.4%; and all of the values were lower than the nominal 5% value suggested by most other reports. What then can account for this discrepancy? This question can be

Table 4–1 Screening Data from the Dallas Independent School District

Tester	No. Children Screened	Percent Failing Test (%)
1	10,129	1.0
2	8,525	3.4
3	9,680	1.4
4	7,997	2.1
5	9,351	1.2
6	8,688	.9
Total	54,370	
Mean		1.7

answered on the basis of data gathered from epidemiological studies of auditory disorders in children.

Epidemiology is technically defined as the study of frequencies and distributions of disorders, and the relationship between the various factors that contribute to their occurrence.[21] When an epidemiological study is conducted, all of the factors that relate to a particular disease process are considered, including age, sex, social and cultural characteristics, climate, and so on. Once an epidemiological study is completed, it is possible to assess how the factors studied affect the incidence of the disorder and its severity.

The generalizations we are able to make now about auditory disorders include: hearing loss and ear disease are more prevalent in young children and in certain populations, such as American Indians[22] and Eskimo children[23]; low socioeconomic status may increase the incidence of hearing loss and ear disease[19]; the incidence of hearing loss and ear disease changes with climate and specific seasons of the year[24]; and high-frequency sensorineural hearing loss is more prevalent in older males in the grades 9 to 12.[25,26] A summary of literature dealing with screening in special populations has been published by Northern.[27] These factors make it impossible to estimate the expected incidence of hearing loss or ear disease in a population of school age children on an a priori basis, no matter what screening techniques are used.

HEARING SCREENING IN THE SCHOOLS—IDENTIFICATION OF HEARING LOSS

General considerations for any hearing conservation program, whether it be designed for preschool or school age children, include the test environment; the personnel supervising and administering the testing; the equipment; the contributions of school personnel, such as the teacher and school administrator, the periodicity of testing, the tests to be used, and the pass-fail criteria and follow-up.

Test Environment

The test environment should be well lighted, adequate in size to accommodate the tester and equipment, well ventilated, and have low ambient noise levels. One of the most critical requirements

of the test environment is the ambient noise level, because false-positive identifications will occur in hearing screening if the background noise levels are too high. The most desirable space for hearing screening in any school is located as far away as possible from heating units, air conditioners, and other mechanical equipment, and away from the cafeteria, shop areas, music rooms, rest rooms, and other high traffic areas. The best areas for hearing screening in the schools typically include the auditorium stage with the curtains drawn, the nurse's office, or the teachers' lounge. But the exact location depends entirely on the school building itself and the schedule of daily activities.

The problem with testing in environments having high ambient noise levels is that the noise in the environment has the potential to mask or block out the test stimulus itself. High ambient noise levels have a limiting effect on the frequencies and intensity at which hearing screening can be performed and are the reason for imposing many of the recommended guidelines for hearing screening. Most noise found in a typical school environment will have its main energy concentrated in the frequencies below 1000 Hz. This one factor is the primary reason why guidelines for school screening programs have recommended testing at 1000 Hz and above, even though some important data can be obtained at 500 and 250 Hz. Moreover, screening tests performed at intensities of 10 to 15 dB HL can be severely affected by noise, even though these intensities are more sensitive to marginal hearing loss.

It has been reasoned by some that if the background noise level is too high, simply increasing the intensity level of the test stimuli will solve the problem. However, this solution is not acceptable because by increasing the intensity level, the sensitivity of the screening test is reduced and those children who actually have hearing loss at the screening level optimally chosen may pass at the higher level. In no case should the levels of the test stimuli be increased above those specified by the screening program, and an alternate test site should be selected.

One solution to resolve the problem of ambient noise is the use of sound-isolated rooms. The National Conference on Identification Audiometry recommended that all schools purchase and install commercial sound-treated booths.[28] This recommendation is ideal because it would ensure that acceptable background noise levels would be present all of the time. However, with the constant demands and limitations on school finances, such equipment is beyond the scope of most school budgets. Mobile test vans or trailers are commercially available with sound-isolating booths installed and do provide adequate test environments. However, mobile test vans also represent a sizeable financial investment in both purchase and maintenance.

Small, portable hearing test booths have been developed, which are economical and can be effective in reducing ambient noise levels. Fisher[29] has shown that the use of a portable sound room can provide significant benefit in school hearing conservation programs. In this study, data obtained from the portable rooms were compared with those obtained in an open environment and in an audiometric sound-treated booth. Results from the portable sound-treated enclosure correctly identified a significantly larger percentage of students with and without hearing impairment than the open environment. The major advantage of using the portable sound room appears to be that the number of false-positive identifications is reduced significantly, saving a considerable amount of time and money in retesting. The use of the portable sound rooms in school screening is not widespread at this time, but results from Fisher's study indicate that their use definitely deserves additional consideration.

A final solution for eliminating unwanted background noise is the use of noise-excluding earphone enclosures and insert-type earphones (described in Chapter 2). Certain types of these enclosures are generally more effective in reducing background noise than the standard headsets (see Chapter 2).[30-32] Furthermore, laboratory and field studies on their use with children have proven their overall effectiveness.[33-34] Despite these studies supporting their use, noise-excluding headsets do present inherent problems, such as earphone placement. Thus, they should be utilized only by highly experienced examiners who are aware of the difficulties that may occur with their use. Noise-excluding headsets should not be used routinely in hearing conservation programs. Insert-type earphones not only attenuate background noise, but also reduce ear canal collapse and have higher interaural attenuation. An excellent use of insert-type earphones is to perform threshold screening tests after the child has failed the pure tone screening and before referring for follow-up testing and treatment.

A simple biologic check should always be made prior to screening to assess the appropriateness of the test environment before any testing is performed. The biologic check is performed by screening several subjects (as an example, the tester and one other person) with known normal hearing sensitivity. Obviously, if both of these individuals fail to perceive the test stimuli at the same frequency, the environment most likely is not satisfactory, provided that the equipment is known to be in proper calibration. For those who may have access to a sound level meter, Table 4–2 provides allowable decibel sound pressure levels (SPL) for conducting screening.

Personnel

Two levels of personnel may be utilized in school hearing conservation programs, one supervisory and one technical.[28,35] The supervisor of the program should be an audiologist holding the Certificate of Clinical Competence from the American Speech-Language-Hearing Association (ASHA). As the supervisor of the program, the audiologist is responsible for selecting the screening procedures to be used, training and monitoring the technical staff, ensuring proper equipment calibration, referring certain children for diagnostic audiological testing or performing the tests, discussing test results with medical personnel, and generally carrying out the higher administrative functions of the program.

Resources may not be available in smaller school systems to have a full-time audiologist to supervise the hearing conservation program. In

Table 4–2 Allowable Octave-Band Ambient Noise Levels (SPL; 20 μPa) for Threshold Measurements at 0 dB HL (ANSI 1969) and for Screening at the ASHA-Recommended Levels (ANSI 1969)*

Test frequency	500	1000	2000	4000
Octave-band cutoff	300	600	1200	2400
Frequencies	600	1200	2400	4800
Octave-band levels: Ear covered with earphone mounted on MX-41/AR cusion (ANSI 3.1, 1977)	21.5	29.5	34.5	42.0
Plus ASHA screening level (ANSI 1969)	20	20	20	20
Resultant maximum ambient noise level allowable for ASHA screening	41.5	49.5	–54.5	62

*Reprinted with permission from

such cases it is possible in most areas of the country to have a part-time audiologist consultant who will monitor the activities just listed. The consultant's primary role is to set up the program and train the technical staff as thoroughly as possible. Only when special problems arise is the consultant required to be available in the school system itself.

The technical or support personnel perform the screening tests and carry out the day to day activities of the program, such as performing daily calibration checks and filling out statistical reports. Many school systems use nurses or speech-language pathologists in this role. Because of their training, such professionals are effective, but still require in-service training to familiarize them with the general area of hearing, hearing disorders, and audiometric testing. Such sessions should be held for no less than one full day before the individual begins to perform in the program. A very helpful way to avoid any confusion in the program, and to keep it uniform, is to develop a manual describing the screening program and procedures used.

When paraprofessionals or professionals with no training in auditory disorders and screening are used for technical support, additional training is mandatory. The National Conference on Identification Audiometry recommended that for such persons the training course be conducted over a 2- to 6-week period, with at least one half of the time devoted to supervised practice in testing.[28] Since the success of the entire hearing conservation program rests on the support personnel, the need for adequate training cannot be stressed enough. The absolute minimum training period for the paraprofessionals should be 5 days, with one half of the time in supervised practicum. As a guide, topics that should be included in the training program are listed in Table 4-3.

Table 4-3   Topics to be Included in Paraprofessional Training Programs for Auditory Screening Schools

1. Basic physical principles of sound
2. Anatomy and physiology of the auditory system
3. Disorders of the ear and types of hearing loss
4. Use, care, maintenance, and calibration of audiometers
5. Screening procedures
6. Threshold measurement and referral procedures
7. Record keeping

Four organizations that currently have training manuals for audiometric technicians are listed in Table 4-4. Although these manuals were not

Table 4-4   Organizations That Have Training Manuals for Audiometric Technicians

1. Council for Accreditation in Occupational Hearing Counservation
   1619 Chestnut Avenue
   Haddon Heights, NJ 08035
2. Audiometric Assistant Trainee's Workbook
   US Department of Education
   Division of Manpower Development and Training
   Washington, DC
3. American Association of Industrial Nurses
   79 Madison Avenue
   New York, NY 10016
4. American Association of School Nurses, Inc.
   P.O. Box 1300
   Scarborough, ME 04070-1300

designed specifically for school hearing conservation programs, they can be adapted for use in training school personnel.

Speech versus Pure-Tone Stimuli

Two choices of test stimuli are available for assessing hearing. Speech has the advantage of being less abstract than pure tones, so tests using speech can generally be administered more successfully to younger children. Based on this one principle, several tests using speech stimuli were developed and are still in use today in some school systems.

The Verbal Auditory Screening for Children (VASC) test is one of the more popular hearing screening procedures using speech.[36] Although there is some variability in the procedures used in the VASC test,[37] in the classic test four recorded randomized lists of 12 spondaic (bisyllabic) words, such as "cowboy" and "airplane," are used as stimuli. The initial level of presentation is 51 dB HL, and each stimulus deceases in intensity 4 dB. During the test, the child points to a picture representing the stimulus after each presentation.

Early reports on the VASC screening procedure were encouraging, suggesting a very low rate of false-positive identifications.[36] However, the major limitation of using speech as a stimuli for any hearing screening procedure is that it is not sensitive to mild or high-frequency hearing impairment, causing the false-negative rate to be unacceptably high. Studies that have compared both speech and pure-tone tests have reported false-negative rates between 50 and 58% for speech tests, primarily because they were not sensitive enough to detect mild and high-frequency hearing losses.[38-40] Mencher and McCullock[40]

Table 4–5 Summary of Group Hearing Screening Tests

Name of Test	Stimuli	Method of Response	Maximum No. Children Tested Per Session
Fading Numbers Test or Western Electric 4-A Phonographic Recording Test	Recordings of spoken single or paired digits	Written	40
Pulse Tone Test	Pure tones (250, 1000, 2000, and 4000 Hz)	Written (record the number of pulses heard)	40
Massachusetts Test	Pure tones (500, 4000, and 8000 Hz)	Written (circle "yes" or "no")	40
Bennett Test	Phonetically similar words	Pointing	—*
Johnston Group Screening Test	Pure tones	Hand raise	10
Modified Massachusetts Test	Pure tones (500, 1000, 2000, and 8000 Hz)	Written (circle "yes" or "no")	40

*Maximum number not specifically stated.

state that the high false-negative results occur with speech stimuli due to the high-intensity cues in speech, which provide clues to the child, resulting in positive responses. Because of their insensitivity, the use of speech stimuli alone in school screening programs must be considered inadequate and, at least with children in grades 1 and above, the use of tests utilizing pure tones is recommended.

Group versus Individual Testing Procedures

At one time, group hearing screening procedures were advocated as a means of screening hearing in the schools. The group test was a means of saving time; several children, as many as 40 at a time, are screened with each administration of the test. Following the initial group screening, children who fail are seen for either a second group test or an individual test. Table 4–5 summarizes the most popular group hearing screening procedures that have been advocated throughout the years.

Even though studies have documented the efficacy of group tests as a means of saving time, when other considerations are taken into account, group tests are less desirable overall than individual tests (described later). Limiting factors include the calibration and maintenance problems of multiple earphones, finding an appropriate test environment, increased set-up time, the level of training of the personnel administering the test, and the inherent problem of using speech as a stimulus.[41] Because of these factors, individual screening tests have been recommended over the use of group tests.[35,42]

The Individual Pure-Tone Sweep-Check Test

The most widely preferred individual pure-tone test is the sweep-check screening test,[42,43] originally described by Newhart.[44] The pure-tone sweep-check test is the screening procedure recommended by the ASHA Committee on Audiometric Evaluation.[35,42] In the pure-tone sweep-check test stimuli at predetermined frequencies are presented at fixed intensity levels, and the child is instructed to respond by raising a hand, raising a finger, or responding in some other manner. Earphones are placed over both ears of the child and a practice tone is presented at a level above the test tone (ie, 40 dB HL) to acquaint the child with the type of signal to be heard. All of the test stimuli are first presented to one ear and then the other, and a record is made as to the presence or absence of a response at each frequency; no attempt is made to alter the attenuator dial to determine the threshold level when the child fails to respond. The sweep-check procedure can be successfully administered to both school age and preschool children in about 2 minutes per child.[43]

Frequencies and Intensitities. Differences exist concerning the frequencies and intensities to test in the individual pure-tone sweep-check test. In general, the frequencies recommended have been in the 500 to 6000 Hz range. Tones at and below 500 Hz are not recommended because they are more easily masked by room noise and do not provide significant information to the testing procedure; most recent guidelines do not recommend using frequencies at and below 500 Hz.[35,42] The use of 6000 Hz in screening has also been questioned due to its variability.[45]

At one time, it was believed that limiting the test frequency to one or two tones would significantly reduce the time required for the individual sweep-check test without affecting the overall test results. House and Glorig[46] first suggested screening only at 4000 Hz. This recommendation was made after careful examination of 5000 records and observing that 98 to 99% of the subjects with hearing loss at lower frequencies had the same or greater loss at 4000 Hz. Although the test was initially suggested as a screening tool for industrial workers, it was thought to be suitable for screening in the schools. Other investigators have suggested screening with two tones, using 2000 and 4000 Hz[41]; 500 and 4000 Hz[47]; and 1000 and 4000 Hz.[48]

Although data are available to support limited frequency screening,[49] conclusive data suggest that limited frequency screening procedures are not as effective as the pure-tone sweep-check test. Siegenthler and Sommer[47] evaluated the audiometric test results of more than 19,500 children and estimated that 35% of those failing the sweep-check test did not demonstrate losses at 4000 Hz. Stevens and Davidson[50] report similar observations on 1784 audiograms. These findings suggest that limiting the screening to a single frequency, or even to two frequencies, significantly reduces the sensitivity of hearing screening, at least in school children. In light of these data, it is apparent that screening should be performed at three or four frequencies.

The recommended intensity or intensities at which screening should occur has generally varied between 20 and 30 dB HL (ANSI, 1989). In selecting the screening level, two factors should be considered. First is the effect of the background noise and second is the sensitivity of the test in detecting even slight hearing loss. Background noise was discussed previously in this chapter. However, as the screening level decreases, the ambient noise will have a greater effect on the test signal. This one factor has prevented schools from screening at or below 15 to 20 dB HL.

By decreasing the level at which the test is performed, the sensitivity of the test can be increased and children with even slight hearing loss can be identified. Since audiologists believe that even slight hearing loss affects the development of speech and language, the goal of many programs is to reduce the intensity at which the screening is performed to identify children with minimal hearing loss. However, we are forced into accepting screening levels of 20 to 25 dB HL because of the conditions under which most screening is performed. It is unfortunate, but reduction of the screening level to 10 or 15 dB HL would significantly increase the number of overreferrals because of false-positive identification due to background noise.

Pass-Fail Criteria. The specific pass-fail criteria used in the program will depend entirely on the frequencies and intensities at which the screening is performed. However, results from several studies make it quite clear that referral should be based on failure of two screening tests given several hours apart on the same day or several days apart. In this procedure the child is referred for follow-up only if he fails the second screening test. The reason for requiring the second test is that temporary factors, such as noise in the test environment, nervousness, and transient conductive hearing loss, can be allowed to abate, thus reducing the number of overreferrals. Melnick et al[3] found that the inclusion of a second screening reduced the number of overreferrals by 23%. Wilson and Walton[8] rescreened 411 children in grades K to 5 who failed an initial screening test and found that slightly more than 50% passed the rescreening. Results from these two studies certainly support the need for rescreening before referral.

Table 4–6 summarizes seven recommended pure-tone sweep-check procedures. Although these seven protocols in no way exhaust the possible screening guidelines that have been suggested, they represent the wide range of screening procedures used in the schools. The procedures outlined by the American Speech-Language Hearing Association[42,43] were developed after many years of careful study; they appear to represent the most acceptable hearing screening procedures available to date. As shown in Table 4–6, the recommended frequencies are 1000, 2000, and 4000 at a level of 20 dB HL (the 1975 ASHA standard recommended increasing the level to 25 dB at 4000 Hz if no

Table 4–6   Comparison of Recommended Test Frequencies, Intensity Levels, and Pass-Fail Criteria for School Hearing Screening

Source	Test Frequencies	Intensity Level (ANSI, 1969)	Pass-Fail Criteria
American Speech and Hearing Association Committee on Identification Audiometry[35] (1975)	1000, 2000, and 4000 Hz	20 dB at 1000 and 2000 Hz 25 dB at 4000 Hz	Fail to respond to any frequency in either ear
American Speech and Hearing Association[64] (1985)	1000, 2000, and 4000 Hz	20 dB	Fail to respond to 1 tone in either ear
Anderson[2]	1000, 2000, and 4000 Hz	20 dB	Fail to respond to any 1 signal in any ear
Downs[52]	1000, 2000, 4000, and 6000 or 8000 Hz	15 dB	Fail to respond to either 1000 or 2000 Hz or to both 4000 and 6000–8000 Hz in either ear
National Conference on Identificiation Audiometry[28]	1000, 2000, 4000, and 6000 Hz	20 dB at 1000, 2000, and 6000 Hz 30 dB at 4000 Hz	Fail to hear any signals at these levels in either ear
Northern & Downs[11]	1000, 2000, 3000, and/or 4000 and 6000 Hz	25 dB	Fail to Respond to 1 tone at 1000 or 2000 Hz; or Fail to respond to 2 of 3 tones at 3000, 4000, and 6000 Hz
State of Illinois Department of Public Health[51]	500, 1000, 2000, and 4000 Hz	25 or 35 dB	Fail to respond to 1 tone at 35 dB in either ear or respond to any 2 tones at 25 dB in the same ear

response was recorded at 20 dB HL); not responding to any frequency in either ear is considered a failure.

The ASHA procedures are intended to detect those children with educationally significant hearing loss. However, unless the loss is in the severe range and also affects 3000 Hz, those who fail at 4000 Hz only should not experience significant auditory problems in the classroom; 4000 Hz falls outside of the speech range (see Chapter 2). Detecting high-frequency hearing loss is important because there are medical and audiological conditions that need to be identified. As an example, noise-induced hearing loss first manifests itself in the 4000 to 6000 Hz range. Children failing only at 4000 Hz need to be referred for a complete audiological follow-up and appropriate treatment and counseling be provided.

A limiting factor of the ASHA guidelines is that they do not detect minimal hearing loss (see Chapter 9); the relatively high noise levels in the

schools prevents screening at lower levels. The most effective program for identifying a child with an abnormal auditory system is to perform immittance screening, as well as hearing screening, since minimal hearing loss is typically associated with conductive pathologic conditions having associated middle ear disease.

Pitfalls to Avoid in Hearing Screening

The following factors are often found in hearing screening programs and can have a detrimental effect on the results of the screening and steps must be taken to avoid them.

1. *Child observing the equipment.* This should be avoided at all times, because children will respond to the visual cues. The appropriate position to seat the child is at an oblique angle, so the tester and audiometer are out of the child's peripheral vision.

2. *Examiner giving visual cues* (such as facial expression, eye or head movements).

3. *Incorrect adjustment of the headband and earphone placement.* Care must be taken to place the earphones carefully over the ears so that the protective screen mesh of the earphone diaphragm is directly over the entrance of the external auditory canal. Misplacement of the earphone by only 1 inch can cause as great as a 30 to 35 dB threshold shift.

4. *Vague instructions.*

5. *Noise in the test area.* False-positive identifications will result from excessive noise in the test environment. If there is a question about the noise levels present, the examiner should perform tests on individuals with known normal hearing (the examiner's hearing, if it is normal). If they do not pass the test, the noise levels are too high.

6. *Overlong test sessions.* The screening should require only 3 to 5 minutes. If a child requires significantly more time than this, the routine screening should be discontinued and a short rest taken. If the child continues to be difficult to test, play conditioning should be used.

7. *Too long or too short a presentation of the test tone.* The test stimulus should be presented for 1 to 2 seconds. If the stimulus is presented for a shorter or longer time than this, inaccurate responses may be obtained.

IMMITTANCE SCREENING IN THE SCHOOL—IDENTIFICATION OF MIDDLE EAR DISORDERS

The literature is now replete with studies showing the advantages and disadvantages for immittance screening in the schools. The most notable support for immittance screening is unanimous documentation that pure-tone screening tests are not sensitive to middle ear disorders. The advantage of immittance screening is an increase in the overall accuracy of the screening program, reduction in the number of children needing retests prior to referral, and increased probability in identifying children with otologic problems.[53] In addition to these factors, there is compelling evidence that significant delays in speech and language development and educational retardation are related to chronic ear disease in children, especially during the early years.

Holm and Kunze[54] were among the first to document the effects of middle ear disorders on speech and language development. The performance of two groups of 16 children each, an experimental group with documented histories of otitis media and a matched normal control group, ages 5 to 9 years, was evaluated using standardized tests of language and speech. Findings revealed the experimental group was significantly delayed when compared with the control group in all language skills requiring auditory reception or speech production, but no significant differences were observed on tests of visual or motor skills. This study provided the first formal documentation on the detrimental effects of middle ear disorders on the development of speech and language. Although there continues to be some debate regarding the association of middle ear disease and permanent delays in speech and language, compelling data from longitudinal and cross-sectional studies are available to support a direct relationship between the decreased hearing sensitivity resulting from middle ear disease and delays in speech and language development.[55,56]

The desire to detect middle ear disorders in school children is clear. However, the extreme sensitivity of the immittance measures and their transient nature has caused high false-positive rates for a large number of programs. For example, studies have found poor agreement between otoscopy and immittance results.[57-59] Since otoscopy is the ultimate procedure used by most physicians to diagnose middle ear disease, many children referred with negative middle ear pressure would be judged normal (false-positive results).

In a classic study, Tos[60] performed immittance screening on 2-year-old children at 3-month intervals. Of 51 ears found to have flat (type B) tympanograms initially, 27 (53%) improved spontaneously during the first 3 months, and spontaneous improvement was found in 45 (84%) within 9 months. This finding not only raises the question of when to refer following the immittance screening, but also questions the nature and course of medical treatment when abnormal results are found. The findings just given, combined with the lack of definitive research on the specified referral criteria and benefits for immittance measures and the sometimes transient nature of middle ear disorders,[60] have significantly affected the widespread use of immittance in screening programs.

National guidelines do not recommend universal mass screening with immittance on a routine basis for the detection of middle ear disorders.[61] However, it should be emphasized that regular screening using immittance is not discouraged for special populations of children. Because of the effects of middle ear disease on speech and language development and the high incidence of middle ear disorders in special populations, immittance screening should be performed routinely on these children. Included are Native Americans; those with sensorineural hearing loss, developmental delay, and mental impairment; and craniofacial anomalies, including cleft palate and Down's syndrome.[62]

Test Environment

Unlike screening for hearing loss, there are no background noise level requirements needed to perform immittance screening because the test stimuli are presented well above normal threshold sensitivity. This factor has prompted many to state that sound-treated environments are not necessary when immittance is used.[7] Although this statement is valid, as will be pointed out later, immittance screening must be performed in conjunction with hearing screening if the identification program is to be effective. Therefore, when hearing and immittance screening are performed in the same testing area, it is necessary to have background noise levels that meet the minimum requirements necessary for hearing screening.

Personnel

The personnel used in the hearing screening program may be those used in the immittance screening program, but more extensive training is necessary. The technical personnel must be thoroughly familiar with the mechanics of the instrumentation used in the program, the proper use of the instrumentation, and the problems that can be encountered with the instrument and how to troubleshoot such problems. They must also be familiar with interpretation of test results and thoroughly knowledgeable about disorders of the ear.

Training seminars have been developed that cover the basic procedures used in immittance screening in 1 or 2 days. This type of seminar is appropriate for those who have had exposure and experience with hearing loss and screening procedures (speech pathologists and school nurses), but does not meet the necessary requirements for those who have had no past training in this area. There are no guidelines for training paraprofessionals in the use of immittance. However, it is believed that 2 or 3 days of specific training in immittance, beyond the training in hearing screening, is required. As with hearing screening, an emphasis on supervised practicum is needed. Because the addition of immittance screening requires more technical expertise, there is a far greater need for a certified audiologist to be available to the program.

Pass-Fail Criteria and Follow-Up

Several sets of guidelines have been established for immittance screening. The most notable are guidelines from the 1977 Nashville conference,[61] the 1979 ASHA guidelines,[63] and the 1990 ASHA guidelines.[64]

The 1990 ASHA recommendations described in Table 4–7 have several novel components: case history information is obtained and tone screening is performed in addition to immittance testing. With the exception of the recommendations of Roeser and Northern,[65] all prior guidelines based referral criteria *either* on pure-tone *or* immittance test results. In addition, the 1990 ASHA guidelines use physical, rather than descriptive immittance measures (see Chapter 2). Table 4–8 lists each component of the 1990 ASHA screening guidelines and presents referral criteria; the following is a summary.

Case History

A complete case history is typically not possible, but information on otalgia (ear pain) and otorrhea (ear discharge) should be obtained. The most appropriate respondent should be used (the child in some cases or the parent in others), and the information can be obtained at the time of the screening or requested in advance of the screening.

Visual Inspection of the Ear

Visual inspection of the ear includes gross examination of the pinnae and external ear canal, and otoscopy. Medical referral should be made for any gross defects of the ear and ear canal because structural defects may suggest the presence of other otologic abnormalities that may

Table 4–7   Summary of Procedures and Suggested Interim Norms from the 1990 ASHA Screening for Hearing Impairment and Middle Ear Disorders Document[64]

Procedure	Method/ Description/Norms
Case history	Acquisition from most appropriate respondent
Visual inspection of the ear canal	Inspect pinnae and outer ear—use of an otoscope
Hearing screening (identification audiometry)	Pure-tone sweep-check test at 1000, 2000, and 4000 Hz at 20 dB HL
Static admittance (peak Y) (mmho or cm³/ml) Children	
Mean	0.5
90% range	0.2–0.9
Adults	
Mean	0.8
90% range	0.3–1.4
Equivalent ear canal volume (V_{ec}) (cm³/ml) Children	
Mean	0.7
90% range	0.4–1.0
Adults	
Mean	1.1
90% range	0.6–1.5
Tympanometric width (gradient) (daPa) Children	
Mean	100
90% range	60–150
Adults	
Mean	80
90% range	50–110
Tympanometric peak pressure (daPa)	Not used as a referral criterion
Acoustic reflex	Not used as a referral criterion

Table 4–8   Referral Criteria from the 1989 ASHA Guidelines for Screening for Hearing Impairment and Middle Ear Disorders

I.   History
   A. Otalgia
   B. Otorrhea

II. Visual Inspection of the ear
   A. Structural defect of the ear, head or neck
   B. Ear canal abnormalities
      1. Blood or effusion
      2. Occlusion
      3. Inflammation
      4. Excessive cerumen, tumor, foreign material
   C. Eardrum abnormalities
      1. Abnormal color
      2. Bulging eardrum
      3. Fluid line or bubbles
      4. Perforation
      5. Retraction

III. Hearing Screening—Fail air conduction screening at 20 dB HL at 1, 2, or 4 kHz in either ear (ASHA, 1985; these criteria may require alteration for various clinical settings and populations)

IV. Tympanometry
   A. Flat tympanogram and equivalent ear canal volume (V_{ec}) outside normal range
   B. Low static admittance (peak Y) on two successive occurrences in a 4- to 6-week interval
   C. Abnormally wide tympanometric width (TW) on two successive occurrences in a 4- to 6-week interval

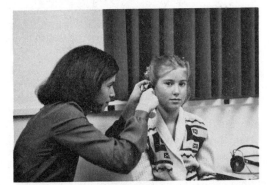

Figure 4–6.   Otoscopic inspection of the external ear.

need attention. Examples are abnormal position or structure of the external ear, ranging from complete absence of the pinna and atresia of the ear canal to more subtle abnormalities, such as malpositioned pinnae or preauricular pits and tags. Discharge from the ear canal may be seen as dry crusty material and needs immediate referral.

Otoscopy is the process by which the ear canal and tympanic membrane are inspected by an examiner, with an otoscope (see Fig. 4–6). The purpose of the inspection is to assess the condition of the outer ear and tympanic membrane. The value of otoscopy is highly dependent on the training and skill of the examiner; accordingly, the procedure should be administered by individuals with supervised training and experience in visual examination of the ear. The examiner should note any blockage due to a foreign object or cerumen in the ear canal and the following eardrum conditions: abnormal color (red, yellow, or dull gray), bulging eardrum, fluid line or bubbles behind the eardrum, perforation, and retraction pockets.

Until recently, the use of otoscopes by audiologists has been somewhat equivocal; many audiologists have routinely used otoscopes for years and others have not. However, in 1991 the ASHA legislative council passed a resolution that specifically states that otoscopy, as well as cerumen management, are within the scope of practice of audiology.[66] It is now clear that audiologists not only should, but must, perform routine otoscopic examination on their patients. In addition, audiologists are sanctioned by ASHA to manage cerumen (see later).

Musket and Dowraczyk[67] state that otoscopic inspection can be frightening to school children, especially preschoolers. They describe the modification of an otoscope in which it is disguised as a puppet, so it will be acceptable to younger children. Figure 4–7 shows this innovative modification.

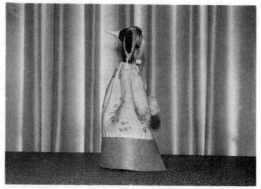

Figure 4–7. Modification of an otoscope to disguise it as a puppet (after Musket and Dowraczyk)[67]

Until recently, children with excessive or impacted cerumen present in the earcanal in the pretest otoscopic inspection, a condition that occurs between 3 and 10% in normal school age children,[68] were referred for medical management. However, in many cases these children were not treated properly or, even worse, were not treated at all. Roeser, et al[69] describe an innovative program for cerumen management in the public schools. Cerumen management was conducted as part of the school hearing conservation program for children failing hearing screening. The cerumen management procedures described by Roeser and Roland[68] were used. Over the period 1982 to 1989, a total of 2156 ears were managed and the program was found to be safe and effective; 92% of those who failed the testing prior to cerumen management passed the retest and there were no complications. The value of the

program is that it saves families from having to make an office visit and, more importantly, it assures that the procedure will be carried out. There are excellent written materials[70,71] and a videotape[72] for those who would like more information on cerumen management procedures.

Acoustic Immittance Measurement (Tympanometry)

The possible acoustic immittance measures specified in the 1990 ASHA standard are: static admittance (peak Y), equivalent ear canal volume, tympanometric width (gradient), tympanometric peak pressure, and acoustic reflex. Chapter 2 describes these measures in more detail.

Static admittance (peak Y) measures the height of the tympanogram in either mmho or cm³/ml; static admittance is a more objective way of classifying the tympanogram than the A, B, and C system. As shown in Table 4–7, the suggested norms are 0.5 mmho or cm³/ml for children and 0.8 mmho or cm³/ml for adults, with a range of 0.2 to 0.9 and 0.3 to 1.4, respectively.

Equivalent ear canal volume is an estimate of the equivalent volume of air in front of the immittance probe when an air pressure of +200 daPa is present in the external ear canal; this procedure was previously called the "physical volume test." The mean values in Table 4–7 for children and adults are 0.7 and 1.1 cm³/ml, respectively. Values that exceed the 90% range shown in Table 4–7, when accompanied by a flat tympanogram, suggest perforation of the tympanic membrane and should be referred immediately for medical follow up. Equivalent ear canal volume measures do not detect all tympanic membrane perforations; however, other procedures (history, pure-tone screening, and otoscopy) should help in detecting them.

Tympanometric width (gradient) is used to describe the shape of the tympanogram in the vicinity of the peak quantitatively. The gradient is associated with the width of the tympanogram and the 1990 ASHA standard uses as a criterion the 50% reduction in peak (static) admittance. The mean values for children and adults are 100 and 80 daPa with 90% ranges of 60 to 150 daPa and 50 to 110 daPa, respectively. Since there are no firm data on the efficacy of tympanometric width in identifying middle ear disease, only abnormally large values should be used as a criterion for medical referral.

Tympanometric peak pressure is an indirect measure of the air pressure in the middle ear. Abnormal tympanometric peak pressure in the absence of other abnormal findings is not used as a criterion for audiological or medical referral.

Acoustic reflex is an indirect measure of stapedial muscle contraction to an intense stimulus. Because the acoustic reflex contributed to unacceptably high false-positive rates reported in previous assessments of screening protocols, this measure is not used as a criterion for referral.

Roush et al[73] compared the efficacy of the 1990 ASHA immittance guidelines[64] to the traditional procedure based on tympanometric peak pressure and acoustic reflexes.[61,63] Immittance findings from 374 ears were compared to pneumatic otoscopy. Results are given in Table 4–9.

Table 4–9 Comparison of Immittance with Pneumatic Otoscope in 374 Ears

	Traditional Procedures[61,63] (%)	1990 ASHA Immittance Guidelines[64] (%)
Senstivity	95	84
False-negative results	5	16
Specificity	65	95
False-positive results	35	5
Positive predictive value	27	69
Negative predictive value	99	98

The 1990 ASHA guidelines resulted in a lower sensitivity and higher false negative rate (5 of 44 children passed by the immittance screening who were judged to be abnormal by otoscopy [false-negative identification]). However, the 1990 ASHA guidelines also resulted in a significant improvement in specificity and related reduction in false-positive identifications (97 of 330 children who were judged to be otoscopically normal would have been incorrectly referred for medical treatment). The negative predictive values for the two procedures were high and essentially identical, but the 1990 ASHA guidelines resulted in better positive predictive values. Only through similar studies will it be possible to establish the effectiveness and efficiency of established guidelines.

GENERAL CONSIDERATIONS FOR BOTH HEARING AND IMMITTANCE SCREENING

The specifications for the equipment that should be used in the screening program are described in Chapter 2. One additional criterion in selecting equipment for use in the screening program is the quality and availability of maintenance service. All audiometric equipment must be serviced on a regular basis, and the location and efficiency of the service center should be considered before making a purchase. It would not be advisable to purchase an instrument from the dispenser 1000 miles away, when a local dealer who provides direct service is available.

Teacher Contribution

There are many behaviors that have been associated with auditory impairment in children, and it is important that school personnel become familiar with signs of classroom behavior or physical symptoms of hearing loss that might give them clues as to children in need of audiologic examination. Behaviors and physical symptoms that may indicate auditory impairment in a child are listed in Table 4–10. Although these signs may also be associated with other types of school problems, any child exhibiting one or more of them should be referred for audiometric screening, and diagnostic evaluation when indicated.

Several studies have been conducted on the efficacy of teacher identification of school children with hearing loss. Early studies reported that teachers were able to identify only one of four to six children with significant hearing loss.[74,75] Nodar[76] compared teachers' identifications with audiometric and immittance screening data. Results from this study indicated that teachers were able to identify almost 50% of the children in the hearing loss group. This study showed that, although not always accurate, classroom teachers can play a valuable role in detecting children with hearing problems, and their observations should definitely be considered as an adjunct to the screening process. However, in no way should these data be interpreted to imply that teachers are an adequate substitute for auditory screening procedures.

Periodicity of Testing

Few would argue that the ideal screening program would test every child every year. However,

Table 4–10   Behaviors and Physical Symptoms in Children That May Indicate Hearing Loss

Behaviors

a. Frequently asks to have this repeated
b. Turns one side of head toward speaker
c. Talks too loudly or too slowly
d. Shows strain in trying to hear
e. Watches and concentrates on teacher's lips
f. Is inattentive in classroom discussion
g. Makes frequent mistakes in following directions
h. Makes unusual mistakes in taking directions
i. Tends to isolate self
j. Tends to be passive
k. Is tense
l. Tires easily
m. Has a speech problem
n. Is not working up to apparent capacity
o. Has academic failure following severe illness

Physical Symptoms

a. Mouth breathing
b. Draining ears
c. Earaches
d. Dizziness
e. Reports of ringing, buzzing, or roaring in ears (tinnitus)

screening all children annually is not practical most of the time and many compromises have been suggested. Virtually all published guidelines support two general principles with regard to periodicity of testing.[36,61]

1. There is a greater need for screening children in the lower grades than in higher grades.
2. There are populations of children with a higher incidence of hearing loss and ear disorders who warrant testing outside of the routine schedule.

The need to concentrate screening on the lower grades is based on two observations. First, during the early school years there is a higher prevalence of transient hearing loss due to middle ear disease; second, mild and frequency-specific hearing losses are many times undetected in the early school years.[11] Based on these principles, annual screening of all preschool children and children in grades K, 1, 2, and 3 is highly recommended.[35]

Controversy exists on the cost-benefit ratio of screening after grade 3. After analyzing the data from 14,800 10th graders, Downs and Doster[1] concluded that audiometric screening programs should be relaxed in the upper grades. This conclusion is based on the low yield of previously undetected hearing impairment in the upper grades.

Although there is a general reduction in the incidence of hearing loss in the upper grades, studies have shown that the incidence of high-frequency loss significantly increases in the 4000 to 6000 Hz region beyond grade 8, especially in males. Weber et al[25] reviewed the audiometric configurations from 1000 students failing the screening procedures performed by the Colorado Department of Health. Thirty percent of the losses identified were in the 4000 Hz region, with 24.9% in males and 5.1% in females. As age increased to 16 years or older, there was a significant increase in the losses at 4000 Hz. Hull et al[26] report data from 38,568 children in grades 1 through 12. In comparing all grade levels across frequencies, the highest incidence of hearing loss exceeding 25 dB HL (ISO, 1964) was at 4000 Hz in the male population in the 11th and 12th grades.

Woodford and O'Farrell[77] documented the high noise levels in school band rooms and vocational education areas, and found that students involved in high sound level activities are more likely to have high-frequency hearing loss. In addition, they, unfortunately, found that few industrial arts programs furnish hearing protection or are aware of the need for such protection. A survey by Allonen-Allie and Florentine[78] found similar results in 27 schools, but also revealed that teachers desired training in hearing conservation.

Since the losses are typically greater in males who engage in noisy activities, implementing a hearing conservation program for the students exposed to high noise levels in the schools (band and industrial arts programs) is important, because these students most likely are those who will be exposed to high noise levels in later life. In addition to identifying existing hearing loss, through education, these students will become aware of the effects of noise on their hearing, which may prevent occupational hearing loss from noise exposure in later years.[79]

With respect to special populations and high-risk children, the following guidelines should be applied. Annual hearing conservation should be performed on students:

1. Who are new to the school or to the school district
2. Who repeat a grade
3. With delayed or impaired speech and language before they are enrolled in therapy
4. Returning to school after a serious illness
5. Who appear to be delayed
6. Having emotional or behavior problems

7. Who were absent during a previously scheduled screening examination
8. Who are involved in course work that places them at risk for noise exposure (band, woodworking, and auto mechanics).

Regardless of grade level, annual testing should also be performed on pupils discovered by previous tests to have hearing impairment and on pupils enrolled in adjustment or remedial classes.

Follow-up and Record Keeping

The exact procedures used for follow-up will vary considerably from district to district, but provisions for three areas of concern must be made: audiologic, medical, and educational.

Audiological Follow-up. In many traditional school hearing conservation programs, all children who fail the screening are immediately referred for medical follow-up. Such referral is important to identify significant medical problems, but might be considered premature in the sequence for some categories. The screening tests administered in the schools must be considered only as a preliminary indication of the presence of hearing loss or a middle ear disorder. Before the exact nature and extent of the loss can be determined, additional audiological testing must be performed under acceptable testing conditions.

It would be ideal for all failures to be referred to a clinic where both medical and audiological facilities are available. In that way the physician and audiologist will work together in assessing the nature and extent of the problem and in providing appropriate treatment and follow-up. Many of the larger metropolitan areas have such facilities. However, where such facilities are not available, follow-up audiological threshold testing should be performed and the results evaluated by a senior member of the school's testing staff. In this way the physicians will have necessary audiological data available to provide the appropriate treatment.

The ASHA guidelines[35,63] support the need for audiological follow-up before medical referral. In addition, the 1975 ASHA guidelines[35] give the following priority for audiological evaluation for those children failing the hearing screening and rescreening procedures.

1. Binaural loss in both ears at all frequencies tested
2. Binaural loss at 1000 and 2000 Hz only
3. Binaural loss at 1000 or 2000 Hz only
4. Monaural loss at all frequencies

5. Monaural loss at 1000 and 2000 Hz only
6. Binaural or monaural loss at 4000 Hz only

Medical Follow-up. Traditional medical ethics require that children failing screening be referred to the family physician. Typically, the family physician is a general practitioner or pediatrician. The general medical practitioner plays a very important role in the overall management of the family's medical needs, but often does not have the expertise required in the diagnosis and management of otologic problems. For this reason, those children failing the screening program will be served best if referred directly to an ear specialist (otologist). With the entry of Health Maintenance Organizations and Preferred Providers into the health care delivery system, decisions regarding who to refer those who fail the screening is becoming less of an issue.

Whenever referral is made for medical follow-up, the parents must be contacted. Initially, contact can be made by telephone, but written recommendations also should be made. In addition, feedback from the physician should be requested and records kept on all medical referrals. Anderson[2] and Barrett[80] provide examples of forms that can be used for follow-up purposes.

School systems need a formal mechanism to communicate with the medical community; a very useful way to establish a liaison with the medical community is through a School Medical Advisory Board. Having the expertise of several of the community physicians available to the school allows for direct and frequent interaction with them, resulting in a better understanding of the procedures that are used in the schools. Many physicians will also welcome such an opportunity to serve the school.

Educational Follow-up. Teachers must be notified when hearing loss is found so that special provisions can be made in the classroom. In many cases, the hearing loss will be transient and the extent and duration of the impairment will depend on the nature of the abnormal condition. However, even for these children, the teacher must take into account the effect of the loss and make special provisions in the classroom.

Effective follow up requires well organized, up-to-date, and accurate records. Computerized database management would be an excellent way to organize and store records efficiently.

REFERENCES

1. Downs MP, Doster MF, Weaver M: Dilemmas in identification audiometry. *J Speech Hear Disord*, 30 (1965), 360–364.

2. Anderson CV: Conversation of hearing, in Katz J, ed: *Handbook of Clinical Audiology*, ed 2 (Baltimore: Williams & Wilkins, 1978).

3. Melnick W, Eagles EL, Levine HS: Evaluation of a recommended program of identification audiometry with school-age children. *J Speech Hear Disord*, 29 (1964), 3–13.

4. Books DN: A new approach to identification audiometry, *Audiology*, 10 (1971), 334–339.

5. Eagles EL: Hearing levels in children and audiometer performance. *J Speech Hear Disord* (Monogr), suppl 9 (1961), 1–274.

6. Cooper JC, Gates GA, Owen JH, et al: An abbreviated impedance bridge technique for school screening. *J Speech Hear Disord*, 40 (1975), 260–269.

7. Frankenberg WK: Selection of diseases and tests in pediatric screening. *Pediatrics*, 54 (1971).

8. Wilson WR, Walton WK: Identification audiometry accuracy: Evaluation of a recommended program for school-age children. *Lang Speech Hear Serv Sch*, 5 (1974), 132–142.

9. Frasier GR: The genetics of congenital deafness. *Otolarygol Clin North Am*, 4 (1971), 227–247.

10. Stewart J: HRS screening. Paper presented at the annual meeting of the Western Society for Pediatric Research, Carmel, CA, 1974.

11. Northern JL, Downs MP: Hearing In Children, ed 4 (Baltimore: Williams & Wilkins, 1991).

12. Berg F: Definition and incidence, in Berg F, Fletcher SG: The *Hard of Hearing Child* (New York: Grune & Stratton, 1970).

13. Klein JO: Epidemiology or otitis media, in Harford ER, Bess TH, Bluestone D, et al, eds: *Impedance Screening for Middle Ear Disease in Children* (New York: Grune & Stratton, 1978).

14. Jerger J: Dissenting report: Mass impedance screening. *Ann Otol Rhinol Laryngol*, 89 suppl 69 (1980), 21–22.

15. Brooks DN: Impedance in screening, in Jerger J, Northern J, eds: *Clinical Impedance Audiometry* (Acton, MA: American Electronics Corp, 1980).

16. Silverman RS, David H, eds: *Hearing and Deafness* (New York: Holt, Rinehart, Winston, 1978).

17. Eagles EL, Wishik SM, Doerfler LG: Hearing sensitivity and ear disease in children: A prospective study. *Laryngoscope* (Monogr), 1967, 1–274.

18. Connor LE: Determining the prevalence of hearing impaired children. *Except Child*, 27 (1961), 337–344.

19. Fay TH, Hochberg I, Smith CR, et al: Audiologic and otologic screening of disadvantaged children, in Glorig A, Gerwin K, eds: *Otitis Media* (Springfield, IL: Charles C Thomas, 1972).

20. Robinson CG, Anderson DO, Mogohodam HK, et al: A survey of hearing loss in Vancouver school children: In Methodology and prevalence, *Can Med Assoc J*, 97 (1967), 119–207.

21. Newman MH: Hearing Loss, in Strom M, ed: *Differential Diagnosis in Pediatric Otolaryngology* (Boston: Little, Brown, 1975).

22. Weit P: Patterns of ear disease in the Southwestern American Indian. *Arch Otolarngol*, 105 (1979), 381–385.

23. Kaplan GY, Fleshman JK, Bender TR, et al: Long-term effects of otitis media: A ten year cohort study of Alaskan Eskimo children. *Pediatrics*, 52 (1973), 577–585.

24. McEldowney D, Kessner PM: Review of the literature: epidemiology of otitis media, in Gloria A, Gerwin KS, eds: *Otitis Media* (Springfield, IL: Charles C Thomas, 1972).

25. Weber HJ, McGovern FJ, Fink D: An evaluation of 1000 children with hearing loss. *J Speech Hear Disord*, 32 (1967), 343–354.

26. Hull FM, Mielke PW Jr, Timmons RJ, et al: The national speech and hearing survey: Preliminary results. *ASHA*, 13 (1971), 501–509.

27. Northern JL: Impedance screening in special populations: State-of-the-art, in Harford E, Bess F, Bluestone CD, et al, eds: *Impedance Screening for Middle Ear Disease in Children* (New York: Grune & Stratton, 1978).

28. Darley FL: Identification audiometry for school-age children: basic procedures. *J Speech Hear Disord* (Monogr), suppl 9, (1961), 26–34.

29. Fisher LI: Efficiency and effectiveness of using a portable audiometric booth in school hearing conservation programs. *Lang Speech Hear Serv Sch*, 7 (1976), 242–249.

30. Roeser RJ, Glorig A: Pure tone audiometry in noise with auraldomes. *Audiology*, 14 (1975), 144–151.

31. Roeser RJ, Seidel J, Glorig A: Performance of earphone enclosures for threshold audiometry. *Sound & Vibration*, 10, No. 9 (1975), 22–25.

32. Roeser RJ, Musket CH: Noise attenuating earphone systems. Maico Aud Library, Series 15, Report 4, 1976.

33. Stark EW, Borton TE: Noise excluding earphone enclosures for audiometry. *Audiology*, 14 (1975), 232–237.

34. Musket CH, Roeser RJ: Using circumaural enclosures with children. *J Speech Hear Res*, 20 (1977), 325–333.

35. American Speech and Hearing Association (ASHA) Committee on Audiometric Evaluation Guidelines for Identification Audiometry. *ASHA*, 17 (1975), 94–99.

36. Grifing TS, Simonton KM, Hedgecock LD: Verbal auditory—screening for pre-school children. *Trans Am Acad Ophthalmol Otolaryngol*, 71 (1967), 104–111.

37. Ritchie BC: Review of the literature: Verbal auditory screening of children, in Gerwin KS, Glorig A, eds: *Detection of Hearing Loss and Ear*

Disease in Children (Springfield, IL: Charles C Thomas, 1974).

38. Ciocco A, Palmer CE: The hearing of school children. Society for Research in Child Development (Monogr 4), National Research Council, 1941.

39. Johnson KO, Newby H: Experimental study of the efficiency of two group hearing tests. *Arch Otolaryngol*, 60 (1954), 702–710.

40. Mencher GT, McCullock BF: Auditory screening of kindergarten children using the VASC. *J Speech Hear Disord*, 35 (1970), 241–247.

41. Norton MC, Lux E: Double frequency auditory screening in public schools. *J Speech Hear Disord*, 26 (1961), 293–299.

42. American Speech-Language-Hearing Association (ASHA). Guidelines for identification audiometry. *ASHA*, 27 (1985,May) 49–52.

43. Hood B, Lamb LE: Identification audiometry, in Gerwin KS, Glorig A, eds: *Detection of Hearing Loss and Ear Disease in Children* (Springfield, IL: Charles C Thomas, 1974).

44. Newhart HA: A pure tone audiometer for school use. *Arch Otolaryngol*, 28 (1938), 777–779.

45. Villchur E: Audiometer-earphone mounting to improve intersubject and cushion-fit reliability. *J Acoust Soc Am*, 48 (1970), 1387–1396.

46. House HP, Glorig A: A new concept in auditory screening. *Larygoscope*, 67 (1957), 661–668.

47. Siegenthaler BM, Sommers RK: Abbreviated sweep check procedures for school hearing testing. *J Speech Hear Disord*, 24 (1959), 249–257.

48. Maxwell WR, Davidson GD: Limited frequency screening and ear pathology. *J Speech Hear Disord*, 26 (1961), 122–125.

49. Ventry I, Newby H: Validity of the one-frequency screening principle for public school children. *J Speech Hear Res*, 2 (1959), 147–151.

50. Stevens DA, Davidson GD: Screening tests of hearing. *J Speech Hear Disord*, 24 (1959), 258–261.

51. Illinois Deptartment of Public Health: A Manual for Audiometrists. (Springfield, IL, 1974).

52. Downs MP: Auditory Screening. *Otolaryngol Clin North Am*, 11 (1968), 611–629.

53. Northern JL: Impedance screening: An integral part of hearing screening. *Ann Otol Rhinol Laryngol* 89, suppl 68, (1980), 233–235.

54. Holm VA, Kunze LH: Effect of chronic otitis media on language and speech development. *Pediatrics*, 43 (1969), 833–839.

55. Finitzo-Hieber T, Friel-Patti S: Conductive hearing loss and ABR. In Jacobson J, ed: *The Auditory Brainstem Response*. (San Diego, CA: College-Hill Press, 1985).

56. Friel-Patti S, Finitzo T: Language learning in a prospective study of otitis media with effusion in the first two years of life. *J Speech Hear Res*, 33 (1990), 188–194.

57. Roeser RJ, Soh J, Dunckel C, Adams RM: Comparison of tympanometry and otoscopy in establishing pass/fail referral criteria. *J Am Audiol Soc*, 3 (1977), 20–25.

58. Lucker J: Application of pass-fail criteria to middle ear screening results. *ASHA*, 22 (1980), 839–840.

59. Roush J, Tait CA: Pure tone and acoustic immittance screening of preschool aged children: an examination of referral criteria. *Ear Hear*, 6 (1986), 245–250.

60. Tos M: Spontaneous improvement of secretory otitis and impedance screening. *Arch Otolaryngol*, 106 (1980), 345–349.

61. Bess FH: Impedance screening for children: A need for more research. *Ann Otol Rhinol Laryngol*, 89, suppl 68, (1980), 228–232.

62. Bluestone, CD, Fria Tj, Arjona SK, et al: Controversies in screening of middle ear disease and hearing loss in children. *Pediatrics*, 77 (1986), 57–70.

63. American Speech-Language-Hearing Association (ASHA) Committee on Audiometric Evaluation Guidelines for acoustic immittance screening of middle ear function. *ASHA* 21 (1979), 283–288.

64. American Speech-Language-Hearing Association (ASHA). Guidelines for screening hearing impairment and middle ear disorders. *ASHA*, 32, suppl 2, (1990), 17–24.

65. Roeser RJ, Northern JL: Screening for hearing loss and middle ear disorders. in Roeser, RJ and Downs MP eds: *Auditory Disorders in School Children*, 2nd ed (New York, Thieme Medical Publishers, 1988).

66. American Speech Language Hearing Association (ASHA). External auditory canal examination and cerumen management. *ASHA*, 35 (1991, May), 64–66.

67. Musket CH, Dowraczyk RD: Using an otoscope with preschoolers in acoustic immittance screening programs. *Lang Speech Hear Serv Sch*, 11 (1980), 109–111.

68. Roeser RJ, Roland PW: What audiologists must know about cerumen and cerumen management. *Am J Audiol*, 1, (November 1992), 27–35.

69. Roeser RJ, Adams RM, Watkins, S: Cerumen management in hearing conservation: The Dallas Independent School District Program. *J Sch Health*, 61 (1991), 47–49.

70. Mechner F, Saffioti LJ, Holman J: Patient assessment: Examination of the ear. *Am J Nurs*, 75 (1975), 19–24.

71. Ballachanda BB, Peers CJ: Cerumen management-instruments and procedures. *ASHA*, 34 (1992, Feb), 43–46.

72. Roeser RJ, Roland P, Carver W: Otoscopic examination of the earcanal and cerumen management. (St. Louis: C & R Video Productions, 1992).

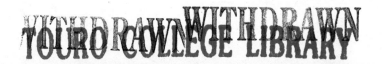

73. Roush J, Drake A, Sexton JE: Identification of middle ear dysfunction in young children: A comparison of tympanometric screening procedures. *Ear Hear*, 13 (1992), 63–69.

74. Curry ET: The efficiency of teacher referrals in a school hearing testing program. *J Speech Hear Disord*, 15 (1950), 211–214.

75. Kodman F: Identification of hearing loss by the classroom teacher. *Laryngoscope*, 66 (1956), 1346–1349.

76. Nodar RH: Teacher identification of elementary school children with hearing loss. *Lang Speech Hear Serv Sch*, 9 (1978), 24–28.

77. Woodford CM, O'Farrell ML: High-frequency loss of hearing in secondary school students: An investigation of possible etiologic factors. *Lang Speech Hear Serv Sch*, 14 (1983), 22–28.

78. Allonen-Állie N, Florentine M: Hearing conservation programs in Massachusetts' vocational/technical schools. *Ear Hear*, 11 (1990), 237–251.

79. Roeser RJ: Industrial hearing conservation programs in the high schools. *Ear Hear*, 1 (1980), 119–120.

80. Barrett K: Hearing and immittance screening of school-age children; in Katz J, *Handbook of Clinical Audiology* (Baltimore: Williams & Wilkins, 1985).

TESTS OF CENTRAL AUDITORY PROCESSING

Robert W. Keith

> *Since the measuring device has been constructed by the observer...we have to remember that what we observe is not nature in itself but nature exposed to our method of questioning.*
>
> —Werner Karl Heisinberg, 1901–1976

DEFINITION OF CENTRAL AUDITORY PROCESSING

In this chapter, approaches to the assessment of central auditory processing (CAP) skills and identification of children with central auditory processing disorders (CAPD) will be discussed. Currently, the term "central auditory processing" is used interchangeably with other terminology that includes, for example, central auditory ability, central auditory function and auditory processing abilities. A deficiency in processing auditory information is called by several terms, including CAPD, auditory perceptual disorder, and sometimes an auditory language-learning disorder.

There are several definitions of CAP and CAPD. My early work in CAP was influenced by the Association of Children and Adults with Learning Disabilities (ACLD)[1] quote of the Education of the Handicapped Act of 1975, which defined specific learning disabilities as "a disorder in one or more of the basic psychological processes involved in *understanding* or in using language...which may manifest itself in an imperfect ability to *listen....*" The ACLD further described specific learning disabilities as "a chronic condition of presumed neurologic origin which selectively interferes with the development, integration, and/or demonstration of verbal and/or non-verbal abilities." Subsequently I defined an auditory processing disorder as:

> The inability or impaired ability to attend to, discriminate, remember, recognize, or comprehend information presented auditorily even though the person has normal intelligence and hearing sensitivity. These difficulties are more pronounced when listening to low-redundancy (distorted) speech, when there are competing sounds or poor acoustic environments. In the normal child, auditory processing abilities develop in a parallel or

reciprocal relationship with language abilities. Children with auditory processing disorders are a subset of children with receptive and/or expressive language disorders.[2]

An American Speech-Hearing-Language Association (ASHA) ad hoc committee on CAP[3] defined CAPD as deficits in information processing of audible signals not attributed to impaired hearing sensitivity or intellectual impairment. Specifically, the committee stated that CAPD refers to limitations in the ongoing transmission, analysis, organization, transformation, elaboration, storage, retrieval, and use of information contained in audible signals. At the time of this writing, another ASHA task force on CAP is attempting to arrive at a consensus definition of CAP and CAPD. Musiek et al[4] stated simply that auditory processing is: "The utilization of acoustic information by the auditory system." This definition of Musiek et al included both peripheral and central auditory systems as being critical to auditory processing. What is suggested in all of these definitions is the construct that CAPD contributes to developmental language disorders and interferes with academic achievement in the classroom.

Another simplified definition of an auditory processing disorder is any breakdown in the child's auditory abilities that result in diminished learning through hearing, even though peripheral auditory sensitivity is normal. In an effort to be systematic, various authors have attempted to identify and define those auditory processing abilities that may be important to a child's learning through hearing. Some abilities commonly listed by authors are shown in Table 5–1, although other auditory processing abilities can be identified. Even though central auditory abilities can be categorized, a direct cause and effect relationship between the abilities listed in Table 5–2 and

Table 5–1   Auditory Processing Abilities Important to the Learning Process

Descriptive Term	Ability
Discrimination	To differentiate among sound of different frequency, duration, or intensity
Localization	To localize the source of sound
Auditory attention	To pay attention to auditory signals, especially speech, for an extended time
Auditory figure ground	To identify a primary speaker from a background of noise
Auditory discrimination	To discriminate among words and sounds that are acoustically similar
Auditory closure	To understand the whole word or message when part is missing
Auditory blending	To synthesize isolated phonemes into words
Auditory analysis	To identify phonemes or morphemes embedded in words
Auditory association	To identify a sound with its source
Auditory memory; sequential memory	To store and recall auditory stimuli of different length of number in exact order

Table 5–2   Information Model for Taking a Case History

Area	Information Needed
Family history	History of the family's difficulty in school achievement. The language spoken in the home
Pregnancy and birth	Unusual problems during pregnancy or delivery. Abnormalities present at the birth of the child
Health and illness	Childhood illnesses, neurological problems, psychological trauma, head trauma or injury, middle ear disease, allergies. Drugs or medications prescribed by a physician
General behavior and social-emotional development	Age-appropriate play behavior, social isolation, impulsiveness, withdrawal, aggression, tact, sensitivity to others, self-discipline
Speech and language development	Evidence of articulation, voice, or fluency problems. Ability to communicate ideas verbally. Ability to formulate sentences correctly. Appropriateness of verbal expression to subject or situation
Hearing and auditory behavior	Ability to localize sounds auditorily. Ability to identify sound sources. Ability to listen selectively in presence of noise. Reaction to sudden, unexpected sound. Ability to ignore environmental sounds. Tolerance to loud sounds. Consistency of response to sound. Need to have spoken information repeated. Ability to follow verbal instructions. Ability to listen for appropriate length of time. Ability to remember things heard. Ability to pay attention to what is said. Ability to comprehend words and their meaning. Ability to understand multiple meanings of words. Ability to understand abstract ideas. Discrepancies between auditory and visual behavior
Nonauditory behavior	Motor coordination: gross, fine, and eye-hand. Hand dominance. Visual perception. Spatial orientation. Any unusual reaction to touch
Educational progress	Reading ability, mathematical ability, and art ability

achievement in language acquisition, reading, or academics has not been established. Many children who fail to achieve in these areas have auditory processing problems, but some children who achieve normally also have poor auditory processing skills, and some poor readers and students with low achievement have normal auditory processing abilities.

As with learning disabilities that are multidimensional, CAPD can exist in combination with or as a result of other disorders. For example, auditory perceptual problems may stem from neurological problems, such as seizure disorders or agenesis of the corpus callosum. Other factors may include conductive or sensorineural hearing loss, brain injury from many different causes, including, for example, head trauma, meningitis,

or other viral infections. Drug and alcohol abuse may also result in CAPD. There are undoubtedly genetic factors involved because many family members have similar educational histories of auditory learning problems.

PREVALENCE OF AUDITORY LANGUAGE—LEARNING DEFICITS

According to the ACLD, between 8,000,000 and 12,000,000 children in the United States are learning disabled. Many of these children have CAPD. One difficulty in establishing the number of children with CAPD is that no standard definition of terminology is used. Thus, estimates of prevalence will vary, depending on definitions used in different localities. Another problem with prevalence studies is that mild cases of auditory processing disorders are inconspicuous or easily compensated for when educational demands are at a minimum. With increased pressure for academic achievement, however, mild disorders can become educationally significant. The fact is, that until consensus is reached on a definition of CAP and CAPD and validity research conducted, prevalence estimates are just that, informed guesses.

BEHAVIORS OF CHILDREN WITH CENTRAL AUDITORY PROCESSING DISORDERS

When asked what behaviors were typical of children with CAPD, a teacher noted that they often seem to be "in a fog" and to say "Huh?" frequently. The teacher explained that such children often do not do their schoolwork, do not follow directions, and do not respond to auditory stimuli. She remarked, "When I talk to children with that kind of problem, they just look at me."

The following observations appear to be characteristic of children with auditory processing problems:

1. Most are male.
2. They have normal pure-tone hearing thresholds.
3. They generally respond inconsistently to auditory stimuli. They often respond appropriately, but at other times they seem unable to follow auditory instructions.
4. They have short attention spans and fatigue easily when confronted with long or complex activities.
5. They are distracted by both auditory and visual stimulation. Brutten el al[5] describe these children as being at the mercy of their environment. Unable to block out irrelevant stimuli, they must respond immediately and totally to everything they see, feel, or hear, no matter how trivial.
6. They may have difficulty with auditory localization skills. This may include an inability to tell how close or far away the source of the sound is and an inability to differentiate soft and loud sounds. There have been frequent reports that these children become frightened and upset when they are exposed to loud noise, and often hold their hands over their ears to stop the sound.

7. They may listen attentively but have difficulty following long or complicated verbal commands, or instructions.
8. They frequently request that information be repeated.
9. They are often unable to remember information presented verbally for both short-term and long-term memory. They may have difficulty in counting or in reciting the alphabet, or in remembering the days of the week and months of the year or addresses and telephone numbers.
10. They may be allergic to various factors in the environment.
11. They sometimes have a significant history of chronic otitis media.

Other behavioral characteristics of children with CAPD include poor listening skills, taking a substantial amount of time to answer questions, having difficulty relating what is heard to the words seen on paper, and being unable to appreciate jokes, puns, or other humorous twists of language.

Cohen[6] points out that in addition to specific auditory behaviors, many of these children have significant reading problems, are poor spellers, and have poor handwriting. They may have articulation or language disorders. In the classroom they may act out frustrations that result from their perceptual deficits, or they may be shy and withdrawn because of the poor self-concept that results from multiple failures.

These examples are only a few of the behaviors that are associated with CAPD. Not every child with an auditory processing problem will exhibit all of the behaviors mentioned. The number of problems experienced by a given child will be an expression of the severity of the auditory learning disability. A child with problems in only a few auditory areas will have only a mild auditory learning problem. If the CAPD is profound, affecting many auditory perceptual skills, affecting language comprehension severely, and persisting for years, it is called receptive aphasia, central deafness,[6,7] or auditory agnosia.

The reader will recognize that the behaviors just listed are not unique to children with CAPD. They are common to children with peripheral hearing loss, attention deficit disorders, allergies, and other problems. It should not bother clinicians to find similar behaviors among children with various-language learning disorders. Children (and adults) are capable of a limited repertoire of responses to the problems of life. However, children with similar behaviors may have very different underlying causes and do not represent a homogenous group. It is the clinician's task to determine the true underlying deficit or deficits among children with similar behaviors and to recommend the appropriate remediation approach for each child.

IDENTIFICATION AND ASSESSMENT OF AUDITORY PROCESSING PROBLEMS

Peripheral Hearing Loss

Before any attempt is made to diagnose a child as having CAPD, it is necessary to rule out the presence of a peripheral hearing loss of the conductive or sensorineural type. A conductive hearing loss results from damage or disorders to the sound-conducting mechanism, including the external ear canal, eardrum, middle ear space, or the bones of the middle ear (see Chapter 2). Examples of a conductive loss include foreign body or wax (cerumen) occluding the ear canal, a perforated eardrum, or fluid in the middle ear from a cold or allergy. A hearing loss in the cochlea (inner ear) is called a sensorineural hearing loss (SNHL) (see Chapter 2). SNHL is caused by genetic factors, viral infections, noise, head trauma, and other factors. When a SNHL is severe, it is relatively easy to identify because the child will not respond to sound or develop speech and language. When a SNHL is mild the diagnosis may be more difficult.

Mild flat peripheral hearing loss at all frequencies and sloping high-frequency hearing losses are likely to result in inconsistent auditory responses, poor auditory attention, and other behaviors that indicate difficulty in learning through the auditory channel. Therefore, any child who exhibits these behaviors, or any child with speech or language delay needs to be tested to rule out a peripheral hearing loss. It is vitally important to recognize that pure-tone hearing screening tests done in the schools are not sensitive to the presence of fluid in the middle ear, and fail to identify mild conductive hearing loss. Tympanometry gives additional information about middle ear function, and is a necessary component of school hearing screening programs.

It is also important to keep in mind that a single hearing test performed on a child may not be adequate. Fluctuating hearing loss associated with allergies or colds, or the possibility that a sensori-neural hearing loss is progressive, makes it unwise to plan a child's long-term educational experience on the basis of a single hearing test.

A final word about conductive hearing loss. Until recently, little information was available on the long-term effects of early and prolonged otitis media with static or fluctuating hearing loss on central auditory abilities. There is growing evidence that otitis media can cause auditory learning problems and is not the innocuous disease that it was once considered to be.[8-15] The residual effects can be CAP problems that may cause language and learning delays long after the middle ear disease has been resolved. Therefore, children with histories of frequent colds or chronic middle ear disease should be carefully watched for signs of auditory language-learning problems. This subject is covered in detail in Chapters 3 and 9.

ASSESSMENT PROCEDURES

When a peripheral hearing loss has been ruled out in a child with a language or learning disability and when behaviors indicate that an auditory processing problem is present, a thorough evaluation of central auditory abilities should be performed.

History

The assessment should begin with careful observation of the child, with particular attention to the auditory behavior patterns described previously in this chapter. Care should be taken to identify strengths as well as weaknesses, and to note performance in other modalities, including vision, motor coordination, tactile response, and speech.

When possible, an in-depth history from the child's caregiver should be taken. Rosenberg[16] called the case history "the first test" because of the value of the information obtained. He pointed out that a carefully taken history can be extremely useful in differentiating among various problems, can supplement results from auditory tests, and can help in making decisions about the child's educational management.

The case history should be taken systematically to avoid missing important information. The person taking the history should provide an opportunity for the caregiver to state their concerns about the child, to describe the child's behaviors, and to express any other related concerns. Specific information that should be requested includes: (1) information about the family; (2) the mother's pregnancy; (3) conditions at birth, the child's growth and development, health, and illnesses; (4) general behavior and socioemotional development; (5) speech and language development; (6) hearing and auditory behavior; (7) nonauditory behavior; and (8) educational progress. The specific questions asked of parents will depend on the setting in which the testing is being done and the purpose of the examination. Areas to be investigated in the history when a CAPD is suspected are given in Table 5–2. A format for taking a case history of CAPD was published by Willeford and Burleigh.[17]

Check Lists of Central Auditory Processing

Several check lists exist to assist school personnel in identifying children who may benefit from central auditory testing. They include the Fisher[18] auditory problems checklist. Although that checklist is frequently cited, it has poor norms and has never been subjected to validation studies. Willeford and Burleigh[17] refer to a checklist that involves a rating scale for ranking behaviors associated with CAPD, but their checklist has never been validated. Sanger et al[19] developed a Checklist of Classroom Observations for Children "At Risk" for Auditory Processing Problems. This 23 item questionnaire was devised for educators to record and rate their observations of children's behavior throughout a typical day. Teachers rate the behaviors according to the frequency observed. Behaviors addressed include inattentiveness, reading or spelling problems, and recurring ear infections.

One tool useful in reviewing children's behavior is the Childrens Auditory Processing Performance Scale (CHAPPS) developed by Smoski et al[20] to systematically collect and quantify the observed listening behaviors of children. CHAPPS is a questionnaire-type scale consisting of 36 items concerning listening behavior in a variety of listening conditions and functions. According to the authors, the clinical applications of this scale are to identify children who should be referred for a CAP evaluation and to prescribe and measure the effects of therapeutic intervention.

Tests of Central Auditory Processing

There are at least two difficult approaches to tests of central auditory abilities that depend in part on the examiners understanding of CAPD. Butler[21] pointed out that there is a traditional audiological perspective, a speech-language pathologist's perspective, and a teacher's perspective. Fundamentally, the audiologist's past "anatomic" perspective has led to development of an assessment approach based on the processing of auditory signals along the auditory pathway leading to the language center of the brain. This approach has differed from the speech-language pathologist's cognitive perspective, which stresses information processing strategies. Teachers often view the problem in terms of the child's ability to follow oral directions, comprehend academic instructions, etc.

Speech-language pathologist's are familiar with nonstandardized auditory receptive language samples. Lasky and Cox[22] describe a systematic approach to observation of the child's auditory behavior in their SPERS remediation model: They recommend observational evaluation of the child under different conditions of Signal, Presentation, and Environment, while evaluating the child's Responses, and Strategies.

Some of the auditory abilities that are assessed during formal testing include the following.

Auditory Attention. The ability to sustain attention over time can be assessed by observing the child in comparison with his or her peers. The child should have the ability to direct attention toward a relevant acoustic signal, whether speech or music, and to sustain that attention for an appropriate length of time. When a child is not tuned in to listen, the child cannot learn auditorily. Preliminary research in our laboratories indicated that tests of auditory vigilance may be useful in describing a child's auditory attention.[23] The Auditory Continuous Performance Test (ACPT)[24] contains a list of 100 monosyllable words presented at the rate of 1/s. Within each word list is embedded 20 random presentations of a target word "dog." The list is repeated six times without interruption, making a test of approximately 10 minutes. Measurement of performance decrements in identifying the target word over the duration of the test is a way of objectively determining a child's auditory vigilance. Keith and Engineer[25] found that performance on the ACPT was significantly better in children with attention deficit disorder (ADD) when on methylphenidate (Ritalin) compared with their performance when not on that medication. Additional studies by Riccio et al,[26] Herrod and Shapiro,[27] Burk and Smaldino,[28] and Weingart[29] have validated the use of the ACPT in assessing children with ADD. Further validation studies will confirm whether the ACPT or other similar tests will help separate children with disorders of attention from those with auditory figure-ground problems.

Auditory Figure Ground. Auditory figure ground is the ability to understand speech in the presence of a competing background noise. The ability to understand speech in noise varies widely among individuals. However, some children experience extreme problems understanding speech in the presence of background environmental noise that have adverse affects on their academic achievements. Observation of the child can help determine behavior changes that occur when it is quiet and when in the presence of competing speech and other environmental noise. When observing these changes, it is necessary to determine whether a child's decreased ability to perform in noise is due to diminished auditory abilities or to a more generalized ADD. Formal testing under standardized conditions can help differentiate between these problems. Because of the wide range of individual abilities to resist background noise, the examiner should have adequate normative data with adequate numbers of subjects to define ranges of performance in a normal population for the test conditions used. Informal observations of figure ground performance must be made carefully because an observation is subjective.

Tests of auditory figure ground are usually administered using recorded speech in the presence of competing background speech or environmental noise. The test must be recorded with the speech at a favorable signal-to-noise (S/N) ratio. When the speech is presented at levels equal to or below the background noise, masking occurs and the listening situation becomes one of auditory closure. Tests that use competing speech ranging from a single talker to a speech babble background are preferable to those that use white or "speech" noise.

Auditory Discrimination. Auditory discrimination can be assessed at many levels. For example, when a child repeats a monosyllable word correctly, the child has demonstrated an ability to discriminate speech sounds at the imitative level. When syllables or word pairs are presented orally and the child is asked to report whether they were exactly the same or different (eg, the Wepman Auditory Discrimination Test,[30]) another level of discrimination is introduced. In that case, the child must understand the concept of the same and different, and a cognitive aspect to auditory discrimination is introduced. When children can repeat words correctly but cannot tell whether the sounds are the same or different, the problem is cognitive and not auditory discrimination. Another test difficulty is that there is no assurance that the child is listening to all parts of the word pairs and not simply to the initial, middle (usually the "stronger" vowel), or final part.

Some tests of auditory discrimination require the child to point to a picture in response to stimulus words. The conceptual difficulty with any picture-pointing test is that it is cross-modality, requiring visual recognition of all of the pictures and an auditory-visual association between word and picture. Because these tests rely on visual perception and auditory-visual integration, it is difficult to attribute any breakdown to auditory discrimination in the narrow sense. Nevertheless, because they are common behaviors asked of a child, an inability to respond appropriately to a picture-pointing task indicates a possible delay in the child's development.

Another level of auditory discrimination testing is demonstrated by the Lindamood Auditory Conceptualization test.[31] In this test, the child is asked to associate sounds with colored blocks and to manipulate them to demonstrate their ability to discriminate one speech sound from another; and their ability to perceive the number, order, and sameness or difference of speech sounds in different sequences. This highly cognitive task is on the opposite end of the continuum of auditory discrimination abilities that range from imitation to cognition. In the assessment of auditory discrimination abilities, the examiner should determine the level at which the child's auditory discrimination abilities break down.

Auditory Closure. Auditory closure is the ability to understand the whole word or message when the part is missing or missed. Being a linguistically based cognitive ability, auditory closure can be assessed using tasks that require the child to fill in missing parts of a word. One example is the auditory closure subtest of the Illinois Test of Psycholinguistic Abilities (ITPA).[32] In this test the child fills in missing parts of a word. For example, the examiner will say "airpla__," or "ea__ter __unny"; the correct responses are airplane and Easter bunny.

A different approach to testing auditory closure is to eliminate certain frequency components of spoken words by electronic low-pass filtering. Eliminating the high frequencies of speech results in a signal that sounds muffled. Research has shown that low-pass filtered speech effectively separates children with learning problems from those who are normally achieving.[33] According to Costello,[34] depressed scores on the Central Auditory Abilities Test, which contains a filtered speech subtest, are often found in children with language or learning problems.

Auditory Blending. Sometimes called auditory synthesis or phonemic synthesis, this auditory ability is considered by many to be a fundamental requisite to learning to read by a phonic method.[35,36] According to Bannatyne,[37] a child may sound out the phonemic units of a word successfully, but may be unable to approximate a normally spoken word. Bannatyne states that auditory blending and closure abilities are significantly correlated. Several standardized tests assess auditory blending abilities by presenting isolated sounds that make up a word.[32,38,39] The child must combine those sounds to tell what the word is. Examples of stimuli are: f-oot (foot), t-oa-st (toast), and k-e-tch-u-p (ketchup). Schneider[40] and Katz[35] discuss phonemic training in their chapters on audiologic management of CAPD.

Auditory Analysis. The ability to identify phonemes, syllables, or morphemes embedded in words requires both auditory processing and linguistic processing abilities.[41] Some diagnostic reading tests contain subtests of auditory analysis abilities.[42,43] The Auditory Analysis Test[44] requires the subject to form a new word when a phoneme or syllable is removed from a larger word. For example, gate without "g" is ate, trail without "t" is rail, glow without "l" is go.

Auditory Memory. As is the case with auditory discrimination, memory exists at many levels, including perceptual or echoic memory, short-term memory, long-term memory, and episodic memory. Many parents do not recognize these several levels, and it is difficult for them to reconcile the fact that a child can remember an incident from the distant past, but cannot remember a spelling lesson between the time of the previous evening's practice to the next day's test. Therefore, innumerable tests have been designed to assess auditory memory using all kinds of speech stimuli, including phonemes, sentences, paragraphs, and short stories. Two aspects of memory that are typically assessed are memory span[45,46] and sequential memory.[32,47] The Memory for

Content subtest of the GFW Auditory Memory Test[48] uses a different test approach. A picture-pointing task is used in which the child is asked to indicate the two pictures that were not *named*.

CELF-R Screening Test and Clinical Evaluation of Language Fundamentals—Revised. The CELF-R Screening test is a measure designed to screen students for language disorders, whereas the CELF-R is used to assist in the diagnosis of the language disorder and to identify areas of relative strength and weakness (Semel et al[49,50]). These tests are mentioned here because they assess the highest levels of auditory processing. For example, the receptive language subtests include (depending on age of the subject) word structure, formulated sentences, recalling sentences, and sentence assembly. Professionals should use all levels of assessment of auditory perceptual and auditory language skills to determine the child's abilities and disabilities before embarking on a remediation program.

Comment. In these paragraphs, many different auditory abilities have been discussed as if they each occurred in isolation. It may be possible to describe the components of auditory perception, but it is virtually impossible to actually test auditory abilities independent of each other. A number of specialists have noted that each of these skills overlap and that they are inseparable.[51-53] Nevertheless, attempts to describe auditory processing subskills in a child who is having problems with language and learning can be important for developing an effective remediation program.

Dilemmas of the Auditory Processing Test Battery

Uncertainty exists whether the specific auditory skills, as they have been defined, form the basis of learning language, or whether these skills are acquired as a result of having learned the language. Some experts state that auditory perception is fundamental to learning language and that auditory processing deficits cause disorders in areas of language, reading, and learning.[54] These experts further state that auditory perception can be readily broken down into specific deficits that are amendable to training,[41,55] that a hierarchy of auditory perceptual skills exists with processes moving from simple to complex, and that remediation should follow the same order.[31,41,56-58] Others[59-61] believe that poor performance on auditory skills may result from a language disorder because these children do not have sufficient linguistic, semantic, and cognitive skills to enable them to develop strategies for dealing with the auditory tasks.

These different positions are discussed here because the selection of remedial techniques will depend directly on which philosophy is adopted. If one holds that specific auditory deficits, such as auditory closure, auditory blending, and so forth, are responsible for the language deficit, then remediation would proceed via training of those specific skills on a hierarchical basis. If, on the other hand, one takes the position that central auditory problems result from a language disorder, then remediation would proceed on a language basis, in which the therapist would use intervention strategies such as those described in Chapter 16.

A further point is that many of the tests purported to measure specific auditory skills are actually measures of language. That is, to perform on these tests, the child must have developed relatively sophisticated language skills, and the more advanced the child's language, the better the child will perform. For example, the following three tests of auditory discrimination are heavily linguistically based. They include: (1) the Flowers-Costello CAA Sentence Completion task, which is a cognitive-based language task ("On Halloween we carved a _____."); (2) the auditory closure tasks ("tele_____ one is telephone"); and (3) the auditory analysis task (gate without "g" is ate). In addition, the GFW auditory memory test requires more than basic auditory abilities when a child is asked to point to the two pictures that were not named. And in the GFW Auditory Discrimination Test[62] when the word stimulus is "big," the correct response is to point to the picture of the elephant and mouse, which is a cognitive response.

To assess auditory abilities, therefore, it is critical to evaluate each test for prelinguistic and linguistic or precognitive and cognitive language content. A prelinguistic task is one in which a stimulus sound is simply imitated, without the need to understand it, define it, or associate a visual object with it. For example, to repeat the nonsense syllables "ba" and "da" is the simplest form of imitation and is a prelinguistic skill, but to know whether these two sounds are the same or different requires higher linguistic competence. Repetition of syllables or words heard in the presence of a background noise at a favorable signal-to-noise (S/N) ratio is a low-level cognitive imitative speech task. When the intensity of the noise is equal to or exceeds the intensity of the speech, direct masking occurs, and the task becomes a higher-level cognitive task of auditory closure. Repeating nonsense syllables or simple words presented simultaneously to opposite ears is a low-level language task. Repeating a string of unrelated syllables, digits, or words is a simple low-linguistic memory task; but remembering groups of related words becomes a complex cognitive task, since the person is required to see relationships among words, develop categories, and through a cognitive process increase recall abilities.

The purpose of this discussion is simply to raise the issue of differences between low linguistic auditory perceptual and cognitive-based tests of auditory processing. They are important concepts when considering whether a child's problem is one of auditory perception or receptive language.

THE AUDIOLOGICAL EVALUATION

A second and different approach to assess CAP is used by audiologists. This approach evaluates the child's ability to respond under different conditions of signal distortion or competition. Most of these tests require an imitative speech response and are not cognitive based tasks. The principle of this approach assumes that a person who has a normal auditory system can tolerate mild distortions of speech and still understand it. A listener with an auditory processing deficit will encounter difficulty with the distorted speech due to added "internal distortion."[63] Results of distorted speech tests can be used to infer the development status of the child's central auditory nervous system and to help determine whether CAPD may form a basis for language or reading problems. Although the cause and effect relationship between auditory perception and language has not been established, there is reason to believe that growth of language is related to progressive maturation of the cerebral cortex.[64] When it is shown that prelinguistic auditory processing abilities are poorly developed, the child may not have the neurologic potential necessary to organize and develop a linguistic system, or development may be slower than normal. The more severe the auditory abnormalities, the greater the effect on acquisition of language. When auditory abnormalities occur in combination, problems of other sensory systems (for example, a visual perceptual disorder), or when associations among auditory, visual, tactile, vestibular sensory systems are not established, the effect is more devastating, and the child will have difficulty in overall learning.

There are a few screening tests available to identify children with auditory processing disorders. These tests were designed to be administered in the schools, and do not require two channel diagnostic audiometers. Tests introduced in the 1970s include the Goldman-Fristoe-Woodcock Test of Auditory Discrimination[62] and the Flowers-Costello Test of Central Auditory Abilities.[65] More recently, the Pediatric Speech Intelligibility Test[66] is a well-designed and normed diagnostic test that can be administered to children as young as 3 years.

One test marketed as screening test for CAPD is the Selective Auditory Attention Test (SAAT).[65] The SAAT obtains speech recognition scores in quiet and in the presence of a semantic distractor in the same ear at 0 dB signal-to-noise ratio. Children point to pictures using the Word Intelligibility by Picture Identification Test plates. Normative data for the test was obtained from 325 children ages 4 to 9 years. Children in the standardization study fell into three groups: normal-achieving, learning-disabled, and teacher concerned with school progress. Results found that children in the normal group scored substantially better than the other groups. According to Cherry,[67] this test is an efficient screening device to help identify children with learning difficulties resulting from a CAPD for deciding when to administer a lengthy battery of CAP tests.

SCAN Screening Test for Auditory Processing Disorders[2] has three subtests, including monosyllable words that are low-pass filtered at 1000 Hz, auditory figure ground with monosyllable words presented in speech babble background noise at +8 dB speech-to-noise ratio, and competing words. The two subtests tapping auditory perception of low redundancy speech (filtered words and auditory figure ground) are representative of functional auditory abilities in everyday listening situations. The other subtest is a dichotic speech test (competing words) that reflect the development of the auditory system, auditory maturation, and hemispheric specialization. The test requires approximately 25 minutes to administer. SCAN was normed on 1034 children between 3 and 11 years of age. In addition to mean and standard deviation of subtest and composite test results, the SCAN normative data includes standard scores, percentile ranks, age equivalents, and standard score confidence levels.

Subsequent research has validated the use of the SCAN test in various populations.[68-71]

Recently an upward extension of SCAN was normed on subjects between the age of 12 and 50 years. SCAN-A: Test for Auditory Processing Disorders in Adolescents and Adults[72] contains four subtests: monosyllable words low-pass filtered at 500 Hz, auditory figure ground with words presented with speech babble background noise at 0 dB S/N ratio, the competing words test, and a competing sentence test. SCAN-A requires approximately 30 minutes to administer. As with SCAN, standardization data include mean and standard deviation of subtests, composite test results, standard scores, percentile ranks, and cut-off scores for normal, questionable, and abnormal performance. The standardization results are also analyzed for content and construct validity.

Temporal ordering or sequencing tasks are potentially valuable screening tests because of the underlying processes they tap. The Frequency Pattern Test[73,74] requires the child to listen to a series of three tones and report the pitch pattern that was heard, such as low-high-low, low-low-high. Conceptually, the tones are initially processed in the nondominant right hemisphere. Interpretation of pitch perception is transferred through the corpus callosum to the language areas of the left hemisphere where a verbal response is sequenced.[74] The test takes approximately 10 minutes to administer. According to Musiek et al,[4] low scores have been shown to be sensitive to auditory dysfunction related to various learning disabilities and to defined lesions of the auditory areas of the cerebrum.

Many other diagnostic central auditory tests exist, and description of them is beyond the scope of this chapter. The diagnostic tests can be categorized in different ways. For example, the ASHA Committee on Disorders of Central Auditory Processing[75] used the following outline:

Monotic (signals presented to one ear)
    Filtered speech (eg, low-pass filtered)
    Time altered speech (eg, time compressed speech)
    Pattern recognition (frequency patterns)
    Ipsilateral competing signals (eg, auditory figure ground)
Dichotic (signals presented simultaneously to two ears, binaural separation tasks)
    Digits
    Syllables
    Words and sentences
Binaural (signals presented simultaneously to two ears, binaural integration tasks)

Binaural fusion

Selective listening and rapidly alternating speech

Masking level differences

As a group, central auditory tests all share certain characteristics. They are applicable only after the emergence of language, since they require either verbal repetition of syllables, words, or sentences or pointing to pictures that represent the stimulus words. Most of the tests show substantial maturation effects. When given to children at an early age, the results of tests are highly variable, with average performance improving remarkably up to 12 years of age. By about 12 years of age, the auditory system of normal children has matured to the point where their responses approximate those of adult listeners. Children with speech, language, reading, and learning problems have been reported to perform poorly on central auditory tests, although some children with language or reading problems yield normal scores.

Although there is no lack of approaches to assessment of central auditory function in children, the problems with many of the measures is that they are poorly normed, have poor quality recordings, and are difficult to obtain. For example, Keith[76] reported that neither of two popular tests, the Colorado State University Central Auditory Test Battery[77] and the Staggered Spondee Word Test[77] had standardization data available on children for whom they were intended to be used. By contrast, the SAAT[67] was normed on 325 children ages 4 to 9 years in three groups and SCAN[2] was standardized on 1034 normally achieving children between the ages of 3 and 11 years.

It is also difficult to get a sense of the sensitivity and specificity of various audiological measures that are available. Matkin and Hook[78] reported that 4 of 10 measures used in their central auditory test battery identified more than half of the children in their at-risk children. Those tests included simultaneous sentences, binaural fusion, filtered speech, and dichotic words. Musiek et al[79] evaluated a test battery on 22 children with CAPD and found that the pitch pattern sequence test and competing sentences were the most sensitive followed by the dichotic digits and SSW. Similarly, Ferre and Wilber[80] studied normally achieving and learning-disabled children ages 8 to 12 years. They found that low-pass filtered words were the most sensitive, with binaural fusion the next most sensitive, and time compressed speech and dichotic monosyllables equally

sensitive to disorders. Ferre and Wilber found that low-pass filtered words had the lowest false-positive rate of identification.

One other issue is the relationship that exists between central auditory and language measures administered to children. For example, in the development of SCAN Keith[2] reported a validity study conducted by Sanger and Deshayes on 31 grade 1 through 3 regular classroom students. The students were suspected of having auditory processing problems but were not previously identified. SCAN was concurrently administered with subtests of CELF, GFW Auditory Subskills Battery, the GFW Test of Auditory Discrimination, and the SSW. The pattern of correlations between SCAN subtests and general measures of language were positive but low. Similar findings are reported by Keith et al[71] who found significant correlations between SCAN and both the SSW and the Willeford battery but no significant correlations among SCAN and CELF scores. Matkin and Hook[78] found one significant correlation among 52 possible comparisons between a central auditory test battery and an auditory-language battery. They concluded that audiologists and speech-language clinicians investigate different functions. Sanger et al[81] studied students with auditory language or language-processing disorders and found no significant correlations between the SSW scores and the auditory-language battery.

Not all studies find a lack of significant correlation between central auditory and language measures. For example, Harris et al[82] reported that the SSW and a test of speech discrimination in noise were significantly correlated to the total scores of the Token Test for Children, the Test for Auditory Comprehension of Language and each subtest of the Del Rio Language Screening Test. Keith and Novak[83] studied 205 children between the ages of 6 and 8 years as part of a multicenter collaborative study investigating the effects of phototherapy treatment. The children all had normal hearing, and the WISC-R full scale IQ of the group reported was 102.1 =/−14.6. In addition, Keith and Novak[83] found that children who had normal receptive language as measured by results of the Token Test for Children did significantly better on the SSW and Dichotic CV tests than children who had below average receptive language. It would appear that outcomes of studies of central auditory and language abilities are affected by the types of tests used. Nevertheless, findings of low correlation between central auditory and language measures are to be expected. They simply indicate that tests of auditory processing that are less linguistically loaded (eg, require a simple imitative response by repeating words) measure different aspects of auditory processing abilities than those that are more linguistically loaded (eg, require knowledge of the vocabulary, knowledge of rules of syntax, etc).

The use of central auditory tests is increasing although there is a great deal to learn about interpretation of obtained results. However, well-designed central auditory tests show reveal some of the following information about the child being tested:

1. The test results describe the maturation level of the central auditory pathways, and through longitudinal studies on a given child demonstrate development of central auditory abilities.
2. The test results provide data to document the neurological origin presumed to exist in children with specific learning disabilities.
3. The test results can be used to assess the effect of medication on auditory abilities.
4. The test results can aid in ruling out abnormalities or the central auditory pathways as contributing to a language-learning problem.
5. The test results help to describe whether cerebral dominance for language has occurred.
6. The test results describe whether the auditory channel is "weak" or "strong," and whether classroom, tutoring, or remedial material should be modified to account for auditory processing abilities.
7. The tests are useful in research on auditory processing abilities.

Tests of central auditory function cannot be expected to indicate specific language, learning, or reading deficits. To describe these specific problems, the examiner needs to administer tests that are appropriate for that purpose. The central auditory test battery does provide information that can be used to develop remedial strategies for language-learning-disordered children. These strategies include both classroom management suggestions to teachers and parents and direct intervention techniques that are generally administered by speech-language pathologists.

REMEDIATION

In general, remediation for children with central auditory disorders falls into three categories, including compensatory training to strengthen basic perceptual processes and teach specific academic skills; management of the environment, including classroom placement; and cognitive therapy in which the clinician assists the subject in learning auditory strategies for dealing with their auditory processing disorder. Management of the environment includes altering the psychological environment to modify negative attitudes and habits of the subject and those around the subject. For adults, much of the remediation process is in the form of counseling, and development of coping strategies, including management of the auditory environment.

When an auditory figure-ground deficit has been identified, recommendations for remediation should be directed toward management of the environment to enhance listening opportunities. Although direct intervention to help achieve better listening skills in noise through cognitive training and focusing of auditory attention may be beneficial, there is no evidence to support the improvement of auditory-figure-ground perceptual deficits through such training. When auditory-figure-ground problems are severe, attempts to compensate for the deficit with FM auditory training systems may be useful.[84-87] However, trials with FM systems should be carefully monitored to be sure that the child, teachers, and parents understand the device, and that real, not imagined, benefits accrue from its use.

Specific recommendations for remediation of central auditory disorders can be found in several sources, including Kahn,[88] Keith,[89] Katz et al,[90] Levinson and Sloan,[91] Willeford and Burleigh,[18] Lasky and Katz,[92] Chermak and Musiek,[86] and in Part III of this book.

Finally, diagnosis of a central auditory processing disorder and recommendations for remediation/rehabilitation must be made as part of a transdisciplinary team decision to assure that different aspects of the individual's speech, language, auditory, psychological, emotional, and physical function have been evaluated. Only after all these aspects have been examined can a CAPD be diagnosed and appropriate recommendations for treatment can made. This is especially true when evaluating children and adolescents with learning problems and developing Individualized Education Plans.

CASE HISTORIES

The following case studies provide examples of *SCAN • A* performance by two individuals. In Case 1, the adolescent exhibits difficulties with specific subtests on *SCAN • A* (Fig. 5–1). Case 2 shows *SCAN • A* results for an adolescent who exhibits poor performance across all subtests (Fig. 5–2).

Case Study 5–1

NN is a 13-year-old boy with normal hearing and intelligence. He was in an ungraded special education program for children with learning disabilities. He scored at the 16th percentile on the *Peabody Picture Vocabulary Test* (PPVT) and the 9th percentile on the *Test of Language Competence—Expressive* (TLC-E). On the *Detroit Test of Learning*, NN scores were 9.3 years on the Oral Directions subtest, 5.9 years on the Auditory Attention subtest, and 9.6 years on the Verbal Opposites subtest. Current *SCAN • A* results are shown in Figure 5–1.

SCAN • A results indicate difficulty with functional auditory processing skills (resisting distortion, speech in noise) but not with dichotic word tasks (Competing Words and Competing Sentences). These results indicate a delay in auditory maturation with functional difficulties of interpreting distorted speech or speech in the presence of background noise. *SCAN • A* results for NN do not indicate a damaged central auditory nervous system.

Recommendations for remediation for NN included continued placement in small, structured classroom settings rather than the open concept public school classes that predominate in his county system. NN should be seated away from air conditioning units and other competing noise sources. His teacher was advised that his comprehension is reduced when she paces while instructing or turns away from him to write on the backboard. She was advised to check his understanding of material from time to time because the small class size and her teaching style permits individual attention. NN used earphones when tape recorders and videotape equipment were used in the classroom. Use of the earphones minimized distortion and reduced ambient noise interference. NN was reluctant to uses an FM system, even on a trial basis.

NN received language therapy services on a regular basis. His speech-language pathologist introduced concepts/skills in a quiet environment, then systematically introduced competing steady-state noise, music, and competing voices. This procedure helped NN to develop listening and attending strategies that will enable him to cope with the demands of processing auditory information in competing signal environments. In addition, his parents were counseled about his need for structured communication to assist them in communicating rules and expectations at home.

SCORING SUMMARY

Age 13	Raw Score	Standard Score	Standard Score Confidence Range 68% Confidence Level		Percentile Rank
Filtered Words	29	4	2	to 6	2
Auditory Figure-Ground	26	1	1	to 3	1
Competing Words	51	8	6	to 10	25
Competing Sentences	19	9	8	to 10	37
Sum of Standard Scores		22			
Total Test Standard Score		65	61	to 69	1

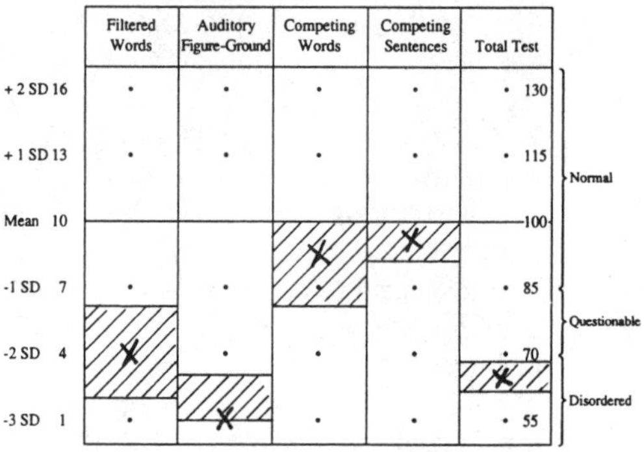

Competing Words Ear Advantage	
Right Ear Total	27
Left Ear Total	−24
Ear Advantage	3
Right Ear Advantage ✓ Left Ear Advantage ____	

Figure 5–1. *SCAN • A* results for NN.

Case Study 5–2

BJ is a 14-year-old boy with normal intelligence who is enrolled in a program for individuals with learning disabilities. BJ scored at the 9th percentile on the *Peabody Picture Vocabulary Test—Revised*. Receptive, Expressive, and Total Language scores on the *Clinical Evaluation of Language Fundamentals—Revised* were at the 68th percentile. Scores on the *Test of Written Language—Revised* ranged from the 50th to the 75th percentile. *SCAN • A* results are shown in Figure 5–2.

BJ scored in the "Questionable" range (between 1 and 2 standard deviations below the mean) on the Auditory Figure-Ground subtest. BJ scored in the "Disordered" range on the other three subtests. His performance on the Filtered Words and Auditory Figure-Ground subtests suggests that he has difficulty understanding in non-optimum listening conditions and cannot cope with distortions of the acoustic environment or when background noise levels are high relative to the speech signal. The poor performance on the Competing Words and Competing Sentences tests suggests that there is a neurophysiological basis for this young man's learning problems. His auditory system appears to be disordered, not delayed. For example, his scores on the Competing Sentences subtest indicate that he cannot direct his attention to one ear and listen to the other. He is unable to attend to the right ear and ignore the left, an ability that is present in children who are 6 years old.[17] BJ frequently mixes the words in sentences presented to different ears. This mixing of sentences is common among children with learning disabilities, less common among children with delays in auditory maturation, and uncommon among young normal children.

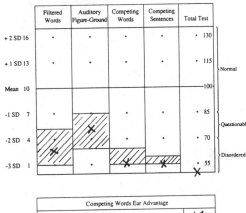

SCORING SUMMARY

Age 14	Raw Score	Standard Score	Standard Score Confidence Range 68% Confidence Level	Percentile Rank
Filtered Words	28	3	1 to 5	1
Auditory Figure-Ground	33	5	3 to 7	5
Competing Words	33	1	1 to 3	1
Competing Sentences	1	1	1 to 2	1
Sum of Standard Scores		10		
Total Test Standard Score		42	38 to 46	1

Competing Words Ear Advantage	
Right Ear Total	14
Left Ear Total	−19
Ear Advantage	−5
Right Ear Advantage ____ Left Ear Advantage ✓	

Figure 5–2. For the test items presented to the right ear, BJ frequently combined words heard in both sentences. For example, on item 4 ("People are going home" and "The lady washed the shirt"), BJ said "The lady walked home." For his age, responses like this indicate a severe auditory perceptual disorder. The pattern of responses suggests that BJ has a damaged central auditory nervous system. When BJ was younger, speech-language pathologic treatment goals focused on auditory processing of linguistic rule systems. In later years, speech-language pathologic treatment focused on expressive phonologic, semantic, and pragmatic rules for reading and writing.

REFERENCES

1. ACLD Newsbriefs: *ACLD Description: Specific Learning Disabilities*, No. 166 (Sept–Oct 1986).
2. Keith RW: *SCAN: A Screening Test for Auditory Processing Disorders* (San Antonio, Psychological Corporation, 1986).
3. ASHA *Current Concepts and Issues in Central Auditory Processing Disorders*. A report from the Ad Hoc Committee on Central Auditory Processing. (1991).
4. Musiek FE, Gollegly KM, Lamb LE, Lamb P. (1990) Selected issues in screening for central auditory processing dysfunction. *Semin Hear*, 11 (1990), 372–383.
5. Brutten M, Richardson SO, Mangel C. *Something's Wrong with My Child* (New York: Harcourt Brace Jovanovich, 1973) p. 29.
6. Cohen RL: Auditory skills and the communicative process. *Speech, Lang Hear*, (1980).
7. Myklebust H: *Auditory Disorders in School Children: A Manual for Differential Diagnosis* (New York: Grune & Stratton, 1954), p 14.
8. Holm VA, Kunze LH: Effect of chronic otitis media on language and speech development. *Pediatrics*, 43 (1969), 833–839.
9. Schleiper A, Kisilevsky H, Mattingly S, Yorke L: Mild conductive hearing loss and language development: A one year follow up study. *Dev Behav Pediatr*, 6 (1985), 65–68.
10. Brandes P, Ehinger D: The effects of early middle ear pathology on auditory perception and academic achievement. *J Speech Hear Disord*, 46 (1981) 250–257.
11. Welsh L, Welsh J, Healy M: Effect of sound deprivation on central hearing. *Laryngoscope*, 93 (1983), 1569–1575.
12. Sak R, Ruben R: Recurrent middle ear effusion in childhood: Implications of temporary deprivation for language and learning. *Ann Otol* 90 (1981), 546–551.
13. Hanson DG, Ulvested RF: Otitis media and child development of speech, language and education. *Ann Otol Rhin Laryngol*, suppl; 60 (1979), 88,pt2.
14. Lehmann MD, Charron K, Krummer A, et al: The effects of chronic middle ear effusion on speech and language development. A descriptive study. *Pediatr J Otolaryngol*, 1,pt 2 (1979), 137–144.
15. Menyuk, P: Relationship of otitis media to speech processing and language development, in Katz J, Stecker, and Henderson, eds: *Central Auditory Processing: A Transdisciplinary View* (St. Louis: Mosby-Year Book, 1992.
16. Rosenberg PE: Case history: The first test, in Katz J, ed: *Handbook of Clinical Audiology*, ed 2 (Baltimore: William & Wilkins, 1978), chap 7.
17. Willeford J, Burleigh J: *Handbook of Central Auditory Processing Disorders in Children* (Orlando, FL: Grune & Stratton, 1985).
18. Fisher LI: *Auditory Problems Checklist* (Bemidji, Minnesota: Life Products, 1976).
19. Sanger DD, Freed JM, Decker TN: Behavioral profile of preschool children suspected of auditory language processing problems. *Hear J*, 38 (1985), 17–20.
20. Smoski WJ, Brunt MA, Tannahill JC: Listening characteristics of children with central auditory processing disorders. *Lang Speech Hear Serv Sch*, 23 (1992), 145–152
21. Butler KG: Personal communication, 1986.
22. Lasky E, Cox C: Auditory processing and language interaction, in Lasky E, Katz J, eds: *Central Auditory Processing Disorders* (Baltimore: University Park Press, 1983), chap 13.
23. Keith RW, Krafft K: The auditory continuous performance test: Unpublished research.
24. Keith RW: *The Auditory Continuous Performance Test* (The Psychological Corporation, San Antonio, TX, 1994).
25. Keith RW, Engineer P: Effects of methylphenidate on auditory processing abilities of children with attention deficit-hyperactivity disorders. *J Learn Disabil*, 24 (1991), 630–636
26. Riccio CA, Cohen MJ, Hynd GW, Keith RW: Central auditory processing disorder and attention deficit hyperactivity disorder: Results of the Auditory Continuous Performance Test. *Ear Hear*, 1994), in press.
27. Herrod LA, Shapiro SK: Diagnostic utility Of visual and auditory tasks in the assessment of attention-deficit hyperactivity disorder. *Ear Hear* (1994), in press.
28. Burk J, Smaldino J: Attention deficits in children. Poster Session Presented to the annual convention of the American Auditory Society. San Antonio, TX, 1992.
29. Weingart AM: The relationship between self-perceived hearing handicap and attention in the elderly. Unpublished Master of Arts thesis, University of Northern Iowa, 1991.
30. Wepman JM, *Auditory Discrimination Test* (Los Angeles: Western Psychological Services, 1973).
31. Lindamood CH, Lindamood PC: *Lindamood Auditory Conceptualization Test* (Revised) (Hingham MA: Teaching Resources Corp, 1975).
32. Kirk S, McCarthy J, Kirk W: *Illinois Test of Psycholinguistic Abilities* (Urbana: University of Illinois Press, 1968).
33. Keith RW, Farrer S: Filtered word testing in the assessment of children with central auditory disorders. *Ear Hear*, 12 (1981), 267–269.
34. Costello MR: Evaluation of auditory behavior of children using the Flowers-Costello test of central auditory abilities, in Keith RW, ed: *Central Auditory Dysfunction* (New York: Grune & Stratton, 1977), chap 8.
35. Katz J: Phonemic synthesis, in Lasky E, Katz J, eds: *Central Auditory Processing Disorders* (Baltimore: University Park Press, 1983).

36. Katz J, Harmon C: Phonemic synthesis testing and training, in Keith RW: *Central Auditory and Language Disorders in Children* (San Diego: College Hill Press, 1981).

37. Bannatyne A: *Language, Reading and Learning Disabilities* (Springfield, IL: Charles C Thomas, 1971).

38. Roswell FG, Chall JS: *Roswell-Chall Auditory Blending Test* (New York: Essay Press, 1963).

39. Goldman R, Fristoe M, Woodcock R: *GFW Sound Symbol Tests: Blending* (Circle Pines, MN: American Guidance Service, 1974).

40. Schneider D: Audiologic management of central auditory processing disorders, in Katz J, ed.: *Central Auditory Processing: A Transdisciplinary View* (St. Louis, MO: Mosby Year Book, 1992).

41. Wiig E, Semel EM: *Language Disabilities in Children and Adolescents* (Columbus, OH: Charles E. Merritt, 1976).

42. Karlsen B, Madden R, Gardner F: *Stanford Diagnostic Reading Test* (New York: Harcourt Brace Jovanovich, 1966).

43. Gates AI, McKillop AS: *Gates-McKillop Reading Diagnostic Tests* (New York: Columbia University Teacher's College Press, 1962).

44. Rosner J, Simon D: The auditory analysis test. *J Learn Disabil*, 4 (1971), 384–392.

45. Wepman JM, Morency A: *Auditory Memory Span Test* (Los Angeles: Western Psychological Services, 1973).

46. Wechsler D: *Wechsler Intelligence Scale for Children* (New York: Psychological Corporation, 1949).

47. Wepman JM, Morency A: *The Auditory Sequential Memory Test* (Los Angeles: Western Psychological Services, 1975).

48. Goldman R, Fristoe M, Woodcock R: *GFW Auditory Memory Test* (Circle Pines, MN: American Guidance Service, 1974).

49. Semel E, Wiig E, Secord W: *Clinical Evaluation of Language Fundamentals- Revised* San Antonia, TX: The Psychological Corporation, 1987).

50. Semel E, Wiig E, Secord W: *CELF-R Screening Test* (San Antonio, TX: The Psychological Corporation, 1989).

51. Williamson DG, Alexander R: *Central Auditory Abilities* (Minneapolis: Maico Audiological Library Series 13, 1970).

52. Sanders DA: *Auditory Perception of Speech* (Englewood Cliffs, NJ: Prentice-Hall, 1977).

53. Witkin BR: Auditory perception. Implications for language development. *Lang Speech Hear Sci* 4 (1971), 31–52.

54. Rampp D: *Proceeding of the Memphis State University First Annual Symposium on Auditory Processing and Learning Disabilities* (Las Vegas, 1972).

55. Butler KG: Auditory perceptual processing and dysfunction, in *Sixteenth International Congress of Logopedics and Phoniatric*. Interlaken, 1974 (Basel: Karger, 1976), pp 65–69.

56. Kirk S, Kirk W: Psycholinguistic learning disabilities, in *Diagnosis and Remediation* (Urbana: University of Illinois Press, 1971).

57. Butler KG: Auditory perceptual training. *Acta Symbolica*, 3 (1972), 123–125.

58. Lasky E: An approach to auditory processing. *Acta Symbolica*, 4 (1973), 51–62.

59. Sanders DA: *Auditory Perception of Speech* (Englewood Cliffs, NJ: Prentice-Hall, 1977), p 187.

60. Rees N: Auditory processing factors in learning disorders, a view from procrusters' bed. *J Speech Hear Res*, 15 (1972), 382–389.

61. Rees N: The speech pathologist and the reading process. *ASHA*, 16 (1974), 155–158.

62. Goldman R, Fristoe M, Woodcock RW: *Test of Auditory Discrimination* (Circle Pines, MN: American Guidance Service, 1970).

63. Teatini GP: Speech audiometry, in Rojskjaer C, ed: *Second Danavox Symposium* (Odense, Denmark, 1970).

64. Chase RA: Neurological aspects of language disorders in children in Irwin J, Marge M, eds. *Principles of Childhood Language Disabilities* (Englewood Cliffs, NJ: Prentice-Hall, 1972).

65. Flowers A, Costello R: *Flowers-Costello Test of Central Auditory Abilities* (Dearborn, MI: Perceptual Learning Systems, 1970).

66. Jerger S: Evaluation of central auditory function in children in Keith, RW, ed *Central Auditory and Language Disorders in Children* (San Diego, College Hill Press, 1981).

67. Cherry R: *The Selective auditory Attention Test (SAAT)* (St Louis: Auditec of St Louis, 1980).

68. Marlowe J, Engels TL, Keith RW: Screening for Auditory Disorders in Psychiatric Hospitals, in Bess F, ed: *Proceedings of the International Symposium on Screening Children for Auditory Function* (Nashville, TN: Bill Wilkerson Center Press, 1992).

69. Katbamna B, Keith RW, Johnson, JL: Auditory processing abilities in children with learning disabilities: A pilot study, *Hearsay, J Ohio Speech Hear Associ* Fall/Winter: 80–87, 1990.

70. Keith RW, Rudy J, Donahue P, Katbamna B: Comparison of SCAN results with other auditory and language measures in a clinical population. *Ear Hear*, 10 (1989), 382–386.

71. Deitrich KN, Succop PA, Berger OG, Keith RW: Lead exposure and the central auditory processing abilities and cognitive development of urban children: The Cincinnati Lead Study Cohort at Age 5 Years. *Neurotoxicol Teratol* 14 (1992), 51–56.

72. Keith RW: *SCAN-A: A Test of Auditory Processing Abilities for Use with Adolescents and Adults. The Auditory Continuous Performance Test* (San Antonio, TX: The Psychological Corporation, 1994).

73. Pinheiro ML: Tests of central auditory function in children with learning disabilities, in Keith RW, ed: *Central Auditory Dysfunction* (New York: Grune & Stratton, 1977).

74. Musiek FE, Pinheiro ML: Frequency patterns in cochlear, brainstem and cerebral lesions. *Audiology*, 26 (1987), 79–88.

75. *ASHA:* Audiological assessment of central auditory processing: An annotated bibliography. Committee on Disorders of Central Auditory Processing.

76. Keith RW: Central auditory testing: Some ongoing questions. *Hum Commun Can*, (1985), 145–150.

77. Katz J: The Staggered Spondaic Word Test, in Keith R, ed *Central Auditory Dysfunction* (New York: Grune & Stratton, 1977).

78. Matkin N, Hook PE: A multidisciplinary approach to central auditory evaluations, in Lasky E, Katz J, eds *Central Auditory Processing Disorders* (Baltimore: University Park Press, 1983).

79. Musiek F, Geurkin K, Keitel S: Central Auditory Assessment of Auditory Perceptual Dysfunction in Children. *Laryngscope* 92 (1982), 251–257.

80. Ferree J, Wilber L: Normal hearing disabled children's central auditory processing skills. An experimental test battery. *Ear Hear*, 7 (1986), 336–343.

81. Sanger D, Keith RW, Deshayes I, Stevens P: A Comparison of SSW abd Language Test Results, *J of Communi Disord*, 23 (1990).

82. Harris V, Keith RW, Novak K: Relationships between two dichotic listening tests and token test for children. *Ear Hear*, 4 (1983), 278–282.

83. Keith RW, Novak K: Relationships between tests of central auditory function and receptive language, *Semin Hear*, 5 (1984), 243–250.

84. Flexer C, Millin JP, Brown L: Children with Developmental Disabilities: The effect of sound field amplification on word identification. *Langu Speech Hear Ser Sch*, 21 (1990), 177–182.

85. ASHA: Amplification as a remediation technique for children with normal peripheral hearing. Committee on Amplification for the Hearing Impaired. *ASHA* 33 suppl 3 (1991), 22–24.

86. Chermak GD, Musiek F: Managing central auditory processing disorder in children and youth. *Am J Audiol* 1 (1992), 61–65.

87. Schneider D: Audiologic management of children with central auditory processing disorders, in Katz J, Stecker, Henderson *Central Auditory Process: A Transdisciplinary View* (St. Louis: Mosby-Year Book, 1992).

88. Kahn MS: Learning problems of the secondary and junior college learning disabled student: Suggested remedies. *J Learn Disabil* 13 (1980), 40–44.

89. Keith RW: *Central Auditory and Language Disorders in Children* (San Diego, CA: College-Hill Press, 1981).

90. Katz J, Stecker, Henderson: *Central Auditory Process: A Transdisciplinary View* (St. Louis: Mosby Year Book, Publishers, 1992).

91. Levinson P, Sloan C: *Auditory Processing and Language* (New York: Grune & Stratton, 1980).)

92. Lasky E, Katz J: *Central Auditory Processing Disorders: Problems of Speech, Language and Learning* (Baltimore: University Park Press, 1983).

6

THE PSYCHO-EDUCATIONAL ASSESSMENT OF CHILDREN WITH HEARING IMPAIRMENT

Robert E. Kretschmer

> *Synergy means behavior of whole systems unpredicted by the behavior of their parts.*
>
> —Richard Buckninster Fuller, 1895–1983

At the heart of most direct services provided by the school psychologist are the psycho-educational evaluation and the *diagnostic-prescriptive* process. The goals of this chapter are to provide relevant definitions of terms connected with the notions of *evaluation and the diagnostic process* and to discuss topics related to the assumptions and prerequisites of conducting any evaluation, especially that of a student with hearing impairment. Issues related to the identification and placement process and the application of various evaluation materials and results to the programming of individual children will also be addressed.

THE DIAGNOSTIC PROCESS

The term "diagnostic process," as used by practicing psychologists, appears to have taken on two meanings or connotations. The first of these relates to the entire sequence of events associated with a child with a handicap moving through the educational system from the point when a handicapping condition is suspected to the actual placement and programming for a child. A second, more limited meaning of this term refers to the sequence of events that any given individual professional within this larger framework goes through to arrive at his or her own conclusions about the functional status of the child suspected of having a disabling condition.

When the diagnostic process is thought of as a movement through the educational placement and programming system, the sequence of events generally involves: (1) the screening of individual children to identify those who possibly need special educational consideration; (2) the actual certification by one or more specific professionals of the disabling conditions; (3) the verification by a team of individuals, including the parents or their representatives, of one or more handicapping conditions; (4) the making and delineating of various placement and programmatic decisions, if any are required; and, finally, (5) the actual implementation of the prescribed program and the subsequent follow-through monitoring evaluations, as required by law.[1]

Although many children with severe and profound hearing impairment will have been certified and verified as disabled before they enter school, they typically will still go through the diagnostic process in order to be placed within the educational system. Many children with mild or moderate hearing loss, high frequency hearing loss, and unilateral hearing loss may initially be identified through auditory screening procedures. Other forms of screening commonly used to identify disabled children are visual screening through the use of such instruments as the Snellen chart, developmental screening during kindergarten or first grade *round-ups*, and school-wide achievement testing programs. Thus, one definition of *screening* is the use of any systematic behavioral observation, checklist, rating scale, or objective test to initially establish the possibility of a disability (see Chapter 2).

Once a child has been screened and a potential disabling condition is suspected, a sequence of events is set into motion. Usually, a referral is made to those individuals within the school system who are responsible for making sure that all the necessary information pertinent to the resolution of the particular child's educational problems is gathered. This would include collecting a social and family history, obtaining informed consent for further diagnostic testing, and scheduling the necessary evaluations with one or more professionals.

The ultimate goal of the diagnostic process is to obtain the necessary information to make appropriate decisions regarding placement and subsequent programming of individual children. Ideally and legally, this process should be performed by a team, which would include the participation of the parents and the child. Deciding whether a child is disabled and in need of special educational consideration is a group process; a disabling condition is verified by the documented "diagnosis" of the disabilities made by a *multidisciplinary team* (M-team) or *transdisciplinary team* (T-team) after reviewing and synthesizing all the pertinent background information, observations, and test materials collected on a child. Although the team of individuals, including the classroom teacher and the parents, verifies the salient disabling conditions, individual members of the team may certify specific disabilities appropriate to their professional specialties and disciplines. Each professional, at the conclusion of his or her evaluation, generally presents a series of recommendations. The *individual education program* (IEP), *individual family service plan* (IFSP), or *individualized transition plan* (ITP) is the composite of the recommendations of all the M- or T-team members with regard to educational placement and programming. These recommendations should be written in behavioral terms or learning outcomes and should address all major aspects of development and the child's specific strengths and weaknesses. In addition to specific recommendations, time frames and performance criteria are to be specified, as well as the person who is to implement each recommendation.

These studies and tests may help in meeting the spirit of the law, which requires that the child be evaluated in his native language or mode of communication unless it is clearly not feasible to do so.[1]

ASSUMPTIONS UNDERLYING TESTING

A number of assumptions underlie any evaluation processs. Newland[2] in considering the case of psychological testing, cites six such assumptions. The first is that the person administering the test is properly trained to do so. Any violation of this assumption could yield results of questionable validity. Recently, several national and regional surveys of psychological services for individuals with hearing impairment have been conducted.[3-8] Each of these studies has indicated

that the majority of the providers of these services do not have formal or special preparation to work with deaf persons. For example, in 1974, Levine[3] in a national survey found that only 10% of her respondents were employed on a full-time basis to work with persons with deafness, and only 17% of the sample had specialized training to do so. Although progress has been made in some areas, in other areas it has not and the majority of school psychologist working with youngsters who are deaf and hard of hearing continue to be ill prepared to do so. For example, in a recent national survey of school psychologists selected from the membership rolls of the National Association for School Psychologist,[8] 54% of all the respondents indicated that they had responsibility of working with students who are deaf and hard of hearing, but only two individuals reported working full-time with these populations. Of those who worked with students having hearing loss, only 41% of the respondents reported having had some form of special training, minimal as it might be, and 75% rated themselves as having poor or no sign language proficiency.

The issue of communication difficulty, and the possible test bias resulting from failure to understand the directions of a test, are at the heart of a number of Furth's studies[9] and a study by Ray.[10] They, as well as Vernon and Brown,[11] note that failure to perform on a task may simply be a function of not understanding the directions, rather than an inherent disability. It is therefore essential that the examiner have experience with clients who are deaf and be proficient in all forms of communication used by people who are deaf. Those tests that have been standardized on persons with hearing loss have usually taken into account the problem of communication and have provided for standardized instructions and procedures. For example, the Hiskey-Nebraska Test of Learning Aptitude has two sets of instructions, one verbal and one pantomime, and the Stanford Achievement Test-Hearing-Impaired, 8th edition, has a series of special instructions and practice items for each battery level. Unfortunately, most of the tests that have not been standardized on hearing-impaired people have verbal directions. Some notable exceptions are the Leiter International Performance Scale and the Chicago Nonverbal Examination, which have essentially pantomime directions. (The references for all the tests can be found in either Salvia and Ysseldyke[12] or Mitchell.[13])

Investigations into the influence of various forms of test administration and modification for the Wechsler Intelligence Scale for Children-Revised (WISC-R) Performance Scale have been conducted by Sullivan,[14] Courtney et al,[15] and Ray.[10] Courtney et al[15] found that when subjects were administered the WISC-R Performance Scale exclusively by means of pantomime gestures, the resulting effect was a 5 intelligence quotient (IQ) point decrement (resulting IQ = 90) when compared to the Anderson and Sissco[16] norms for children and youths with hearing impairment. Likewise, Sullivan,[14] in comparing pantomime, visual aids, and total communication test administration modifications (using a residential school sample of children with genetic, questionable, and multiply disability etiologies) found an even greater decrement when using pantomime gestures (IQ = 88). Although the use of visual aids resulted in slightly better performance, they—with the use of pantomime directions—still resulted in as much as a 15 point poorer performance than when total communication was used, and the use of an interpreter as an intermediary for those psychologists not familiar with manual forms of communication did not seem to be an attractive alternative either.

Ray attempted to investigate the possibility that the Performance Scale scatter profile, often associated with the Wechsler Scales for children with hearing impairments, was a function of misunderstanding the task, due to certain communication variables. Although he was not entirely able to demonstrate this, he did provide the field with a standardized method of administration for the performance section of the WISC-R, which can be used with any child with hearing impairment, whether the child relies on oral communication, simultaneous communication, or gestures/pantomime; and he was able to eliminate the typical overall decrement associated with most forms of test modification. Braden[17] in reviewing a large body of psychometric data found that the Ray procedure yielded a significantly higher mean IQ (103.87) than sign and speech, speech alone, or written directions.

The second assumption noted by Newland[2] is that any test only samples behavior to some statistically satisfactory degree of adequacy. By this, it is meant that the test should be both reliable and valid. These two terms are discussed in detail in Chapter 4. In brief, a reliable test is one that yields similar scores for individuals after repeated administrations over time. Validity, on the other hand, is the degree to which a test actually measures what it purports to measure. A valid test by definition must be a reliable test, but the

reverse is not true. These notions of reliability and validity refer to both norm-referenced and criterion-referenced tests. Thus, even teacher-made tests should demonstrate reliability and validity.

The third assumption underlying psychological testing is that the individuals on whom a particular test is to be used have been exposed to learning experiences or acculturation comparable to the original norming group. This particular point addresses itself directly to the issue of test bias. That is, a test can only be considered valid in relationship to particular individuals or groups of individuals. What may be valid for one group of individuals may not be valid for another group. This notion of test bias has been the point of much discussion and the source of much litigation, which has finally resulted in certain statements being made within the federal mandate governing the rights of all children with disabilities.[1]

This mandate has stated that information concerning cultural and social background, among a number of other variables, must be taken into account when making placement decisions and when planning for any child with a disability. Newland[2] has suggested that validity with respect to acculturation is probably not an all-or-nothing matter, but, rather, there are degrees of validity. Also, the mere fact that a test is normed on a population or that certain subcultures were included in the norming process does not guarantee a nonbiased valid test. The fact that other subgroups were excluded from the norming process does not automatically invalidate a test's use with these subgroups. If the test can be found to perform the same function with a special group as it does with the normed population, then it should be considered valid. In fact, this has been the focus of much of the psychological literature on the population that is hearing impaired, which will be discussed later in this chapter.

This notion of test bias is complicated not only by the issue of hearing impairment, but also by the fact that a large percentage of the population that is hearing impaired is comprised of individuals from backgrounds other than Caucasian, whereby the culture may be different and English may not be the language spoken in the home.

The fourth assumption noted by Newland[2] is that error is associated with all measurement. This means that the instruments used, the conditions under which the individual is examined, and the examinee are not perfect. This is true even under what are seemingly ideal testing conditions. Because of this implicit error, an individual's performance on any particular test is usually reported as a spread of scores, rather than a single score, which increases the chances of being accurate. The more that the testing situation departs from the ideal, the less accurate the obtained scores on a test become.

Finally, the fifth and sixth assumptions noted by Newland[2] are that only present behavior is observed and all future behavior, abilities, and disabilities are inferred. For example, when a youngster "fails a test," all that is observed is that the student did not complete the task as expected. Any statements concerning inability to complete the task or future behavior, although *educated* in nature and based on known relationships (predictive validity), are considered inferences rather than fact. In discussing the nature of psychoeducational evaluations and the diagnostic-prescriptive process, Ysseldyke and Salvia[18] advance four addition assumptions that are fairly self-explanatory. These four assumptions are:

1. Children enter into a teaching situation with identifiable strengths and weaknesses.
2. The strengths and weaknesses are causally related to academic success.
3. Strengths and weaknesses can be reliably and validly assessed.
4. Pupil performance on diagnostic devices interacts with intervention strategies to produce differential instructional gains.

These assumptions are thought to be in operation whether one is concerned with children with normal hearing or children with hearing impairment, and are central to the notion of individualized educational programming.

IDENTIFICATION AND PLACEMENT

Assessment data are collected for a number of purposes.[12] One of these purposes is for the classification and placement of individuals having disabilities in the most appropriate instructional setting possible. Two types of decisions are involved in this process. The first is whether a child should be placed in a special class or left in regular classes. The second has to do with choosing specific methodologies, teaching strategies, or communication modes that should be used with a child. The former decision is, in part, determined by the general philosophy of the school system. That is, if the system's organization is highly predicated on ability or homogeneous grouping the criteria for entrance into or staying within a particular classroom are apt to be very stringent. If, on the other hand, a more heterogeneous grouping philosophy is adopted, less stringent criteria will be used. Typically, though, most school systems have adopted a philosophy of homogeneous grouping and, as a result, have developed local plans that include a variety of placement options, although in recent years this has been challenged by advocates of *inclusion*. If the placement decision is to situate the child in a self-contained classroom, another decision must be made as to which classroom, implying further homogeneous grouping and often decisions as to what communication mode will be used. For the most part, these decisions will be based on the use of some form of norm-referenced test. That is, the child will be *grouped* with other children who perform similarly on a norm-referenced test. In fact, this is one of the primary values of such tests. These tests assist in making various classification, selection, and placement decisions and, when used in this manner, they can serve a legitimate function.

There are some unfortunate side effects of norm-referenced placement, however: (1) once the child is classified, he or she is labeled, and this label then becomes the explanation for all subsequent learning difficulties or behavioral styles; (2) an attempt might be made to use the norm-referenced test to develop diagnostic-prescriptive programs; and (3) there is not unanimity in the criteria used by various professionals in placing children with hearing impairments within the continuum of possible educational options.[19] The first situation is referred to as *nominalism*, and the second assumes that certain children, given a particular aptitude or ability, will learn better under one condition than under another. This situation refers to the second type of placement decision mentioned previously. Although it would be highly desirable to use these tests to develop individual programs, the research into "ability by treatment interactions" has not yet provided support for this notion.[20]

DOMAINS ASSESSED

Myklebust et al[21] have suggested a comprehensive evaluation scheme for individuals with hearing impairment in which information is collected in each of the following areas: (1) general background information and developmental history; (2) sensory functioning; (3) cognition or intelligence; (4) language and academic achievement; (5) psychomotor functioning; (6) social maturity and adaptive behavior; and (7) emotional adjustment. Given the comprehensive nature of this scheme, the same general framework will be adopted in this chapter for discussing the psycho-educational evaluation of individuals with hearing impairment.

History and Background Information

The first area to be considered in the evaluation of any youngster with a hearing loss is the collection of thorough birth, genetic, developmental, educational, familial, social/emotional, work (if applicable), and previous evaluation (including any previous speech and hearing, educational, medical, or psychological evacuations) histories. In addition to these areas of concern, parental expectations, attitudes, observations, judgments, and concerns should be obtained as well. When the referral source is not the parent but another professional, such as the teacher, the professional's expectations, attitudes, observations, judgments, and concerns should be elicited and recorded as well because the referring agents should feel that their concerns are recognized and considered when the evaluation process has been completed. Table 6-1 provides a brief overview of some of the major areas to be covered in a life history interview.

Although it is important to obtain as complete a history as possible on an individual, certain research studies have indicated that not all of these data are equally predictive of academic success or language development, which are often two of the major criteria used in placement decisions for children who are hearing impaired. There have been conflicting reports about the significance of the age at which a hearing disability is identified, the age at which initial training or admission to school begins, or the age at which amplification is initiated on predictions of academic success. However, Laughton[22] and Pressnell[23] found these variables to have an effect on the achievement of certain oral and written language structures and written language productivity. In terms of family characteristics, family size has been found to be related to academic success for integrated oral children, with children from

smaller families achieving more than children from larger families.[24]

Although certain parental attitudes, expectations, and child-rearing practices have been found to have low to moderate correlations with academic success, as defined by scores on tests of academic achievement, for orally integrated children who are hearing impaired, they have not generally been found to predict success, but with a few exceptions.[24] With young children, parental expectations for achievement potential were found to be highly predictive, but as the child became older, the predictive power of parental expectation decreased. Interestingly, the parental assessment of the child's athletic or artistic abilities became increasingly more important as a predictor when the child entered adolescence. Neuhaus[25] also found a definite relationship between the positive and negative attitudes of parents toward their children who are hearing impaired, and their children's subsequent emotion adjustment, which in turn should relate to academic success. Some researchers have noted that parents tend to overestimate the potentials and abilities of their children who are hearing impaired. Also, some parents tend to have unrealistic future expectations that reflect more their own ambitions than the capacities and abilities of their children.[24]

It is often generally assumed that hearing parents of children who are hearing impaired are at risk for psychiatric problems and marital difficulties.[26] Research conducted in this area[26-28] however, does not support these contentions.

It has been found that teacher ratings of intellectual ability correlate well with children's performance on the Leiter International Performance Scale,[29] and a teacher's initial assessment of the academic potential of children has been cited as a significant predictor of future academic success.[30] However, in considering this, one must entertain the possibility that a self-fulfilling prophecy may be in operation as much as a legitimate predictive relationship.

Finally, in terms of integrating children who are hearing impaired into a regular classroom, the regular teacher's attitude toward children with a handicap in general and children who are hearing impaired specifically should be considered. Alexander and Strain[31] have found that regular teachers often have negative attitudes about and may be less accepting of special education children introduced into their classrooms. The regular teacher's attitude toward the number of

Table 6–1 Life History Outline

Medical, Genetic, and Developmental	Clinical Evaluation	Family	Educational	Emotional and Social	Vocational	Familial Observations, Expectations, Judgments, and Attitudes	Teacher Observations, Expectations, Judgments, and Attitudes
Pre-, peri-, post-natal condition of mother and child	When first noticed hearing loss	Genetic basis for hearing loss	When entered school	Method and style of communication and interaction with family members	Vocational and pre-vocational training	Statement of suspected problem	Statement of suspected problem
Medical history of illness	When began to wear a hearing aid	Other disabling conditions	Type of school	Relationships with peers and neighbors	Work history	Cognitive abilities	Cognitive abilities
Genetic milestones	Type of hearing aid used	General family structure	How long in school	Relationship with community	Occupational preferences and goals	Language abilities	Language abilities
Sensory development	Auditory evaluations	Family milieu	Schools attended	Preference for friends (deaf or hearing)		Academic abilities	Academic abilities
Language development	Medical evaluations	Ethnic heritage	Academic achievement, adjustment, progress	Leisure time (play) activities and preferences		Sensory abilities	Sensory abilities
Cognitive development	Psychological evaluations	Extended family		Participation in deaf community		Emotional stability	Emotional stability
Emotional development	Educational evaluations	Religious background		Social interests		Social abilities	Social abilities
Social development	Other evaluations	Family values and belief systems		Marital preference and status		Vocational abilities	Vocational abilities
				Social independence			
				Self-evaluation and attitude toward self and deaf and hearing peers			

children who are hearing impaired that should be enrolled in a single classroom has been found to be predictive of academic success for oral integrated students.[24] The sensitivity of administrators to various individual differences and needs of these children is also predictive of academic success for these children.[24] Haring et al[32] have developed two instruments that may be helpful in determining the attitudes and knowledge of regular education teachers or administrators about various handicapping conditions, including hearing impairment. More recently, Berryman et al[33] revised their Attitudes Toward Mainstreaming Scale, which was meant to evaluate educators attitudes regarding various disabling conditions (particularly low incidence disabilities, including hearing impairment) and various aspects of mainstreaming in general.

Unfortunately, no studies investigating the predictive variables associated with integrating children who use the simultaneous or total form of communication are known to exist.

Sensory Functioning

Although the child possesses five basic senses, only two and possibly three are of concern here.

These are audition, vision, and possibly the tactile sense, given the increased use of tactile devices (see Table 6-2). Obviously, any child who has been identified and certified as hearing-impaired will have had an audiometric evaluation. Generally speaking, one would minimally expect an air conduction and (if possible) bone conduction pure-tone audiogram (aided and unaided), speech threshold, and (if possible) discrimination test results, and some statement or objective test results concerning the youngster's candidacy for amplification. In addition, there may be reports of middle ear functioning, as determined by immittance measures, and the results of any special testing that may be warranted by the child's particular case (see Chapter 2).

Although the child with hearing loss should have undergone a thorough audiological evaluation, the child's functional use of residual hearing may still be unknown. To fulfill a need in this area, the Test of Auditory Comprehension (TAC),[34] and the Developmental Assessment of Successful Listening II (DASL-II)[35] were developed. These tests were designed to evaluate the functional auditory status of children with moderate to profound hearing loss along the continuum of auditory skill development.

Table 6–2   Psycho-educational Assessment: Sensor Functioning

Audition	Vision	Taction
1. Hearing sensitivity	1. Visual acuity	No tests available
a) Pure-tone audiogram (a/c + b/c)	a) Snellen chart	
b) Speech detection/reception	b) Keystone Telebinocular	
c) Word discrimination	c) Bausch and Lomb Orthorator	
d) Tests of middle ear functioning	d) Titmus Vision Screener	
e) Results from hearing aid evaluation	2. Visual-motor perception	
f) Special Tests	a) Bender-Gestalt Test for Young Children	
2. Auditory perception	b) Frostig	
a) Test of Auditory Comprehension	c) Graham and Kendall Memory for Designs Test	
b) Developmental Approach to Successful Listening, II	d) Developmental Test of Visual-Motor Integration	
	e) Rey's Complex Figure Drawing	
	3. Motor-free tests of visual perception	
	a) Embedded Figures Test	
	b) Perceptual Speed Identical Form Test	
	c) Ratner's Test of Visual Perceptual Abilities[36]	
	d) Ratner's Test of Spatial Perception in Sign Language[37]	

More specifically, in the case of the TAC, the test was designed to assess the auditory discrimination of suprasegmentals and segmentals, memory sequencing, story comprehension, and figure-ground discrimination of children with hearing impairments ages 4 to 12 years, 11 months. The test was designed to be used as both a criterion-referenced, curriculum-based test in conjunction with its companion auditory training curriculum, as well as a norm-referenced test.

Although there were some technical problems in the selection of a standardization sample, the reliability and validity data presented in the manual suggest that this test and its associated auditory training curriculum may be useful. Additionally, according to the manual, because substantial and positive correlation were obtained between scores on this test and functioning within different types of educational settings, this test may he useful in making placement decisions.

As a part of the DASL-II, a test is provided that has been designed to place a child within the curriculum and, thus, is to be used as a criterion-referenced, not a norm-referenced test. The curriculum placement test has three parts that correspond to the curriculum against which it is referenced. The three areas evaluated are sound awareness, phonetic listening, and auditory comprehension.

An individual with an auditory sensory impairment is typically required to rely more heavily on the senses of vision and touch. Of these two, more attention has been given to the screening and evaluation of vision, although interest should also be directed toward taction, given the increased interest and use of tactile devices. The reported incidence of visual problems has ranged from 6%[38] to slightly more than 50%.[39] Although this range is large, there exists general agreement that the incidence of visual problems is greater for individuals with hearing impairment than individuals with normal hearing.

Many of these visual problems do not appear to be sensitivity problems. Greene,[40] for example, using a sophisticated in-depth optometric clinical screening program, noted that the combined categories of binocularity problems and pathologic states were greater than all of the categories of refractive errors. Greene also commented on the inefficiency of the typical screening programs that consist of only the Snellen chart. The Snellen chart could account for the identification of only 23% of his sample of children with visual and hearing impairments. He further noted that other typical vision screening instruments, such as the Keystone Telebinocular, the Bausch and Lomb Orthorator, and the Titmus Vision Screener, although improvements over the simple Snellen chart, are still incomplete. Thus, he recommended the establishment of a complete optometric clinical screening program, as do Walters et al.[41]

As noted previously, some children failing vision tests might do so not because of acuity problems, but rather because of some form of "perceptual" problem. Essentially, a perceptual problem is one in which the person is unable to be aware of (as opposed to sense), organize, or understand particular stimuli. Thus, although the sense receptor is intact, the "sensor" is unable to understand or has difficulty in processing the visual stimulus. This difficulty apparently can be a function of the individual, the stimulus structure, or the interaction of the two. Occasionally, the term "visual perceptual problem," as used by some psychologists and other special service providers, refers to difficulty in visual-motor integration. That is, this "perceptual problem" manifests itself in the inability to copy specified designs or figures. Actually, the inability to complete such a task may be due to either difficulties in visually analyzing and organizing stimuli or to the execution of the motor act in making a visual-motor match. In terms of the former, Locher and Worms[42] have suggested that visual perceptual difficulties may actually be due to difficulties in focusing or regulating attention (a type of meta-cognition), rather than an actual visual disability. Such inappropriate scanning of the visual stimulus would not permit the youngster to extract effectively all the necessary information to respond adequately to the task.

Among the most common visual-motor tasks used by psychologists in their assessments of children are the Bender-Gestalt Test for Young Children (Bender-Gestalt), the Graham and Kendall Memory for Designs Test, and the Developmental Test of Visual-Motor Integration (VMI). Salvia and Ysseldyke[12] have indicated that most tests of visual motor perception lack the technical adequacy to be used in making important instructional decisions. Despite this, these tests are often used in the evaluation of most children, including children with hearing impairments, and they have been used in various research projects. Generally speaking, when a child is found to have a deficit in this area, it is usually interpreted to mean that either the child has a legitimate visual-motor or visual-perception problem, possibly symptomatic of "minimal brain damage," or emotional difficulties and anxieties. Unfortunately, there is little empirical evidence to support these claims for most of these tests. This is not to suggest that such "causes," however, are not possible.

A few of these instruments have been used in research projects with individuals having hearing loss with inconsistent results. Although many hearing-impaired individuals are found to perform poorly on the Bender-Gestalt Test, Keogh et al[43] have found the interjudge reliability scoring of these drawings to be very poor. Interestingly, in contrast to the findings of poor visual motor integration, Blair[44] among others, has found subjects with hearing impairments to do well on a memory-for-designs test, which involves a design drawing component in addition to a memory component. Conflicting results have been reported for other such "perceptual" tests, which may be due to the unreliability of the tests themselves. As a result, these tests should probably only be used as a rough screening instrument and only grossly deviant reproductions should be considered abnormal.

The fact that visual perceptual functioning is difficult to assess does not detract from its possible importance. Sharp[45] attempted to isolate the visual perceptual correlates of speech-reading in children by comparing the performance of good and poor speech-readers on various measures of visual perceptual and visual perceptual speed tasks. She found that performances on the Porteus Mazes, the Visual Sequential Memory subtest of the Illinois Test of Psycholinguistic Abilities (ITPA) which is a memory task involving geometric designs, and three tests specially designed by the researcher (Rhythm Patterns: A Test of Movement, the Hidden Figures Test, and the Hidden Objects Test) were all related to good speech-reading ability. The latter two tests essentially were figure-ground tests. These results, then, suggest that visual memory for movement, rhythm perception, speed of visual perception, and figure-ground ability are associated with speech-reading ability. To date, there have been relatively few studies investigating the visual-perceptual correlates of sign language ability and acquisition. Siple et al,[46] in a longitudinal study, investigated the visual perceptual correlates of sign language acquisition by students who were deaf and had hearing at the National Technical Institute for the Deaf. Two different sets of predictors were isolated. For the students who

are hearing impaired, whose initial sign language scores were poor, improvement in sign language ability was significantly associated with initial scores on a rapid visual perceptual discrimination test (Perceptual Speed Identical Form Test) and the Embedded Figures Test. The predictors of the individuals' progress who were hearing in sign language were initial performances on the Flags Test, involving spatial manipulation, and the Visual Closure Speed Test, which assesses the speed at which an individual can recognize or infer a whole from minimal cues. These results suggested to the investigators that the individuals with deafness acquired facility in sign language by attending to details and analyzing the whole, whereas individuals with normal hearing used a process of synthesizing whole patterns and gestalts.

Recently, Ratner[36,37] developed two tests designed to evaluate the visual perceptual abilities of children who are deaf as they might relate to the visual processing of sign language. The Test of Spatial Perception in Sign Language (TSPSL) is a 47 item videotaped test designed to evaluate the ability to discern various dynamic features and aspects of signs. The Test of Visual Perceptual Abilities (TVPA) is divided into two parts: Part I consists of six subtests evaluating various aspects of static visual perception and Part II consists of six subtests designed to evaluate certain dynamic properties associated with visual perception. Both tests were shown to identify individuals with visual perpetual deficits that interfere with sign language comprehension and that each subtest of the TVPA tapped different visual perceptual abilities and contributed separately and differently to performance on the TSPSL.

Cognition (Intelligence)

The intent of testing in this domain is to obtain general and specific measures of intelligence, creativity, and the mode of internalized mediation. The intelligence tests most widely used with individuals with hearing impairments are shown in Table 6-3.

Only the Hiskey-Nebraska Test of Learning Aptitude was specifically designed for and standardized on the population with hearing impairments. Although a few other scales standardized on individuals with hearing impairments are available, the Hiskey-Nebraska and several tests not standardized on persons with hearing impairments

Table 6–3 Psycho-educational Assessment: Cognition (Intelligence)

Tests Available
1. Wechsler Scales
   Adult Intelligence Scale (WAIS)
   Adult Intelligence Scale-Revised (WA1S-R)
   Intelligence Scale for Children (WISC)
   Intelligence Scale for Children-Revised (WISC-R)
   Intelligence Scale for Children-III (WISC-III)
2. Hiskey-Nebraska Test of Learning Aptitude*
3. Harris-Goodenough Draw-A-Man
4. Leiter International Performance Scale
5. Leiter International Performance Scale— Arthur Adaptation
6. Raven's Colored Progressive Matrices
7. Naglieri's Nonverbal Matrix Tests
8. Kaufman Assessment Battery Test for Children
9. Learning Potential Assessment Device[47]
10. Torrance Tests of Creative Thinking
11. Test for Internal Speech

*This is the only intelligence test specifically designed for and standardized on individuals with hearing impairments.

Table 6–4 Subtests of the Wechsler Tests

	Test			
Subtest	*WAIS and WAIS-R*	*WISC and WISC-R*	*WISC III*	*WPSSI and WPPSI-R*
Verbal				
Information	X	X	X	X
Comprehension	X	X	X	X
Similarities	X	X	X	X
Arithmetic	X	X	X	X
Vocabulary	X	X	X	X
Digit Span	X	X	X	X
Sentences				X
Performance				
Picture Completion	X	X	X	X
Picture Arrangement	X	X	X	
Block Design	X	X	X	X
Object Assembly	X	X	X	
Coding	X	X	X	X
Mazes	X	X	X	X
Symbol Search			X	
Geometric Design				X

are in much greater use in this country. Although not standardized on the populations with hearing impairments, the Leiter scales do not require verbal instructions.

The Wechsler Scales probably have been the most researched instrument used with the population with hearing impairments. Presumably because of the popularity of the WISC-R, norms for the population with hearing impairments have been developed.[16] A newly developed version of this test has recently been published, the WISC-III. Although the manual states that 7% of the standardization sample included learning disabled, emotionally disturbed and physically disabled individuals, no individual who is deaf or hard of hearing was included. Because of its newness, separate norms have yet to be developed for this test, if they will be at all.

The Wechsler tests are comprised of two scales, each containing a series of subtests. The two scales are a Verbal Scale, in which sets of verbal questions are posed to the examinee, and a Performance Scale involving various manipulation tasks. More precisely, the verbal scale is comprised of six subtests, (See Table 6–4) These subtests are as follows:

1. *Information*, which requires the subject to answer factual, academic type questions.
2. *Comprehension*, which involves answering open-ended question concerning various social conventions, institutions, practices, and procedures, requiring one to make explicit one's social and cultural awareness and knowledge, social problem solving, practical knowledge, and social judgment.
3. *Arithmetic*, requiring the solution of orally presented story problems.
4. *Similarities*, which asks individuals to induce a superordinate term, such as dishes, when given the two subordinate terms cup and saucer, involving the understanding of semantic, or conceptual, entailments.
5. *Vocabulary*, which asks the individual to define word, involving verbal preciseness and the understanding of and ability to articulate semantic entailments.
6. *Digit span* (optional), in which the subject has to recall a series of digits presented orally.
7. *Sentences* (only on the Wechsler Preschool and Primary Scale of Intelligence [WPPSI] and the revised WPPSI [WPPSI-R]), in which the subject has to repeat sentences of increasing length and syntactic difficulty.

The performance scale is also comprised of six subtest (five in the case of the WPPSI and WPPSI-R and seven in the case of the WISC-III), one of which is optional (two in the case of the WISC-III):

1. *Picture Completion*, requiring the individual to identify missing parts of familiar objects, involving object knowledge and the

ability to recognize and distinguish essential from nonessential details.

2. *Picture Arrangement*, requiring the individual to sequence a series of pictures so as to tell a sensible story involving event knowledge, the understanding of social conventions and cause and effect relationships, and the ability to note details. (Neither the WPPSI nor the WPPSI-R have this subtest.)

3. *Block Designs*, which requires the individual to copy mosaic design utilizing a series of multicolored block cubes involving visual analysis and the ability to note part-to-whole relationships.

4. *Object Assembly*, which is a type of jigsaw picture puzzle tasks of familiar objects involving visual synthesis and the ability to note part-to-whole relationships. (Neither the WPPSI nor the WPPSI-R have this subtest.)

5. *Coding* (called Digit Span in the WAIS and WAIS-R and Animal House in the WPPSI and WPPSI-R), which is a symbol association task whereby the individual is to draw a simple design underneath a series of randomly distributed numbers based on a key that is provided, involving the ability to make rapid symbol associations.

6. *Mazes* (optional), which requires the individual to trace through a series of mazes requiring, reflectivity, forethought, and planning ability.

7. *Symbol Search* (WISC-III only, optional), which requires the individual to determine whether one of two geometric designs is present in an array of four geometric drawings, requiring systematic visual search and speed of processing.

8. *Geometric Designs* (WPSSI and WPSSI-R only), which requires the individual to copy geometric designs, similar to the Bender Gestalt Test of Visual Perception, requiring visual perceptual analysis and visual-motor integration.

Because there are two scales and a number of subtests each yielding their own scores, it is possible to have interscale and subtest comparisons on an individual and to engage in profile analyses to determine relative strengths and weakness. Indeed, this practice was and is so pervasive that the authors of the WISC-III, as a part of their statistical treatment of the normative data, have provided a series of *significant difference*, *frequency*, and *scatter* tables and developed a series of *Index Scores* based on factor analytic models derived from earlier versions of the test. These indexes are: Verbal Comprehension (the composite of Information, Similarities, Vocabulary, and Comprehension), Perceptual Organization (Picture Completion, Picture Arrangement, Block Designs, and Object Assembly), Freedom from Distractibility (Arithmetic and Digit Span) and Speed of Processing (Coding and Symbol Search). Extreme care, however, must be taken when performing such analyses and comparisons, even in the case of the WISC-III in which more rigor is available in interpreting intersubtest differences because serious placement and intervention system decisions may be based on unreliable or chance or error factors. Taking this point into account, however, the Wechsler tests still permit one to observe an individual's performance under several conditions, and it is the only test mentioned in this chapter that permits the comparison of both verbal and nonverbal performances.

In the case of individuals with hearing impairments, it has become almost axiomatic that the verbal sections of these tests are considered invalid as measures of intellectual abilities because they are assumed to be testing language and language functioning opposed to inherent *intellectual* or *cognitive abilities*.[11] (Henceforth, any reference to any of the Wechsler Scales will refer to the Performance section only unless otherwise stated.) Although it may be true that failure to perform on the Verbal Scale of these tests might be caused by a failure to understand specific questions or other related language factors, rather than a lack of more basic cognitive skills required to acquire the necessary information, the ability to score well on this test is still highly correlated with and related to academic achievement. As a result, it would be very helpful to obtain Verbal Scale scores, whenever and however possible, to assess the ability of persons with hearing impairments to compete verbally with hearing peers. Such scores should properly be treated as verbal achievement scores and be reported in the language or academic achievement section of any psycho-educational report. It has been demonstrated that there can be as large as a 16 to 44 IQ point difference between the overall performance scores and verbal scores on these scales for middle childhood to adolescent children who are hard of hearing[48] and adults with congenital deafness.[49,50] Most recently, in a study using the WISC-III, a group of 30 children with severe to profound deafness in which the verbal section of the Wechsler scale was communicated via American Sign Language or Pidgin Signed English, as the case warranted, presented a 25.7 IQ point discrepancy between the Verbal and Performance Scales in favor of the latter.[51] The discrepancy between verbal and performance scores has been noted to be greater for students with congenital deafness than for children who are hard of hearing or have post-lingual deafness,[52] and seems to be related to the degree and type of high-frequency hearing loss in Caucasian children only.[53] It should be pointed out that Hine[48] found the Picture Arrangement subtest correlated best with the results of the Verbal Scale. This correlation, although low, was positive and statistically significant.

A number of studies have attempted to determine whether youngsters and adults with hearing impairments did as well on the Wechsler Performance tests as individuals with normal hearing, and whether a characteristic profile of subtest performance could be identified. The majority of these studies have found little or no difference between the overall performance of the two populations. The composite of the results of these studies suggests that a characteristic profile of subtest performance for the population with hearing impairments may exist. This composite profile seems to have the following characteristics:

1. Performance on the Picture Completion subtest varies from slightly less than the hearing mean to slightly above it.
2. Performance on the Picture Arrangement subtest varies from no difference to slightly less than the hearing mean.
3. Performance on the Block Designs subtest ranges from no difference to slightly above the hearing mean.
4. Performance on the Object Assembly subtest ranges from the hearing mean to slightly above it.
5. Performance on the Coding subtest ranges from no difference to slightly below the hearing mean.

In a meta-analysis of 25 studies using the Wechsler scales, Braden[54] derived weighted mean scale scores of 9.41, 9.26, 9.89, 9.92, and 8.77, respectively, for these subtests. As can be seen, these mean scores tend to mirror the relative profile previously suggested, although only the mean scale score for coding was found to be significantly deviant. Thus, Braden suggested that only poor performance on this subtest should be considered characteristic of the population with deafness. As Braden himself noted, however, these weighted mean scores included the results of four studies that used the WISC-R deaf norms that would "wash out" any characteristic profile information and would serve to depress the overall differences. No information is available on the general performance of deaf persons and persons with hearing impairments on the Symbol Search subtest of the WISC-III, as of yet.

The previously mentioned profile appears to be more evident with the younger children with deafness and is statistically controlled for in the norms provided by Anderson and Sissco[16] for the WISC-R. Ray[10] has challenged the utility of these norms because they were compiled post hoc and no attempt was made to control for standardization of the administration procedures. Sullivan[14] argued that the previously mentioned profile was an artifact of test administration modifications. Thus, norms are available, but they are not standardized. Some investigators have attempted to determine the reliability, validity, and utility of the Wechsler scales with individuals with hearing impairments. In general, the WISC and the WISC-R have been found to correlate moderately well to well with such other measures of intelligence as the Hiskey-Nebraska,[55,56] and the WISC-R has been found to be a reliable instrument when used with persons with deafness.[57] The overall performance IQ of the WISC has been found to be predictive of academic success,[30,58] and performance on all of the subtests (with the exception of Mazes) of this test has been found to discriminate between high and low academic achievers. The Picture Arrangement, Block Design, and Coding subtests in particular discriminate well between high and low achievers,[59] and it has been noted that these same three subtests correlate significantly with speech-reading ability.[60] (The WISC is no longer in print and not now used, so the reader is cautioned to be conservative and tentative in generalizing these specific findings to subsequent versions of the WISC even though each version of this test shares much of the same item pool.)

Similarly, scores on the WISC-R PIQ correlate moderately well and, thus, predicts to some degree scores on the Stanford Achievement Test for the Hearing-Impaired (SAT-HI).[61] Correlations between WISC-R PIQ and percentile ranks on the SAT-HI ranged from 0.33 (spelling) to 0.57 (concept number). Reading Comprehension on the SAT-HI correlated 0.39 with the WISC-R PIQ. It has been also been noted that comparable result are obtained when youngsters at the upper-age limits of the WISC-R are subsequently evaluated using the WAIS-R.[62] Thus far, only one study using children who are deaf has been conducted utilizing the WISC-III and that was a study reported in the manual itself. This study of 20 students who were severely and 10 who were profoundly deaf were administered the WISC-III via American Sign Language or Pidgin Signed English and yielded a mean performance IQ of 105.8, a mean Perceptual Organization Index score of 106.0, and a mean Processing Speed Index score of 101.4.

The Hiskey-Nebraska Test of Learning Aptitude is the only commonly used test of intelligence designed specifically for the population in this country who are hearing impaired. Because of this, some individuals have used it as the standard against which other tests are measured. The test has 12 subtests, many of which involve visual memory, and two sets of directions and norms (ie, verbal directions and hearing norms, and pantomime directions and hearing-impaired norms). Salvia and Ysseldyke,[12] in reviewing the technical adequacy of the test, note several limitations and suggest that the results should be interpreted with caution. Watson[63] established moderate test-retest reliability even after a 5-year interval ($r = 0.65$). Watson and Goldgar[64] found high concurrent validity when the Hiskey was compared to the WISC-R, except that the Hiskey yielded a greater number of subjects with extreme upper and lower limits scores. It has also been reported that the Hiskey-Nebraska scores correlate highly with such various measures of academic success as the Stanford Achievement Test, the Gates Reading Test, the Metropolitan Achievement Test, teacher ratings of academic achievement in the early elementary years but not during the middle school and adolescent years (eg, grades 5 to 9)[65] and the Peabody Individual Achievement Tests.[66] Also, the Hiskey Learning Quotient (LQ) score and those subtests stressing visual memory have been found to be moderately predictive of performance on the Test of Language Development and the Reynell Developmental Language Scales administered via total communication.[67] Finally, it has been noted that the Block Patterns, Paper Folding, Picture Association, and the Visual Attention Span subtests, in particular, are predictive of academic achievement with 6- to 12-year-old orally trained children with deafness.[68]

The Leiter International Performance Scale and its Arthur adaptation have also been used to assess the individual with hearing impairment and have been found to be highly predictive of academic achievement, as defined by teacher ratings and performance on tests of reading, despite their technical inadequacy.[12] This relationship has even held up longitudinally over an 11- to 13-year period.[58,68] Bonham[69] found the Leiter, in combination with the WISC, to be an exceptionally good predictor of success in the reading comprehension subtests of the Metropolitan Achievement Test. The Leiter was designed to be used with individuals with speech and language difficulties, ages 2 to 18 years, and was standardized on a hearing sample. The Arthur adaption is identical to the original Leiter but is only appropriate for children ages 2 to 12 years. There are no subtests to these tests; instead, they are comprised of a series of graduated but essentially unrelated tasks. To facilitate test interpretation, Levine et al[70] have suggested an item classification scheme. In a series of concurrent validity studies, the Leiter has been found to correlate well with numerous other tests, including the Hiskey-Nebraska,[71] the Ravens Colored Progressive Matrices,[72] the WISC[72] and the ITPA.[73] Although the Leiter has been found to be predictive of academic achievement, and appears to be sensitive to learning problems, Ratcliffe and Ratcliffe[74] warn that caution should be exercised when using this instrument in decisions of placement, since a few studies using both hearing and youngsters with hearing impairments have found as much as an 11 to 20 or more point discrepancy between scores on this and other tests. Also, Mira[71] found that the test-retest reliability for young children with deafness was low (with a reliability coefficient of 0.36).

The Standard Ravens Progressive Matrices and its revision, the Ravens Colored Progressive Matrices, have been used in a few research projects with individuals with hearing impairments, despite the fact that at the time that those research studies were conducted no norms were available in the United States (only European norms were available). As of 1986, however, norms have been available in the United States.[75] In essence, the test involves the pattern completion of a number of items. The Ravens Colored Progressive Matrices have been described as tapping a special aspect of intelligence, and some believe that it measures pure g (pure global or general intelligence). Carlson,[76] however, provides data on children with hearing that suggest that on the Colored Progressive Matrices, sets A and Ab test perceptual pattern completion, whereas set B actually evaluates the ability to solve analogies by operations or rules. The composite picture from studies using the Ravens Colored Progressive Matrices with individuals who are hearing impaired suggests that younger children have difficulty with the test, but that by the time they become young adults, performance improves.[77] Goetzinger and Houchins[78] and Ritter[72] found essentially normal performance with younger children who are deaf and children with hearing impairments. Ritter also found the Colored Progressive Matrices to correlate well with the Leiter and moderately well with the WISC, and James[79] found a high correlation with the WISC-R.

In recent years, a newly developed, well-constructed performance test involving the completion of various matrix analogies similar to the Raven Matrices Tests has been developed (ie, the Matrix Analogies Test-Expanded form [RMT-EF]).[80] Unfortunately, few studies have been conducted with this test, although it does seem to hold promise. Naglieri and colleagues[81] have found that for children with severe to profound deafness, performance on this test correlates well with the performance scale of the WISC-R ($r = 0.71$)[81] and for children 11 to 16 years old who are severely and profoundly deaf, performance on this test correlated well with performance on the Standard Progressive Matrices whether using European or United States norms (ie, $r = .79$ for both).[82] Additionally, performance on this test did not differ from performance on the Standard Progressive Matrices using United States norms but both differed from scores derived from the European norms. Mean average performance on these tests were as follows: 84.5 (RMT-EF), 84.7 (Raven's United States norms), and 89.7 (Raven's European norms). The lower overall performance on these tests is consistent with earlier studies and may be related to difficulty in handling multiple sources of information simultaneously, as suggested by Ottem.[83]

Historically, the use of the Standford Binet for individuals who are hearing impaired was considered ill advised, given that it was ostensively a test of verbal knowledge. Also, like the Leiter, earlier versions of the Binet contained no subtests, but rather were comprised of a series of graduated but, essentially, unrelated tasks. The most recent edition, the fourth, however, represents a substantial departure from this approach in that it is organized according to a series of verbal and performance subscales. Although no research has been conducted investigating the utility of this instrument with individuals with hearing impairments, it does hold promise given its technical

adequacy (eg, a short form reliability of 0.95 for a composite score of all the performance scales [Bead Memory, Pattern Analysis, Copying, Memory for Objects and Matrices] and a 0.91 correlation with the entire composite score).

The last two tests of intelligence that have received some attention from researchers in hearing impairment are the Harris-Goodenough Draw-A-Man test and, more recently, the Kaufman Assessment Battery for Children (KABC). Although early studies using the Draw-A-Man test found children with hearing impairment to do poorly on this test, more recent studies have found that children with hearing impairments perform within average limits up to 13 years of age.[49] After this age, decrement of performance to below average was found. As for the KABC, Porter and Kirby[84] established that children with deafness who were 7 to 12 years of age did not differ in their performance from the normative sample, nor was performance affected by the use of pantomime directions or directions communicated via American Sign Language. High correlations have been obtained between KABC scores and performance on the WISC-R, although KABC scores tend to be slightly lower than those on the WISC-R.[84-86] Moderate correlations have been obtained between KABC scores and scores on the Metropolitan Achievement Test[84] and on the Wide Range Achievement Test and the KABC reading subtests.[86] Similar findings were obtained by Gibbins[7] (ie, mean score = 100.3 on the KABC and a correlation of 0.84 with corresponding IQ scores derived from the WISC-R for youngsters born in the United States).

The Learning Potential Assessment Device, although using standard instruments or "tools," is not a standard test in the traditional sense. Rather, it is a collection of commercially available tests and some specially designed instruments for which no norms are reported or available. It is one of the newer instruments out of the growing trend away from "static" norm-referenced tests toward dynamic measures of learning ability or potential.[87] The 16 (5 verbal and 11 largely performative) instruments are to be used in a Test-Teach-Test paradigm, wherein the "teaching phase" is to follow the tenants of the author's theory of mediated learning, which is similar to and borrows heavily from the work and theory of Vygotsky.[88]

Mediated learning in this context emphasizes that the role of the examiner is one of assisting the child to regulate metacognitively in a clear and accurate manner the input, elaboration, and output phases of the child's information processing, and to guide and provoke the use of appropriate learning strategies that will, it is hoped, generalize or transcend to other stimuli and events. (Pedagogically and in terms of language development, this has been referred to as *scaffolding*.) The extent to which this can be done is a measure of the child's modifiability and potential for learning. Keane and Kretschmer[89] reported on the application of this technique and noted its superiority in assessing the learning potential of children with deafness over that of traditional psychometric approaches and even dynamic approaches that provide feedback.

The Torrance Test of Creative Thinking is a test of cognitive functioning. More precisely, it purports to measure an individual's flexibility, fluency, originality, and elaborative skills of thinking. Both verbal and performative tasks are available. Laughton[87] recommended that the Torrance Thinking Creatively with Pictures, Form A be included with the routine battery used to evaluate children with hearing impairments, because in her study of children who had hearing loss, several scores derived from this measure were found to predict the development of morphological, phrase structure, and transformation rule usage. The originality score in particular predicted usage of all the linguistic structures studied, and the elaboration score aided in the prediction of morphological rule development. Kaltsounis[90] has demonstrated in a number of studies that children with hearing impairments did as well on this test as did children who can hear. Average to superior performance on the nonverbal form has been supported by several other studies.[91,92]

One of the implicit purposes in formal testing of intelligence and cognition is to gain some insights into the thinking and problem-solving abilities of the examinee. Of particular interest are insights into the examinee's ability to handle symbolic material because they may reveal information about the examinee's mediational processes and capacity to handle symbols in general. Occasionally, the results of some of the more symbolically oriented nonverbal subtests on intelligence tests (eg, the Picture Arrangement and Coding subtests on the Wechsler tests and the Picture Analogies or Picture Association subtests on the Hiskey-Nebraska test) are used for this purpose, and we already discussed the Learning Potential Assessment Device. Although these tests give us insight into the child's ability to deal with symbolically oriented materials, they do not directly assess the mode of internal symbolic representation. Mode of internalized representation must be inferred from behavioral observations and tests.

Recently, however, attempts have been made by some researchers to determine empirically the nature of the mediating process. Odom et al[93] and Bellugi et al[94] have suggested that with children with deafness, the mediating process involves the use of signs. Locke and Locke[95] made the alternative suggestion that children who can hear and many children who are deaf but with intelligible speech tend to recode internally certain visually presented symbolic material phonetically. Children with deafness without intelligible speech were found to prefer a dactylic (finger spelling) or visual recoding system. Conrad[96] reported on a series of studies he had conducted and argued that the use of a phonetic internal coding system probably is not an all or nothing matter, but exists in degrees. The use of a phonetic code by individuals with hearing impairments, according to Conrad, is strongly associated with their use of external intelligible speech, although he noted that many youngsters who are profoundly deaf and whose speech would be considered unintelligible use this code form. He concludes this from observing that their speech, although unintelligible to a listener, is consistent and probably *intelligible* to the speaker.

Lichtenstein[97] reporting on some of his unpublished research, stated that "syntactic skills (proper use of free functors) were related to WM [working memory] capacity and to the ability to efficiently use a speech-based coding strategy" (p.113; brackets mine) and that those individuals who failed to recode morphological endings to speech generally demonstrated lowered general knowledge of morphology. This seems logical, given that the orthographic regularities of written words are highly related (but not exactly correspondent) to the phonological regularities of written words. Precisely because of this overlap or confound, however, it is totally possible that some of the time, or at least for some individuals who are deaf, a visual orthographic strategy of encoding may be in operation. Indeed, it may be totally possible that at least a portion of those individuals previously identified as speech-based encoders are actually visual encoders exploiting certain visual and spelling orthographic regularities without recourse to speech and the graphophonemic correspondence between print and speech.[98,99] Lichtenstein[97] noted that skill in the use of English morphology was positively related to the ability to use a visual code.

Lichtenstein,[97] again reporting on unpublished data, noted that "for both speech and sign recoding, students who tended not to recode the function words during reading had poorer syntactic skills than those who consistently recoded functors. Thus, while the tendency to be selective in the recoding of free functors may be an adaptive strategy for coping with a limited WM (working memory) it may also effectively limit exposure to English grammatical information so as to cause serious gaps to develop in the students' knowledge of English syntax" (p. 113). Unfortunately, Lichtenstein did not elaborate on these points nor did he publish his stimuli, data, or analyses. Given his general description, however, it entirely possible that among the "functor" and morphological markers not recoded were critical cohesion devices, markers of new information, specifiers, modulators, deictic markers, adjuncts and disjuncts, all of which serve to bind text together, gives it its richness, and which serve to signal various pragmatic functions.

Conrad,[96] as a result of his work, has developed a testing procedure that he believes can discriminate between children who use a phonetic coding system and those who use a visual coding system. However, his test does not discriminate among individuals who might use other possible coding strategies (ie, those who might prefer finger spelling, signs, or a combination of all possible internal codes). Currently, Kretschmer and Martello[100] are in the process of developing a screening test designed to identify the preferred mode of encoding (speech, sign, visual) of young individuals with hearing impairments. Obviously, there is a need for such tests and for further research into what determines mediation preferences. Such knowledge should help in the decision-making process regarding placement and programming for children with hearing impairments.

Language and Academic Achievement

Although this is probably one of the most important areas to be assessed, few studies have been conducted using formal assessment techniques with the hearing-impaired (Table 6-5) As noted in the Cognition (Intelligence) section of this chapter, the verbal scale of the Wechsler test

has been used with hearing-impaired children and adults under limited circumstances. The results on this test, although very helpful in providing an index of the hearing-impaired child's verbal understanding of the world, do not specify more precisely the particular linguistic structures or lexical items (with a few exceptions) that the child knows. Ideally, in a full-language evaluation, all aspects of language functioning should be considered. This would include: (1) communication modality preference; (2) articulation skills in terms of speech and signs; (3) knowledge and use of morphological rules of English and American Sign Language, if appropriate; (4) knowledge and use of the syntactic rules of English and American Sign Language, if appropriate; (5) vocabulary or semantic aspects of the language used; (6) pragmatic uses of language; and (7) ability to engage in metalinguistic behaviors such as making judgments of grammaticality and being able to paraphrase, dealings with the metaphorical use of language and in the case of bilingual bicultural youngsters, preferences for, dominance, and abilities in a language other than English or signs.

To review all the possible issues and procedures associated with these topics is beyond the scope of this chapter. As a result, the reader will be referred to other resources when appropriate, for example, Ling[101] describes in detail a procedure for assessing speech. Recently, however, two very interesting approaches to assessing speech intelligibility have been developed by Monsen[102] and Monsen et al,[103] which are based on listener responses to speech uttered by individuals who are deaf rather than ratings of intelligibility. Although the technical adequacy of these evaluative procedures have not been fully established, the work that has been done on them is encouraging in that interrespondent reliability is high (ie, correlations above 0.9) as is concurrent validity (also correlations above 0.9 with a second measure of speech intelligibility).

In terms of certain aspects of speech, Pflaster[24] has emphasized the importance of suprasegmental control (eg, speech rhythm) over actual articulation ability, in that this factor significantly entered into a prediction equation of success for orally integrated children up to age 10 years. After that age, apparently, the oral receptive skills of the children were more important. Although there undoubtedly exists an entire range of articulation ability in terms of finger spelling and signing, no formal testing procedure for school age children is known to exist. Taking a lead from assessment procedures for oral speech,

Table 6–5 Psycho-educational Assessment: Language and Academic Achievement

Ability Rated	Test
Articulation/ intelligibility	Ling Speech Articulation Assessment CID Picture SPINE

Morphology and syntax	Berko Test of Morphology
	Grammatical Closure Subtest of the Illinois Test of Psycholinguistic Abilities
	Berry Talbot Exploratory Test of Grammar
	Test for Examining Expressive Morphology
	Northwestern Syntax Screening Test
	Carrow Elicited Language Inventory
	Test for Auditory Comprehension of Language-Revised
	Miller-Yoder Language Comprehension
	Boehm Test of Basic Concepts
	Bare Essentials in Assessing Really Little Kids—Concept Analysis Profile*
	Grammatical Analysis of Elicited Language*
	    Presentence
	    Simple
	    Complex
	Teacher Assessment of Grammatical Structures*
	Rhode Island Test of Language Structure*
	SKI-HI Receptive Language Test*
	Test of Expressive Language Ability*
	Test of Receptive Language Ability*
	Maryland Syntax Evaluation Instrument*
	Test of Syntactic Abilities*
	Analysis of Spontaneous Language Sample Procedures

Lexical development	Peabody Picture Vocabulary Test-Revised Word Recognition Subtests of Achievement Test Vocabulary Subtest of the Wechsler Scales Boehm Test of Basic Concepts Bare Essentials in Assessing Really Little Kids—Concept Analysis Profile* SKI-HI Receptive Language Test* Carolina Picture Vocabulary Tests Total Communication Receptive Vocabulary Test Test of Word Knowledge
Pragmatics	Communication Intention Inventory Dore's List of Primitive Speech Acts Interpersonal Language Comprehension Test Dore's Taxonomy of Conversational Acts Test of Pragmatic Skills
General verbal ability and knowledge	Verbal Scale of the Wechsler Scales Test of Problems Solving

Interactive Language	*Informal*
	    Parent interviews
	    Naturalistic observations
	    Standardized observations
	    Contained observations
	Formal
	    Bales Interactive Process Scales
	Flanders Interactive Scales
	Craig and Collins Analysis of Communicative Interaction
	Cognitive Verbal/Nonverbal Observation Scale

Academic achievement	Stanford Achievement Test Battery Hearing-Impaired edition

*Tests and procedures designed for the hearing impaired.

though, various rating systems and articulation tests might be devised by utilizing the information reported by Wilbur[104], contained in Coulter[105], and reported by and others concerning the "phonology" of finger spelling and signs.

A number of evaluation instruments and techniques currently are available for the assessment of syntactic and morphological rule knowledge of English. Cooper[106] successfully administered the Berko test of morphology to a group of children with hearing loss. The Berko test attempts to assess the child's ability to generalize the use of certain inflectional endings and markers, such as the plural [s] or the regular past tense marker [ed].

The grammatical closure subtest of the Illinois Test of Psycholinguistic Abilities and the Berry Talbot Exploratory Test of Grammar are adaptations of this test and are commercially available. Three other tests that have been used with individuals with hearing loss are the Northwestern Syntax Screening Test (NSST), the Carrow Elicited Language Inventory, and the Boehm Test of Basic Concepts.

The NSST, as the name suggests, is a screening test of receptive and expressive language abilities. Only 40 syntactic structures are used in the test. The Carrow Elicited Language Inventory is meant to evaluate a slightly wider scope of linguistic constructions. The Boehm Test of Basic Concepts was developed to be a criterion-referenced test of certain beginning, academically related concepts (lexical items), and it involves concept identification, statement repetition and comprehension, and pattern awareness. No attempt was made by the author of the test to specify the specific linguistic constructions that are being evaluated, but a visual inspection of the items by the user can easily reveal their nature. As might be expected, studies using these instruments have shown that individuals with hearing loss perform more poorly than their hearing counterparts.[23,107,108] These tests may be used as a type of criterion measure to identify specific language structures with which the individual may be having difficulty. It should be pointed out, however, that these instruments test only a very limited number of possible constructions, and, thus, give only a very narrow picture of the child's linguistic understanding and capacity. Other useful tests might be the Miller-Yoder Language Skills Assessment, the Preschool Language Assessment Instrument, the Test of Auditory Comprehension of Language-Revised, and the Test for Examining Expressive Morphology.

The tests just mentioned have been standardized on and for a hearing population. In recent years, a number of formal instruments have been developed for the population with hearing loss. As with tests normed on those with normal hearing, these tests either emphasize receptive abilities or expressive abilities. Those emphasizing receptive abilities follow the format whereby the child is to identify an appropriate picture or to perform some action with manipulatives in responses to what the examiner says. The expressive tests follow a format that either involves generating utterances after observing the manipulation of various objects or the completion of sentence stem in response to a picture or some verbal print stimulus.

The receptive tests/scales are:

1. Bare Essentials in Assessing Really Little Kids-Concept Analysis Profile Summary,[109] a spoken/signed criterion-referenced test of certain lexical and semantic relational concepts for children with hearing loss ages 1 year, 6 months to 5 years.

2. The Rhode Island Test of Language Structure,[110] a test of receptive understanding of various syntactic constructions designed for hearing-impaired individuals ages 3 to 20 years, to be administered via total communication, and youngsters with normal hearing, ages 3 to 6 years.

3. SKI-HI Receptive Language Test,[111] a criterion-referenced test designed to assesses 3- to 6-year-old children with hearing loss for the ability to understand various semantic relationships that increase one element at a time.

4. Teacher Assessment of Grammatical Structures,[112] a series of criterion-referenced checklists designed to assess the receptive and productive use of various morphological and grammatical structures of children with hearing loss ages 0 to 9 years.

5. Test of Receptive Language Ability,[113] a normed referenced test designed to assess 7- to 12-year-old children with hearing loss for the ability to understand 12 morphological and grammatical structures via print.

6. The Test of Syntactic Abilities,[114] a normed and criterion-referenced paper and pencil test designed to screen and test in depth 10- to 19-year-old children with hearing loss for the understanding of nine major areas of syntactic structure in English (ie,

negation, conjunction, determiners, question formation, verb processes, pronominalization, relativization, complementation, and nominalization). From a technical standpoint, this test is the most well-constructed of all those normed on the hearing-impaired. Norms for normally hearing youngsters are also available.

The tests of expressive ability designed for individuals who are hearing impaired are:

1. The Grammatical Analysis of Elicited Language—Presentence,[115] Simple Sentence,[116] and Complex Sentence Levels,[117] a set of three normed referenced tests on orally taught children with hearing impairments, ages 3 to 5 years, 11 months, 5 to 8 years, 11 months, and 8 to 11 years, 11 months, respectively, with norms available for the Simple Sentence Level when administered via total communication, using a format similar to that of the Carrow Elicited Language Inventory, with the exception that the various activities or tasks are structured so that they are a natural consequence of the object manipulation or pictorial context.
2. The Maryland Syntax Evaluation Instrument,[118] a normed referenced test for children who are deaf, ages 6 years to 11 years, 11 months, wherein individuals are to write sentences to in response to pictures presented on a filmstrip.
3. Test of Expressive Language Ability,[119] a normed referenced test for 7- to 12-year-old children who are hearing impaired, designed to assess the written control of 13 morphological and grammatical structures.

Of the three, the Grammatical Analysis of Elicited Languages tests are the most technically adequate.

Another procedure that has gained acceptance is the use of analysis of spontaneous language samples. In this procedure, a corpus, or sample, of spontaneous language is elicited from the child and a grammatical, semantic, or pragmatic analysis of the production is made using some *a priori* classification scheme. A number of these schemes are available.[120,121]

Unlike syntax, which is thought to be comprised of a finite number of rules that, hypothetically, could be evaluated exhaustively, lexical development is in principle infinite. As a result, it would be virtually impossible to obtain a complete inventory of the child's vocabulary. A number of receptive vocabulary test that have been standardized on the population with normal hearing are available. One such test is the Peabody Picture Vocabulary Test (PPVT) and its revision PPVT-R. All of these tests generally follow the same format. A word is spoken and the examinee is expected to select the appropriate corresponding picture. When administered to individuals with hearing impairments in the prescribed fashion, the test becomes as much a test of speech-reading and auditory processing as a test of vocabulary. If a simultaneous form of communication is used, inflated scores may often result, given the iconic nature of the signs that may induce a correct response without actual lexical knowledge of the English word. Similarly, problems arise if the items are administered via finger spelling or presented in a written format, since the tests were not intended to be used this way. As a result, tests like the PPVT and the PPVT-R have limited value with many individuals who are hearing impaired. Presumably for this reason, two tests of signed vocabulary following the PPVT/PPVT-R format have been designed for use with children who are deaf: the Carolina Picture Vocabulary Test[122] designed for use with children who are deaf, ages 4 years to 11 years, 6 months, and the Total Communication Receptive Vocabulary Test,[123] designed for 3- to 12-year-old children who are hearing impaired. Of the two the former is more technically adequate.

Yet another index of vocabulary development that does not involve any task modification is the use of word recognition subtests of various achievement tests, such as the SAT-HI. Such tests, however, tap only one aspect of lexical knowledge—knowledge of the printed word. A relatively new test on the market, the Test of Word Knowledge,[124] alternatively, attempts to evaluate eight different aspects of word knowledge (Expressive Vocabulary, Receptive Vocabulary, Word Definitions, Word Opposites, Synonyms, Multiple Meanings, Figurative Usages, and the understanding of language structure through the use of Conjunctions and Transition Words).

Interest in pragmatics is of only recent vintage, relatively speaking. Pragmatics has to do with the uses to which language is put and the manner in which it is organized in discourse for social purposes, whereas mathetics has to do with those uses of language for learning about the world.

For the most part, the area of pragmatic assessment is dominated by: (1) various assessment inventories of communicative intent with little attention being given to assessing the appropriateness of these intents in meeting various felicity conditions, (2) assessments of discourse structure, and (3) the use of cohesion devices as defined by Halliday and Hasan.[125] One problem associated with assessments of discourse structure, is that there exists a plethora of possible discourse genres that have not been fully explored or developed into various taxonomies or inventories.

With regard to the communication inventories and assessment techniques, the following are most notable: the Communicative Intention Inventory[126], an inventory designed to assess young children's (8 months to 2 years) nonverbal and verbal intents; Dore's list of Primitive Speech Acts[127]; the Interpersonal Language Skills Assessment, designed to assess 8- to 14-year-old children's use of 16 different communication intents during a card game; the Test of Pragmatic Skills[128]; and, Dore's[129] Taxonomy of Conversational Acts.

In terms of mathetics, much interest has focused on meta processes. Technically, practically all formal tests involve some form of metacognitive ability in that the examinee is usually required to reflect on some aspect of his or her knowledge. More specifically and with respect to language and culture, this is exemplified in the Vocabulary (defining words), the Similarities (inducing superordinate terms), and Comprehension (answering questions about social and cultural conventions) subtests of the Wechsler tests, and with respect to study skills it is exemplified by the work of Peverly and Brobst.[130] Although in name the Test of Problem Solving[131] was meant to be a test of problem-solving achievement, it is as much a test of one's ability to understand, solve, and talk about daily social problems.

Language learning, for children with normal hearing and those with hearing loss, at least in part, involves an interactive process, and, as a result, the child's participation in these interactions needs to be assessed. The interactive patterns of the primary caretaker and the child, or the interaction between a classroom teacher and the students, are examples of interactions that could he used for assessment. One could also assess the interaction patterns of a group of children who are hearing impaired among themselves or in an integrated situation.

The methods used to investigate these interactive patterns are of several types—verbal statements gathered from interviews with parents, naturalistic observation, standardized observation, and containing observation, which is the limiting of one's observation to a specifically prescribed behavior.[132] In terms of mother-child, as well as teacher-child interactions, the behaviors of most interest are those that would most promote intellectual development, psychosocial attachment and development, academic achievement, and language development. A good review of the current studies and strategies in observing normal mother-infant interaction is provided by Ramey et al[132] and Feuerstein.[47] The need for considering these interactions is amply demonstrated by Collins and Rose[133] and Goss,[134] who have shown that hearing mothers of children who are deaf respond differently and less effectively as teachers of language than hearing mothers of hearing children. (See Caissie and Cole[135] for an alternative consideration of this matter.)

Similarly, a number of interaction scales are available to investigate classroom and teacher-child interactions. Among these are the Bales Interaction Process Analysis,[136] the Flanders Interactive Scale, Craig and Collins Analysis of Communicative Interaction,[137] and the Cognitive Verbal/Nonverbal Observation Scale.[138] Recent studies using these scales have shown that, at least in some classes for students with hearing loss, the conversations tend to be teacher dominated (with few student-initiated communications),[137] the activities center around memory work as opposed to inference building,[138] and the children lack the ability to ask for information, make suggestions, provide orientations, or clarify other's opinions in group problem-solving situations.[139]

Each of these approaches, however, involve the use of some *a priori* categorization system emphasizing an *etic* approach to caretaker-child and classroom interaction. A growing trend in the field, however, is the use of ethnographic and microethnographic approaches, which do not specify *a priori* any categorical system but attempt to induce them by describing the internal *emic* structure of events and activities. Such an approach might require, however, the psycho-educational evaluator to abandon certain professional orientations in favor of a more social-psychological perspective.

Historically, there have been several academic tests available that were either normed on students who are deaf or had empirical data available to assist in their interpretation. Only one test presently exists that possesses the technical adequacy to warrant its use. That test is the eighth edition of the SAT-HI, which consists of a series of eight screening tests to assist the examiner determining which of the eight test batteries is most appropriate for administration, ranging from Primary 1 (typically for grades 1.5 to 2.5) to Advanced 2 (typically for those at grade 8.5 to 9.9). Indeed, it is technically an outstanding test. Not only are norms available for the combined group of individuals who are hearing impaired (those who are hard of hearing and severely to profoundly deaf) but also separate norms for only those with severe to profound losses and a series of specialized norm tables based on degree of loss, type of education program (special schools for the deaf, partial mainstreaming or mainstreaming, mainstreamed), presence or absence of additional handicaps, ethnic background, and region location. One advantage that the Stanford tests have is that they are both norm-referenced and criterion-referenced, and, thus, in principle are amenable to direct translations into an educational program (instructional objectives associated with each item on the screening test and the test batteries themselves are available).

Given that most diagnostic reading tests are phonically based, their utility with the population that is hearing impaired is limited. Obviously, these tests would be limited to use with children who are hard of hearing or phonically oriented children with deafness. However, Ewoldt[140] has discussed the application of the Goodman-Burke Reading Miscues Inventory, which is a test of oral reading fluency, to children with hearing loss who used simultaneous communications. Her findings have suggested that children with hearing loss make the same kinds of reading errors that children who hear make, and that the reading processes of the two groups are in many ways similar. A similar approach to that of the Miscues Reading Inventory has been devised by Mory Clay[141] and has been referred to as the *running record*. Its advantage over the Miscues Reading Inventory is reported to be its simplicity and the fact that it is adaptable to the teacher's day-to-day activities and routines. In addition to the running record and as a part of the entire diagnostic survey, Clay also developed a letter identification component, an evaluation of young children's concepts about print, a word identification task, and a series of free and dictation writing tasks. Although no literature is known to exist reporting

results of using this diagnostic approach with individuals with hearing impairments, the approach is being used in the field and it holds good promise in providing additional insights into the reading process of children with hearing impairments.

Unfortunately, little research has been done in the area of diagnostic assessment of mathematical ability or the processing of mathematical information in recent years. The reader, however, may find the Sequential Assessment of Mathematics Inventories[142] to be a useful diagnostic test in this area. This test evaluates the individual in the following areas: Number and Notation, Computation, Math Language, Ordinality, Geometric Concepts, Measurement, Math Applications, and Word Problems.

Although a great deal of the research on the English language abilities of children who are hard of hearing and deaf has involved the analysis of their written language, few formal tests are available in this area. One notable instrument that has not been reported on in the literature in a number of years is the Picture Story Language Test.[143] Although this instrument attempts to assess syntax in terms of traditional notions of errors of addition, omission, substitutions, and word order, rather than using more sophisticated linguistic analyses (which were not available at the time), it does have a very interesting approach to evaluating the ideational component of narratives referred to as the Abstract-Concrete Scale. A story is ranked along a 25 level continuum of ideation ranging from meaningless stories to abstract imaginative stories.

Although not totally systematized, as of yet, other considerations that need to be taken into account when evaluating the written language of individuals, or any child, are the developmental stages and processes that children typically go through (eg, as described by Calkins[144], Applebee[145] and others), notions of coherence and cohesion,[125,146] and the role of various forms of writing genres.[146] Recently, Yoshinaga-Itano and Downey[147] have suggested an approach that incorporates some of these notions.

Finally, the last area to be considered in the assessment of academics is that of study skills. Although no studies have been conducted in this area with youngsters with hearing impairments to my knowledge, it is an area gaining increased attention within the psycho-educational literature in general. One promising approach is that offered by Peverly and Brobst[130]. Their approach is to have a student read and study one of a series of gradated pieces of expository text, after which the examinee is to summarize what he or she has read and, then, the examinee is asked some comprehension questions. While reading, the examinee is encourage to use whatever methods he or she wishes to study for this examination, which the examiner notes. The examinee also undergoes a structured interview concerning his or her use of study skills.

Psychomotor Functioning

Although the psychomotor integrity of the individual may provide the examiner with one more piece of information concerning the total development of the child with hearing impairment, few studies have been performed in this area and few tests of psychomotor ability are available. The studies that have been conducted have suggested that some individuals with hearing impairments have difficulties in terms of static balance (standing on one foot) and psychomotor speed (doing a manual task with speed), with lesser but still significant difficulties in maintaining balance while in motion (dynamic balance). These identified motor difficulties are the result of a study using the Oseretsky Test of Motor Proficiency.[49]

Social Maturity and Adaptive Behavior

Social maturity essentially is the ability to take care of oneself and to assist in the care of others. The related concept of adaptive behavior is defined by the American Association on Mental Deficiency (AAMD) as the "effectiveness with which the individual copes with the natural and social demands of the environment."[148] The AAMD further explains that the definition has two major facets: (1) the degree to which the individual is able to function independently, and (2) the degree to which she or he meets satisfactorily the culturally imposed demands of personal and social responsibility. The importance of including measures of this kind in a total assessment is emphasized by the official position of both the AAMD and the Office of Civil Rights.[148] Both organizations have stated that an individual can be classified as mentally retarded only if the individual is found to be subnormal in both intelligence and in adaptive behavior.

Although a number of adaptive scales are available, only one has been used with individuals with hearing impairments in research studies— the Vineland Social Maturity Scale and its most recent revisions the Vineland Adaptive Behavior Scale, the Survey form, the Expanded Form, and the Classroom form. Both sets of instruments are administered in a structured interview situation with someone who is familiar with the child being rated. The original scale is comprised of eight clusters of items: self-help general, self-help eating, self-help dressing, locomotion, socialization, occupation, communication, and self-direction; whereas the revised versions are comprised of 11 clusters of items: receptive language, expressive language, written language, personal daily living skills, domestic daily living skills, community living skills, interpersonal relationships, use of play and leisure time, coping skills, gross motor skills, and fine motor skills. These tests were intended to assess the social competency of individuals from birth to adulthood.

Myklebust[49] and others have used the Vineland Social Maturity Scale with residential school students and have found that in the early years, very little difference existed between youngsters with normal hearing and those with hearing impairments, except in items directly evaluating communication skills related to English and interacting with society at large. However, as the children matured, the pervasiveness of problems associated with reduced English proficiency and interacting with individuals with hearing at large was found to have serious effects in other areas, so that by age 15 years, the mean social quotient was in the low 80s (the original version calculated a ratio social quotient similar to an intelligence quotient in that 100 was considered the average. The revised versions yield standard deviation scores similar to deviation IQ with a average standard score being 100 with a standard deviation of 15).

An investigation by Quarrington and Solomon[149] studied the social maturity of three groups of children with hearing impairments, ages 5 to 16 years. The groups studied were day students in a public school setting, students attending a residential school but who had numerous trips home, and residential students who rarely went home. The first two groups had social quotients in the mid 80s, as might be expected, whereas the latter group had a mean social quotient in the mid 70s, which is distinctly below average. Although no rationale was given for the procedure, the revised versions of this test include supplemental norms for students with deafness placed in residential facilities. These norms, however, are virtually impossible to interpret and border on being meaningless because an individual's adaptive levels is to be judged adequate, above average, or below average based on data collapsed over an age span of 6 years (ie, 6 to 12 years, 11 months). The survey form of this test has been shown to be useful in classifying persons with hearing impairments according to their ability to acquire independent living skills and, thus, providing some evidence for construct validity when used with adolescents and young adults with hearing loss.[150]

Emotional Adjustment

In terms of the child's emotional development, the psycho-educational assessment team needs to be concerned with the child's overall mental health and behavioral functioning and the child's motivation to learn. The need to consider the former is emphasized by the fact that several surveys have suggested that the incidence of emotional disturbance and behavioral disorders in the population with hearing loss is greater than in the population with normal hearing.[151] In terms of the latter, the psycho-educational evaluator should also he interested in those behaviors that, although not pathologic, do affect learning and functioning within the classroom.

A number of studies have been conducted to examine the personality characteristics of those with hearing-impairment. Many of these investigations have been based on the use of projective techniques (Table 6-6). Unfortunately, a few of the instruments require extensive verbalization on the part of the examinee, which limits their use to a portion of the population with hearing impairments and calls into question the conclusions derived from the use of such instruments. These criticisms are in addition to those leveled against all projective and most personality tests—that they generally lack the necessary technical adequacy to be considered highly valid or reliable. Despite the technical inadequacy of these tests and the clinical or subjective nature of their interpretations, researchers having access to previous studies have tended to come to somewhat similar conclusions regarding certain personality characteristics using different tests.[152] The fact that these clinical impressions may be socially constructed interpretations in and of themselves may not invalidate them, although care has not been take in these cases to authenticate (validate) these findings through some process of corroboration and "triangulation" as required by this approach.

Table 6–6 Psycho-educational Assessment: Emotional Adjustment Tests Available

1. Rorschach
2. American Sign Language version of the Rorschach
3. Make-A-Picture-Story-Test
4. Draw-A-Person Test
5. Mosaic Test
6. Id-Ego-Superego Test
7. Missouri Children's Picture Series
8. Rotter Incomplete Sentences
9. Meadow/Kendall Social-Emotional Assessment Inventory for Deaf Children[153]
10. Meadow Assessment of Social-Emotional Adjustment In Hearing-Impaired Preschoolers[154]
11. Hand Test
12. Sixteen Personality Factor Questionnaire, Form E
13. Behavior Problem Checklist
14. Leigh et al's adaption of the Beck Depression Inventory, Sociotropy-Autonomy Scale, and the Parental Bonding Instrument

The general pattern obtained from these studies is emotional immaturity, adaptive rigidity, sociocultural impoverishment, egocentricity, dependency, short attention span, poor impulse control, and aggression. Hogan[155] has likened these characteristics to an authoritarian personality, whereas Levine and Wagner[152] have suggested that these characteristics are similar to those of culturally deprived individuals. Although the personality profiles obtained from projective tests give the impression of severe maladaptive behavior, in all probability, they actually reflect good coping skills, considering the impact of the physical disability, the psychosocial reactions to it, and society's reactions to "it" as well. Leigh et al[156] have shown a higher prevalence of mild depressive symptoms with college students with deafness than college students who hear, but a lower prevalence of severe depression.

Only recently have attempts been made to address the assessment concerns already expressed in the area of the affective domain. For example, Schwartz et al[157] investigated the effects of mode of administration (written vs American Sign Language) on the responses elicited on the Rorschach using the Exner's Comprehensive System[158] (the current standard); Brauer[159] investigated aspects of an American Sign Language version of the Minnesota Multiphasic Personality Inventory (MMPI); Ouellette[160] attempted (successfully) to investigate the external validity of certain findings obtained on the House-Tree-Person (ie, aggression, impulsivity, immaturity, egocentricity and dependency); and, Leigh et al[156] have developed modified versions of the Beck Depression

Inventory, the Sociotropy-Autonomy Scale, and the Parental Bonding Instrument.

The results of the Schwartz et al[157] study indicated that only a few difference existed between the two administration procedures of the Rorschach (written and signed) and that individuals with deafness tended to score more than 1 deviation from the mean in terms of perceptual accuracy, perceptual complexity, and self focus, each of which were interpreted with respect to the biosocial impact of deafness, (ie, the former two being the result of the visual orientation of the deaf clients and the latter the result of normal and expected reactions to societal reactions to deafness). Although a tendency toward ''rigidity'' was noted, the results were interpreted in terms of qualitative differences with respect to affect expression and modulation. Finally, Brauer[159] established the possibility of insignificant signer effect on an ASL version of the MMPI.

Of recent years, several investigators have investigated various aspects of these personality traits as they relate to the academic setting. More specifically, interest has been expressed in the interrelated notions of impulsivity, external versus internal locus of control, learned helplessness, and the need for achievement. Impulsivity refers to the tendency to make fast decisions with many errors, whereas its opposite, reflection, refers to the tendency to react slowly with relatively few errors. According to Harris,[161] reflectivity is associated with age, reading ability, adjustment, social class, high motivation to achieve, persistence, and long attention spans. Similarly, the bipolar dimensions of external versus internal locus of control have also been associated with several of these variables, as has field dependency.[162] For example, locus of control has been associated with greater or lesser information learning, information seeking, academic achievement, and motivation to achieve.[163] Some of these ideas have been investigated with individuals who are hearing impaired. Both Altshuler et al[164] and Harris[161] have found persons with hearing impairments to be less reflective and, thus, more impulsive than their counterparts who hear. Harris[161] also found children with deafness of parents with deafness to be more reflective than children with deafness born to parents with hearing.

Apparently, the nature of the home environment in terms of the quality of the parent-child interactions and communication patterns has a bearing on the extent of the child's reflectivity

or impulsivity. Similarly, Stinson[165] found that the motivation of children with hearing loss to achieve, their persistence, and their actual achievement were a function of the mother's interaction with her child in a learning/teaching situation and Kampfe[166] found that children's reading achievement may be related to the signing skill levels of mothers who used manual communication. Thus, the quality of the mother-child interaction and the extent of the actual external (locus of) control placed on the child has an effect on immediate achievement and probably on the child's eventual perception of locus of control. To the extent that children with hearing impairments are actually overprotected, controlled, and directed, they may not learn to take responsibility for their behavior, and thus develop what McCrone[167] has identified as *learned helplessness*. (See Caissie and Cole[135] for an alternative consideration of the role of directiveness in mother-child interactions.) Learned helplessness is characterized by: (1) an external locus of control; (2) underachievement; and (3) reduced performance when faced with failure. These are characteristics that are common in many children with hearing impairments.

Because these behaviors appear to be modifiable,[47,89,168] it would seem important to include various measures of impulsivity and locus of control within a standard battery, if possible. Some instruments that could be used are shown in Table 6-7.[169,170]

Table 6–7   Psycho-educational Assessment: Measures of Impulsivity and Locus of Control

Materials available
1. Matching Familiar Figures Test
2. Timed Draw-A-Man Test
3. Porteus Mazes
4. Wechsler Mazes
5. Id-Ego-Superego Test
6. Rotter Test of Internal/External Control

SPECIFIC CRITERIA FOR INTEGRATION

In this chapter instruments and procedures have been described that have been used in identifying and programming for the academic and language needs of the child with hearing impairments. No attempt was made to discuss minimal competencies needed to integrate children with hearing impairments into a regular classroom either on a full- or part-time basis. There are few studies of this problem. Reich et al[171] on the basis of a study of 195 integrated children with hearing impairments, suggested several sets of minimal criteria that depend on the type of program and the age of the child. Criteria were derived for elementary age children who were candidates for either full integration (EFI) or integration with itinerant help (EIH), and secondary age children who were candidates for full integration, integration with itinerant help (SIH), or partial integration (SPI). The minimum requirements for full integration at the elementary level were:

1. No greater than a moderate (70 dB HL) pure-tone average hearing loss.
2. No greater than a severe (90 dB HL) high-frequency average (the average of the thresholds at 4000 and 8000 Hz).
3. Aural functioning of 62% or better correct response to a specially designed test of sentence and paragraph understanding.
4. Oral functioning of 78% or better on a test similar to that used to assess aural functioning.
5. An English language background.
6. Parents who had no less than a high school education.
7. Parents who had aspirations for their child of high school graduation or college.
8. Some degree of help at home, and good parental contact with the school.
9. An IQ of no less than 90.
10. Diagnosis of hearing impairment no later than age 7 years a hearing aid being fitted no later than age 8 years.

Almost identical criteria for the other four groups were reported, with the exception of permitting:

1. Severe hearing losses in the case of pure-tone averages for the EIH and the SPI children.
2. Profound high-frequency average losses for all four groups.
3. Slightly lower aural functioning (58%) for the EIH children.
4. Slightly higher oral functioning (86%) for all the secondary groups.
5. Slightly lower intelligence for the EIH children, but slightly higher intelligence for the SIH and SPI children (IQs of 97 and 95, respectively).
6. Slightly later age of diagnosis (9 years) for the SIH and SPI children.
7. Slightly younger age (5.5 years) for a hearing aid fitting for the EIH children, but slightly older for all the secondary children (age 9 years).

Rudy and Nance[172] also have developed criteria whereby an individual's candidacy for integration can be estimated. The procedure is based on ratings in the areas of intelligence, academic achievement, social adjustment, and degree of loss. These ratings yield a composite score that can be compared with a decision-making cutoff point provided by the researchers to determine eligibility for integration. Although these minimal criteria can be very useful, it should be remembered that they have not been tested beyond the initial populations studied. Thus, they should only be used as guidelines.

ASSESSMENT OF TRANSITION COMPETENCE

There has been long-standing interest in the adult population with deafness and the transition from school to the work world in the field of deafness. Given recent legislation, increased attention is being paid to this critical event of transition in the lives of individuals with disabilities. Although a number approaches have been taken to assess transition skills, the approaches often do not effectively address certain crucial skills needed by individuals with hearing impairments or the content necessary to succeed independently at work or in the community.[173] As a result, the Transition Competence Battery for Deaf Adolescents and Young Adults was developed, which according to Bullis and Reiman[173] was designed to be a "language-appropriate, content-relevant and psychometrically sound measure of transition skills for deaf persons" (p.13), standardized on adolescents and adults with deafness from both mainstream and residential settings. The two multiple choice versions of the test, a written and a signed version, consist of six subtests covering various aspects of Job-Seeking, Work Adjustment, Job-Related Adjustment, Money Management, Health and Home Skills, and Community Awareness. An interesting feature of this test is it attention to assessing subtle aspects of the examinee's conscious (meta) awareness of social and work ethic conventions, in general, and as it relates to adult deafness issues in particular (eg, where an interpreter should sit during a job interview). Another interesting point is that, based on pilot data and feedback from their examinees, the videotape version was signed in Pidgin English rather than American Sign Lananguage. Although difficulties exist with the norming sample, the instrument does hold some promise, particularly if the psychometric properties and norms could be enhanced and further demonstrated.

FUTURE DIRECTIONS AND NEEDS

There are a number directions in which I believe that the area of psycho-educational assessment that have to do with the diagnostic process, in general, and with assessment, in particular, is or should be moving.

To begin, there seems to be two parallel, but seemingly contradictory trends occurring simultaneously at the present time. The first trend has to do with the consequences of certain sociopolitical acts that have resulted in a heuristic, over bureaucratized approach to the evaluation process that emphasizes reliance on strict adherence to static measures. The second trend is essentially in the opposite direction. It is more academic and theoretically oriented and involves the movement toward ecological, process oriented, and dynamic assessment procedures. The former trend seems to be a reaction to the increasing regulations (real, imagined, or interpreted) associated with current legislation, mounting litigation, and fears thereof. It may also be a reflection of the on-going tradition of the positivist's philosophical orientation within school psychology. Although well-intentioned and of merit, PL94-142, PL99-457, and Americans with Disabilities Act have had some profound unintended consequences in many situations and locales—most notably, for our purposes, is the over reliance on a rigid, minimal, normed referenced battery of tests, the restricting of psychological services to evaluative functions for purposes of placement and monitoring, and the trivialization of the individual education, family plan, and transition planning process and products themselves.

The alternative trend operating out of a (social) constructivist philosophical orientation is more theoretically oriented and views teaching, learning, comprehension, intervention, and decision making (even about placement of disabled children[174]) as dynamic processes. As a result, various models and approaches to process testing have been devised operating out of various social psychological or information processing models (eg, Feuerstein's[47] Learning Potential Assessment Device and Brown and Campione's[175] Dynamic Assessment approaches in terms of cognitive function; Ewoldt's,[140] Clay's,[141] and Schirmer's[176] approaches in terms of reading process and comprehension; Garrison et al[177]

work in terms of reading comprehension test item difficulty; and Locher and Worms's[42] work in terms of visual-motor functioning). Indeed, this trend toward putting theory into practice is reflected in various aspects of the reform movement and, interestingly enough, in the professional literature in that a special section of the *Journal of School Psychology* has been created entitled the "Scientific Practitioner."

Consistent with this approach has been the growing trend and interest in the nature and construction of knowledge, including social knowledge and social competence,[178] various metaprocesess and thought processes, including those relating to the affective domain as discussed within the framework of rational emotive therapy,[179] social psychological processes,[180] and attributional processes. Even within the framework of traditional testing, the impact of this approach has been felt in that, more and more, school psychologists are using testing the limits procedures and are incorporating various type of informal testing techniques based on various theoretical notions and constructs when the working conditions are conducive to it. Additionally, traditional methods of interpreting test results are being augmented by what we know about learning, language, and culture, (eg, the interpretations associated with the Comprehension, Similarities and Vocabulary tests of Wechsler tests as discussed before, which differ from that originally proposed by Wechsler). Finally, this approach advises and encourages more ecologically oriented approaches examining actual behavior and learning in real contexts (eg, school, the work place, the home).

Clearly, another trend, which was only touched on in this chapter, is and will be of interest in the future: the assessment of infants and toddlers and those in transition from school to work.

As for the needs within the field, the following are cited:

1. Large-scale studies investigating the various components of successful mainstreaming, successful learners who are deaf or hard of hearing, and various encoding, comprehension, social variables (including cultural and familial issues) and strategies used by individuals with hearing impairments.

2. Large-scale studies of the psychometric properties of various cognitive, linguistic, academic, social, and emotional evaluative techniques, taking into account the

pluralistic and heterogeneous nature of the population with hearing impairments.

3. Continued research into the specifics of the structure of knowledge within various domains.

4. Better accounts of the structure of emotions and the affective domain as it relates to personal well-being, literature, and the understanding of others.

5. Continued work in understanding the relationship between thought, language, social behavior, and affect.

6. The pre- and in-training training of psychologists to work with individuals with hearing impairments with a firm foundation in information processing and social psychological approaches to knowing, comprehension, learning, and instruction.

REFERENCES

1. Rules and Regulations for Implementation of the Individual Disabilities Education Act of 1975. U.S. Dept of Health, Education, and Welfare. *Fed Reg*, 42 (1977), 42474–518.

2. Newland TE: Assumptions underlying psychological testing. *J Sch Psychol*, 11 (1973), 316–322.

3. Levine ES: Psychological tests and practices with the deaf: A survey of the state of the art. *Volta Rev*, 76 (1974), 298–319.

4. Spragins AB, Schildroth AN, Karchmer MA: Profile of psychological service providers to hearing-impaired students. *Am Ann Deaf*, 126 (1981), 94–105.

5. McQuaid ME, Alovisetti M: School psychological services for hearing-impaired children in the New York and New England area. *Am Ann Deaf*, 126 (1981), 37–42.

6. Trott LA: Providing school psychological services to hearing-impaired students in New Jersey. *Am Ann Deaf*, 129 (1984), 319–323.

7. Gibbins S: Use of the WISC-R performance scale and K-ABC Non-Verbal Scale with deaf children in the USA and Scotland. *Sch Psychol Int*, 10 (1989), 193–197.

8. Weaver CB, Bradley-Johnson S: A national survey of school psychological services for deaf and hard of hearing students. *Am Ann Deaf*, 138 (1993), 267–274.

9. Furth HG: A review and perspective on the thinking of deaf people, in Hellmuth J, ed: *Cognitive Studies* (New York: Brunner/Mazel, 1970).

10. Ray S: *An Adaptation of the Wechsler Intelligence Scales (Performance) for Children Revised*, dissertation (Knoxville, TN, University of Tennessee, 1979).

11. Vernon M, Brown DW: A guide to psychological tests and testing in the procedures evaluation of deaf and hard of hearing Children. *J Speech Hear Dis*, 29 (1964), 414–423.

12. Salvia JA, Ysseldyke JE: *Assessment*, ed 5. (Boston: Houghton Mifflin, 1991).

13. Mitchell J, ed: *Eleventh Mental Measurement Yearbook* (Lincoln, NB: Buros Institute of Mental Measurement, University of Nebraska-Lincoln, 1992).

14. Sullivan PM: Administration modification on the WISC-R Performance Scale with different categories of deaf children. *Am Ann Deaf*, 127 (1982), 780–788.

15. Courtney AS, Hayes FG, Couch KW, Frick M: Administration of the WISC-R Performance Scale to hearing-impaired children using pantomimed instructions. *J Psychoeduc Assess*, 2 (1984), 1–7.

16. Anderson RJ, Sissco FM: *Standardizations of the WISC-R: Scale for Deaf Children*. Office of Demographic Studies. Series T, No 1 (Washington, DC: Galluadet College Press, 1977).

17. Braden JP: Intellectual assessment of deaf and hard-or-hearing people: A quantitative and qualitative research synthesis. *Sch Psychol Rev*, 21 (1992), 82–94.

18. Ysseldyke JE, Salvia JA: Diagnostic-prescriptive teaching: Two models. *Except Child*, 41 (1974), 181–185.

19. Spear BS, Kretschmer RE: The use of criteria in decision making regarding the placement of hearing impaired students. *Spec Serv Sch*, 4 (1987), 107–122.

20. Ysseldyke JE: Diagnostic-prescriptive teaching: The search for aptitude-treatment interactions, in Mann I, Sabatino DA, eds: *The First Review of Special Education*, vol 1 (Phil: JSE Press, 1973).

21. Myklebust HR, Neyhus A, Mulholland AM: Guidance and counseling for the deaf. *Am Ann Deaf*, 107 (1962), 370–415.

22. Laughton J: *Nonverbal Creative Thinking Abilities a Predictors of Linguistic Abilities of Hearing-Impaired Children*, dissertation, (Kent State University, 1976).

23. Pressnell L: Hearing impaired children's comprehension and production of syntax in oral language. *J Speech Hear Res*, 16 (1973), 12–21.

24. Pflaster G: *A Factor Analytic Study of Hearing-Impaired Children Integrated into Regular Schools*, dissertation (New York: Teachers College, Columbia University, 1976).

25. Neuhaus M: Parental attitudes and the emotional adjustment of deaf children. *Except Child*, 35 (1969), 721–727.

26. Henggeler SW, Watson SM, Whelan JP, Malone CM: The adaptation of hearing parents of hearing-impaired youths. *Am Ann Deaf*, 135 (1990), 211–216.

27. Freeman SF, Malkin RD, Hastings JD: Psychosocial problems of deaf children and their families. *Am Ann Deaf*, 121 (1975), 391–417.

28. Calderon R, Greenberg MT: *Social Support and Stress in Hearing Parents with Deaf Vs. Hearing Children*. Paper Presented at the Western Psychological Association, San Francisco, 1983.

29. Birch JR, Birch JW: Predicting school achievement in young deaf children. *Am Ann Deaf*, 101 (1956), 348–352.

30. *Hard of Hearing Child in the Regular Classroom*. Pontiac, Michigan. Oakland County School, final report, Eric Number ED 145646, 1975.

31. Alexander C, Strain PS: A review of educators attitude toward handicapped children and the concept of mainstreaming. *Psychol School*, 15 (1978), 390–396.

32. Haring N, Cruickshank WM, Stern G: *Attitudes of Educators Toward Exceptional Children* (Syracuse, NY: Syracuse University Press, 1981).

33. Berryman JD, Neal WR, Berryman JE: *Attitudes Toward Mainstreaming Scale-Revised* (Athens, GA: University of Georgia, 1989).

34. *Test of Auditory Comprehension*. Office of Los Angeles County Superintendent of Schools (North Hollywood: Foreworks, 1976).

35. Stout GG, Windle EVJ: *The Developmental Approach to Successful Listening, II* (Houston, TX: Houston School for the Deaf, 1992).

36. Ratner V: New tests for identifying hearing-impaired students with visual perceptual deficits: Relationship between deficits and ability to comprehend Sign Language. *Am Ann Deaf*, 133, (1988), 336–343.

37. Ratner V: *Test of Visual Perceptual Abilities-Revised* (South Salem, NY: Visual Perceptual Abilities, 1988).

38. Wolff AB, Harkins JE: Multihandicapped students, in Schildroth AN, Karchmer MA, ed: *Deaf Children in America* (San Diego, CA: College Hill Press, 1986).

39. Lawson LJ, Myklebust HR: Ophthalmological deficiencies in deaf children. *Except Child*, (1970), 17–20.

40. Greene HA: Implications of a comprehensive vision-screening program for hearing-impaired children. *Volta Rev*, 80 (1978), 467–475.

41. Walters JW, Quintero S, Perrigin DM: Vision: Its assessment in school-age deaf children. *Am Ann Deaf*, 127 (1982), 418–432.

42. Locher PJ, Worms PI: Visual scanning strategies of neurologically impaired, perceptually impaired, and normal children viewing the Bender-Gestalt Designs. *Psychol Sch*, 14 (1977), 147–157.

43. Keogh BK, Vernon M, Smith CE: Deafness and visuo-motor function. *J Spec Educ*, 4 (1970), 41–47.

44. Blair F: A study of the visual memory of deaf and hearing children. *Am Ann Deaf* 102 (1957), 254–263.

45. Sharp EY: The relationship of visual closure to speech reading. *Except Child*, 38 (1972), 729–734.

46. Siple P, Hatfield N, Caccamise FF: The role of visual perceptual abilities in the acquisition and comprehension of Sign Language. *Am Ann Deaf*, 123 (1978), 852–856.

47. Feuerstein R: *The Dynamic Assessment of Retarded Performers* (University Park Press: Baltimore, MD, 1979).

48. Hine WD: The abilities of partially hearing children. *Br J Educ Res*, 39 (1969), 171–178.

49. Myklebust HR: *Psychology of Deafness* (New York: Grune & Stratton, 1960).

50. Ross DR: A Technique of Verbal Ability Assessment of Deaf Adults. *J Rehab Deaf*, 3 (1970), 7–15.

51. Wechsler D: *Wechsler Intelligence Scale for Children—III* (San Antonio, TX: Psychological Corporation, 1991).

52. Smith CS: The assessment of mental ability in partially deaf children. *Teacher Deaf*, 60 (1962), 216–224.

53. Roach RE, Rosencrans CJ: Intelligence test performance of Black children with high frequency hearing loss. *J Audiol Res*, 11 (1971), 136–139.

54. Braden, JP: Do deaf persons have a characteristic psychometric profile on the Wechsler Performance Scales? *J Psychoeduc Assess*, 8 (1990), 518–526.

55. Hiskey M: *Hiskey-Nebraska Test of Learning Aptitude*. (Lincoln: Union College Press, 1966).

56. Hirshoren A, Hurley A, Hunt JT: The reliability of the WISC-R and the Hiskey-Nebraska Test with deaf children. *Am Ann Deaf*, 122 (1977), 392–394.

57. Hirshoren A, Kavale K, Hurley OI, Hunt JT: The reliability of the WISC-R Performance Scale with deaf children. *Psych School*, 14 (1977), 412–415.

58. Fiedler M: *Developmental Studies of Deaf Children* (Washington, DC: ASHA, 1969).

59. Lavos G: WISC psychometric patterns among deaf children. *Volta Rev*, 64 (1962), 547–552.

60. Jeffers J: The process of speechreading viewed with respect to a theoretical construct, in *Proceedings of International Conference on Oral Education of the Deaf*, vol II (Washington, DC: Alexander Graham Bell Association, 1965), pp 1530–1561.

61. Kelly MD, Braden JP: Criterion-related validity of the WISC-R Performance Scale with the Stanford Achievement Test-Hearing Impaired Edition. *J Sch Psychol*, 28 (1990), 147–151.

62. Braden JP, Paquin MM: A comparison of the WISC-R and WAIS-R Performance Scales in

deaf adolescents. *J Psychoeduc Assess*, 3 (1985), 285–290.

63. Watson BU: Test-retest stability of the Hiskey-Nebraska Test of Learning Aptitude in a sample of hearing-impaired children and adolescents. *J Speech Hear Dis*, 48 (1983), 145–149.

64. Watson BU, Goldgar DE: A note on the use of the Hiskey-Nebraska Test of Learning Aptitude with Deaf Children. *Speech Hear Serv Sch*, 16 (1985), 53–57.

65. Giancreco C: The Hiskey-Nebraska Test of Learning Aptitude (Revised) compared to several achievement tests. *Am Ann Deaf*, 111 (1966), 556–577.

66. Watson B: Nonverbal intelligence and academic achievement in the hearing impaired. *Volta Rev*, 88 (1986), 151–158.

67. Humphrey JM: *Performance of Deaf Children on Tests of Cognitive, Linguistic, and Academic Achievement*, dissertation (Houston: University of Houston, 1976).

68. Birch JR, Stuckless ER, Birch JW: An eleven year study of predicting school achievement in young deaf children. *Am Ann of Deaf*, 108 (1963), 236–240.

69. Bonham SJ: Predicting achievement for deaf children. *Psychol Serv Cent J*, 14 (1974), 34–44.

70. Levine MN, Allen RM, Alker LN, et al: Clinical profile for the Leiter International Performance Scale. *Psych Serv Cent J*, 14 (1974), 45–51.

71. Mira MP: The use of the Arthur adaptation of the Leiter International Performance Scale and the Nebraska Test of Learning Aptitude with preschool deaf children. *Am Ann Deaf* 107 (1962), 224–228.

72. Ritter DR: Intellectual estimates of hearing-impaired children: A comparison of three measures. *Psychol Sch*, 13 (1976), 397–399.

73. Taddonio RO: Correlations of Leiter and the Visual Subtests of the Illinois Test of Psycholinguistic Abilities with deaf elementary school children. *J Sch Psych*, 11 (1973), 30–35.

74. Ratcliffe KJ, Ratcliffe MW: The Leiter Scales: A Review of validity findings. *Am Ann Deaf*, 124 (1979), 38–45.

75. Raven JC: *Manual for Raven's Progressive Matrices and Vocabulary Scales*. (London: H.K. Lewis, 1986).

76. Carlson JS: A note on the relationship between Raven's Colored Progressive Matrices Test and operational thought. *Psychol Sch*, 10 (1973), 211–214.

77. Goetzinger CP, Wills RC, Dekker Wills RC: Nonlanguage IQ tests used with deaf pupils. *Volta Rev*, 69 (1967), 500–506.

78. Goetzinger MR, Houchins RR: The 1947 Raven's Colored Progressive Matrices with deaf and hearing subjects. *Am Ann Deaf*, 114 (1969), 95–101.

79. James RP: A correlation analysis between the Raven's Matrices and WISC-R Performance Scale. *Volta Rev*, 86 (1984), 336–341.

80. Naglieri JA: *Matrix Analogies Test—Expanded Form* (New York: The Psychological Corporation, 1985).

81. Naglieri JA, Bardos AN: Canadian children's performance on the Matrix Analogies Test. *Sch Psychol Int*, 9 (1988), 309–313.

82. Naglieri JA, Welch JA: Use of Raven's and Naglieri's Nonverbal Matrix Texts. *J Am Deafness Rehabil*, 24 (1991), 98–103.

83. Ottem E: An Analysis of cognitive studies with deaf students. *Am Ann Deaf*, 125 (1980), 564–575.

84. Porter LJ, Kirby EA: Effects of two instructional sets on validity of the Kaufman Assessment Battery for Children-Nonverbal Scale with a group of severely hearing impaired children. *Psychol Sch*, 23 (1986), 37–43.

85. Phelps L, Branyan BJ: Correlations among the Hiskey, KABC Nonverbal Scale, Leiter and WISC-R Performance Scale with public-school deaf children. *J Psychoeduc Assess*, 8 (1988), 354–356.

86. Phelps L, Branyan BJ: Academic achievement and nonverbal intelligence in public school hearing-impaired children. *Psychol Sch*, 27 (1990), 210–217.

87. Laughton J: Nonlinguistic creative abilities and expressive syntactic abilities of hearing-impaired children. *Volta Rev*, 81 (1979), 409–420.

88. Vygotsky LS: *Mind in Society: The Development of Higher Psychological Processes* (Cambridge, MA: Harvard University Press, 1978).

89. Keane K, Kretschmer RE: The effect of mediated learning intervention on task performance with a deaf population. *J Educ Psychol*, 79 (1987), 49–53.

90. Kaltsounis B: Differences in verbal creative thinking abilities between deaf and hearing children. *Psychol Rep*, 26 (1970), 727–733.

91. Pang H, Harrocks C: An exploratory study of creativity in deaf children. *Percept Mot Skills*, 27 (1968), 844–846.

92. Silver RA: The question of imagination, originality, and abstract thinking by deaf children. *Am Ann Deaf*, 122 (1977), 349–354.

93. Odom PB, Blanton RL, McIntyre CK: Coding medium and word recall by deaf and hearing subjects. *J Speech Hear Res*, 13 (1970), 54–58.

94. Bellugi U, Klima E, Siple P: Remembering in signs. *Cognition*, 3 (1975), 93–125.

95. Locke SL, Locke VL: Deaf children's phonetic visual and Daylic coding in a grapheme recall task. *J Exer Psych*, 89 (1971), 142–146.

96. Conrad R: *The Deaf School Child*. (London: Harper & Row, 1979).

97. Lichtenstein E: Deaf working memory processes and English Language Skills, in Martin DS ed: *Cognition, Education, and Deafness* (Washington, DC: Gallaudet University Press, 1985.

98. Quinn L: Reading skills of hearing and congenitally deaf children. *J Exp Child Psych* 31 (1981), 139–161.

99. Kretschmer RE: Reading and the hearing-impaired individual: Summary and application, *Volta Rev*, 84 (1982) 107–122.

100. Kretschmer RE, Martello A: Developing a screening test and follow-up procedure for identifying encoding preference. Presented at the Convention of American Instructors of the Deaf (1993).

101. Ling D: *Speech and the Hearing Impaired Child: Theory and Practice* (Washington, DC: AG Bell Association, (1976).

102. Monsen RB: A Usable test for the speech intelligibility of deaf talkers. *Am Ann Deaf*, 126 (1981), 845–852.

103. Monsen R, Moog JS, Geers AE: *CID Picture SPINE* (St. Louis: Central Institute for the Deaf, 1988).

104. Wilbur RB: *American Sign Language* (San Diego, CA: College Hills Press, 1987).

105. Coulter GR, ed: *Phonetics and Phonology: Current Issues in ASL Phonology* (San Diego: Academic Press, 1983).

106. Cooper R: The ability of deaf and hearing children to apply morphological rules. *J Speech Hear Res*, 10 (1967), 77–86.

107. Davis J: Performance of young hearing impaired children on a test of basic concepts. *J Speech Hear Res*, 17 (1974), 342–351.

108. Geers AE, Moog JS: Syntactic maturity of spontaneous speech and elicited imitations of hearing impaired children. *J Speech Hear Dis*, 43 (1978), 380–391.

109. Hasenstab MS, Laughton J: Bare Essentials in Assessing Really Little Kids: An approach, in Hasenstab MS, Horne JS, ed: *Comprehensive Intervention with Hearing-Impaired Infants and Preschoolers* (Rockville, MD: Aspen Park Publishers, 1982).

110. Engen E, Engen T: *Rhode Island Test of Language Structure* (Baltimore: University Park Press, 1983).

111. Longhurst TM, Briery D, Emery M.: *SKI-HI Receptive Language Test* (Logan, UT: Dept. of Communication Disorders, Utah State University, 1975).

112. Moog JS, Kozak VJ: *Teacher Assessment of Grammatical Structures* (St. Louis, MO: Central Institute for the Deaf, 1983).

113. Bunch GO: *Test of Expressive Language Ability* (Toronto: G.B. Services, 1981).

114. Quigley SP, Steinkamp MW, Power DJ, Jones B: *Test of Syntactic Abilities* (Beaverton, OR: Dormac, 1978).

115. Moog JS, Kozak VJ, Geers AE: *Grammatical Analysis of Elicited Language: Pre-Sentence Level* (St. Louis: Central Institute for the Deaf, 1983).

116. Moog JS, Geers AE: *Grammatical Analysis of Elicited Language: Simple Sentence Level* (GAEL-S) (St. Louis: Central Institute for the Deaf, 1979).

117. Moog JS, Geers AE: *Grammatical Analysis of Elicited Language: Complex Sentence Level* (St. Louis: Central Institute for the Deaf, 1980).

118. White AH: *Maryland Syntax Evaluation Instrument* (Sanger, TX: Support Systems for the Deaf, 1981).

119. Bunch GO: *Test of Receptive Language Ability* (Toronto, Ontario: G.B. Service, 1981).

120. Bloom L, Lahey M: *Language Development and Language Disorders* (New York: John Wiley & Sons, 1978.)

121. Kretschmer RR, Kretschmer LW: *Language Development and Interaction with the Hearing Impaired* (Baltimore: University Park Press, 1978).

122. Layton TL, Holmes DW: *Carolina Picture Vocabulary Test* (Tulsa, OK: Modern Education Corporation, 1985).

123. Scherer P: *Total Communication Receptive Vocabulary Test* (Northbrook, IL: Mental Health and Deafness Resources, 1981.

124. Wigg EH, Secord W: *Test of Word Knowledge* (New York: The Psychological Corporation, 1993).

125. Halliday MAK, Hasan R: *Cohesions in English* (London: Longman Press, 1976).

126. Coggins TE, Carpenter RL: The Communication Intention Inventory: A system for observing and coding children's early intentional communication. *Appl Psycholinguist*, 2 (1981), 235–351.

127. Dore J: Holophrase, speech acts and language universals. *J Child Lang*, 2 (1975), 21–40.

128. Shulman BB: *Test of Pragmatic Skills—Revised* (Tucson, AZ: Communication Skill Builders, 1985).

129. Dore J: Conversational acts and the acquisition of language, in Ochs E and Schiefelin BB, ed: *Developmental Pragmatics* (New York: Academic Press, 1979).

130. Peverly S, Brobst K: *Inventory and Assessment of Study Skills* (New York: Teachers College, Columbia University, 1989).

131. Zachman L, Jorgensen C, Huisingh R, Barrett, M: *Test of Problem Solving* (Moline, IL: LinguiSystems, 1984).

132. Ramey CT, Farran DC, Campbell, FA, et al: Observations of mother-infant interactions: implications for development, in Minifie FD, Lloyd LL, eds: *Communicative and Cognitive Abilities—Early Behavioral Assessment* (Baltimore: University Park Press, 1978).

133. Collins JL, Rose S: Communicative interaction patterns in an open environment for deaf high school students. *Am Ann Deaf*, 121 (1976), 497–501.
134. Goss RN: Language used by mothers of deaf children and mothers of hearing children. *Am Ann Deaf*, 115 (1970), 79–85.
135. Caissie R, Cole EB: Mothers and hearing-impaired children: Directiveness reconsidered. *Volta Rev*, 95 (1993), 49–59.
136. Bales RE: *Interaction Process Analysis* (Reading, MA: Addison-Wesley Press, 1950).
137. Craig WN, Collins JL: Analysis of communication interaction in classes for deaf children. *Am Ann Deaf*, 115 (1970), 79–85.
138. Wolff S: Cognitive and communication patterns in classrooms for deaf students. *Am Ann Deaf*, 122 (1977), 319–327.
139. Pendergrass RA, Hodges M: Deaf students in group problem solving situations: A study of the interactive process. *Am Ann Deaf*, 121 (1976), 327–330.
140. Ewoldt C: Reading for the hearing or hearing impaired: A single process. *Am Ann Deaf*, 123 (1978), 945–948.
141. Clay MM: The Early Detection of Reading Difficulties, 3 ed (Birkenhead, New Zealand: Heinemann, 1979).
142. Reisman FK: *Sequential Assessment of Mathematics Inventories* (San Antonio, TX: Psychological Corporation, 1985).
143. Myklebust HR: *Picture Story Language Test* (New York: Grune and Stratton, 1965).
144. Calkins LM: *The Art of Teaching Writing* (Portsmouth, NH: Heinemann Educational Books, Inc., 1986).
145. Applebee AN: *The Children's Concept of Story* (Chicago: University of Chicago Press, 1978).
146. Kretschmer RE: Pragmatics, reading, and writing: Implications for hearing impaired individuals. *Top Lang Dis*, 9 (1989), 17–32.
147. Yoshinaga-Itano C, Downey M: A process analysis of the written language of hearing-impaired children. *Volta Rev*, 94, 2 (1992), 131–158.
148. Oakland T: *Psychological and Educational Assessment of Minority Children* (New York: Brunner/Mazel, 1977).
149. Quarrington B, Solomon B: A current study of the social maturity of deaf students. *Can J Behav Sci Rev Can Sci Comp*, 7 (1975), 70–77.
150. Dunlap WR, Sands DI: Classification of the hearing impaired for independent living using the Vineland adaptive behavior scales. *Am Ann Deaf*, 135 (1990), 384–388.
151. Schlesinger HS, Meadow KP: *Sound and Sign Childhood Deafness and Mental Health* (Berkeley: University of California Press, 1972).
152. Levine ES, Wagner EE: Personality patterns of deaf persons: An interpretation based on research with the hand test. *Percept Mot Skills*, 31 (1974), 1167–1236.
153. Meadow KP, Karchmer MA, Petersen LM, Rudner L: *Meadow/Kendall Social-Emotional Assessment Inventory for Deaf Students* (Washington, DC: Gallaudet College, Pre-College Programs, 1980).
154. Meadow KP: An instrument for assessment of social emotional adjustment in hearing-impaired preschoolers. *Am Ann Deaf*, 128 (1983), 826–834.
155. Hogan HW: Authoritarianism among white and black deaf adolescents: Two measures compared. *Percept Mot Skills*, 31 (1970), 195–200.
156. Leigh IW, Robins CL, Welkowitz, J, Bond RN: Toward greater understanding of depression in deaf individuals. *Am Ann Deaf*, 134 (1989), 249–254.
157. Schwartz NS, Mebane DL, Malong HN: Effects of alternate modes of administration on Rorschach performance of deaf adults. *J Pers Assess*, 54 (1990), 671–683.
158. Exner JE: *The Rorschach: A Comprehensive System* (New York: Wiley-Interscience, 1986).
159. Brauer BA: The signer effect on MMPI performance of deaf respondents. *J Pers Assess*, 58 (1992), 380–388.
160. Ouellette SE: The use of projective drawing techniques in the personality assessment of prelingually deafened young adults: A pilot study. *Am Ann Deaf*, 133, 3 (1988), 212–218.
161. Harris RI: The relationship of impulse control to parent hearing status, manual communication and academic achievement in deaf children. *Am Ann Deaf*, 123 (1978), 52–67.
162. Davey B, LaSasso C: Relations of cognitive style to assessment components of reading comprehension for hearing-impaired adolescents. *Volta Rev*, 87 (1985), 17–27.
163. Chan KS: Locus of control and achievement motivation—critical factors in educational psychology. *Psychol Sch*, 15 (1979), 104–110.
164. Altshuler KZ, Deming WE, Vollenweider J, et al: Impulsivity and profound early deafness: A cross-cultural inquiry. *Am Ann Deaf*, 121 (1976), 331–345.
165. Stinson M: Deafness and motivation for achievement: research with implications for parent counseling. *Volta Rev*, 80 (1978), 140–148.
166. Kampfe CM: Reading comprehension of deaf adolescent residential school students and its relationship to hearing mothers' communication strategies and skills. *Am Ann Deaf*, 134 (1989), 317–322.
167. McCrone WP: Learned helplessness and level of underachievement among deaf adolescents. *Psychol Sch*, 16 (1979), 430–434.

168. Chandler TA: Locus of control: A proposal for change. *Psychol Sch*, 12 (1975), 335–339.

169. Kagan J: Impulsive and reflective children: Significance of conceptual tempo, in Krumbolid JD, ed: *Learning and the Educational Process* (Chicago: Rand McNally, 1965).

170. Rotter JB: Generalized expectancies for internal versus external control of reinforcement. *Psychol Monogr*, 80 (1966), 1–28.

171. Reich C, Hambleton D, Houldin: The integration of hearing impaired children in regular classrooms. *Am Ann Deaf*, 122 (1977), 534–544.

172. Rudy JP, Nance JG: A Transitional instrument, in Northcott WH, ed: *The Hearing Impaired Child in a Regular Classroom* (Washington, DC: The Alexander Graham Bell Assoc., 1973).

173. Bullis M, Reiman J: Development and preliminary psychometric properties of the transition competence battery for deaf adolescents and young adults. *Except Child*, 59 (1992), 12–26.

174. Davidow J, Levinson EM: Heuristic principles and cognitive bias in decision making: Implications for assessment in school psychology. *Psychol Sch*, 30 (1993), 351–361.

175. Brown, AL, Campione JC, Weber LS, McGilly K: *Interactive Learning Environments: A New Look At Assessment and Instruction* (Berkeley: University of California, Commission on Testing and Public Policy, 1992).

176. Schirmer BR: Constructing meaning from narrative text. *Am Ann Deaf*, 138 (1993), 397–403.

177. Garrison W, Long G, Dowliby F: Reading comprehension test item difficulty as a function of cognitive processing variables. *Am Ann Deaf*, 137, 1 (1992), 22–30.

178. Bye L, Jussim L: A Proposed model for the acquisition of social knowledge and social competence. *Psychol Sch*, 30 (1993), 143–161.

179. Bernard ME: Rational-emotive therapy with children and adolescents: Treatment strategies. *Sch Psychol Rev*, 19, 3 (1990), 294–303.

180. Tingstrom DH, Little SG: School consultation from a social psychological perspective: A review. *Psychol Sch*, (1990), 43–50.

7

PSYCHO-EDUCATIONAL ASSESSMENT OF CHILDREN WITH AUDITORY LANGUAGE LEARNING PROBLEMS

R. Ray Battin

> *Auditory space has no point of favored focus. It's a sphere without fixed boundaries, space made by the thing itself, not space containing the thing.*
>
> —Edmund Carpenter and Marshall McLuhan,
> *Explorations in Communication*, Beacon Press, 1960, p. 67

Auditory verbal language disturbances can range from the severely involved, as seen in children with aphasia, auditory agnosia, or autism, to the more mildly involved children with auditory imperceptions or learning disabilities.

For the child with severe auditory-verbal language problems, psycho-educational assessment will, by necessity, consist of a modified test battery tailored to the perceptual and communicative skills of the child. Test instruments typically used for evaluating the severely hearing impaired are also applicable to this population (see Chapter 2).

Children with auditory language-learning problems are more difficult to identify than those with peripheral hearing loss or impaired vision. Their behaviors may be misunderstood. As a result, these children are frequently labeled immature or inattentive. Their performance in school worsens each year, and by grades 3 or 4 they are either making failing grades or significantly underachieving for their level of abilities. At this point, the teacher or parent may seek further evaluation of these children.

The child is referred to the educational diagnostician, counselor, or school psychologist because of school or behavioral difficulties. It is the responsibility of the examiner to assess the child's general abilities, how he or she learns, and how he or she perceives and deals with new situations. The examiner must also present an extensive analysis of independent responses and test scatter. Specific test data, if properly analyzed, may delineate the child with an auditory perceptual problem.

This chapter will deal with the selection and interpretation of psycho-educational tests and their use in evaluating the child with an auditory-verbal processing or perceptual disturbance. It will attempt to demonstrate how the child's test profile can be used in educational planning and in establishment of a remedial program directed to specific deficits.

VALIDITY AND RELIABILITY

Care must be taken when choosing an assessment instrument. With the proliferation of tests (they sprout like leaves on a tree), the examiner must know how to choose appropriately.

Standards, as recommended by the Committee on Standards of the American Psychological Association, apply to any published test used in evaluation, diagnosis, or prognosis. Each test should have data available on validity and reliability, directions for administration and scoring, and qualifications required to administer and properly interpret the test.

INFORMAL VERSUS FORMAL TESTING

Increasing criticism has been directed toward formal testing. Intelligence tests have come under critical review because they have been used to classify children for placement in classes for the mentally retarded. It was found that blacks tended to score lower on the Wechsler Intelligence Scale

Case study 7-1.   John was referred for comprehensive evaluation when he was 13 years 9 months of age because of behavior problems at school. He was getting into trouble; he was in detention hall for talking, being late, and fighting with students both on and off campus.

Behavior during the evaluation revealed a quiet youngster who was somber, cooperative, and had fair eye contact. He was inconsistent in his effort and frustration to task. Questions had to be repeated throughout the session. Gross and fine coordination fell withing normal limits.

Audiological findings were within normal limits with pure-tone averages of 3 dB for the left ear and 0 dB for the right, speech reception thresholds of 5 dB for the left ear and 0 dB for the right, and word discrimination scores of 100%, bilaterally. Impedance audiometry provided type A tympanograms bilaterally.

The Staggered Spondaic Word Test showed a moderate to severe disturbance in central auditory processing. He had a significant ear effect as well as a significant order effect. He experienced his greatest difficulty when the competing message was in the right ear, suggesting involvement in the auditory reception area of the left temporal lobe.

The Clinical Evaluation of Language Fundamentals-Revised was administered and John failed the test, falling 5 points below the criterion score for his age. He had problems in auditory association and in reconstructing sentences.

This young man was performing in the average range of abilities, slightly on the low side, with performance skills in the average range and verbal skills in the low average range. He showed severe auditory processing problems and mild to moderate auditory memory problems. Academically, he was performing at the level of his ability, with the exception of mathematical computation, but below grade placement. Emotionally, he showed a poor self-concept and poor coping skills. His responses to the Rorschach indicated a thought disorder, although not of the bizarre type. His responses to the Thematic Appreciation Test were constricted with anxiety, sadness, anger, and a parting of the ways between mother and son present in his responses. He was concerned about his father's alcoholism. He was somewhat guarded and distant in regard to what precipitated his suicidal thoughts. The suicide potential was still present and needed to be explored further. In addition, it was recommended that he receive therapy for the severe auditory processing disturbance. The problem in processing what he received auditorially may have been a contributing factor to the observed thought disorder.

John met the criteria for 296.22 Major Depression, 300.40 Dysthymia and 313.81 Oppositional Defiant Disorder.

for Children (WISC) and the Stanford-Binet tests, and thus were overrepresented in these classes. As a result, a moratorium on the use of formal psychological testing for special education placement has been declared in many school districts. (1–3) To discontinue the use of generalized intelligence tests, however, is to throw out the good with the bad. The error comes when examiners use such tests as the Wechsler Intelligence Scale for Children-III (WISC-III), the Wechsler Preschool and Primary Scale of Intelligence-Revised (WPPSI-R), or the Stanford-Binet Intelligence Scale, fourth edition, to compute a single composite score, rather then analyzing the components. As will be pointed out in later sections of this chapter, the WISC-III, WPPSI-R, and the Stanford-Binet Intelligence Scale, fourth edition, can provide information on auditory-verbal and visual-motor skills.

Informal assessment may provide insight into the child's problems, but with the present concern over accountability, it does not provide an adequate base on which to build a treatment or educational program. The generalized assessment utilizing well-standardized tests provides the examiner with more reliable and valid data against which treatment gains versus maturational gains may be checked. By using the child as the control, a learning and abilities profile can be plotted and used to determine if significant strengths and weaknesses exist and whether therapeutic intervention is indicated. Classification can be made according to independent learning skills, as opposed to a more global labeling.

UNIMODAL, BIMODAL, OR MULTIMODAL ASSESSMENT

It is extremely difficult to dissect learning by modality. Jastak and Jastak[4] theorize that the three sensory modalities—hearing, vision, and kinesthesia (touch)—are "involved in the formation of lexigraphic and other linguistic communication codes."

With increasing specialization, learning disorders are divided into discipline-specific disabilities.

As we test in our specialty and see what we are trained to see, we become like the proverbial blind men describing the elephant. Rarely is a child with a learning disability depressed in only a single modality. Furthermore, if we look only at a single modality when we assess a child's capabilities, we may label as deficient areas in which the child is depressed across all modalities and is performing within his level of ability. To reemphasize, a child must be used as his or her own control if we are to understand the learning potential as well as the disabilities of that child.

HISTORY AS A PART OF THE ASSESSMENT

A detailed birth, health, family, social, educational, and behavioral history are a critical part of any comprehensive assessment. A preinterview questionnaire, which the parents can complete at home with the help of the baby book, and which is returned prior to the testing, allows the examiner some insight into the problems presented by the child.[5] A comparison of the behaviors described in the questionnaire with test behavior and performance provides the examiner with some support for the interpretation drawn from the assessment.

In addition to specific questions, the questionnaire should contain several open-ended questions that allow the parents to describe the child's behavior and personality. Methods of discipline used by the parents should also be explained in detail. The examiner will want to review the responses to questions on birth, health, and development carefully, as well as scrutinize the behavioral responses.

Behaviors that point to a disturbance in the auditory-verbal area include inattentiveness, short attention span, daydreaming, and a tendency to play with younger children. The child may also be withdrawn, unable to follow directions, and forgetful. The child may misunderstand instructions or directions, be disruptive in school and at home, fail to bring homework home, or be unable to remember assignments. For example, the child might know spelling words or other material at home, but fail a test on the material at school. Teachers may label the child as a "smart aleck" or one who "refuses to conform."

SPECIFIC TEST INSTRUMENTS

A comprehensive psycho-educational test battery for children suspected of an auditory-verbal learning disturbance should include tests that fall under five general categories: general abilities, auditory-verbal behavior, visual-motor behavior, academic behavior, and personality. Table 7-1 summarizes the psychological tests that should be considered for assessment in these five areas.

Table 7-1 Psycho-educational Test Battery

Type of Assessment	Sequence of Tests
	Appropriate Instruments
I. General Abilities	1. Stanford-Binet Intelligence Scale: Fourth Edition
	2. Wechsler Intelligence Scale for Children (WISC-III)
	3. Wechsler Preschool and Primary Scale of Intelligence-R (WPPSI-R)
	4. Kaufman Assessment Battery for children
	5. Kaufman Brief Intelligence Test (KBIT)
II. Auditory-Verbal Behavior	1. Illinois Test of Psycholinguistic Abilities (ITPA; selected subtests)
	2. Detroit Tests of Learning Aptitude-3 (DTLA-3; selected subtests)
	3. Goldman Fristoe Woodcock Test of Selective Attention
	4. Peabody Picture Vocabulary Test-Revised (PPVT-R)
III. Visual-Motor Behavior	1. Illinois Test of Psycholinguistic Abilities (ITPA; selected subtests)
	2. Detroit Tests of Learning Aptitude-3 (DTLA-3 selected subtests)
	3. Bender-Gestalt Test
	4. Slosson Drawing Coordination Test for Children
	5. Primary Visual Motor Test
	6. Goodenough-Harris Draw-A-Person
IV. Academic Behavior	1. Peabody Individual Achievement Test-R
	2. Woodcock Johnson Tests of Achievement-R
	3. Wechsler Individual Achievement Test
	4. Wide Range Achievement Test-R
	5. Myklebust Written Language Test
	Selected Tests
V. Personality	1. Rorschach Test
	2. Thematic Apperception Test
	3. Children's Apperception Test
	4. Incomplete Sentences Test
	5. House-Tree-Person Test
	6. Kinetic Family Drawing
	7. Others as needed

General Abilities Assessment

The most widely used tests of general abilities are the Stanford-Binet and the Wechsler Scales.

The first scale of intelligence, the Binet, was published by Binet and Simon in 1905. It was developed to help separate the uneducable from the educable in the schools of Paris. In 1916, while at Stanford University, Terman revised the Binet test—thus, the name Stanford-Binet.[6] Since that time, it has gone through several additional revisions. In 1960, the best items from the L and M forms of the 1937 scale were combined into a single scale. This revision was restandardized in 1972.[7] Thorndike et al[8] introduced the fourth edition in 1986.

The present revision covers the same age range. It requires the examiner to establish a basal age and includes many of the same types of test items, All other aspects of the test differ significantly from previous editions. Items of the same type are now grouped into 15 tests, with each test tapping different cognitive skills and different funds of information.

Four broad areas, Verbal Reasoning, Abstract/Visual Reasoning, Quantitative Reasoning, and Short-Term Memory, are assessed by the 15 tests. The tests provide a composite standard age score of general reasoning ability and standard age scores for the four areas. Standard age scores are also available for any combination of the four areas as well as for individual test scores for the 15 tests. This edition was constructed to better identify individuals who are mentally retarded, have specific learning disabilities, or are gifted. Once an examiner becomes familiar with the new test, he or she will find it is much more flexible than earlier editions. The new edition can be adapted more readily to the child undergoing the test, and it provides information in both the auditory-verbal and visual-motor modalities. This information can then be used in the development of a treatment program.

The complete battery consists of 8 to 13 tests and takes 1 hour to 90 minutes to administer. A screening battery composed of the Vocabulary, Bead Memory, Quantitative, and Pattern Analysis can be administered in 30 to 40 minutes. A six subtest battery, which requires less testing time than the complete battery, can be assembled by adding Memory for Sentences and Comprehension to the original screening test. The authors recommend that assessment of students experiencing difficulty in school includes tests that have the greatest diagnostic value and a balance of verbal and abstract/visual reasoning tests. The test manual provides recommendations for abbreviated batteries.[8]

The revised, restandardized WISC-III was published in 1991 (See Case Study 7-1). It was developed for use with children between 6 to 16 years, 11 months. The lower limit overlaps with the WPPSI-R and the upper limit with the WAIS-R. In addition to the 12 subtests that made up the 1949 WISC and 1974 WISC-R, the publishers have added a new optional subtest, Symbol Search. Six subtests make up the Verbal Scale and seven subtests, the Performance Scale. As with earlier editions, 10 of the WISC III tests are considered mandatory; the Digit Span, Symbol Search, and Mazes subtests are supplementary tests and were not included in establishing the IQ tables. In addition to the verbal, performance, and full-scale IQ scores, four-factor based scores can be calculated for verbal comprehension, perceptual organization, freedom from distractibility, and processing speed.

The WISC-III has improved subtest content, administration, and scoring rules. An effort was made to minimize content bias and to refine and update the artwork. Easier as well as more difficult items were added to various subtests. Although many of the test items were retained and unchanged in the verbal subtests, other items were modified and new items were added. On the performance scale, the pictures have been redrawn, color has been added, and there is an increase in the number of items. The Picture Completion subtest has been increased from 12 to 14 items. There are 12 items instead of 11 on the Block Design subtest and a new item has been added to both the Object Assembly subtest and the Mazes subtest. Symbol Search is a new optional subtest with levels A and B.

The new order for presenting subtests, plus the improved drawing and addition of color, makes the test more interesting and less tiring, both for the child and the examiner. The subtests most relevant to auditory-verbal dysfunction are the verbal ones; however, they only reveal a disturbance within a particular child when they are compared with that child's scores on the performance subtests.[10]

Analysis of a child's performance on the individual subtests of the WISC-III will indicate whether further testing in specific modalities is needed.[11] The Information subtest indicates how well the child stores information gained from education and experience and how well this information can be retrieved on command. By comparing responses on the Information, Arithmetic, and Digit Span subtests, the examiner can observe the effectiveness of the child's delayed recall as opposed to immediate recall, auditory attention, and mental control. The ability to provide practical solutions to everyday problems and social adjustment may be seen through the Comprehension subtest, with the Vocabulary subtest providing an estimate of verbal fluency, word knowledge, and expressive skills. The Similarities subtest provides information on the child's logical and abstract verbal reasoning ability.

By careful observation of the child's behavior during the verbal subtests, an understanding of how the child processes auditorily emerges. Questions that indicate auditory processing function include:

1. Does the child need frequent repetitions or restatement of questions?
2. Does the child tend to reauditorize the material or are there long response latencies?
3. How are the numbers on the Digit Span Subtest retrieved?
4. Are the problems on the Arithmetic Subtest forgotten before they can be solved?
5. Are there difficulties in perceiving the questions or following directions on the Information, Comprehension, and Similarities subtests?
6. Does the child appear to confuse words (eg, pail for nail) on the Vocabulary subtests?

Similar analysis of the subtests of the Performance Scale can pinpoint problems in visual closure, gestalt, praxis, short-term memory, scanning, and left-right tracking. Problems with delayed visual recall, visual problem-solving inability, and fine motor control can also be delineated.

The Revised WPPSI (WPPSI-R) was published in 1989.[12] Like the WPPSI, the revision is an individually administered test of intelligence for children. However, the age range has been extended to cover children age 3 through 7 years, thus overlapping the WISC-III. In this test, the mean IQ is 100, with a standard deviation of 15. The subtests have a mean scaled score of 10 and a standard deviation of 3. Comparison of the WPPSI and WPPSI-R scores places the WPPSI full scale IQ 8 points higher than the WPPSI-R, with the WPPSI verbal scale IQ 9 points higher and the performance scale 5 points higher than the WPPSI-R. Comparing the WISC-R with the WPPSI-R revealed similar findings. When the

WPPSI-R was compared with the Stanford-Binet Intelligence Scale, fourth edition, the composite score of the Stanford-Binet fell 2 points higher, suggesting the two tests yield similar IQs for normal children ranging from 4 to 7 years of age. Similar results were obtained for the WPPSI-R and the McCarthy Scales of Children's Abilities. The Kaufman Assessment Battery for Children (KABC) showed a difference, with the WPPSI-R full scale IQ falling approximately 6 points lower than the Mental Processing Composite of the KABC.

Data for the WPPSI-R were also collected from various populations of exceptional children, including children who were identified as gifted, mentally deficient, learning disabled, and speech/language impaired. The samples for these groups were small. Although the data indicate that the WPPSI-R is a useful diagnostic instrument with these populations, more extensive research is needed.

With the exception of Arithmetic, the subtests begin with items on which the correct response is demonstrated or taught, thus ensuring that the child understands the directions. This would be especially helpful for those children with auditory processing difficulties. The preferred order for administering the test starts with Object Assembly and follows with Information, Geometric Design, Comprehension, Block Design, Arithmetic, Mazes, Vocabulary, Picture Completion, Similarities, Animal Pegs, and Sentences. The examiner is allowed to vary the order if a child experiences difficulty with a particular subtest. The WPPSI-R takes approximately 60 to 90 minutes to administer and may have to be broken into two testing sessions if the child becomes unduly fatigued. As with the WISC-III, the WPPSI-R uses 10 subtests—five verbal and five performance—to determine IQ. A review of the child's performance on individual subtests does give the examiner a pattern of strengths and weaknesses in auditory-verbal and visual-motor learning. In my opinion, the WPPSI-R does not provide sufficient additional information over the Stanford-Binet to warrant the added time it takes to administer. For the child under 5 years of age, the time would be more profitably used by administering a language test in conjunction with the Stanford-Binet.

The KABC was published in 1983[13] as an individually administered measure of intelligence and achievement for children 2.5 thorough 12.5 years of age. Administration time is approximately 45 minutes for preschool children and 75 minutes for school age children. The test is made up of the following 16 subtests: Hand Movements, Number Recall, Word Order, Magic Window, Face Recognition, Gestalt Closure, Triangles, Matrix Analogies, Spatial Memory, Photo Series, Expressive Vocabulary, Faces and Places, Arithmetic, Riddles, Reading/Decoding, and Reading/Understanding. Seven subtests are administered to 2.5-year-old children, 9 subtests to 3-year-old children, and the maximum (13) to children 7 years old and older. It provides standard scores (mean, 100; standard deviation, 15) in four areas: Sequential Processing, Simultaneous Processing, Mental Processing Composite (obtained from Sequencing Processing and Simultaneous Processing, which provides and IQ equivalence), and Achievement. Supplemental sociocultural norms assist in interpreting the tests of children from minority groups. In addition, a nonverbal scale made up of selected subtests that can be administered and responded to through gestures provides assessment of the general abilities level of children with auditory processing problems, speech and language delay, or hearing impairment.

The Kaufman was developed from neuropsychological theory, but does not claim to be a neuropsychological test. However, those examiners who look at brain dysfunction, as it relates to performance and developing a therapy plan, will find the test fits well into their assessment battery.

An examiner may need an estimate of cognitive skills if he or she is evaluating central auditory processing or language-learning ability, or if a standard test of intelligence was administered by another agency and the examiner wants to assess present functioning. The Kaufman Brief Intelligence Test (KBIT) published in 1990 is an excellent instrument to use.[14] The KBIT is an individually administered test that measures both verbal and nonverbal intelligence. Verbal and crystallized abilities are measured by a vocabulary test, and nonverbal and fluid abilities are measured by a matrices subtest. The KBIT has an age range of 4 to 90 years and is easy to administer. The authors state that it may be given by technicians or allied health professionals not licensed in administering standard intelligence tests. The test takes from 15 to 30 minutes to administer and was developed as a screening instrument that provides an estimate of intelligence. Care must be taken to not use this test for diagnosis, placement, or neuropsychological evaluation.

The Test of Nonverbal Intelligence, second edition (TONI-2), published in 1990, was developed for use with individuals who require a language-free, motor-reduced and culture-reduced test format.[15] It measures abstract, visual problem solving with an age range of 5 through 85 years, 11 months. It takes approximately 15 minutes to administer and has no reading, writing, listening, or speaking requirement. Gestures are used for giving instructions and there are six training items. The individual indicates his or her response by pointing. School psychologists have used the TONI-2 to qualify a student for services when unable to obtain the required discrepancy between achievement and IQ from standard intelligence tests.

Other intelligence tests that test special abilities are the Hiskey-Nebraska Test of Learning Aptitudes,[16] Leiter International Performance Scale,[17] Arthur Point Performance Scale,[18] Slosson Intelligence Test for Children and Adults-R,[10] Raven Progressive Matrices,[20,21] and the Columbia Mental Maturity Scale.[22]

Auditory-Verbal Behavior Assessment

Although speech pathologists have laid claim to the Illinois Test of Psycholinguistic Abilities (ITPA) as a language test, it was designed as a diagnostic test of psychological and linguistic function (see Case Study 7–2).[33] Although the test is in need of revision, it continues to be a useful tool in assessing children with learning disabilities, particularly those children who experience difficulty processing information received auditorily. The test assesses specific ability strengths as well as weaknesses, and thus allows a plan for remediation to be developed. The experimental edition of the ITPA was published in 1961, with the present revision published in 1968. The revised ITPA extended the age range and covers children from 2.5 years through 10 years, 3 months of age. Clinically, the test is more effective for those over 4 years of age. For children who are learning disabled whose age is above the test ceiling, the full test or selective subtests provide useful information on developmental lags.

The 10 main and two supplementary subtests of the ITPA are divided into two categories: auditory-verbal and visual-motor. Scaled scores, which are a linear transformation of raw scores, are used to express the child's functioning level on each subtest. There is a mean of 36 and a standard deviation of 6. Psycholinguistic age scores may provide information on the child who falls

Case study 7–2. Testing was requested by David's pediatrician to rule out a possible attention deficit hyperactivity disorder. David was enrolled in the fourth grade and was experiencing difficulty in all his classes, especially social studies. School behavior was described as having poor work habits, not paying attention, not using time and materials effectively, and not disciplining himself. Grades had been inconsistent.

Birth history placed weight at 6 pounds, 8 ounces with delivery at term. No complications were reported. A hernia was observed and operated on at 3 months of age. Motor development was within normal limits.

Speech and language development was significantly delayed. First words did not occur until 2 years of age, with connected discourse at 3 years of age. At age 3 years he was tested by the School District and placed in an early childhood education program for speech and language.

No childhood diseases were reported; however, he has had many problems in early childhood with ear infections.

David lives with his father, stepmother, a brother age 20 years, and a stepsister age 18 years. His social adaptation skills were described as excitable; he sometimes threw temper tantrums and talked back to his parents. He generally was personable, congenial, had a pleasant personality, and willing to change to get approval.

The Fisher's Auditory Problems Checklist was completed by the father. The results where borderline significant for auditory processing problems.

David was a friendly and playful child who was very hyperactive. He was out of his seat and sometimes lying on the floor. He was impulsive and tried to grab test materials as well as to start the task before the appropriate time was given. He was inattentive and needed to be refocused to task using verbal and visual cues. At times he verbalized his problem-solving.

Gross and fine motor coordination fell within normal limits, slightly on the low side. Responses to the Reitan Finger Oscillation Test were age-appropriate.

Audiological evaluation placed hearing within normal limits, with a pure-tone average of 3 dB for the left ear and 0 dB for the right ear. Speech reception thresholds of 5 dB for the left ear and 0 dB for the right were obtained with word discrimination scores of 100%, bilaterally.

The Goldman-Fristoe-Woodcock Test of Selective Attention was administered, with David getting all of the items correct in quiet and dropping to below the 1st percentile when competing messages were introduced. He had trouble on all three of the competing messages subtests, which suggests he would experience difficulty handling classroom noise. He would benefit from preferential seating to the front of the room so that competing messages are behind him rather than between him and the primary sound source (teacher).

David was performing in the average range, slightly on the low side, as reflected on the WICS-III and the Detroit Tests of Learning Aptitude-3. He had a significant split between his Verbal Scale and his Performance Scale, with verbal skills falling in the low average range and performance skills falling in the average range. His strengths were alertness to visual detail, visual praxis, learning a meaningless code and rapidly transferring it to paper, and understanding social relationships when presented through pictures. His weaknesses were the ability to attend to a message presented auditorially when there was background noise, word knowledge, verbal concept formation, auditory decoding, practical knowledge, and social judgment. David met the criteria for 314.01 Attention Deficit Hyperactivity Disorder. Academically, he was performing at or above the level of his ability.

Emotionally, David was anxious and depressed. The Revised Children's Manifest Anxiety Scale showed that he was experiencing significant anxiety. His Thematic Apperception Test stories indicated that he was depressed, angry, having suicidal thoughts, and had low motivation to achieve. He was also having problems with his self-image and his ability to perform.

It was recommended that the parents seek a medical consultation with their family physician. Classroom modifications consisted for preferential seating, the use of a study buddy, and reducing the amount of written work. Visual cues as well as auditory signals needed to be used to help David focus on the task. It was recommended that David receive remediation therapy to address his deficits as well as psychotherapy to address the emotional issues. It was also recommended that class placement be discussed at the parent conference.

above the age ceiling of the ITPA, but they do not provide the data available in the scaled scores, which takes into consideration variability of performance for different ages on the various subtests. The scaled scores allow for comparison of test-retest data. An overall psycholinguistic age as well as a psycholinguistic quotient is available from the total score of the 10 main subtests.

A mental age estimate and IQ equivalent are also available by using the IQ conversion tables of the Stanford-Binet form L-M.

There are five main tests and two supplementary tests under the auditory-verbal area of the ITPA. They assess the ability to gain meaning from auditorily received stimuli (auditory reception), the ability to see the relationship between stimuli received auditorily (auditory association), and the ability to convey ideas in words (verbal expression). Grammatical closure uses visual clues together with auditory clues for assessing the child's retention of syntax and grammatical form. It also assesses the child's ability to complete or close out an incomplete sentence. The auditory sequential memory test uses digits that are presented two per second to assess immediate sequential recall. The two supplementary tests consist of auditory closure for assessing the ability to complete or *fill in* the missing parts or part of a word, and sound blending for testing the ability to synthesize or resynthesize words or nonsense words. Both the auditory closure and the grammatical closure subtests tap long-term memory.

Although the auditory reception and association tests tap the specific skills set forth by the test, they are dependent on a child's vocabulary and are somewhat culturally biased. At times, due to the child's shyness or lack of comprehension of the task, it is difficult to obtain sufficient responses on the verbal expression subtest to estimate expressive skills adequately. However, it has been observed clinically that there is a close relationship between performance on this subtest and the written expression skills observed on the Myklebust Test of Written Expression.[24]

Each subtest of the ITPA was to measure only one discrete function through a single modality or channel without contamination by using another channel. As was seen in the discussion of the grammatical closure subtest, it is difficult to isolate a single channel or modality when developing any test. This is particularly true on the visual subtests that utilize pictures to elicit a response. Only one of the five main tests that propose to test the visual-motor skills is free of auditory-verbal contamination. The visual sequential memory test uses discrete abstract figures that restrict verbal labeling to evaluate the ability to reproduce a sequence of designs. The test provides the examiner with information on attention span, visual scanning, and directionality, as well as immediate recall of a visual sequential pattern.

The ability to recognize the whole from parts or to *close out* an incomplete visual pattern is assessed through the visual closure subtest. It also provides the examiner with information on visual recall, visual scanning, left/right tracking, and how organized the youngster is in visual problem solving. Simple line drawings of common objects (fish, shoes, bottles, hammers, and saws) are used in the four separate scenes. Although the child is able to label the pictures, this auditory-verbal response minimally assists in the visual closure task. Both the visual reception subtest, which assesses the ability to decode visual stimuli, and the visual association subtest, which assesses the ability to see the relationship between visual stimuli, receive some contamination from the auditory channel. Children who are severely depressed in auditory verbal skills also score low on the visual association subtest of the ITPA, even though visual problem-solving tests that are not language-contaminated, such as the Raven Progressive Matrices, are well executed.

The remaining subtest of the ITPA is manual expression. This subtest deals with communicating ideas through gestures. It provides some insight into the child's inner language, particularly when there is a delay in verbal expression.

The Detroit Tests of Learning Aptitude was revised by Hammill[25] in 1985 (DTLA-2) and again in 1991 (DTLA-3)[26]. The DTLA-3, like its predecessor, is a flexible, comprehensive test containing 11 subtests that assess interrelated mental abilities. The test takes from 50 minutes to 2 hours to administer. The age range for the battery is 6 through 17 years. The test was normed on 2587 individuals from 36 states. The author describes the third edition as: "a battery that measures a variety of developed abilities. Depending on the orientation or need of the test user, DTLA-3 results can be used to estimate general cognitive functioning (intelligence), predict future success (aptitude), or show mastery of particular content and skills (achievement)." It can be used to verify areas of difficulty and to supplement the WISC-III and Stanford-Binet, or in place of the ITPA for children over 10 years, 3 months of age. In addition to providing a general mental ability quotient and three domain composites (linguistic, attentional, and motoric), the DTLA-3 provides an optimal level composite. This is an important feature for evaluating children with auditory processing problems. The four largest standard scores are combined to obtain the optimal level composite, providing an estimate of the individual's potential (Case Study 7–3).

Case study 7–3.   Timmy was initially evaluated in July 1993 to screen for language-learning problems. Testing at that time revealed a significant depression in articulation, problems with gross and fine coordination, and a significant delay in language development. Nonverbal skills fell in the average or above range with the exception of visual-spatial abilities. Academically, he was performing at beginning first grade level in reading and spelling and at beginning of second grade level in mathematics. The diagnosis at the time of the initial evaluation was severe auditory processing disorder and developmental expressive-receptive language disorder, as well as a developmental articulation disorder. We also observed a developmental coordination disorder.

The reevaluation was ordered by his physician to assess growth. Following the initial evaluation, Timmy was enrolled in a private school.

During the first day of testing, Timmy was very quiet. He was cooperative, smiled occasionally, and put forth good effort. Questions needed to be repeated constantly. He did not understand the intent of the questions or instructions. He could not remember or hold onto directions or instructions long enough to complete them. He was unable to hold onto the words long enough on the word association task of the Clinical Evaluation of Language Functions-Revised (CELF-R) to pick out the two that were alike. He was unable to reorder the phrases to construct sentences. He appeared lost in trying to figure out how to do it. Spelling was extremely poor when writing his story for the written expression subtest of the PIAT-R.

During the second day of testing, Timmy was friendly and cooperative and put forth good effort. He showed good frustration to task. Many times, he looked lost and did not understand the intent of the instruction or the question. The examiner used visual cues to aid in his understanding questions.

Audiological assessment placed hearing within normal limits, with a pure-tone average of 0 dB for the left ear and 2 dB for the right. Speech reception thresholds of 5 dB, and word discrimination scores of 100% were obtained bilaterally. Masking level differences were mildly depressed at both 1 KHz and 500 Hz. Impedance audiometry provided type A typanograms bilaterally, indicating normal middle ear function.

During the second day of testing, the Screening Test for Auditory Processing Disorders was administered. Timmy obtained a composite age score of 5 years, 2 months, with severe difficulty observed when he had to listen to competing words or filtered words. Auditory figure ground was in the low average range. Timmy continued to show a significant delay in articulation consistent with a dysarthric disorder.

Timmy fell 24 criterion points below score for his age on the CELF-R. This is a gain of two criterion points over the testing in July. He experienced severe difficulty with word association, auditory memory, and decoding. He was unable to construct a sentence. Written language was severely depressed with ''hr'' for ''her,'' ''neny'' for ''money,'' and 'pec'' for ''pick.

Timmy continued to show a highly significant difference between verbal and performance skills, with verbal skills falling in the mildly retarded range and performance skills in the average range of abilities. He showed above average abilities in visual gestalt and object assembly on the WISC-III with average skills observed in visual praxis, the ability to copy an abstract design from a pattern, understanding social relationships when presented through pictures, and alertness to visual detail. Poor ability was observed in range of knowledge, long-term memory, the ability to learn a meaningless code and rapidly transfer it to paper, verbal abstract reasoning, verbal concept formation, mathematical reasoning, verbal fluency, word comprehension and practical knowledge and social judgment. Low-average ability was observed in immediate auditory recall.

On the DLTA-3, Timmy fell in the average range when required to sequence designs as well as when required to construct a story. Low average ability was observed in understanding symbolic relationships and in handling reversed letters. Above average skills were observed in recognizing picture fragments.

This shows he has good visual closure skills, with results of this subtest consistent with the strengths observed on the WISC-III. Timmy's performance on the Bender-Gestalt, while below age level, showed better than a 2-year gain over the initial evaluation.

Emotionally, Timmy has a very low self-esteem. He sees poor peer acceptance and poor success as a student, and he does not feel good about his emotional state. His stories on the Thematic Apperception Test had running themes of sadness and unhappiness.

In summary, Timmy continued to show a severe language delay, with the results of the testing suggestive of a congenital aphasia. Articulation was also disturbed, with performance consistent with a dysarthric pattern. Academic skills were in line with his verbal rather than his nonverbal skills. Emotionally, he had begun to internalize a sense of failure, and of being different and unable to succeed as a student. He demonstrated a severe auditory processing disorder and poor auditory memory. This further exacerbated his problem. Emotionally, he was showing some depression and a sense of helplessness. Timmy met the criteria of 315.00 Developmental Expressive-Receptive Language Disorder, 315.39 Developmental Articulation Disorder, and 315.40 Developmental Coordination Problem under Axis II. He showed indications of an Attention Deficit Disorder (314.00) under Axis I.

It was recommended that Timmy continue in a one-on-one learning situation. Consideration should be given to providing him with sign language as a way of helping him develop communication skills. Since he showed strong right hemisphere function, sign language might provide him with a mnemonic device for word retrieval. Timmy does meet the criteria for special education through the public schools and they should accomodate his need for one-on-one placement.

Hammill has retained subtests from the DTLA-2, dropped items, and added new ones. The subtest that measures verbal-language learning skills is the word opposites subtest, which was originally called verbal opposites and was one of the subtests in the 1935 edition of the DTLA. It taps the ability to understand word meaning as well as word retrieval. The sentence imitation subtest was previously called auditory attention for related syllables; it measures the ability to retain and recall correct English sentences. Word sequences (auditory attention span for unrelated words) has been retained from the original test. The scoring procedure has been simplified and a few items have been added. The reversed letters subtest measures auditory memory, integration, and fine motor skills. The ability to conceptualize and express oneself orally is measured by the story construction subtest. The basic information subtest is new to this edition and measures knowledge acquired from everyday situations.

There are five nonverbal subtests. Symbolic relation, which measures nonverbal reasoning ability, uses items included in the TONI-2. Design reproduction, retained from the original DTLA, measures visual spatial and visual memory ability. Design sequences is new and is similar to the visual sequential memory subtest of the ITPA, It measures visual sequential memory and discrimination. Story sequences is a new subtest, which is similar to the picture arrangement subtest of the WISC-III. Picture fragments is also a new subtest, replacing the word fragments subtest. It is similar to the gestalt closure subtest of the Kaufman.

The oral directions subtest was omitted from the DTLA-3. However, for children with auditory processing or auditory memory problems, observation of how a child handles this subtest provides information on compensatory behavior. For example, do they repeat the direction, do they attempt to anchor the pictures or letters as the directions are presented or do they gesture to themselves. I recommend this subtest be added to the test battery. It takes very little time and provides insight into the child's behavior.

The DTLA-Primary (DTLA-P) was designed to measure intellectual abilities of children 3 to 9 years of age.[27] The test is organized developmentally from easiest to most difficult, and uses a Binet-type format. The examiner establishes a basal (that point where 10 items in a row are passed) and a ceiling (that point where 10 items in a row are missed). An articulation test and eight subtests, which may be used in the identification of specific abilities, are included in the DTLA-P. A general intelligence or aptitude score is also provided.

Individual assessment places the child in an optimum testing learning situation. Children who have problems with auditory figure ground or selective attention may do well in the one-to-one situation, but have extreme difficulty attending in the classroom. The Revised Goldman-Fristoe-Woodcock (GFW) Test,[28] or discrimination tests presented both in quiet and with competing noise, should be given. Clinically, it has been found that children who have difficulty selectively attending in the classroom are depressed on the cafeteria and/or voice noise subtests of the GFW. Children who are depressed on the fan noise subtest, but who fall at or above the 50th percentile on the other two subtests (cafeteria and voice noise), show emotional rather than auditory perceptual problems.

Picture vocabulary tests are often used to assess receptive language. The results are reported by mental age or IQ, implying that these test results are comparable to results from more comprehensive tests of general ability. The most frequently used vocabulary test is the Peabody Picture Vocabulary Test-Revised (PPVT-R).[39]

IQs obtained from the PPVT-R are not interchangeable with the IQ scores obtained from either the WISC-III or the Stanford-Binet, fourth edition. The PPVT "may be useful in measuring extensiveness of vocabulary and degree of cultural assimilation of children."[30] Costello described the PPVT as a screening instrument for children who have a limited expressive vocabulary or who are verbally inhibited. PPVT scores should not be used in measures of general abilities.[31]

Visual-Motor Behavior Assessment

A complete evaluation should include one or more tests of visual perception, integration, and execution. The Bender-Gestalt Test has been widely used since it was developed by Loretta Bender in 1938. Koppitz[32] revised the scoring system in 1963 and again in 1975, and her scoring system has been adopted by most individuals administering the Bender-Gestalt Test. She has developed an objective scoring system as well as age norms for ages 5 through 10 years, 11 months. In addition, she has delineated indicators of brain injury for children ages 5 to 10 years.

Two other tests of visual perception and eye/hand coordination are the Slosson Drawing Coordination Test for Children[33] published in 1975, and the Primary Visual Motor Test published in 1970.[34]

The Goodenough-Harris Draw-A-Person Test[35,36] allows the examiner to compare the youngster's spatial, size, and shape orientation, as well as the child's sequencing ability when drawing freehand without a pattern, as opposed to copying designs. It also provides insight into a child's body imagery and emotional state. The youngster is asked to draw a picture of a person, then a picture of the opposite sex, and then a self drawing. New norms were established for the test in 1970 for ages 6 to 11 years by the Department of Health, Education, and Welfare.[37] The test is nonthreatening and serves as a good introduction to the total test battery. It should be observed which hand the youngster uses to write and draw as well as how the pencil is held.

Academic Assessment

Some estimate of academic performance should be made during the comprehensive evaluation. This allows the examiner to observe how well the child handles academic material in a one-to-one testing situation as opposed to the group, timed achievement test administered in the classroom. The report of results should describe how the child handles different types of problem-solving, as well as areas in which there is difficulty. Difficulties should be analyzed in light of deficits observed in auditory, verbal, and visual motor areas. For example, one might report the results of testing as follows:

The memory problems did not overly hamper her academic achievement. She worked slowly in reading; however, her performance fell in the same range as her intellectual ability. The youngster seemed to perform better when given ample time to consider her response. The memory problems did not interfere with her spelling, but did appear to hamper long-term retention of academic facts.

A popular individual achievement test used by school psychologists and educational diagnosticians is the Woodcock Johnson Tests of Achievement-Revised that was published in 1989 (See Case Study 7–2).[38] It is divided into two parts: a standard battery and a supplementary battery. The standard battery is made up of nine tests that measure basic reading skills, reading comprehension, basic mathematics skills, mathematical reasoning, basic writing skills, and written expression. In addition, broad cluster scores in reading, mathematics, writing, knowledge, and skills are provided. Most examiners use six of the nine tests when administering the Woodcock Johnson Tests of Achievement—Revised.

With the exception of the written expression subtest, the Peabody Individual Achievement Test-Revised (PIAT-R) is an untimed power test of achievement published in 1989.[39] The test takes approximately 60 minutes to administer. Some children will take less time to complete the test; however, the examiner must not make the subject feel hurried. It is advised to give the test in one uninterrupted session. The test instructions should be followed precisely. The examiner may repeat an item when requested by the child being tested or if the child does not respond. However, the items must be repeated in their entirety without any change in the wording. An item cannot be readministered once a response has been given. The examiner must note carefully whether the child seems to misperceive the instructions or does not know the material.

The order of subtest administration was changed to increase interest and motivation. General information is administered first, followed by reading recognition, reading comprehension, mathematics, spelling, and written expression. The total test score does not include the written expression subtest, allowing the examiner the option to omit it from the test battery. A computer scoring system is available for the PIAT-R. It provides the examiner with a printout of age level and grade level standard scores and percentiles. It also graphs the results.

A new individual achievement test has been published in 1992 by the Psychological Corporation.[40] The Wechsler Individual Achievement Test (WIAT) consists of a screener that evaluates basic reading, mathematics reasoning, and spelling, and a comprehensive test, which evaluates reading comprehension, numerical operations, listening comprehension, oral expression, and written expression in addition to the items on the screener. Results are reported in standard scores and percentiles. The WIAT assesses children in grades kindergarten through 12 and ages 5 through 19 years, 11 months. The test was normed on a sample equivalent to the sample used in standardizing the WISC-III. A sample of 5-year-old children was administered both the WIAT and WPPSI-R and a sample of 17 through 19-year-old adolescents was administered the WIAT and WAIS-R.

An estimate of ability-achievement discrepancies can be calculated when the WIAT is used with the Wechsler scales. The test should become a useful tool in evaluating for learning disabilities, including the child with an auditory learning disability.

The Wide-Range Achievement Test-3 (WRAT-3) was published in 1993 and has returned to a single level format with an age range of 5 to 75 years.[41] The revised test has two scales that cover the entire age range. The two forms can be used together or individually. Each form takes 15 to 30 minutes to complete. The academic skills are measured by converting the raw scores into standard scores, grade scores, absolute scores, and percentiles. As with the revised WRAT, the new edition measures basic skills in reading, spelling, and arithmetic. The time limit on the arithmetic subtest has been extended to 15 minutes. As with the earlier edition, additional informa-

tion can be obtained if the examiner records what the child has completed at the 15-minute limit and then allows the youngster to continue until he or she can no longer work the problems.

Both the WRAT and the PIAT tend to overestimate when the results are compared with teacher-administered achievement tests. Williamson[42] questioned whether this was due to the diagnostician, who tests on a one-to one basis, being in a more supportive role and thus obtaining much higher scores. It may be that group (classroom) testing underestimates the ability of the child with a learning disability.[43] It would also tend to punish the easily distracted, or children with problems in selective attention or attention span. Therefore, the individually administered achievement test may give a more accurate estimate of academic achievement of a child with auditory-verbal problems.

The Myklebust Picture Story Language Test,[24] or a similar test of written expression, allows comparison of written language with verbal expression and reading. Children who are depressed in verbal expression frequently are also depressed in the number of words or sentences that they use to write a story, even though the content may be age-appropriate or above. Children who are poor readers or who score low in reading comprehension often do poorly on content. Grammar and punctuation disturbance on the written test tends to reflect how well a child has acquired the rules of language.

Personality Assessment

Whether or not children are disabled, they will acquire a distinct manner of handling different situations and dealing with their environment and people. They are individuals with distinct personalities. Personality tests provide information about the *inner workings* of individuals, their perceptions of their world, how they cope, their social skills, their self-concept, and their frustration tolerance level. Such tests give the examiner some understanding of the child's attitudes toward self, family, and the outside world—how the child perceives that he "fits into the scheme of things." Personality assessment utilizes projective tests and personality inventories.[44] Many test instruments are available, and each examiner has favorites. The most popular are the Rorschach Test,[45,46] the Thematic Apperception Test and Children's Apperception Test,[47] the Incomplete Sentences Test,[48] the House/Tree/Person Test,[49] and the Kinetic Family Drawings.[50]

One or two personality tests should be a part of the comprehensive evaluation. The examiner should be qualified to administer and interpret projective instruments. It is important that information on the perceptual disabilities be available at the time of interpretation of the projective tests. When a child's misperceptions of the environment result from an auditory perceptual disturbance, the child's responses to the projective instrument will be affected. If a child constantly misperceives what is said by improper coding, or if the child cannot hold information in short-term memory long enough to rescan it and interpret and act on the message, or if selective attention is disturbed, the child's environment will be constantly punishing. Frustration, poor self-worth, and a sense of failure, as well as feelings of anger, aggression, and hostility, are bound to develop. These feelings are secondary to the primary disorder of disturbed auditory perception and processing. Clinically, it has been found that when specific deficits are remediated, the emotional components tend to resolve themselves. When an emotional disturbance does remain beyond specific treatment of deficits, it responds quickly to psychotherapy.

EDUCATIONAL PLANNING AND REMEDIATION

The primary purpose of a comprehensive psycho-educational evaluation is to provide the parents, school, and remediation specialists with a better understanding of the child and the child's general abilities, disabilities, and academic strengths and weaknesses. Test results should also provide an explanation of nonconforming behavior and allow for the development of an individualized educational, behavioral, and remediation plan. The test profile may dictate such things as:

1. Modifications in the home and school environment to allow the child to attend selectively to what is being said.
2. Reinforcement of auditory instruction by visual and kinesthetic means.
3. Allowing the child to record written work on a tape recorder and then transcribe from his or her own dictation.
4. Modifying the length and sequence of orally presented material.
5. Placement in a resource program.
6. Individualized therapy directed to remediating specific deficits.[51]

The case evaluations in this chapter show how information relating to intellectual, academic, and behavioral factors is obtained from the history and how this information may be interpreted.

SUMMARY

A comprehensive psycho-educational assessment of a child with auditory language-learning problems should use the child as his or her own control. It should evaluate general abilities as well as specific auditory, language, and learning areas. The examiner should be concerned with the child's optimum performance level at the time of testing as well as abilities when the child is under stress or fatigued, and in a variety of learning situations. Examiners should also look to specific deficits, as well as strengths, in the auditory, visual, haptic-kinesthetic, and language areas. How the child performs in a quiet, nonstimulating environment, as well as when distractions or competing messages are introduced, needs to be determined. Some understanding of family health should be a part of the assessment, as should a comprehensive history that explores birth, health, behavior, developmental milestones, academic performance, and peer and family relationships. Furthermore, the examiner must be an astute observer of behavior, noting how a child perceives questions, whether the child asks for repetition, whether restatement is necessary, how environmental noises affect him or her, and what type of response latency is present.

A profile of the child should be drawn to show strengths as well as deficits so that an individualized educational plan and a comprehensive remediation program can be developed. The child's strengths should be utilized for ego building, while the deficits are being remediated, thus improving the child's ability to function in the classroom, at home, and with peers.

REFERENCES

1. Jackson GD: On the report of the Ad Hoc Committee on Education Uses of Tests with Disadvantage Students: Another psychological view from the Association of Black Psychologists. *Am Psychol*, 30 (1975), 88–92.
2. Mercer J: Sociocultural factors in labeling mental retardates. *Peabody J Educ* 48 (1971), 188–203.
3. Zimmerman IL, Woo-Sam JM: Intellectual testing today—relevance to the school-age child, in Oettinger L, Majowski LV, eds: *The Psychologist, the*

School, and the Child with MBD/LD (New York: Grune & Stratton, 1978), p 51.

4. Jastak JF, Jastak SR: *The Wide Range Achievement Test: 1976 Revised Edition* (Wilmington: Guidance Associates of Delaware, 1986), pp 46, 65.

5. Fox DR, Battin RR: Private practice in audiology and speech pathology, in Battin RR, Fox DR, eds: *The Clinical Aspects of Speech and Language Pathology* (New York: Grune & Stratton, 1978), chapter 5.

6. Terman L, Merrill M: *Measuring Intelligence* (Boston: Houghton-Mifflin, 1937), p 461.

7. Terman L, Merrill M: *Stanford-Binet Intelligence Scale: Manual for the Third Revision Form L-M* (Boston: Houghton-Mifflin, 1962), p 362.

8. Thorndike RL, Hagen EP, Sattler JM: *The Stanford-Binet Intelligence Scale, ed 4* (Chicago: Riverside Publishing, 1986).

9. Wechsler D: *Manual for the Wechsler Intelligence Scale for Children—III* (New York: Psychological Corp, 1991).

10. Paul N, Westerly O, Wepfer JW: Comparability of the WISC and the WISC-R. *J Learn Disabil,* 12 (1979), 348–351.

11. Vance H, Wallbrown FH, Blaha J: Determining WISC-R profiles for reading disabled children. *J Learn Disabil,* 11 (1979), 657–661.

12. Wechsler D: *Manual for the Wechsler Preschool and Primary Scale of Intelligence—R* (New York: Psychological Corporation, 1989).

13. Kaufman AS, Kaufman NL: *Kaufman Assessment Battery for Children* (Circle Pines, MN: American Guidance Service, 1983).

14. Kaufman AS, Kaufman NL: *Manual for the Kaufman Brief Intelligence Test* (Circle Pines, MN: American Guidance Service, 1990).

15. Brown, L, Sherbenou, RJ, Johnson, SK: *Test of Nonverbal Intelligence, Second Edition: A Language-Free Test of Cognitive Ability* (Austin, TX: Pro-ed, 1990).

16. Hiskey M: *Hiskey-Nebraska Test of Learning Aptitude* (Lincoln, NE: Union College Press, 1966).

17. Leiter RG: *General Instructions for the Leiter International Scale* (Chicago: Stoelting Company, 1969).

18. Arthur G: *Arthur Point Scale of Performance* (New York: Psychological Corporation, 1947).

19. Slosson RL: *Slosson Intelligence Test for Children and Adults* (East Aurora, NY: Slosson Educational Publications, 1963).

20. Raven JC: *Guide to Using the Standard Progressive Matrices* (London: H.K. Lewis, 1960).

21. Raven JC: *Guide to Using the Colored Progressive Matrices* (London: H.K. Lewis, 1965).

22. Burgemeister BB, Blum LH, Lorge I: *Columbia Mental Maturity Scale, ed 3* (New York: Harcourt, Brace, Jovanovich, 1972).

23. Kirk SA, McCarthy JJ, Kirk WD: *Examiner's Manual: Illinois Test of Psycholinguistic Abilities, Revised Edition* (Urbana: University of Illinois Press, 1968).

24. Myklebust HR: *Development and Disorders of Written Language: Picture Story Language Test* (New York: Grune & Stratton, 1965).

25. Hammill DD: *Detroit Tests of Learning Aptitude-2* (Austin, TX: Pro-Ed, 1985).

26. Hammill DD: *Detroit Tests of Learning Aptitude, Third Edition, Examiner's Manual* (Austin, TX: Pro-ed, 1991).

27. Hammill DD, Bryant BR: *Detroit Tests of Learning Aptitude—Primary* (Austin, TX: Pro-ed, 1986).

28. Goldman R, Fristoe M, Woodcock RW: *GFW Auditory Selective Attention Test* (Circle Pines, MN: American Guidance Service, 1974).

29. Dunn LM: *Peabody Picture Vocabulary Test—Revised Manual* (Circle Pines, MN: American Guidance Service, 1970).

30. Cole A: A study of preschool disadvantaged Negro children's Peabody Picture Vocabulary results, in *Child Study Center Bulletin,* (Buffalo, NY: New York State University at Buffalo, 1966), p 66.

31. Costello J, Ali F: Reliability and validity of Peabody Picture Test scores of disadvantaged preschool children. *Psychol Rep,* 28 (1971), 755–760.

32. Koppitz EM: *The Bender Gestalt Test for Young Children* (New York: Grune & Stratton, 1963), p 195.

33. Slosson RL: *Slosson Drawing Coordination Test for Children and Adults* (East Aurora, NY: Slosson Educational Publications, 1975).

34. Haworth MR: *The Primary Visual Motor Test* (New York: Grune & Stratton, 1970).

35. Harris D: *Children's Drawings as Measures of Intellectual Maturity: A Revision and Extension of the Goodenough Draw-A-Person Test* (New York: Harcourt, Brace & World, 1963).

36. *Intellectual Maturity of Children as Measured by the Goodenough-Harris Drawing Test.* National Center for Health Statistics Series 11, No. 105. Deptartment of Health, Education and Welfare, Public Health Service, 1970.

37. *School Achievement of Children 6–11 Years as Measured by the Reading and Arithmetic Subtests of the Wide Range Achievement Test.* National Center for Health Statistic Series 11, No. 103. Deptartment of Health, Education and Welfare, Public Health Service, 1970.

38. Woodcock RW, Maither, N: WS-R Tests of Achievement: Examiner's Manual. In RW Woodcock and MB Johnson: *Woodcock-Johnson Psycho-Educational Battery-Revised* (Allen, TX: DLM Teaching Resources, 1989).

39. Markwardt FC, Jr: *Peabody Individual Achievement—Revised Manual* (Circle Pines, MN: American Guidance Service, 1989).

40. *WIAT Manual* (New York: Psychological Corporation, 1992).

41. Wilkensen GS: *WRAT-3 Administration Manual* (Delaware: Wide Range, 1993).

42. Williamson WE: The concurrent validity of the 1965 Wide Range Achievement Test with neurologically impaired and emotionally handicapped pupils. *J Learn Disabil*, 12 (1979), 201–202.

43. Miller WH: A comparison of the Wide Range Achievement Test and the Peabody Individual Achievement Test for educationally handicapped children. *J Learn Disabil*, 12 (1979), 65–68.

44. Molish HB: Projective methodologies. *Annu Rev Psychol*, 23 (1972), 577–614.

45. Exner JE Jr: *The Rorschach: A Comprehensive System* (New York: John Wiley & Sons, 1974).

46. Rorschach H: *Psychodiagnostics, ed 2*, Lemkan P, Krononberg B, trans. (Berne: Huber, 1942).

47. Bellak L: *The Thematic Apperception Test and the Children's Apperception Test in Clinical Use, ed 2* (New York: Grune & Stratton, 1971).

48. Murstein, BI, ed: *Handbook of Projective Techniques* (New York: Basic Books, 1965).

49. Buck JN: The H-T-P technique: A qualitative and quantitative scoring manual. *J Clin Psychol*, 4 (1948), 317–396.

50. Burns RC, Kaufman SH: *Actions, Styles, and Symbols in Kinetic Family Drawings: An Interpretive Manual* (New York: Brunner/Mazel, 1972).

51. Bradley PE, Battin RR, Sutter EG: Effects of individual diagnosis and remediation for the treatment of learning disabilities. *Clin Neuropsychol*, (1979), 23–35.

Remediation | III

INTRODUCTION

The term "auditory disorder" represents a wide spectrum of problems within the auditory system, ranging from hearing loss due to abnormal mechanical conditions in the peripheral hearing mechanism (conductive loss), to disruption in the sensory end organ and/or auditory neural pathway (sensorineual loss), to a possible disruption of the neural system(s) responsible for the encoding of neural events (central auditory disorder). The remedial processes that have been espoused for the educational management of children with auditory disorders can vary depending on the severity of the disorders.

However, if one takes the perspective that the educational management of auditory disorders should be based on the nature of the disorder, as well as the severity, it is possible that a hierarchy of confidence levels can be put on the management strategies to be employed. Looking at auditory disorders in this way provides a unique viewpoint that may clarify the remedial process. In order of degree of confidence, these disorders range as follows.

(1) Congenital hearing loss, present at birth or shortly thereafter, may be sensorineural or conductive (see Chapter 2). The language learning deficits resulting from congenital hearing loss are well documented and are directly proportional to the degree of loss, intellectual potential of the child, and environmental factors such as family interrelationships, and the amount and quality of stimulation. There is little question that congenital hearing loss, even when it is mild, significantly affects auditory language learning skills.

(2) Acquired hearing loss may also be sensorineural or conductive in nature. This type of loss may also be fluctuating or permanent. As with congenital hearing loss, the language deficits resulting from acquired hearing loss are proportional to the degree and duration of the loss, intellectual potential of the child, and environmental factors. More and more, evidence is being reported suggesting that even mild fluctuating conductive hearing loss due to middle ear disorders results in language learning problems (see Chapter 9).

(3) Inefficient auditory language learning skills can be due to environmental factors. Factors that may result in inefficiency of auditory language learning skills include a lack of adequate language stimulation, sensory overloading, and malnutrition. Even psychological trauma is suspect in this regard. Although it is documented that auditory language learning disorders may result from factors such as these, this observation is only recent and the exact way in which these factors affect auditory language learning has yet to be established firmly.

(4) Central auditory processing disorders are thought to be unrelated to hearing loss caused by mechanical and sensory end organ problems in the auditory system, and in fact seem to exist in the absence of hearing loss. This type of auditory problem has been discussed and bandied about for a considerable time, but the etiological factors accounting for central auditory disorders remain elusive. There is a presumption that minimal brain damage of some sort is present in a child who is classified as having a central auditory processing disorder. However, this presumption has never been documented by histologic or neurologic evidence, or by radiologic or encephalographic techniques, except in cases of diagnosed neurological disorders where organicity is evident.

From an educational perspective, children who are classified as having central auditory disorders are indistinguishable upon examination from those children in the preceding categories. This observation provides enough evidence to argue that children classified as having central auditory processing disorders have some form of auditory language learning problem that may be related to developmental factors, such as conductive hearing loss, or environmental factors. Because of the paucity of information on the etiology of central auditory disorders, the remedial strategies have yet to be standardized. However, it is reasonable to assume that remediation for children who are thought to manifest central auditory disorders should follow the same basis as for all categories; that is, intervention strategies should be based on normal language development and auditory training.

Part III of our book follows the above philosophy of remediation. Intervention using a collaborative framework is covered in Chapter 8. The effect of mild hearing loss on auditory language learning is covered in Chapter 9. How can the teacher keep the child's hearing aid functioning in the classroom? What is the best acoustic environment, and how should amplification systems, individual and group, be managed? What new technological advances are there to assist students with hearing impairment in specific listening situations? Readers will find answers to each of these specific questions and more in Chapters 10 to 13.

Chapter 14 covers remedial strategies for the child with profound deafness through recent technological innovations: cochlear implants and tactile instruments. With this new technology, some children with profound deafness have the potential to develop auditory skills that a decade ago were incomprehensible.

Specific language intervention should be based on results from psychoeducational assessment (described in Chapters 6 and 7). Chapters 15 and 16 apply this philosophy to auditory training and speechreading and language remediation. The explosion of printed material makes it difficult for therapists and teachers to keep up with what is available. Chapter 17 reviews a variety of materials that are available, gives information on where to find them, and provides examples of how the materials can be used in the classroom and in individual intervention programs. Finally, once a child with a disability is identified and placed in the mainstream, all aspects of the family and the child need to be considered. These areas are covered in our last two chapters on family counseling and enhancing the self image of the child who is mainstreamed.—*RJR, MPD*

A COLLABORATIVE FRAMEWORK FOR INTERVENTION

8

Karen A. Clark and Diana L. Terry

I would help others, out of a fellow-feeling.

—Robert Burton, 1577–1640

An ultimate goal for the education of young children who are deaf is the development of their full potential as happy, healthy individuals, who are responsible members of society, confident and capable in their ability to communicate with others. Speech, language, and listening are each important dimensions of the communication process, but it is the spontaneous, appropriate and integrated use of this communication within all aspects of life that are the true measures of success. This real-life definition of success suggests the need for intervention programs in which long- and short-term therapeutic goals reflect the relationship between communication and daily life. When intervention is viewed in this context, it can only be considered effective when it is designed to facilitate communication that is relevant and integral to the lives of children and families, utilizing strategies that support total child development. This comprehensive approach to integration is best achieved through the combined efforts of many people. A collaborative framework for intervention begins with some basic assumptions about child learning and communicative competence.

HOW CHILDREN LEARN

Young children who are deaf, like all young children, learn through interaction with their immediate world and with the people who live in that world. For young children, learning is an interactive, cyclical process through which they become aware, explore, inquire, and ultimately begin to utilize new ideas and abilities.[1] The best opportunities for learning occur during play and through daily routine experiences. As children develop, they are at different stages of the learning cycle as they experience the same daily events. As they begin to explore one concept more fully, they may concurrently become aware of another. Stacking blocks provides an opportunity to learn that blocks are hard, that they fit together in certain ways, that the big blocks fall off the top of the tower and that blocks make a loud sound when they fall. Taking a bath provides an opportunity to learn that water can feel hot or cold, that slapped water splashes and sloshes, that soap tastes awful and that you sit in the water but your duck sits on the water.

When children are in the early developmental stages, they acquire and internalize knowledge through their physical actions and their observations of what happens as a result of these actions.[2] Through repeated experiences that involve interactions with people and materials, children actually construct their own knowledge.[3] These constructions involve both physical and social knowledge. The child who plays with the floating bathtub duck may decide that small things float until he puts his small car in the tub. Then he must struggle to incorporate this new piece of information into his hypothesis. When his mother says, "That car is too heavy; try this little boat," he has even more information. This process of refining our ideas, based on new information is one that continues throughout our lives.

The role of caregivers and other significant adults is important to successful child development. Adults set the stage and provide the environment in which learning and development will take place. At times, adults take the lead and at times they respond to actions and ideas initiated by the child. Adult and child interactions, both verbal and nonverbal, significantly influence all aspects of development, including physical, cognitive, social, emotional, and language.

COMMUNICATIVE COMPETENCE

Communication and language development occurs concurrently and as an integral part of the process of overall child development. During the early stages of development, children begin to learn first words as they hear them repeatedly in connection with experiences that are important to them and that happen frequently. At later stages, language, itself, becomes a tool for learning more about the meaningful events occurring in their lives. At all times, language and communication connect children with their world and with the people in their lives.

To understand language as a versatile, multidimensional system that facilitates interaction with people and acquisition of information, one must understand its various components. As described by Bloom and Lahey,[4] language development can be understood and observed within three dimensions. These are described as content, form, and use. Content, the meaning of language, reflects knowledge of objects and people and the relationship among these objects, people, and events in the environment. Form refers to word order, or syntax, as well as the sounds of spoken language and the configuration of signed language. Language use includes reasons for speaking or signing and knowledge of the situation or other person that helps one determine the form of the message.

Each component of language may begin developing as separate strands in early infancy and merge in the form of early words around age one.[5] Communicative competence depends on the continued integration and interconnection of these three aspects of language as children mature. In a broader perspective, communication is viewed as an integration or composite of social and individual factors, encompassing grammar, cognitive knowledge, social context, and cultural learning.[6] In each communication interaction or event, important variables that influence communication might include the environment or setting, the communication partner, experiential history, current knowledge constructs, current needs, personal motivation, and expectation of results.

Every aspect of language and true competence in its use reflects its dynamic and fluid nature. One might best take a "kaleidoscopic" view of communication. Each of the factors that has been noted represents a bit of colored glass within the kaleidoscope; each communicative interaction finds those factors rearranged in a different relationship and presenting a different composite. For children to be considered competent in language, they must eventually adapt to the ever changing patterns. They must be able to use language spontaneously and appropriately in a wide variety of contexts and with a wide variety of communication partners. For therapists to be effective in facilitating this competence, the parameters of therapy must be expanded beyond a single therapy setting. Homes, playgrounds, preschool classrooms are all potential therapy settings. Parents, teachers, day-care providers are all potential language facilitators. The speech-language clinician or aural habilitation specialist becomes a partner in a collaborative team.

COMPONENTS OF COLLABORATION

In contemporary literature, one definition of the process of collaboration is widely accepted:

> Collaboration is an interactive process that enables people with diverse expertise to generate creative solutions to mutually defined problems. The outcome is enhanced, altered, and produces solutions that are different from those that the individual team members would produce independently.[7]

In collaborative assessment and intervention settings, the parents, teachers, and habilitation specialists work together to identify needs and to develop the child's intervention plan in an atmosphere of mutual respect. All collaborators have similar responsibilities for the plan's implementation and success. The key elements of collaboration include participant interaction, the availability of diverse expertise, the development of creative solutions, and mutually defined goals. These components of collaboration can enhance the ultimate goal of therapeutic intervention by assisting children to develop and improve skills necessary for optimal functioning and achievement within the educational and social contexts encountered throughout each day. The key elements of collaboration facilitate capitalizing on the linguistic opportunities provided in particular environments and thus the development of communicative competence. The communicative competence of children is effectively addressed when there are beliefs that pooling the talents and resources of everyone who is a part of the child's environment is mutually advantageous, that naturalistic settings are appropriate contexts for language intervention, that language change can be implemented in a variety of ways, and that effectively addressing the needs of a child merits an expenditure of time, energy, and resources. An important feature of collaboration is that it allows all participants a feeling of ownership within the process because they are actively involved in identifying the needs and generating the plans.

Abelson and Woodman[8] identify four developmental phases of collaboration. The first phase is the forming stage when members are defining limits and roles and establishing a framework for communication. The second phase is the storming stage in which members develop and display their skills. Existing leadership roles are often tested during this time. The third phase is the norming stage in which members begin to emerge as a cohesive group. Roles may still be revised but are done so in an effort to increase the effectiveness of the team. The final phase is the performing stage in which team roles and conflicts have been settled and the team is able to work together effectively and communicate in the problem solving process.

As part of the development of a collaborative team, it is often helpful to identify the various characteristics that lead to effective communication and subsequently successful collaboration. The range of characteristics each team member possesses may also contribute to the process of defining team roles and responsibilities. Tables 8–1 and 8–2 list behaviors that may enhance or inhibit a team's problem-solving process of collaboration. The characteristics identified provide the foundation for collaboration and should be considered prior to beginning the process of identifying and addressing a child's specific needs.

A FRAMEWORK FOR COLLABORATION WITH FAMILIES

Legislative Mandates that Support Collaboration

The Individuals with Disabilities Education Act (IDEA) Amendments of 1991, Part H, outlines the requirements for early intervention services for infants and toddlers. Two key assumptions of the Part H requirements are a focus on interdisciplinary services and a recognition that the child is part of a family system rather than an isolated service recipient.[9]

The concept of interdisciplinary services recognizes that any child with disabilities, including one who is deaf, may have diverse needs that can be best met by the integrated services

Table 8–1   Actions That Facilitate the Problem-Solving Process of Collaboration

Working together with other adults
Offering information and opinions
Answering questions from others
Devoting time to the problem-solving process
Observing others in a variety of settings, such as the classroom or home setting
Evaluating and identifying strengths and needs of a child
Sharing concerns with others
Committing to addressing targeted objectives within the child's daily routines and activities
Working as an information seeker
Acting as a summarizer
Sharing ideas that have and have not worked
Asking for help
Giving help
Asking questions
Acting as a recorder
Describing observable behaviors
Encouraging participation
Being flexible
Listening to others viewpoints that might be different from your own
Acknowledging other's perspectives
Being available to meet with other team members
Building bridges to other team members
Understanding change is difficult and often times slow

Table 8–2   Actions That Inhibit Successful Collaboration

Using "you" messages
Criticizing other's opinions
Talking without listening
Giving incomplete information
Using sarcasm
Using jargon or terminology that other team members do not understand
Being argumentative
Being uninvolved, unresponsive, inflexible
Being territorial
Possessing narrow role perceptions

of several professionals. It also recognizes that no aspect of child development, including communication, emerges independently from any other aspect of child development. The focus on the family acknowledges that the child is part of a family system. Quality early intervention supports the family and is aware of family needs and capitalizes on family strengths as the optimum way to assist the developing child. Both interdisciplinary strategies and family services are more readily achieved through collaborative programming for infants and toddlers who are hearing impaired.

Another aspect of Part H is the Individual Family Service Plan (IFSP). The IFSP outlines child strengths and needs, family strengths and needs, intervention outcomes that are desired by and family, and strategies designed to facilitate these desired outcomes. As the title of the plan implies, the needs of the child are considered within the context of the family. Outcomes and strategies chosen for an IFSP may encompass a wider range of issues and will be written in broader terms than behavioral objectives. For example, if the parent needs day care services, location of quality day care services may be included in the family service plan as a desired outcome. Strategies would outline the plan to be used in finding day care services, including ways to ensure that the day care personnel would work with and be receptive to the needs of a child who is deaf.

Partnerships with Families

One of the first collaborative partnerships in the education of young children who are deaf is that of the parent and professional. Throughout this chapter, the term parent is used to encompass both the parent and any other adult who is a primary or significant caretaker. The role of the parent in a child's language development is significant. It is the parent who best understands what is meaningful for the child, and it is the parent who observes and interprets communication signals from the child, and it is the parent who is in the best position to provide the consistency of interaction on a daily and routine basis. The professional can contribute a vast amount of technical knowledge about communication, language, hearing aids, and auditory development. The professional can share experience and expertise for the design of strategies that best facilitate this development. The professional can help parents access a variety of resources and services. These professional contributions help to form a framework or plan in which the parent contributions can be directed and enhanced.

When the partnership between parents and professionals is fully developed, there is mutual respect, sharing, and flexibility.[10] The parent and the professional may not agree on every aspect of the service delivery, but they respect each other's viewpoints and are willing to listen to another opinion. Each recognizes the unique contributions of the other partner. Individual family values as well as cultural differences have a significant impact on the partnership. Basic parent and child communication patterns, child care practices, family structure and roles, and ex-

pectations for children may vary across cultures. Assumptions and decisions based on the cultural background and family values of the professional, rather than that of the family, are rarely successful. Professionals who develop collaborative relationships with parents and others, who are members of a particular culture, have an opportunity to become knowledgeable about that cultural. Sensitivity to cultural issues facilitates a successful partnership.[11]

Successful parent and professional partnerships undergo many transitions. Transitions are inevitable and occur throughout the lifetime of any family. As the child gets older, expectations and educational environments change. Family needs also change over time. Maintaining the partnership of the parent and professional requires planning, commitment, and collaboration.

Role of the Professional

The specific role of a professional within parent and professional partnership can be viewed in in several ways, depending on the philosophy of the service delivery program or service provider. Dunst[12] identifies four separate family oriented models: Professional-Centered, Family Allied, Family-Focused, and Family-Centered. In each of these models, the professionals assume different roles in their relationship to parents.

In the professional-centered model, families are clients of professionals. The professionals make the majority of the decisions and implement the program with little family involvement. For the family of a child with deafness, this might mean, for example, that the professional recommends a specific mode of communication to be implemented within a specific therapy regimen.

In a family-allied model, families are agents of professionals. The professionals still determine the interventions, but families are taught to implement specific aspects of the plan. For the family of a child who is deaf, examples might include giving the parents lessons in hearing aid care or communication skills, with the family having no part in the process of selecting what lessons were to be taught.

In a family-focused program, families are viewed as the consumer of professional services. Both the parents and the professionals may contribute goals and objectives to the plan, but these goals and objectives focus on family needs related to specific program services. In a program providing services to families with children who are deaf, professionals would only include speech/ language/listening and related educational goals in the service delivery plan even though they might assist families to access additional services.

In a family-centered program, professionals are the agents of families. The role of the professional is determined by the family's needs and lifestyle. Concerns addressed may extend beyond issues directly related to the child's hearing loss. Nothing is written on the service plan without the family's agreement. In addressing the needs of the family of a child who is deaf, a single plan may encompass the services provided by many professionals and agencies. Goals are not limited to communication aspects of development or even limited to the needs of the child alone.

The view of collaboration, as described in this chapter, encompasses both the family-focused and the family-centered model. In a collaborative model, both parties contribute their individual skills and talents in a way that establishes mutual respect and supports the development of the child. Whether the parent and professional partnership is family-focused or family-centered may be more determined by program rather than individual philosophy. Programs that comply with the Part H legislative guidelines will provide services that are more family-centered.

In a collaborative program, the aural habilitation professional providing the primary service delivery to the family will fulfill a variety of roles. Whether the collaboration is between parent and professional only or among the parent and several service providers, the habilitation specialist role encompasses multiple aspects. When several professionals are involved, role emphasis may shift but the mutliple aspects of the role are maintained. Table 8–3 outlines the roles of the habilitation professional within a collaborative early intervention framework. It also outlines personal and professional characterisitics and skills that may be associated with successful service provision within the collaborative framework.

ASSESSMENT PROCESS

Assessment within a collaborative model has very broad parameters. Emphasis in early intervention programs will be on family assessment as a way to determine child and family needs within the family context. This assessement process is congruent with the legal requirements to develop a family service plan. It also recognizes that the child is part of a family and that the family needs and concerns, as well as family strengths,

Table 8–3 Multiple Roles of the Habilitation Professional Within a Collaborative Early Intervention Framework

Gathers information for the multiple purposes of assessment of family and child needs, development of an intervention plan, documentation of progress and subsequent modification of the intervention plan

Provides information and resources to the family both directly and through provision of additional contacts so families can develop their own knowledge base

Implements intervention strategies, directly or through modeling, that facilitate the desired outcomes or goals for language/listening as outlined on the Individual Family Service Plan or individual education plan

Provides ongoing family support during identification, assessment, service delivery, and transition from the program

Role-related characteristics or skills
  Understands and accepts family values and culture
  Understands emotional aspects of family concerns
  Values/respects parent opinions, viewpoints and decisions
  Values/respects other professional opinions and viewpoints
  Demonstrates knowledge of typical child development and learning theories
  Demonstrates knowledge and competence in all specialized areas related to service provision for children who are deaf
  Demonstrates good interpersonal communication skills
  Understands own limits, both personally and professionally
  Understands potential impact of own culture and personal values on service provision
  Understands potential impact of own professional values on service provision
  Differentiates habilitationist's role from that of psychologist or counselor

will have a definite affect on the intervention process. As children enter preschool and primary school programs, the assessment emphasis shifts to provide more focus on child skills within a variety of contexts. The assessment process is congruent with the legal requirements to develop an individual education plan. In a collaborative model, the knowledge, concerns, and desires of the family remain an important aspect of the assessment process.

Identifying Family Needs— The Early Years

A great deal of recent research in the area of family assessement is concerned with best practices for gathering information related to family needs and concerns. Surveys and questionnaires, as well as interview formats, are available to help the professional and family as they try to identify significant issues related to establishing family and child goals. Bailey and Simmeonsson[13] provide a good overview of a wide variety of these measures. Their review includes measures for functional assessment of family needs as well as measures that provide information in related areas, such as family members' roles and support systems, critical life events, and family environments.

Parental surveys and questionnaires provide a framework for gathering basic information related to family concerns. More extensive and individualized information can be obtained through open discussion or personal family interviews. Winton[14] suggests one format for a family-focused interview that serves the dual purposes of gathering information and establishing collaborative goals. Winton has also identified several specific communication strategies necessary to the information gathering process. Effective listening includes both verbal strategies, such as simply following the parents lead if they bring up a topic, and nonverbal strategies such as natural eye contact and attentive body posture. Reflecting feelings and content allows the family to know that you understand how they perceive the problem and may help them to clarify their own feelings or thoughts. Effective questioning includes the use of open-ended questions as well as several other question forms that are designed to explore an idea or concept in greater depth and to help generate possible solutions. Without effective communication strategies, and experience in incorporating those strategies into actual practice, the interview process will not be successful.

Whatever method of needs identification is chosen, it is important to remember that identification of family needs is not something that can be completed and checked off a list. The value of determining family needs is in utilizing that knowledge to enhance services to the family. Frequent discussions and attentiveness to parent concerns will ensure that the services remain congruent with family needs over time.

Another significant aspect of family needs assessment is an awareness of the emotional impact that the diagnosis of hearing loss has on a particular family. In the parent and professional partnership, all members are concerned about the welfare of the child, but it is the parent who has the deep emotional tie to the child and the myriad of feelings about what it means to have a child who is deaf. Most parents of children who are deaf are hearing people who never expected to be the parents of a child with a hearing loss. It is important that the service provider understand as clearly as possible the emotional impact that may be experienced by some parents as they attempt to deal with this new direction in their life.

An attitude of acceptance of parents' emotions and empathy for the range of their feelings are perhaps the most effective responses that service providers can have. The listening skills described earlier will again be valuable as we struggle to understand and meet the wide variety of emotional needs reflected in the families we encounter. The ability to deal with families in an open and honest way and to recognize when referral for additional counseling might be helpful are significant aspects of early intervention services.

Identifying Child Competencies and Needs—The Early Years

Identification of overall family needs is just one part of the diagnostic and assessment process. Identification of child competencies in communication, listening, and other areas of development also is a significant responsibility of the habilitation specialist. In traditional diagnostic assessment of children who are deaf, professionals often focused on a product rather than a process. The assessment phase was complete when the professional identified deficit skill areas, made specific recommendations, and the family agreed with the recommendations. This approach to assessment has several limitations. First, by not recognizing the importance of multiple sources and contexts for information gathering, a narrow view of the child's abilities is obtained. Second, families are involved in information gathering in a peripheral way, so they have limited ownership in decisions based on that information. Third, focus on assessment as product does not emphasize information gathering as an ongoing process that provides the basis for many future decisions.

In planning an assessment process that identifies child abilities and needs, information is gathered in three major areas: communication/language, auditory development (including hearing aid use), and cognitive, physical, and social development. In a collaborative family and professional assessment process, there are differences in the type of information gathered, in the number and range of information sources and contexts, and in what happens to the information after it is gathered. In a collaborative process, parents and professionals participate fully, with both parties providing information and both parties gaining a better understanding of the child's abilities and needs.

If we focus on communicative competence as a goal, then diagnostic measures selected will be varied and provide a multidimensional picture of the child's development. It is not enough to know how a child responds to a word or a sound in an isolated setting; we must also know how he responds at home, in the park, or at the babysitters. Traditional, professionally administered, norm-referenced tests generally record what a child does in one setting, with a certain set of materials, at a given moment in time. To obtain real-life information, we need the help of the child's caretakers. Measures that incorporate parental reporting provide a broader view but do not necessarily give the professional an opportunity to observe directly the way in which the child uses communication within his daily life. Interview type assessments also provide little information about the communicative interaction between parent and child. Additional observational data are needed to help round out our picture of the child as communicator.

Two examples of organized observation systems of this type are the SKI-HI Communication Assessment Forms[10] and the Checklist for Caregivers: Communication Promoting Behaviors.[15] The SKI-HI procedure is completed in four stages. The observer looks at parent initiated communication, child initiated communication, nonverbal communication factors, and verbal communication factors. During the observation period, the parent and child are engaged in any activity chosen by the parent. The observation setting is the usually the child's home. The Checklist for Caregivers recommends a videotape process in which the parent and child interact during an activity or event that the parent has chosen or feels comfortable in doing. Again, the home is a preferred setting. There are 22 communication behaviors on the caregiver's checklist designed to include both affective and interactive components of optimal caregiver behavior. Observational data, when utilized effectively, can provide a broader picture of the child's system of communication.

The child's auditory abilities are measured quantitatively during audiological assessment to provide aided hearing levels and eventually speech reception and discrimination abilities. Again, observational data in a variety of settings are needed to supplement and give information about the child's ability to use his early hearing in meaningful ways. Each of four auditory curricula outlined in Table 8–4, provide a framework on which to base beginning and ongoing observations.

Since communication is one aspect of the whole child, information gathered while observing language behaviors will also yield much information about the child's cognitive, physical, and social development. Again, formal and informal developmental measures are available. Ideally, several professionals from different disciplines, as well as family members, pool their observational information so that a realistic picture of the child's development begins to emerge.

In a family-focused, collaborative program, professionals and parents share in both the information-gathering process and in subsequent decisions on how the information will be used in developing an educational plan. The sharing of roles does not suggest that professionals ignore their own knowledge, skills, or opinions, but rather that they blend the family's perspective with their own.

Identifying Family and Child Needs—The Early School Years

Parent and professional partnerships may undergo many transitions as the child gets older and family and child needs change. When the child enters a school program, the focus still includes the family, the child, and the professionals who work with them. Parents are encouraged to continue to function as observers, informers, describers, and evaluators as a part of the collaborative team. Parents provide valuable information about family and community culture, identify meaningful contexts for communication, describe changes in the child and his environment, and help to interpret assessment information.

During the early school years, the diagnostic process continues to rely on collaborative input and thus is individualized to meet the specific needs of the child, family, and professionals. Before utilizing specific diagnostic measures for assessing the speech, language, and listening skills of preschoolers, it is important to have an overall plan for assessment. A collaborative model provides multiple options for identifying characteristics and needs of children and their

Table 8–4   Auditory Skills Hierarchy

SKI-HI Model Resource Manual	Foreworks: Auditory Skills Curriculum	Developmental Approach to Successful Listening (DASL)	Pollack's Curriculum Outline for Auditory-Verbal Communication
Phase one Awareness	Awareness	Awareness	*Level one* Awareness Early vocalization
Attending	Attending	Attending	
Early vocalizing			*Level two* Attention More vocalizations
Phase two Recognizing			*Level three* Recognition Localization
Locating			Distance hearing
Vocalizing with inflection			*Level Four* Vocal play
Phase three Hearing at distances and levels	Distance hearing	Distance hearing	
Producing some vowels and consonants	Environmental discrimination and comprehension	Environmental discrimination and comprehension	*Level five* Discrimination Auditory feedback
Phase four Environmental discrimination and comprehension	Imitates vocal production		*Level six* Discrimination
	Vocal discrimination and comprehension	Vocal discrimination and comprehension	Short-term memory
Vocal discrimination and comprehension			Sequencing
	Short-term memory		
	Sequencing		
Speech discrimination and comprehension	Speech discrimination and comprehension	Speech discrimination and comprehension	*Level seven* Processing patterns Symbolic language Understanding
Speech use	Speech use and modification		
	Distance hearing in noise	Distance hearing in noise	

families. The nature of the information to be obtained and the methods used to obtain it are influenced by why the information is needed. The plan for assessing the child's skills is defined by a combination of who is to be involved, why the skills are being assessed, what information is being assessed, in which contexts the skills are to be assessed, how the skills will be assessed in the various contexts, and how that information will be utilized.

When considering who is to be involved in the assessment, it is advisable to consider anyone who has questions to be answered or issues they want resolved as part of the collaborative assessment plan. Most often, the child's family and the professionals who serve the child and his family are the ones who are involved in the assessment process. Recent findings show that parents demonstrate proficiency in accurately assessing their children when collaborating with other professionals.[16]

Case Study 8-1.   Toby and his family have been in an early intervention home-based program since he was 13 months old. Both parents have been actively involved in all aspects of Toby's assessment and intervention program and are pleased with his speech, language, and listening development. They feel very comfortable working and planning with Toby's early intervention case manager, Joan. Toby's mother expressed concerns that when Toby enters the school-based program in 2 months she will not know what he's learning or what to do with him at home. She also expressed anxiety over who would be his teachers and his classmates. She really wishes that Joan could teach his class.

As part of the Individual Family Service Plan (IFSP), the early intervention case manager and Toby's family identified the steps to be taken to support Toby's transition from his home-based to a school-based setting. The IFSP designated the early intervention case manager as the person who would be primarily responsible for introducing Toby's family to all of the school based professionals who would be working with him. Additionally, the IFSP identified Toby's current strengths and needs as seen by the family and his early intervention case manager and included a suggested timeline to meet and share information with school personnel.

Within the next month, Toby's family was invited to attend new student orientation to meet the teachers, other parents, and tour the school. They also received a packet of school related information. The early intervention case manager attended the orientation and arranged a meeting for the next week with Toby's teachers and his parents. At that meeting, an initial plan was developed for gathering and sharing information. The parents requested that Joan continue to come to their house once a month until they felt comfortable with Toby's transition.

The methods and tools of assessment are often influenced by why the assessment is being made. Perhaps the habilitation specialist needs information to determine additional steps to take in the intervention plan or a way to document progress, or the assessment is necessary to qualify the child for or to continue specific services. Sometimes the parents need more information about their child to help them make a decision about class placement. The reasons why an assessment is being made will also be a factor in determining if norm-referenced measures should be used or if organized observation systems and interview type assessments are appropriate.

As mentioned previously, there are many diagnostic tools available for gathering information ranging from family interviews to standardized measures. The assessment plan defines what type of information is being gathered and determines if the focus is to be on communication skills, language development, auditory development, or other developmental areas. The focus might be on overall development in an area or on specific skills within the area.

In the assessment plan it is important to discuss how the observance or nonobservance of skills will be documented and who will be responsible for that documentation. A decision also needs to be made as to whether qualitative judgments are appropriate or whether the documentation needs to follow standardized guidelines. Additional considerations include whether the skills are to be assessed in isolated settings such as a therapy room or in naturalistic settings, including the home environment. Inventories and checklists that are completed by more than one person in the child's environment provide a wider range of information than information obtained from one isolated setting. For example, completion of listening and speech skill development checklists by the habilitation specialist, parent advisor, classroom teacher, and parent provide a more complete picture of the child's skill development in a variety of settings than a single measure in only one environment. The focus is not on who is "right," but rather on which behaviors are seen in different environments and how they might be generalized to all settings.[17]

The manner in which the assessment results are interpreted and utilized is partially dependent on the purpose of the assessment. The information will be used differently if the purpose is to determine additional steps to take in the intervention plan than if the information is being used to evaluate the educational placement for the child. A variety of assessment team members may bring their perspectives and competencies to the interpretation process. These perspectives provide related and overlapping information that will help to ensure that a child's specific needs are accurately assessed and that an intervention program is relevant to the child's language and learning environment across contexts. These varied perspectives allow for focus on establishing meaningful skills and outcomes for parents, caregivers, professionals, and the child.

Collaborative Communication Methodology Decisions

To understand a collaborative approach to methodology decisions, it may first be helpful to apply the principles of professional-centered and family-focused program philosophies to the communication methodology issue. In a traditional, professional-centered model, the recommendation for communication methodology is the responsibility of the professional. In making a recommendation, the aural habilitation professional may review child assessment data that includes amount of hearing loss, age of identification, additional handicapping conditions, and other factors. The resulting recommendation is usually heavily influenced by the educational philosophy of the professional or the program making the recommendation. The recommendation often conveys to the family, either directly or through implication, that there is a "right" choice. The role of the family is to accept or reject the recommendation. In a family-centered program, the choice of communication methodology is determined by the family. Family values and experiences, child and family needs and strengths, and information and resource availability may all be factors in the decision. The role of the professional within the decision process is determined by the needs of the family at any given time.

In the collaborative approach presented here, the family remains the primary decision maker. The collaborative approach still recognizes the need for professional input, but also recognizes the importance of a wider range of family, community, and cultural issues. The professional continues to want what is best for the child but understands that there may be more than one "right" answer. The role of the professional shifts from the supplier of the right answer to the supplier of information and information resources. The range of information resources may be broader than in the past, encompassing a varied mix of communication professionals as well as adults who are deaf and other families with children who are deaf. The role of the professional is to assist the family by gathering information, identifying and providing potential information resources, and by providing ongoing support to the family.

Providing access to information about communication methodologies is a central part of the professional's responsibility. Ongoing availability of information presented in many formats in a nonbiased manner is recommended. Listening and following the family's lead will allow the professional to have information resources available when the family is ready. Available resources for the family might include: (1) opportunities to read about or discuss a wide variety of aural and sign-based methods, including auditory-verbal, auditory-oral, total communication using manually coded English and American Sign Language; (2) opportunities to meet older children and adults who are deaf, and who, collectively, have a wide variety of opinions about and experiences with the various methodologies; (3) opportunities to explore fully and understand the advantages and limitations of new technologies that support auditory methodologies; (4) opportunities to explore fully and understand the concept of bilingualism as it applies to children who are deaf; (5) opportunities to meet parents who have selected various methodologies for their children; and (6) opportunities to visit school programs which offer various methodologies.

An additional role of the professional is to gather ongoing child information through the assessment and documentation process described earlier in this chapter. This information is also shared with the parents so that they, in making their decisions, have the opportunity to reflect on what is known about the development of their child's communication and language system over time.

A family's decision about communication methodology is often a process rather than a single decision. Early choices about communication systems may be based on parents' personal or family experiences, their dreams for themselves and their children, and currently available information. New information, experiences, and perspectives may influence their later choices. Case study 8–2 reflects the ongoing decision process of one family.

COLLABORATIVE INTERVENTION

The Early Years

The assessment process and the development of the IFSP yield a set of outcomes and strategies that provide the basis for subsequent intervention. The parents and all the professionals who are involved in service provision contribute to the development of this plan. Although a wide range of needs may be included in the plan, it usually incorporates a certain number of communication-

Case study 8–2. When Emily was 4 months old, her parents noticed that she did not wake up when the dog barked or seem disturbed when her 2-year-old brother had a tantrum in the middle of her nap time. After frustrating attempts to convince the family doctor that something was wrong, referral was made to an audiologist, and Emily was diagnosed as having a severe to profound bilateral auditory brainstem response hearing loss. Auditory brainstem response (ABR) testing showed no response at the limits of the equipment; sound field behavioral observation indicated possible response to speech at 60 to 70 dB. Emily was fit with hearing aids at the age of 7 months. Her parents were relieved that someone had listened to their concerns and overwhelmed by the final diagnosis. There was no history of hearing loss in the family and no personal experiences of any kind with deafness. In seeking initial services, they looked to the audiologist for guidance. Emily's parents were referred to both a private therapist and their local public school program for services. Both the private therapist and the original audiologist recommended that Emily's parents begin with an auditory approach. The public school program offered both auditory and total communication options and readily agreed to the parents request for an auditory option. During the first year after Emily's diagnosis, a parent advisor made weekly home visits and Emily's family also chose to enroll Emily in private speech and language therapy. Emily's parents were very involved in therapy and home visits. They suggested and implemented many communication and auditory strategies within their home and daily life. Emily, however, was not an avid fan of her hearing aids and hearing aid wearing time was not consistent and became an ongoing struggle between parent and child for more than 6 months. Although Emily demonstrated little response to sound during therapy or in any other setting, Emily's parents remained committed to an auditory approach to communication development. During the next 12 months, additional audiological data was obtained, revealing that Emily's hearing loss was profound across all frequencies. Aided hearing results revealed limited responses of 75 and 80 dB at 250 and 500 Hz, respectively. Receptive and expressive language scores remained near the 10-month level, although typical developmental progress was seen in social, cognitive, and motor skills. During the course of the weekly home visits, the parent advisor shared information with the family about a wide variety of communication options; the family remained committed to an auditory option. The parent advisor also discussed and provided information about cochlear implants as another alternative to be investigated. Educational services to the family at this time included two center-based weekly therapy sessions and a weekly home visit, both provided through the public school and coordinated so that all those involved in the family service plan agreed with and were working toward the same outcomes, using similar strategies. The family had access to, but rarely attended, parent support group meetings offered through the school. When Emily was 2 years old, her receptive and expressive language remained constant at the 10-month level and she demonstrated little awareness of auditory information. By this time, Emily's parents had investigated vibrotactile devices and requested more information on cochlear implants. Emily's father began asking more questions about sign language and requested books about American Sign Language and total communication options. Emily's mother remained adamantly committed to an auditory-only option. When Emily was 2 years, 3 months old, her parents attended a parent support meeting where the topic of social and emotional development of children who are deaf was discussed. The main speaker was a psychologist who was deaf. During the next home visit, the parents began asking many more questions about sign language. They had been impressed both by the content of the presentation and by the fact that the speaker was deaf, well educated, articulate, and used sign language. Emily will soon be 3 years old. Her parents have begun taking sign language classes, are using some signs with Emily and have requested that her educational program be changed to a total approach. They have begun attending more parent meetings and are interested in the opinion and point of view of the parents who are deaf. Concurrently, the family continued to investigate cochlear implants and Emily has been approved to receive an implant. Emily is enrolled part time in the school's integrated preschool program where total communication is used. Her parents have discussed enrolling her brother as a private, hearing student so that he can have more access to sign language as well. If Emily does receive an implant and her parents see auditory progress, they have indicated that they may consider a return to an auditory educational approach. For now, the development of a functional communication system and a way to communicate with Emily is their highest priority.

related outcomes. The individual communication, language, listening, and speech objectives that are part of the plan are also part of a broader developmental sequence. Specific communication targets are only valuable as they relate to the developmental whole. There are commercially available resources that can be used as a reference in designing intervention plans to meet targeted outcomes. Table 8–4 outlines the auditory skills hierarchy of four different resources, the SKI-HI Model Resource Manual,[10] Foreworks: Auditory Skills Curriculum,[18] Pollack's Curriculum Outline for Auditory Verbal Communication,[19] and the Developmental Approach to Successful Listening (DASL).[20] A comparison of these resources reveals that the overall developmental sequence is similar, particularly for the early stages of development.

The selection of targets and resource guides is only the beginning step in program implementation. Other critical issues include a recognition of the support that various environments can provide, the division of responsibilities among the collaborative partnership, and a determination of the best strategies to facilitate learning.

A child's environment has a significant influence on the learning process and deserves critical consideration in the design of a service plan. Environmental issues directly relate to the cultural and social context dimensions of communicative competence.

A child's home often provides one of the best and most natural locations for service delivery. Many excellent opportunities for learning and communication arise from the ordinary routines of a family's day. Daily events such as eating and getting dressed are important and functional for children. Needs arising from these activities provide motivation for children's communication attempts.

A wide variety of contexts specific not only to the child's developmental level, but also to the family's lifestyle can be accurately identified. Working in the home allows the professional to be more aware of the family's culture and to design or adapt a service plan to reflect that lifestyle accurately and to support family values. Working in the home often makes it easier to understand and incorporate neighborhood or community context into the plan as well.

Although home programs often provide the most appropriate setting for early intervention, they are not always possible. Schedules may be impossible to work out or families may prefer an alternate location. Because the most effective intervention is embedded within daily routines and experiences, selection of alternate locations should reflect this philosophy. When a school-based approach is used with infants and toddlers, a great deal of care must go into providing an environment in which age-appropriate routines may be utilized.

The school or clinic can usually be adapted to support play-based learning. Low shelves or tables, carpeted floors, and a controlled, carefully selected array of materials are needed. Arrangement and design of the setting should be influenced by strategies that facilitate learning in general.

It is difficult to structure a school-based setting to provide the broad range of natural contexts found in the home. Certain routines such as diapering and toileting, washing hands, eating a snack, or bundling into coats can easily be incorporated into school facilities. To provide broader availability of contexts, some programs have attempted to provide a more homelike setting, including a "kitchen," and "living/play area." These settings may be used to some advantage in providing appropriate environments if professionals and families are aware of their real limitations in accurately reflecting cultural or family-specific contexts. Care should be taken that communication developed in this context will have some functional relevance outside the school setting.

When naturally occurring environments cannot be utilized in the early intervention process, the parent and professional collaboration becomes even more important. Family-focused intervention gives parents greater self-determination in deciding what role they will play in the intervention process. It is the responsibility of the professional to be sure that parents make the decision about their role in the collaborative partnership with the knowledge of the importance of parents in children's communication development. A family-focused program may provide parental support in a broad range of areas so that parents have the opportunity to develop the personal resources that will allow them to assume an active role in the collaboration.

After desired family and child outcomes have been determined for the IFSP, strategies for their achievement may define the parent and professional roles. In a plan designed to promote communicative competence, the professional often models specific child communication strategies for the parent. The parent may suggest the context or multiple contexts in which the strategy

---

Case study 8–3. Justine and her family have been in the early intervention program for 10 months. Justine's family includes her mother, Susan, her father, Ray, her older sister, Kathryn, and an older brother, Jeff. Justine, who is 15 months, and her older brother, who is 6 years old, both have a hearing loss. Justine's bilateral hearing loss is moderate through 1000 Hz and drops to severe at 2000 Hz and 4000 Hz. Aided responses range from 15 dB at 500 Hz to 50 dB at 4000 Hz. Susan and Ray had decided on an auditory communication method with Jeff and are continuing to use an auditory method with Justine. The family's current Individual Family Service Plan emphasizes auditory and communication strategies for the family to use with Justine. The early intervention case manager, Beth, is a deaf educator (parent advisor) who makes weekly visits to the home. In this parent and professional partnership both the parents and the parent advisor have a great deal of knowledge and experience to share and utilize. As the parents identify additional areas of interest and need, such as a recent interest in cued speech, the parent advisor's responsibility is to find books, conferences, meetings, and people to contact. The early intervention program has its own library as well as a list of resources and established contacts in the community. The family already provides a good language and listening environment. Some highlights of a typical home visit are provided to illustrate better how this partnership works. At the beginning of the visit, Beth and the parents discuss the past week's activities. The parents relay information about Justine's communication attempts, which include pointing and vocalizing to get milk and vocalizing to gets Mom's attention when she wanted something she dropped. Ray and Susan agree that they would like to continue developing strategies to encourage vocalizations and back-and-forth exchanges with Justine. Beth reviews some information and ideas about encouraging and reinforcing vocalizations. She begins playing with Justine, modeling some of these techniques, and asks Ray and Susan to observe what she does and to look for additional opportunities that she misses. During the next 15 to 20 minutes, each of the adults takes a turn as observer or communication partner for Justine, always following Justine's lead. Since Kathryn is at home, she is also an active participant throughout the session. Parents and parent advisor discuss results of the activity. Before Beth leaves, they outline a plan for the coming week. Ray and Susan rely on the parent advisor for feedback and suggestions about their communication interaction with Justine. The parent advisor, in turn, relies on Ray and Susan for ideas and strategies that work for Justine and that can be naturally incorporated into their daily life.

---

may be implemented. The professional may provide feedback and suggestions. The ways in which the parent continues to implement these strategies when the professional is not present is very important. Watkins and Clark[10] outline one possible model of parent and professional collaboration designed for a home visit format. Case study 8–3 provides an overview of one parent and professional partnership.

The emphasis on natural environments and the collaborative strategies of the parent and professional partnership are compatible with strategies that best support child development and facilitate learning. The issues of child learning and communicative competence discussed earlier in this chapter have a direct and often parallel relevance in the selection of strategies to promote infant and toddler communication development. Strategies that promote communication development are most beneficial to the child when they facilitate overall development.

Effective learning strategies encourage exploration and movement. For young children to have the maximum opportunity to acquire and internalize knowledge, they need the freedom to move. Activities that routinely limit children to table and chairs or a highchair are not conducive to a full range of learning. Effective learning strategies also allow children choices and permit their decisions and actions to change the direction of the activity or influence the outcome. Learning strategies that encourage the child to influence the direction of the activity require a higher degree of flexibility on the part of the professional but are worth the effort. Opportunities to make decisions and choices not only provide additional motivation for communication, they promote cognitive development as well. Effective learning strategies recognize play as a major avenue for development of a wide variety of skills and competencies. Nearly any targeted aspect of communication can be incorporated into a wide range of child-initiated or child-directed play. Allowing children the time to play provides them with an opportunity to develop a stronger conceptual base for their understanding of many abstract and relational language concepts. These abstract concepts are a significant aspect of language mastery and later educational success.

Collaborative Intervention— The Preschool Years

During the early school years, intervention plans continue to rely on collaborative input that is responsive to both home and classroom needs. Objectives are selected to focus on responding to child needs, allowing shared educational roles, emphasizing child strengths, providing real-life success, developing communicative competence, and promoting a child- or student-centered approach. Needs are generally identified in the areas of auditory processing, speech or sign communication, pragmatics, semantics, and syntax. Early school objectives that focus on communicative competence and real-life success might include skills such as requesting objects, help, or information; answering questions; negotiating rules for play or games; participating in show and tell; attending to directions; relaying messages; or expressing a desire or problem.

Objectives can be introduced to educational environments in three ways: provided within the context of existing classroom routines, provided as a concurrent activity imposed on, but consistent with, the context of existing classroom routines, or provided as a separate activity apart from the context of existing classroom routines. Within a collaborative intervention model, team members first consider development, needs, and interests of the child and then purposefully construct opportunities that allow the child to participate actively in and ultimately utilize the targeted objectives. One significant aspect of the intervention process is defining who is to be involved in the process and where the intervention strategies will be implemented. To some extent, anyone in contact with a child in need of speech/language/listening intervention can share in the responsibility for providing input or opportunities for interaction in contexts in which those skills can be used and learned. In the school setting, intervention may include collaborative implementation by the habilitation specialist and the teacher; implementation by the educator or parent, with the habilitation specialist providing consultation; implementation by the habilitation specialist outside the classroom setting; or a combination of these. Within a purposefully prepared environment, learning experiences may be appropriately initiated by the child, parent, habilitation specialist, or teacher.

Providing appropriate organization of the school environment to focus on targeted objectives first requires several observations of the child to determine his level of play and interaction. It is necessary to observe the child as a part of both his social and physical environment. These observations provide an understanding about how the child gives and receives information and how he interacts with his environment. The new information or target objective is then provided so that it is contextually relevant and conforms to the child's social and physical behaviors. Successful intervention strategies involve creating real needs to communicate in routine situations and events that are familiar and meaningful to the child.[21] Providing variety within an environment in which the child is motivated to signify communicative intents, such as requesting, possession, imperative, location, desire, or problem, is essential when planning intervention strategies. Adults provide support for the child's choices and may best respond to the child's initiative by extending and encouraging rather than by directing.

Isolated settings such as therapy rooms can be altered to be more like the natural environments of the child by rearranging the physical attributes of the therapy setting and recreating events that occur naturally in the home or classroom. Therapy becomes more functional when conducted in a variety of settings other than the therapy room, such as the playground, lunchroom, classroom, hallway, or bus room, and using materials that are real, functional, everyday objects. Providing variety in therapy environments is enhanced by moving from one on one settings to interactive small group settings.

When the target objective is introduced into the child's environment, it needs to become a reasonable part of the activity so that the integrity of the child's routine can be maintained. The provider of the new information uses responsive strategies to assure the child's perception that his communicative attempts have had an effect on the listener. It is important to not "take over" the activity, but continue to provide opportunities for the child to be actively engaged and interacting in the activity. Respond as a partner by wondering and questioning with the child. Appropriate organization of the environment enables the child to attend to new information within his social and physical framework and ensures that learning is centered around functional skills that are used to meet the daily demands of communication.

To validate the use of a targeted objective and make it a meaningful part of a child's experiences, the child is first placed in the role of the communicator, not just the recipient of new information. Organizing the environment by allowing the child to be the initiator provides a nonjudgmental, no-risk type of setting in which the child can explore and communicate.

Once opportunities have been provided to allow the child to initiate communication, then it is appropriate to model the targeted objective within the natural environment. This modeling is accomplished by doing, not by telling or directing. The emphasis is on giving meaning and importance, not on setting the modeling as the one and only correct way. This allows the child to attach meaning and function to the new language and the targeted objective is learned through functional use in the environment.

An understanding that it is easiest for a child to learn new skills if he understands the routine and is able to predict what may happen should be a component of intervention strategy planning.

Repetition, routine, and consistency are important in the understanding and development of new skills. Learning experiences are the most beneficial when organized in a continuous and sequential order so that the child can relate one learning experience with another, day after day.

PROVIDING COLLABORATIVE SUPPORT FOR INCLUSION, INTEGRATION, AND MAINSTREAMING

Inclusion, integration, and mainstreaming are terms that have been used to describe programs in which children with identified special needs are educated along with children without identified special needs. The terms are often used interchangeably by educators and authors to describe a wide variety of practices and programs. Because there is little overall consistency in terminology in the literature, it is important to begin with background information and a clear description of the way in which terms are used in this chapter.

The concept of inclusion comes from Part H of IDEA which maintains that, to the extent appropriate to the needs of the child, early intervention services must be provided in natural environments, including home and community settings that include the participation of children without disabilities. For infants and preschoolers, natural settings are often the home, day care, or other community settings. In considering education placement decisions, the education placement team must first identify the educational environment where the child would be educated

if he were not eligible for special services and then determine if special services can be delivered in that setting with the use of modifications and supplementary assistance. Thus, the challenge of identifying and providing the least restrictive environment (LRE), originally associated with school age children, now extends to school programs for very young children. In all situations, the challenge is to identify the most natural environment possible in which the child will experience optimal development.

Providing inclusive services for preschool children who are deaf or have other special needs is especially challenging for public schools because general education programs for children typically do not begin until Kindergarten at age 5 years or, in some schools, with pre-kindergarten at age 4 years. Because there is no general definition of natural environments for children younger than Kindergarten, a wide variety of programs and approaches have developed for this population. As discussed earlier in this chapter, the home environment is often utilized effectively with infants. With older children, school programs may rely on coordination with a wide variety of community-based programs, including private preschools, church schools, and Headstart programs.

The concepts of inclusion and mainstreaming, as discussed here, differ in a significant way. In a traditional mainstream approach children may be assessed to determine if they have the skills necessary to participate in a regular preschool program. Children who do not meet program criteria may be recommended for a self-contained classroom placement. Although programs have varying degrees of flexibility, in a mainstream approach, the child's skills must match the curriculum and the setting to participate in the program. Classroom modifications, curriculum adaptations, and direct or consultative services of an aural habilitation specialist may be offered as support to children in the mainstream setting. In an inclusive approach to education, there is a commitment that, to the maximum extent appropriate, all children will have the opportunity to be in preschool settings similar to what would be available to them if there were no special needs. There is no expectation or requirement that children keep pace with their peers. Placement requires only that children benefit from inclusion in the program.

When selecting community-based programs for preschool inclusion, program philosophy as well as attitude of the administration, staff, and parents are all significant factors to consider. Preschool programs that adhere to a philosophy of developmental appropriateness may be the best programs in which to include any child with a special need. A developmentally appropriate program incorporates knowledge about the predictable growth and sequence of typical child development (age appropriateness) and recognizes the individual uniqueness of each child in learning style, rate and pattern of development (individual appropriateness).[22] This type of program already provides an environment in which individual needs of children are a significant part of the planning process. In addition, successful inclusion programs do not consider remediation of deficits as their only important goal. Successful programs also have an articulated philosophy about the importance of accepting diversity and the importance of accepting each child as a valued and participating member of the peer group.[23]

A true challenge to providing inclusive services for special needs children is to create an environment in which the needs of a wide range children can be effectively met. One way in which to accomplish this mission is through an integrated program. An integrated program, as defined here, combines the professional expertise of both regular and special educators, often through the use of team teaching. The curriculum of the integrated program is developed to meet the needs of all children within the program. Through the development of an integrated setting, true individualization can facilitate the optimal development of each child. This definition of an integrated program requires a high level of professional collaboration.

There is little concrete information and more than a little controversy concerning inclusion for children who are deaf. At either end of the inclusion continuum may be found parents, educators and adults who are deaf who believe that children benefit from placement in education environments that are primarily "hearing" or primarily "deaf." Along the midrange of the continuum are others who believe that a blending of educational philosophies and cultures may be possible and desirable for many children. Most everyone will agree that individual decisions are important and that the LRE is one in which the child will have an opportunity to reach his full potential. The social and linguistic aspects of inclusive settings are important variables in the discussion of opportunities for reaching full potential.

For many parents, educators, and adults who are deaf, the concept of deaf community and deaf cultural identity have gained importance in recent years. Following this view, children who are deaf benefit from the opportunity to communicate and play with other children who are deaf. This view does not preclude the idea that children who are deaf may also experience positive social interaction with hearing peers. Two recent studies of interactions between young children who are deaf and young children who are hearing suggest that although children will interact more frequently with peers of the same hearing status, in educational settings where children are integrated with stable peer groups, interaction and communication with children of other-hearing status will occur.[24,25] Integrated educational placements that have equal or proportionate numbers of children who hear and children who are deaf provide unique opportunities for interaction among all the children.

The concept of least restrictive may also be influenced to some extent by the communication mode of the child. Neither of the two studies just mentioned found any consistent connection between mode of communication and amount of interaction between children who were deaf and children who were hearing. However, for a child to benefit most fully from peer interactions, the optimal situation will provide the opportunity for shared linguistic communication. For children whose primary form of communication includes sign, this means that fully integrated education will facilitate sign language acquisition for hearing peers. Programs that have the capability of providing instruction via total communication for all children eliminate some of the barriers to inclusive education for young children who are deaf.

All evidence considered, it seems that integrated programs for children who are deaf can be beneficial. Case study 8–4 illustrates the collaborative strategies developed by an integrated preschool program that includes children who are deaf.

As a child reaches school age, educational placement teams are once again faced with identifying and providing the most natural school environment possible. An inclusive approach to elementary and secondary school education provides, to the maximum extent possible, regular education classroom settings for children with special needs. Increasingly, regular education teachers in neighborhood elementary and secondary school settings are asked to provide instruction

---

Case study 8–4. The Child Development Preschool utilizes an approach to integration that is highly dependent on the collaborative efforts of many professionals and parents. The program is cooperatively administered by a university center for communication disorders and a public school deaf education program. Both the auditory and total communication classes are fully integrated. Thirty to 50% of the children in each integrated class have hearing loss and entered the program through the public school system; the other children in each class are children with hearing and typical language development who pay private tuition.

A developmentally appropriate philosophy and curriculum and coteaching or team teaching by deaf educators and regular early childhood educators provide the basic program structure. An aural habilitation professional, known as a communication specialist, is an active member of each teaching team. Daily on-site audiological support is available.

Weekly education team planning meetings are the foundation for the entire integration structure. As teachers plan for learning centers that may include art, blocks, dramatic play, reading or writing, science and mathematics or manipulatives, and small group activities and outdoor play, strategies to meet the individual needs of children who are deaf and hearing can be discussed. Documented and shared child observations from the past week provide both accountability data and important planning information for the coming week. Changes in center environments, including the addition or removal of materials, are based on the observations of the past week. The communication specialist has an important role in suggesting specific strategies, materials, and environmental changes that may best facilitate specific language or listening targets.

The curriculum is designed to meet the needs of all children. In addition, each child with a hearing loss has individual language targets that are jointly selected by educators, parents and communication specialists. Implementation strategies emphasize integration of these objectives into the home and classroom environments. The communication specialist provides the majority of individualized therapy within the natural environment during centers, small group activities, field trips or outdoor time.

---

for children with unique needs. Several beliefs are important for successful inclusion within these regular education settings. The first is a belief that regular classroom instruction can be modified and organized so that children with special needs can learn without compromising the learning of their classmates. Inherent in this belief is that technological and instructional supports are currently available to accommodate the unique needs of students in regular classroom settings. According to Rogers,[26] parents, teachers, and special education staff sometimes create barriers to inclusion because they may fear what they do not understand. Teachers frequently express concerns and anxieties related to having a lack of information and training in special needs. They fear they will be asked to do new or difficult tasks without training and support. They are also concerned that too much of their time will be taken away from the other children. These concerns and anxieties if left unchecked can foster resentment toward the child, his parents, and the changing education system. Parents of children who have a hearing loss generally support the concept of inclusion, but voice fears that their children will lose special services and that the classroom teacher may not be able to address fully the educational needs of all the children. Additionally,

parents fear that social rejection and frustration may occur resulting in isolation for themselves and their children. Parents of children who are nondisabled fear their child will be shortchanged because the teacher will need to spend too much time with the special needs child in the class. Some educators of deaf children are hesitant to relinquish their primary responsibility role for children with hearing loss fearing the child's needs cannot be met solely in the mainstream setting.

Another belief consistent with inclusion is that successful placement of a child with special needs in a regular classroom setting provides positive experiences and opportunities for growth for parents, teachers, and all the classroom children. Teachers become more flexible in their teaching and gain experience with collaborative programming for children with a wide range of abilities. Regular and special education staff learn from each other as well as build a cooperative educational setting based on mutual respect. Classmates discover that not all children are the same in their physical attributes nor their learning styles. A belief that placement of children with hearing loss in regular classroom settings provides positive experiences for all those who are involved is often not sufficient to motivate teachers, parents, and support staff to build a collaborative partnership. Each individual within the partnership may react differently to proposed changes in classroom composition, scheduling, and programming. Each individual's needs for support and training may also be different. Parents, educators, and support staff may reflect similar or differing desires for more information about their specific child's special needs, about what type of support will be available, and about what might be the possible consequences of providing services for these children in an integrated setting. Once information is provided about children with impaired hearing, concerns often arise as to how to use that information to provide the most effective intervention. If participants view their intervention strategies as ineffective, then frustration may become apparent. Therefore, the first goal for teachers, parents, and support staff in an inclusive setting is to establish contact and rapport with each other to assist in building a collaborative partnership. Then teachers, parents, and support staff can work together to identify the needs of the adults as well as the children in the setting, to discuss classroom scheduling and management as related to the various needs of both the students and adults, to design plans that address a variety of skill levels within a classroom, and to identify instructional factors that are present or not present within the classroom that are important for children with hearing losses.

As educators, parents, and other team members work together, they become more comfortable with providing support to one another. Regular education teachers bring and share their own unique perspectives of social, academic, and communicative behavior expectations to the education of children with hearing impairment. They are generally knowledgeable about children and teaching strategies for a particular age group and often can share new and innovative techniques with their team members. However, regular education teachers frequently have little training in the area of hearing impairment or other disabilities. Other team members can provide the needed resource, technical, and moral support for the regular education teacher. For support to be real, rather than perceived, the recipient must feel supported.[27] Support means listening to and acting on the needs identified by parents and other team members, acknowledging the efforts of team members, providing assistance in planning classroom organization and management, providing assistance in planning instructional methods to assist the educators and student, providing constructive feedback, providing assistance to individualize the classroom instructional program for all children, and making decisions with ample opportunity for discussion by all team members. Collaborative support among parents, educators, and other staff members contributes to the overall development of successful inclusive educational settings.

REFERENCES

1. Bredekamp S, Rosegrant T: Reaching potentials: Introduction, in Bredekamp S, Rosegrant T, eds: *Reaching Potentials: Appropriate Curriculum and Assessment for Young Children* (Washington, DC: National Association for the Education of Young Children, 1992).
2. DeVries R, Kohlberg L: *Constructivist Early Education: Overview and Comparison with Other Programs* (Washington DC: National Association for the Education of Young Children, 1987).
3. Piaget J: *The Origins of Intelligence in Children* (New York: International Universities Press, 1952).
4. Bloom L, Lahey, M: *Language Development and Language Disorders* (New York: John Wiley & Sons, 1978).
5. Bloom L: Of continuity, discontinuity, and the magic of language development, in Golinkoff RM, ed: *The Transition from Prelinguistic to Linguistic Communication* (Hillsdale, NJ: Lawrence Erlbaum, 1983).
6. Rice ML: Mismatched premises of the communicative competence model and language intervention, in Schiefelbusch RL, ed: *Communicative Competence: Acquisition and Intervention* (1984).
7. Idol L, Paolucci-Whitcomb P, Nevin A: *Collaborative Consultation* (Austin, TX: Pro-Ed, 1986).
8. Abelson MA, Woodman RW: Implications for teams in schools. *Sch Psychol Rev*, 12 (1983), 125–136.
9. Meisels SJ: Meeting the mandate of public law 99-457: Early childhood intervention in the nineties. *Am J Orthopsychiatry*, 59, (1989), 451–460.
10. Watkins S, Clark T, eds: *The SKI-HI Model: A Resource Manual for Family-Centered, Home-Based Programming for infants, Toddlers, and Preschool-Aged Cildren with Hearing-Impairment* (Logan, UT: Hope, 1993).
11. Crago M, Eriks-Brophy A: Feeling right: Approaches to a family's culture. *Volta Rev*, 95 (1993), 123–129.
12. Dunst CJ: A family-centerd approach to early intervention. Paper presented at the Alexander

Graham Bell Association for the Deaf conference, A Sound Beginning: Children with Hearing Impairments Birth to Five, Denver, 1993.

13. Bailey DB Jr, Simmeonsson RJ, eds: *Family Assessment in Early Intervention* (Columbus, OH: Merrill Publishing, 1988).

14. Winton P: The family-focused interview: An assessment measure and goal-setting mechanism, in Bailey DB, Simmeonsson RJ, eds: *Family Assessment in Early Intervention* (Columbus, OH: Merrill Publishing Company, 1988).

15. Cole EB: *Listening and Talking: A Guide to Promoting Spoken Language in Young Hearing-Impaired Children* (Washington, DC: Alexander Graham Bell Association for the Deaf, 1992).

16. Dale PS: The validity of a parent report measures of vocabulary and syntax at 24 months. *J Speech Hear Res*, 34 (1991), 565–571.

17. Crais ER: Families and professionals as collaborators in assessment. *Top Lang Disord*, 14, (1993), 29–40.

18. Head J: *Auditory Skills Curriculum* (N. Hollywood, CA: Foreworks, 1986).

19. Pollack D: *Educational Audiology for the Limited-Hearing Infant and Preschooler* (Springfield, IL: Charles C Thomas, 1985).

20. Stout G, Windle J: *The Developmental Approach to Successful Listening II* (Englewood, CO: Resource Point, 1992).

21. Luetke-Stahlman B: Research-based language intervention strategies adapted for deaf and hard of hearing children. *Am Ann Deaf*, 138, (1993), 404–410.

22. Bredekamp S, ed: *Developmentally Appropriate Practice in Early Childhood Programs Serving Children from Birth Through Age 8* (Washington, DC: National Association for the Education of Young Children, 1987).

23. Peck CA, Furman GC, Helmstetter E: Integrated early childhood programs: Research on the implementation of change in organizational contexts, in Peck CA, Odom SL, Bricker DD, eds: *Integrating Young Children with Disabilities into Community Programs* (Baltimore: Paul H. Brookes Publishing, 1993).

24. Antia S, Kreimeyer K, Eldredge N: Promoting social interaction between young children with hearing impairments and their peers. *Except Child*, 60 (3), (1993) 262–275.

25. Minnett A, Clark K, Wilson G: Play behavior and communication between children who are deaf and hard of hearing and their hearing peers in an integrated preschool. *Am Ann Deaf*, (in press).

26. Rogers J: The inclusion revolution. *Res Bull*, 11 (1993), 1–6.

27. Rainforth B, York J, Macdonald C: *Collaborative Teams for Students with Severe Disabilities* (Baltimore: Paul H Brookes Publishing, 1992).

CONTRIBUTION OF MILD HEARING LOSS TO AUDITORY LANGUAGE LEARNING PROBLEMS

9

Marion P. Downs

It is only with the heart that one can see rightly; what is essential is invisible to the eye.

—Antoine de Saint-Exupery, 1900–1944

The concept of an *educationally handicapping hearing loss* has recently undergone dramatic changes. Traditionally, it has been thought that if a child passed a school hearing screening test at the usual 25 dB hearing level (HL), his or her hearing was adequate for educational purposes. However, in 1964, a large school study[1] found that pure tone screening at 25 dB HL missed ear disorders in 52% of the children tested. Later studies[2-49] are finding that almost all middle ear disorders result in conductive losses that can be educationally handicapping to some degree. This changing concept of a handicapping loss is of immediate concern to educators, school nurses, health service personnel, physicians, and school administrators.

Conductive hearing loss from active ear disease is the most frequently occurring type of loss in school children. Although sensorineural losses are more distressing because of the severity of the handicap, conductive losses should be of more widespread concern because these losses may be responsible for many of the language disorders that are seen in the school population with normal hearing. Often termed "central processing disorders," the language problems may be due to developmental language dysfunction caused by recurrent ear disease. Recognition of this fact will make a difference in the therapeutic techniques used with such children.

What kind of a hearing loss caused by ear disease would result in educational handicap? What decibel level is educationally handicapping? Why should mild losses from common ear disease become learning handicaps? What evidence suggests that ear disease in early life results in language learning disorders? These questions will be thoroughly covered in this chapter because they represent a revolutionary change in our way of looking at hearing loss in school children. In addition, some other environmental deprivations that affect the auditory language learning process will be explored, for almost all of our language is learned through audition.

THE HANDICAP OF CONDUCTIVE HEARING LOSS

Just for a moment, perform a little experiment on yourself. With your index fingers extended, press the tabs in front of your ears into the ear canals, occluding the ear canals completely.

Press tightly. You have just given yourself a 25 dB HL average hearing loss, as shown in Figure 9–1. Try carrying on a normal conversation with this hearing loss, or try listening to someone talk in a crowd. You will find that you have to strain a great deal to catch what people are saying. Yet this kind of hearing loss would have passed the traditional school screening tests, where only 1000, 2000, and 4000 Hz were screened at 25 dB HL. This kind of loss results from the ear disorder called otitis media, extremely common in children. Table 9–1 shows the approximate prevalence of ear disease in children (20% on the average) as delineated in a Washington, DC survey by the National Academy of Sciences.

However, for the benefit of physicians and nurses, we must reiterate which kind of otitis media is the culprit in such hearing losses. As detailed in Chapter 3 there are three types of otitis media:

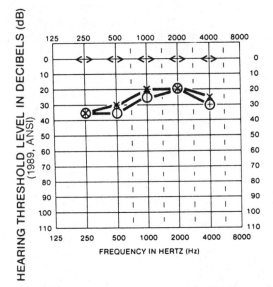

Figure 9–1. Simulation of conductive-type hearing loss obtained when occluding ears with fingers.

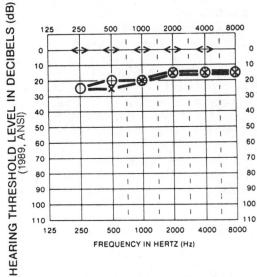

Figure 9–2. Mild conductive hearing loss characteristic of acute suppurative otitis media.

Table 9–1   Distribution of Otologic Examination Results in Children Age 6 Months to 11 Years: Community Sample, Selected Areas in Washington, DC, 1971

Otologic Examination Result*	6 mo–3 yr (%)	4–5 yr (%)	6–7 yr (%)	8–9 yr (%)	10–11 yr (%)	All Ages (%)
Bilaterally normal	68.8	74.3	72.2	81.2	78.8	74.6
Small fibrotic scarring only	3.6	4.6	8.0	5.6	6.7	5.7
Ear pathologic condition	27.6	21.1	19.8	13.2	14.4	19.7
Total percent	100.0	100.0	100.0	100.0	99.9	100.0
Total number	499	411	451	407	390	2158†

*Total chi square (4 df) = 34.132, $p < 0.001$; regression with chi square (1 df) = 30.401, $p < 0.001$.
†Excludes 22 children who could not be examined.
Reprinted with permission from Kessner et al.[66]

1. Acute suppurative otitis media, characterized by fever, pain, redness of the drum, and a significant conductive hearing loss (Fig. 9–2). There is no missing these symptomatic episodes of acute otitis media. Because this disease is caused by bacteria, it may yield readily to antibiotics, so it is easily medically treated.
2. Chronic otitis media, usually characterized by a perforated eardrum accompanied by purulent (pussy) drainage. There may be some pain and the hearing loss can be quite severe.
3. Serous otitis media (sometimes called secretory otitis media), an almost completely asymptomatic disease, unless one is able to identify the mild conductive hearing loss that usually results.

Figure 9–3 shows the mean conductive hearing loss of serous otitis described by Bluestone.[3]

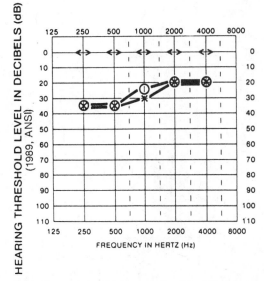

Figure 9–3. Mean conductive hearing loss characteristic of serous otitis media described by Bluestone et al.[3]

There is no pain, no fever, no drainage, no bulging drum, and only a thin fluid behind the eardrum that may be difficult to see in a cursory examination. This is the ear disease that we are particularly concerned with, both in the infant and in the school child, because the child hearing loss that results may be a great deal more educationally handicapping than has been thought.[4] Estimates of its prevalence range from 14% or more in the entire child population to 62% in 7 to 8 year old children.[5,6]

When present, serous otitis media usually affects both ears (see Chapter 3). It may be continuous, causing a constant reduced level of hearing, or it may be recurrent, causing a fluctuating hearing loss. Even when fluctuating, serous otitis media handicaps the overall language learning situation of the child, for acoustic information will be heard sporadically and differently from time to time and cause confusion in the child's learning strategies. Figure 9–4 shows where various speech sounds are heard in relation to the mild conductive hearing loss of otitis media. It can be seen that although the voiced vowel and consonant sounds may be heard at around 40 dB HL on the audiogram, a great many of the unvoiced consonant sounds may be heard faintly or not at all with even a mild conductive hearing

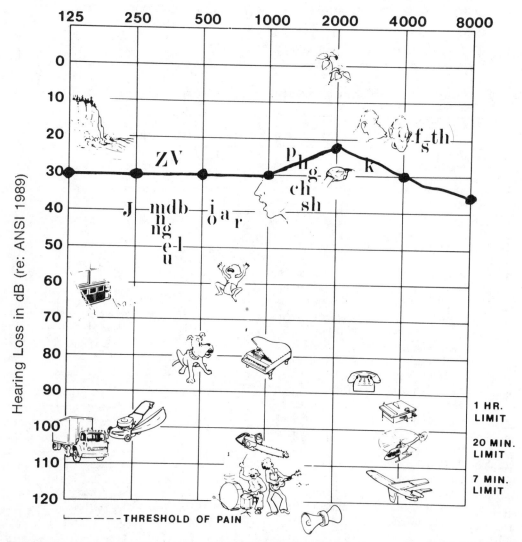

Figure 9–4. Comparison of the frequency and intensity of various environmental and speech sounds in relationship to the mild conductive hearing loss of otitis media. (Reprinted with permission from Northern and Downs.[67])

loss. It is important to understand what this means in terms of the learning strategies of the child.

When you occluded your ears in the exercise above, you found that you could still hear ordinary conversation, even though it was considerably muffled. However, what you may not have realized is that there were some speech sounds that you could not hear at all or could not hear distinctly. You never missed them, for you have been so familiar with the strategies for understanding speech through contextual clues that you were not aware of not hearing some of the sounds. What if you had been a first grader who was learning a variety of words for the first time? It is exceedingly more important for a first grader to hear all of the speech sounds in a new word than it is for you as an experienced listener to hear them. Figure 9–5 illustrates why some of the sounds may be missed. It shows that the voiceless stop consonants and the voiceless fricative consonants are in some cases 30 dB less intense than the vowels and other consonants. Voiceless stop consonants include the /p/ as in *pay*, /t/ as in *to*, and /k/ as in *key*; and the unvoiced fricatives include the /f/ as in *for*, /s/ as in *see*, /th/ as in *thin*, and /sh/ as in *she*. This is illustrated by the word *teak* in Figure 9–5 where the /e/ sound is almost 29 dB more intense than the /k/.

For the child who is still learning language, a mild conductive hearing loss may place an unbearable strain on coping abilities. Only the rare child—one with unusually high intellectual abilities—can surmount this learning hazard without being affected in some way. Thus, when speech sounds are missed entirely or not heard distinctly, or are heard differently from one time to another, the usual learning strategies of the child become disorganized and ineffective.

Moreover, the normal background noise level of our present-day environment can be a most destructive liability when added to a conductive hearing loss. Stop for a moment and do another experiment in hearing. Wherever you are, sit back and listen to the ambient noise in your environment. You will hear noise from air conditioning, fluorescent lights, heating blowers, people talking, etc. According to Skinner,[7] this background noise is usually 10 to 15 dB below the level of speech, giving a +10 to +15 dB signal-to-noise (S/N) ratio (see Chapters 11 and 12). Skinner states that this S/N ratio is not difficult for the normal-hearing adult, because an adult is able to fill in with contextual clues for the missed acoustic signals, but, Skinner says, if children are

to hear all of the acoustic clues clearly, the noise should be 30 dB below the level of speech. Unfortunately, our classrooms do not get a clean bill of health so far as S/N ratio is concerned. Chapters 11 and 12 describe the studies that have shown that there are unfavorable S/N ratios in most school classrooms.

The environmental noise problem in the schools has been exacerbated by open-plan or open area classrooms, air conditioning and heating systems, and by the lack of good acoustic treatment of most classrooms. Even the normal-hearing child may be affected by this rising ambient noise level. A study by Cohen[8] demonstrated that groups of children who lived in high environmental noise backgrounds tend to have more reading difficulties than did children who lived in lower background noise levels. Methods to remedy the background noise situation in the classrooms are described in Chapters 11 and 12. One involves amplifying the teacher's voice through loudspeakers and also using amplification for pupil recitation. The procedures appear to be beneficial both for the child with conductive hearing loss and the normal hearing child.

Results from an investigation by Dobie and Berlin[9] provide dramatic support, confirming the acoustic liabilities of mild conductive hearing loss. Knowing that a child with a 20 dB HL loss would pass a screening test that used 20 dB HL as the criterion intensity level, Dobie and Berlin undertook a study to find out what kind of speech perception problems such a child would have in language learning situation. They treated recorded speech sample utterances, first by recording them through *correcting filters*, which shaped the signal as if it were processed through an ear at about the 40 phon level. They then displayed these utterances oscillographically and attenuated them by 20 dB (to simulate how a 20 dB conductive hearing loss would receive the material). These oscillographic samples were then displayed underneath the unattenuated samples, and spectral analyses of each 600 ms of the speech samples were prepared. A number of readers then read the oscillographs to segment and mark the onsets of the various phonetic utterances.

The readings of these treated utterances revealed the following two observations: (1) there was a potential loss of transitional information, especially plural endings and related final position fricatives; and (2) brief utterances or high-frequency information could conceivably either be distorted or degraded if S/N conditions were

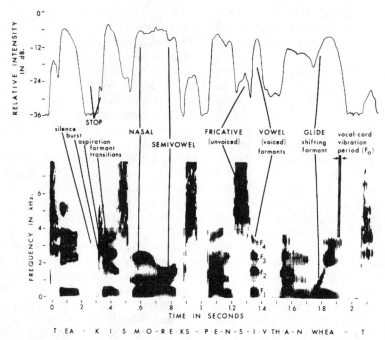

Figure 9–5. Spectrographic analysis and relative intensity of a speech sample showing why some acoustic cues may not be perceived when mild hearing loss is present. (Reprinted with permission from Skinner.[7])

less than satisfactory (remember that the S/N ratios in almost all schools are inadequate).

Dobie and Berlin[9] reasoned that on the basis of their findings, a child with a 20 dB hearing loss from otitis media might be handicapped acoustically in the following ways:

1. Morphological markers might be lost or sporadically misunderstood; for example, "Where are Jack's gloves to be placed?" might be perceived as "Where Jack glove be place?"
2. Very short words that are elided often in connected speech (see "are" and "to" above) will lose considerable loudness because of the critical relationship between intensity, duration, and loudness.
3. Inflections, or markers, carrying subtle nuances such as questioning and related intonation contouring can at the very best be expected to come through inconsistently.

In addition, the authors found that there was a great deal of variability in the acoustic input.

As a result, markers for the beginnings and endings of words and ideas could be inconsistently noted.

This study by Dobie and Berlin[9] completely corroborated the acoustic liabilities that Skinner[7]

had predicted would result from mild conductive loss. She was concerned about the S/N ratios, about the variability of the acoustic input, and about the loss of morphological markers. The study brought scientific evidence supporting her theories.

From the above studies, one would venture predictions that: (1) conductive loss is more devastating to the educational activity of the school child than had previously been suspected; and (2) children who have a history of recurrent otitis media with mild conductive hearing loss might be expected to have central-like symptoms that would masquerade as central processing disorders and language learning problems. There is a great deal of evidence indicating that such is the case. The following will attempt to summarize some of the studies that have demonstrated these conditions.

SEQUELAE OF CONDUCTIVE HEARING LOSSES

A large number of studies have appeared in the literature describing the effect of otitis media on the language functioning of children. The retrospective nature of many of the studies has been severely criticized by Ventry,[10] who believes that only prospective studies will reveal the pathophysiological effects of otitis media on language development in children. However, more recently, prospective, as well as retrospective, studies have appeared indicating that otitis media cannot be overlooked when considering this problem.

A review of the literature on this subject in the past 5 years is shown in Table 9–2.[11–47] Careful perusal will reveal several critical conclusions:

1. When highly discriminating tests are used to identify differences in language skills, school age children who have had histories of otitis media show significant deficiencies. It is only when standard global tests are used that no differences are found. The reason is that by the time school age is reached, speech and language have become so highly redundant, so highly socialized, and so highly global, that it is difficult to see differences in the wide range of normalcy found in these tests. However, in the following areas special distinguishing tests revealed deficiencies in those children with otitis media histories: Morphological ending production; proportional use of compound or complex sentences and prepositional phrases; word production; speech-sound production and auditory perception; ratings of independence, task orientation, attentional skill, and patterns of verbal performance discrepancies in intellectual development; social behavior; and phonological process tests, pitch pattern perception.

2. A recurrent theme, and one that has never been negated, is that attention skills are markedly impaired in children with otitis media. This point was first noted by Feagans et al,[48] who used rating scales to show that in the classroom those children with otitis media histories had twice the amount of distractibility and inattention as children who were normal. Roberts[28,40] has consistently reported the same phenomena, using the Classroom Behavior Inventory. The reason for this problem was originally demonstrated by Jerger et al,[49] who showed that children with otitis media from 2 until 4 years of age had difficulty discriminating words in the presence of background noise (competing sentences). Evidently, the habits formed during periods of mild hearing loss due to otitis media produce listening habits that persist well beyond the episodes of active ear disease. Whether these faulty habits can be remediated is yet to be determined, but it is clear that the mere presence of ear infections may be considered as the presumptive evidence that a hearing disability exists. It follows that it is urgent to establish effective programs to identify middle ear disorders in school screening programs (see Chapter 4).

3. The most significant deficits from otitis media are found in middle class children. Studies by Klein,[14,15] and by Black,[43] have shown that children in low socioeconomic groups have such significant deficiencies in their language and developmental status that any effects from otitis media will be completely screened by the fundamental inadequacies of their speech and language. It is the middle-class children, who have high expectation of accomplishment, that are most affected by the sensory deprivation caused by otitis media. These children are labeled "normal" or "average," but should be achieving in the superior ranges. This fact is particularly poignant because it is those children who hold bright promises for the future, who will not reach their highest potential in productivity. What is particularly significant about all of these reports is that the children studied may be classified as having "central auditory processing deficits, auditory perceptual problems, language learning problems, auditory language deficits, etc." Yet all of their deficits appear to be developmental in origin, caused by early deprivation in a sensory avenue. This calls for a reconsideration of the entire question of labeling children as having central auditory perceptual problems.

The identification of one group of children whose problems are developmental in origin due to early deprivation casts a doubt on the whole concept of *central* problems originating from some congenital brain dysfunction. If auditory deprivation causes central-like disorders, what happens when there is environmental deprivation in language due to reduced or low-quality language stimulation in the home? This, too, is auditory deprivation, whether it is reduced quantity of auditory input or whether the input is of poor quality. An analogy might be drawn to the studies of Dobie and Berlin[9] previously described, in which they showed the auditory

Table 9–2   Studies 1985–1993 on the Language Sequelae of Recurrent Otitis Media*

Study	L/R	No.	Ages	Tests	Results	P/N
Schilder et al[11]	L	47	7–9 yr	Reynell, language, reading, and spelling	The association between OME and language at preschool was no longer present	N
Harsten et al[12]	L	113	B–7 yr	Phoniatric and linguistic examinations—auditory discrimination	Recurrent acute AOM by 3 years: no difference	N
Robb et al[13]	L	1	11–21 mo	Phonetic inventory analyses of child with recurrent otitis media	Consonants fewer. Lack of phonetic complexity in speech	P
Klein et al[14]	L	498	B–3 yr	PPVT, Fisher-Logeman, Goldman-Fristoe, language structure test, articulation scores	Significant association between time with middle ear effusions and language tests	P
Klein et al[15]	L	207	B–7 yr	WISC, Metropolitan Achievement, Articulation, Morphological markers	Difference persisted in all areas tested: intelligence, school achievement, speech and language	P
Updike and Thornburg[16]	R		6–7 yr	Auditory perception, reading ability	OM group: lower scores on all tests	P
Gravel et al[17]	L		B–4 yr	Language and cognitive—pediatric speech intelligibility (PSI)	No difference in groups. OM in 1st year: needed better S/N ratio	N P
Freeark et al[18]	R	56	3–4 yr	Video parent-child interactions; McCarthy Verbal Scale; verbalizing	Active verbilization wih parents buffeted the bad effects of OM	P
Roberts et al[19]	L	30	4½–6 yr	Standard tests and language sample	No relationship between OME and language	N
Knishkowy et al[20]	L	233	B–3 yr	Development quotient; Stanford-Binet	All significantly lower with recurrent OM	P
Teele et al[21]	L	207	B–7 yr	WISC-R; Metropolitan Achievement; Articulation; Morphological markers	Significant differences in all tests for OM before 3 years. After 3 years, no difference	P
Friel-Patti and Finitzo[22]	L	213	B–21 mo	SICD, audiometry	Hearing is related to bouts of OM. Hearing is related to lower scores both expressive and receptive	P
Whiteman et al[23]	R	30	Down's syndrome	Adolescent Basic Skills, Receptive and Expressive Language	Tubed: 100% above mean No OM: 65% above mean OM: 18% above mean	P
Webster et al[24]	R	10	7–11 yr	Auditory, educational, and psychological measures	Matched OM group: lower educational and psycholgical scores	P
Clarkson et al[25]	R		5 yr	Perception of voice onset time (VOT)	OM groups: deficits in identifying and discriminating speech patterns	P
Pearce et al[26]	L	43	B–6 yr	SICD, Bayley, McCarthy Scales at 3 and 6 years	Receptive language and cognitive tests significantly worse in OM group at both 3 and 6 years	P
Rach et al[27]	R	65	Pre-school	Reynell Developmental	Expressive language significantly lower in OM group	P
Roberts et al[28]	L	55	2½–8 yr	Standardized tests of speech	Number of phonological processes lower for OM occurring before 3 years	P

Table 9–2   (Continued)

Study	L/R	No.	Ages	Tests	Results	P/N
Wright et al[29]	L	210	B–2 yr	Speech and language tests	No language delays in the OM children	N
Wallace et al[30]	L	27	12 mo	Bayley, SICD	Lower expressive language in OM children	P
Lous et al[31]	L	463	3–8 yr	Silent Reading Word Test; PPVT; Verbal WISC	No differences between groups but greater variability in OM group	N and P
Wallace et al[32]	L	25	12 mo	ABR and language tests	Lower expressive language and poorer hearing	P
Wallace et al[33]	L	74	B–2 yr	SICD, videos of parent interaction and the Peterson and Sherrod scale	OM group with good parent language had better language	P
Brookhouser and Goldgar[34]	L	1864	9–59 mo	Language battery and developmental tests	More articulation errors and developmental delays in language-delayed OM group	P
Hall and Hill[35]		10		Language development tests	Wide range of disabilities attributable to OM	P
Van Cauwenberge et al[36]	R	1512	2–7 yr	Language, IQ, manual skills, social behavior, tynpanometry	All showed negative influence, greatest under 47 months in speech and language; greatest over 47 months in IQ and activity	P
Fischler et al[37]	L	167	B–8 yr	Battery of language measures	No difference between groups	N
Schlieper[38]	R	26	3–5 yr	Auditory Comprehension of Language test, Northwestern Syntactic Development Sentence Scoring	Highly significant differences between matched groups. Retests a year later showed the same except for Auditory Comprehension	P
Hasenstab et al[39]	R	60	6 yr	Nonsense Syllable test; Phonolgical process test; pitch pattern perception; Kaufman; McCarthy	OM group showed problems in processing, immediate recall, problem-solving strategies, memory, and sequential tasks	P
Roberts et al[40]	L	55 Low SES	3–8 yr	IQ, Achievement scores; Classroom Behavior Inventory	Only Classroom Behavior showed differences: poor attentional skills and Verbal Performance discrepancies	P and N
Friel-Patti et al[41]	L	213	B–3 yr	SICD on OM and non-OM children in 1. Home care 2. Sitter's home 3. Day care center	Number of bouts related to number of children in care. Children in sitter's home had best language (small groups, stimulated)	
Feagans and Blood[42]	L	80	B–2 yr	Early Language Milistone, SICD, attention to language task	High OM group attended less and was more off-task. No effect on receptive or expressive language	P
Black and Sonnenschein[43]	L	31			An inner-city group, low SES, expericned significant decline in their language and developmental status regardless of their history of OM	
Gravel et al[44]	L	39	B–4 yr	Adaptive PSI scores	Significant association between percent visits for OM in 1st year of life	P

Table 9–2   (Continued)

Study	L/R	No.	Ages	Tests	Results	P/N
Lous[45]	R	387	2 y	Silent word reading	Significant correlation between type of typanogram and reading	P
Wendler-Shaw et al[46]	L	105	B–2 yr	PPVT, sound discrimination, sentence repetition, and sentence comprehension	Frequency of OM in 1st year of life and perception or production of words and morphemes	P
Luloff et al[47]	L	138	1–13 mo	Speech sound repertoire	Number of episodes of OM in 1st year equaled reduction in number of consonants	P
Roberts[48]	L	55B	3 mo–8 yr	IQ, Academic performance, Ratings of attention, task orientation, verbal performance discrepancies	No differences found for Academic performance. Early OM predicted all ratings for attention and verbal performance	N P

*L/R: Is the study longitudinal (L) or retrospective (R); P/N: P indicates those studies that found significant differences between otitis groups and nonotitis groups; N indicates those studies in which no differences were found between groups on the measures used; B: birth; OM: otitis media; OME: otitis media with effusions; PPVT: Peabody Picture Vocabulary Test; WISC: Wechsler's Intelligence Scale for Children; S/N: signal to noise ratio; SICD: Sequenced Inventory of Communication Development; SES: socioeconomic status.

deprivation as representing *degraded auditory input*. Reduced, low-quality language input can certainly be considered degraded.

Studies have indeed demonstrated that exposure to low quality language or reduced opportunities for listening have the same effect on language skills as does auditory sensory deprivation. Wachs et al,[50] Uzgiris,[51] Uzgiris and Hunt,[52] and Wachs and Hunt[53] found that infants raised in slum environments will show significantly slower development at a much earlier age than previously suspected. These differences appear as early as 11 months and increase from 18 months on. Messer and Lewis[54] also found that 13-month-old children in the lower class vocalize less than their middle-class peers and are also less mobile in the playroom. They state that understimulation produces apathy and reduced language skills. These are the children who end up in language learning classes.

Not only lack of language stimulation may victimize children; Wachs et al[50] and Uzgiris[51] found that high intensity stimulation and exposure to an excessive variety of circumstances can also be responsible for lower levels of cognitive development. They used the Uzgiris and Hunt[52] infant psychological development scale, and found that stimulus bombardment actually resulted in developmental problems.

Other studies have shown that children raised in noisy environments do not respond as well in a distractive situation as do their peers from quiet homes.[55,57] Thus, these environmental conditions, in effect, may constitute sensory deprivation just as devastating as hearing loss.

DEMOGRAPHIC IMPLICATIONS OF OTITIS MEDIA

The need for remediation may become more and more widespread if the present trends in the demography of otitis media continue. In the general population, Teele et al[58] showed that 71% of children have had at least one episode of acute otitis media by 3 years of age, and 33% have had three or more such episodes. However, this percentage escalates in *day care centers*, where 80% of the children have three or more episodes of acute otitis media by age 3 years.[59] With the proliferation of such centers caring for the children of working mothers, the incidence of recurrent serous otitis will continue to increase alarmingly.

The peak occurrence of otitis media in day care centers is now at 6 months of age, and studies show that such early occurrence places a child at risk for recurrence of the disease.[46] Teele et al[58] reported that the longer the disease process for serous otitis in infants 6 to 12 months of age, the worse the language levels of the children later on. Thus, school systems can expect an escalation of language learning problems with the increase in early otitis.

Unless otitis media is treated vigorously, it can recur repeatedly into the school years, resulting in a growing problem for school health departments. No current figures on the numbers of school children with ear disease are available in the United States, but an in depth study was reported from New Zealand.[6] One hundred children 7 to 8 years old were given audiometry and tympanometry tests every 2 to 3 weeks throughout a school year. An average prevalence of 62% of some ear abnormality was found, with a mean duration of 6 weeks for an episode. A correlation between educational tests and threshold audiometric results was reported, showing that the children with poorer hearing had poorer scores on language and achievement tests. The authors concluded that one audiometric test per school year was not adequate to identify hearing loss and ear disease. They suggested that tympanometry tests three times per year will be the most cost-effective program to detect ear disease, with threshold audiometry once per year. That recommendation was subsequently adopted by the New Zealand Public Health Department for all its schools.

The effects of escalation of otitis media may be felt in the schools within a short time. Feagans and Blood[42] followed a group of school age children with histories of recurrent otitis media beginning by 6 months of age. They were found to have lowered narrative and discrimination skills that were mediated by problems in attentional processes. These children had difficulty in attending to a stimulus, probably due to poor hearing during early critical years.

Another significant finding in the school age child has been that gifted children who have had early recurrent otitis may be misperceived as lower functioning[60] because of poor school performance. Yet, when given in-depth testing, they are found to be highly gifted. Again, deficits in attending seem to be responsible, along with marked weaknesses in sequential processing. Downs[10] has related these problems to auditory processing deficits.

The schools may also find an increase in behavioral problems as a result of early hearing deficits. Silva[63] followed a group of children with early recurrent otitis media through the age of 11 years. In addition to persistent reading and articulation problems, the behavior rating by teachers also were lower in the otitis group than in the normal controls. All the effects were at significant levels at 3, 5, 7, 9, and 11 years of age.

It seems clear that the schools may see a growing number of children with the kinds of deficits that have been described,[64] attributable to early mild hearing losses or present hearing losses from otitis media. Remediating these problems as basic language delays and as problems in attending is the road to follow.

UNILATERAL HEARING LOSS

Hearing loss in only one ear was formerly considered to involve no handicap as long as preferential seating was given in the classroom, with the child sitting near the teacher, and with his or her good ear toward the teacher. However, a new study reported by Bess et al[65] seriously challenges that philosophy and cautions schools not to be sanguine about children with unilateral hearing losses. Bess studied 60 children 6 to 13 years old who had normal hearing in one ear, but sensorineural hearing losses of more than 45 dB in the other ear. Although all of them had been given preferential seating in the classroom, 35% had failed one or more grades in school, and another 13% were in need of special resource assistance—a total of almost 50% with educational problems. Further testing and analysis showed that:

1. Children with unilateral hearing loss exhibited greater difficulty than children with normal hearing in understanding speech in the presence of a competing noise background, even when the good ear was on the side of the speech and the bad ear on the side of the competing noise. Thus, preferential seating in the classroom is not an adequate solution to the problem.

2. Those children who had severe to profound unilateral hearing loss (greater than 61 dB) exhibited significantly lower full scale IQs than those children with milder losses (45 dB to 60 dB). Thus, the degree of loss made a difference in the severity of the effect on the IQ.

3. Teachers consistently rated children with unilaterally hearing-impairment as having greater difficulty in peer relationships, less social confidence, greater likelihood of acting out behavior or withdrawal from social situations, greater frustration, increased need for dependence on the teacher, and more frequent distractibility.

4. Factors in common among those children with unilateral hearing impairment who had greater educational problems included early

age of onset of the hearing loss; perinatal (eg, prematurity) or postnatal (eg, meningitis) complications; severe to profound sensorineural impairment (greater than 61 dB); and right ear impairment. Of the children who failed one or more grades, 63% had right ear hearing losses; and a large mean difference was found between verbal IQ scores of children with left ear hearing impairments and those with right ear impairment: left, 108; right, 99.

Bess[65] concludes that it is no longer appropriate to assume that preferential seating will solve the problems of the child with unilateral hearing loss. Innovative solutions must be devised for these children. Bess offers possible interventions that schools can use, including applying FM wireless systems to the good ear, the use of infrared systems, or simply amplifying the entire classroom to improve the S/N ratio. Special resource assistance is another alternative but is an after-the-fact remedy. Whatever is done for the child with unilateral hearing loss, it must go beyond the traditional recommendations.

SUMMARY

Mild hearing losses of any type or cause (among school children) result in language deficits, lowered academic performance, reduced cognitive skills, or behavioral problems. Many of the problems are due to otitis media, whether incurred in infancy or at school age. Such hearing losses must be zealously identified and remediated, both medically and educationally. The language problems that are found can best be remediated by the comprehensive therapy described in Chapter 16.

REFERENCES

1. Jordon RE, Eagles EL: The relation of air conduction audiometry to otologic abnormalities. *Ann Otol Rhinol Laryngol*, 70 (1961), 819–927.
2. Quigley, SP: Some effects of hearing impairment upon school perfomance. Prepared for the Division of Special Education Services, Office of the Superintendent of Public Instruction, State of Illinois, 1970.
3. Bluestone CD, Beery QC, Paradise JL: Audiometry and tympanometry in relation to middle ear effusion in children. *Laryngoscope*, 83 (1975), 594–604.
4. Friel-Patti S, Finitzo T: Language learning in a prospective study of otitis media with effusion in the first two years of life. *J Speech Hear Res*, 33 (1990), 188–194.
5. Howie VM, Ploussard JH, Sloyer J: The "otitis-prone" condition. *Am J Dis Child*, 129 (1975), 676–678.
6. West SR: Audiometry and tympanometry in children throughout one school year. *N Zealand Med J*, 737 (1983), 603–605.
7. Skinner MW: The hearing of speech during language acquisition. *Otolaryngal Clin of North Am*, 11 (1978), 631–650.
8. Cohen SA: Cause vs. treatment in reading achievement. *J Learn Disabil*, 33 (1970), 163–166.
9. Dobie RA, Berlin CI: Influence of otitis media on hearing and development. *Ann Otol Rhinol Laryngol*, 88, Suppl 60 (1979), 48–53.
10. Ventry IM: Effects of conductive hearing loss: Fact or fiction. *J Speech Hear Disord*, 45 (1980), 143–156.
11. Schilder AG, Van Manen JG, Zielhuis GA, Grievink EH, Peters SA, Van Den Broek P: Long-term effects of otitis media with effusion on language, reading and spelling. *Clin Otolaryngol*, 18 (1993), 234–241.
12. Harsten G, Nettelblandt U, Schallen L, Kalm O, Prellner K: Language development in children with recurrent acute otitis media during the first three years of life. Follow-up study from birth to seven years of age. *J Laryngol Otol*, 107 (1993), 407–412.
13. Robb MP, Psak JL, Pan-Ching GK: Chronic otitis media and early speech development: a case study. *Int J Pediatr Otorhinolaryngol*, 26 (1993), 117–127.
14. Klein JO, Teele DW, Pelton SI: New concepts in otitis media: Results of investigations of the Greater Boston Otitis Media Study Group. *Adv Pediatr*, 39 (1992), 127–156.
15. Klein J, Chase C, Teele D, Greater Boston Otitis Media Study Group: Otitis media and the development of speech, language and cognitive abilities at seven years of age, in Lim D, et al, eds: *Recent Advances in Otitis Media*. (Decker Periodicals, Toronto, 1988).
16. Updike C., Thornburg JD: Reading skills and auditory processing ability in children with chronic otitis media in early childhood. *Ann Otol Rhinol Laryngol*, 101 (1992), 530–537.
17. Gravel JS, Wallace IF: Listening and language at 4 years of age: Effects of early otitis media. *J Speech Hear Res*, 35 (1992), 588–595.
18. Freeark K, Frank SJ, Wagner AE, Lopez M, Olmsted C, Girard R: Otitis media, language development, and parental verbal stimulation. *J Pediatr Psychol*, 17 (1992), 173–185.
19. Roberts JE, Burchinal MR, Davis BP, Collier AM, Henderson FW: Otitis media in early childhood and later language. *J Speech Hear Res*, 34 (1991), 1158–1168.

20. Knishkowy B, Palti H, Adler B, Tepper D: Effect of otitis media in development: A community-based study. *Early Hum Dev*, 26 (1991), 101–111.

21. Teele DW, Klein JO, Chase C, Menyuk P, Rosner BA: Otitis media in infancy and intellectual ability, school achievement, speech, and language at age 7 years. Greater Boston Otitis Media Study Group. *J Infect Dis*, 162 (1990), 685–694.

22. Friel-Patti S, Finitzo T: Language learning in a prospective study of otitis media with effusion in the first two years of life. *J Speech Hear Res*, 33 (1990), 188–194.

23. Whiteman BC, Simpson GB, Compton WC: Relationship of otitis media and language impairment in adolescents with Down syndrome. *Ment Retard*, 24 (1986), 353–356.

24. Webster A, Bamford JM, Thyer NJ, Ayles R: The psychological, educational and auditory sequelae of early, persisten secretory otitis media. *J Child Psychol Psychiatry*, 30 (1989), 529–546.

25. Clarkson RL, Eimas PD, Marean GC: Speech perception in children with histories of recurrent otitis media. *J Acoust Soc Am*, 85 (1989), 926–933.

26. Pearce PS, Saunders MA, Creighton DE, Sauve RS: Hearing and verbal-cognitive abilities in high-risk preterm infants prone to otitis media with effusion. *J Dev Behav Pediatr*, 9 (1988), 346–351.

27. Rach GH, Zielhuis GA, van Baarle PW, van den Broek P: The effect of treatment with ventilating tubes on language development in preschool children with otitis media with effusion. *Clin Otolaryngol*, 16 (1991), 128–132.

28. Roberts JE, Burchinal MR, Koch MA, Footo MM, Henderson FW: Otitis media in early childhood and its relationship to later phonological development. *J Speech Hear Disord*, 53 (1990), 424–432.

29. Wright PF, Sell SH, McConnell KB, Sitton AB, Thompson J, Vaughn WK, Bess FH: Impact of recurrent otitis media on middle ear function, hearing, and language. *J Pediatr*, 113 (1988), 581–587.

30. Wallace IF, Gravel JS, McCarton CM, Ruben RJ: Otitis media and language development at 1 year of age. *J Speech Hear Disor*, 53 (1988), 245–251.

31. Lous J, Fiellau-Nikolajsen M, Jeppesen AL: Secretory otitis media and language development: A six-year follow-up study with case-control. *Int J Pediatr Otorhinolaryng*, 15 (1988), 185–203.

32. Wallace IF, Gravel JS, McCarton CM, Stapells DR, Bernstein RS, Ruben RJ: Otitis media, auditory sensitivity, and language outcomes at one year. *Laryngoscope*, 98 (1988), 64–70.

33. Wallace F, Gravel JS, Ganon EC, Ruben RJ: Two-year language outcomes as a function of otitis media and parental linquistic styles, in Lim D, et al, eds: *Recent Advances in Otitis Media*. (Decker Periodicals, Toronto, 1993).

34. Brookhouser PE, Goldgar DE: Medical profile of the language-delayed child: Otitis-prone versus otitis-free. *Int J Pediatr Otorhinolaryngol*, 12 (1987), 237–271.

35. Hall DM, Hill P: When does secretory otitis media affect language development? *Arch Dis Child*, 61 (1986), 42–47.

36. Van Cauwenberge P, Van Cauwenberge K, Kluyskens P: The influence of otitis media with effusion on speech and language development and psycho-intellectual behaviour of the preschool child—results of a cross-sectional study in 1,512 children. *Auris Nasus Larynx*, 12 (1985), suppl 1, S228–230.

37. Fischler RS, Todd NW, Feldman CM: Otitis media and language performance in a cohort of Apache Indian children. *Am J Dis Child*, 139 (1985), 355–360.

38. Schlieper A, Kisilevsky H, Mattingly S, Yorke L: Mold conductive hearing loss and language development: A one year follow-up study. *J Dev Behav Pediatr*, 6 (1985), 65–68.

39. Hasenstab MS: Auditory processiong and congitive performance of five- and six-year-old children with recurrent otitis media with effusion, in Lim D, et al, eds: *Recent Advances in Otitis Media*. (Decker Periodicals, Toronto, 1993).

40. Roberts JE, Burchinal MR, Henderson F: Otitis media and school age outcomes, in Lim D, et al. eds: *Recent Advances in Otitis Media*. (Decker Periodicals, Toronto, 1993).

41. Friel-Patti S, Finitzo T, Chinn KM, Lindgren MS: Effects of day-care setting on incidence of OME and language development in a cohort of children followed prospectively, in Lim D, et al, eds: *Recent Advances in Otitis Media*. (Decker Periodicals, Toronto, 1993).

42. Feagans, LV, Blood IM: Language and behavioral sequelae of otitis media in infants and young children attending day-care centers, in Lim D, et al, eds: *Recent Advances in Otitis Media*. (Decker Periodicals, Toronto, 1993).

43. Black MM, Sonnenschein S: Early exposure to otitis media: A preliminary investigation of behavioral outcome. *J Dev Behav Pediatr*, 14 (1993), 150–155.

44. Gravel JS, Wallace IF, Ruben RJ: Auditory capabilities of preschoolers with and without a history of otitis media, in Lim D, et al. eds: *Recent Advances in Otitis Media*. (Decker Periodicals, Toronto, 1993).

45. Lous J: Secretory otitis media and reading score in the first grade, in Lim D, et al, eds: *Recent Advances in Otitis Media*. (Decker Periodicals, Toronto, 1993).

46. Wendler-Shaw PD, Menyuk P, Teele DW: Effects of otitis media in the first year of life on language production in the second year of life, in Lim D, et al, eds: *Recent Advances in Otitis Media*. (Decker Periodicals, Toronto, 1993).

47. Luloff AK, Menyuk P, Teele DW: Effect of persistent otitis media on the speech sound repertoire of infants, in Lim D, et al, eds: *Recent Advances in Otitis Media*. (Decker Periodicals, Toronto, 1993).

48. Feagans L, Sangal M, Henderson F, Collier A, Applebaum MI: the relationships of middle ear disease in early childhood to later narrative and attention skills. *J Pediatr Psychol*, 12 (1986), 581–594.

49. Jerger S, Jerger J, Alford BR, Abrams S: Development of speech intelligibility in children with recurrent otitis media. *Ear Hear*, 4 (1983), 138–145.

50. Wachs TD, Uzgiris IC, Hunt IC, Hunt, J McV: Cognitive development in infants of different age levels and from different environmental backgrounds: An exploratory investigation. *Merrill-Palmer Q Behav Dev*, 17 (1971), 288–317.

51. Uzgiris IC: Socio-cultural factors in cognitive development, in Haywood HC, ed: *Social-Cultural Aspects of Mental Retardation* (New York: Appleton-Century, 1970).

52. Uzgiris IC, Hunt J McV: An instrument for assessing infant psychological development. Prepared for the Psychological Development Laboratory, University of Illinois, 1966.

53. Wachs U, Hunt J McV: Cognitive development in infants of different ages and from different environmental backgrounds. *Merrill-Palmer Q Behav Dev*, 17 (1971), 288–317.

54. Messer SB, Lewis M: Social class and sex differences in the attachment and play behavior of the year-old infant. Presented at the Annual Meeting of the Eastern Psychological Association, Atlantic City, 1970.

55. Deutch CP: Auditory discrimination and learning: Social factors. *Merrill-Palmer J Behav Dev*, 10 (1964), 277–296.

56. Clark AD, Richards CJ: Auditory discrimination among economically disadvantaged and non-disadvantaged preschool children. *Except Child*, 33 (1966), 259–262.

57. Nober LW: *A Study of Classroom Noise as a Factor which Affects the Auditory Discrimination Performance of Primary Grade Children*, dissertation, University of Massachusetts, Amherst, 1973.

58. Teele DW, Klein JO, Rosner BA, and the Greater Boston Otitis Media Study Group: Otitis media with effusion during the first three years of life and development of speech and language. *Pediatrics*, 74 (1984), 282–287.

59. Denny FW: Article on otitis media. *Pediatr News*, 18 (1984), 1, 38.

60. Silverman LK, Chitwood DG, Waters JL: Young gifted children: Can parents identify giftedness? *Top Early Child Spec Ed*, 6 (1986), 23–38.

61. Silverman LK: Hunting the hidden culprit in underachievement: Is it ear infections? *Gifted Child Testing Service* (Denver, 1986).

62. Downs MP: Effects of mild hearing loss on auditory processing. *Otolaryngol Clin North Am*, 18 (1985), 337–344.

63. Silva PA: Some long-term psycholgical, educational and behavioral characteristics of children with bilateral otitis media with effusion, in Sade J, ed: *Proceedings of the International Symposium on Acute and Scretory Otitis Media* (Jerusalem, 1985).

64. Davis JM, Elfenbein J, Schum R, Bentler RA: Effects of mild and moderate hearing impairments on language, educational and psychological behavior of children. *J Speech Hear Dis*, 51 (1986), 53–61.

65. Bess FN: Special issue: Unilateral sensorineural hearing loss in children. *Ear Hear*, 7 (1986), 3–54.

66. Kessner DM, Snow CK, Singer J: *Assessment of Medical Care for Children*, vol. 3 (Washington, DC, National Academy of Sciences).

67. Northern J, Downs MP: *Hearing in Children*, 2nd ed (Baltimore: Williams & Wilkins, 1978) p. 12.

MAINTENANCE OF PERSONAL HEARING AIDS

10

Carolyn H. Musket

An ounce of prevention is worth a pound of cure.

—Bracton, *De Legibus*, 1240

BACKGROUND

Hearing aids are the most important resource available for the rehabilitation of children with hearing impairments. However, the instruments are prone to physical and electroacoustic breakdowns. Common defects include clogged earmolds, weak batteries, intermittent controls, cracked tubing, poor frequency response, and excessive distortion. The need for vigilance in hearing aid maintenance is always present. See the case of Ted P in case study 10–1 and Figures 10–1 and 10–2.

Professionals were first alerted to this problem by a study that evaluated hearing aids worn by children in regular school programs. In 1966, after examining hearing aids used by 134 children with hearing impairments, Gaeth and Lounsbury[1] reported that 69% of the aids were inadequate. Subsequent studies throughout the 1970s confirmed that this situation existed in the public schools.[2-4] Identical results were found with hearing aids worn by children in educational programs for those with severe hearing impairments.[5-7] This alarming trend continued in the 1980s: Robinson and Sterling[8] discovered problems with 40% of 97 hearing aids worn by school children; Potts and Greenwood[9] found 25% of the aids malfunctioning in a special school setting before implementing more extensive monitoring; and Elfenbein et al[10] reported, during a 6-week summer program for 10 children, that hearing aids presented an "almost constant problem." In this latter investigation, they found easily remedied hearing aid malfunctions present on 84.6% of treatment days; in addition, 67% of the hearing aids had to be sent away for major repair.

Unfortunately, studies conducted over a 20-year period continue to highlight the fact that consistent hearing aid performance is an issue of major concern. The implications of these findings can-not help but cause dismay for those educational approaches that assume the child's own hearing aid is an integral part of rehabilitation, whether in the classroom or in the home.

One important reason for the repeated high incidence of malfunctioning hearing aids is a generalized lack of knowledge about all aspects of wearable amplification. Many children with hearing loss are being educated today in regular school settings; however, classroom teachers,[11-12] public school nurses,[13] and speech-language pathologists[14,15] have been found to possess limited information about the operation and care of hearing aids, and the educators are not alone. Parents, also, know very little about a hearing aid and its care.[8,16] These recent surveys present a challenge that must not go unanswered if a solution to the dilemma of malfunctioning hearing aids is to be found. This chapter attempts to meet the crucial need for practical, applicable information about hearing aids for those persons in direct daily contact with them—teachers, other school professionals, and parents.[17-19]

THE HEARING AID

No one hears perfectly all of the time. In everyday life, even persons with normal hearing experience difficulty in certain listening situations, such as a large meeting where the speaker addresses a group from some distance away. It would not be possible for those in the audience to hear well without the help of amplification. Some device must be used to intensify the speaker's voice to make it audible to the listener out of normal conversational range. Fortunately, amplification with a public address systems is available. The speaker talks into a microphone; this signal is then carried to an amplifier, where it is intensified greatly and directed to loudspeakers

Case study 10–1. Ted P., a 5-year-old, was seen recently at a university center for communication disorders. Ted, who has been wearing a monaural hearing aid since the age of 2 years, has a severe, flat bilateral sensorineural hearing loss. Figure 10–1 shows his unaided response to warble tones presented through a loudspeaker in the test suite. His average minimal response level was 77 dB HL. However, when wearing a hearing aid his aided responses to these same warble tones occurred at an average hearing level of 45 dB. His aided speech threshold was 40 dB HL. This child has a hearing loss so severe he cannot hear conversational speech at all. With a hearing aid, however, conversational speech is audible, except for sounds in the octave band centered at 4000 Hz. This is a crucial factor for Ted as he strives to acquire speech and language.

One week later, Ted returned to explore his performance with binaural amplification. At the start of the session, the aided results from the week before were rechecked. This time, however, Ted's aided speech threshold was 90 dB HL, not 40 dB HL, and his aided responses to warble tones agreed with this new finding. Ted was not receiving any help whatsoever from the hearing aid. Figure 10–2 displays these second test results. The audiologist soon determined that these discrepancies occurred because Ted's earmold was completely occluded by earwax. Even though the hearing aid was working, the amplified sound could not pass through the earmold into Ted's ear because of the blockage from earwax. Once the earmold was cleaned, Ted's aided scores agreed with those of the previous week.

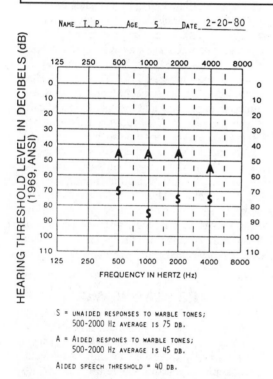

S = UNAIDED RESPONSES TO WARBLE TONES;
500-2000 Hz AVERAGE IS 75 DB.

A = AIDED RESPONES TO WARBLE TONES;
500-2000 Hz AVERAGE IS 45 DB.

AIDED SPEECH THRESHOLD = 40 DB.

Figure 10-1. Unaided (S) and aided (A) responses to sound field warble tones for Ted P (see Case History 1 in this chapter).

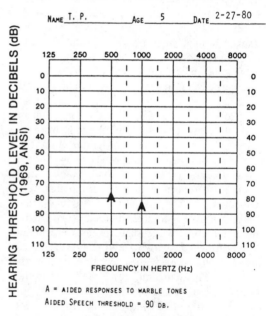

A = AIDED RESPONSES TO WARBLE TONES
AIDED SPEECH THRESHOLD = 90 DB.

Figure 10-2. Aided sound field responses for Ted P, one week after the results shown in Figure 10-1 were obtained (see Case History 1 in this chapter).

strategically placed around the meeting room. From these loudspeakers the magnified voice is delivered to the audience. In addition, this system uses some source of electrical power. The amplification arrangement just described is an accepted feature of auditoriums, stadiums, and theaters.

It is helpful to know that a wearable electronic hearing aid really is a miniature public address system. As shown in Figure 10–3, it has the same components that were just described: microphone, amplifier, loudspeaker (receiver), and power source. Basically, it is designed to accomplish the same goal. The purpose of a hearing aid is to amplify speech so it will be heard as comfortably loud by someone with a hearing impairment. This increased intensity is needed

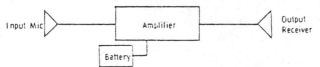

Figure 10–3. A simple block diagram of a hearing aid. Mic: microphone.

not because a great distance exists between speaker and listener, but because the impaired ear has a loss in hearing sensitivity. In hearing aids, the recognizable parts of a public address system are not easily discernible because they are extremely small and packaged together in the unfamiliar form of a hearing aid case. Therefore, instead of being in front of the speaker, the microphone is worn at the ear of the person with a hearing loss (the listener) as a built-in part of the hearing aid. This explains why hearing aids work most effectively in quiet, structured surroundings, where the speaker is at a conversational distance of 3 to 4 feet. When greater distances are involved, the speaker is not within the range of the microphone. When noise is present, it reaches the microphone too, and is amplified, making it difficult for the listener to separate the desired speech signal from this interference.

Hearing Aid Components

Microphone. Sound travels through the air by movement of the molecules of air. This acoustic transmission is cumbersome and difficult to magnify, although it can be done. When one cups a hand behind the ear, more sound waves are collected and directed into the ear, thus enlarging the original signal. An old-fashioned ear trumpet took advantage of this fact. However, the increase in intensity that may be obtained this way is minimal. If the acoustic transmission of sound is converted into electric energy, a much greater increase is possible. This desired energy conversion—acoustic energy into electric energy—is the function of the hearing aid microphone. As the sound waves strike the diaphragm of the microphone, their acoustic energy causes it mechanically to move back and forth. The vibrating motion of the diaphragm in turn causes a change in electric voltage according to principles that vary with the type of microphone used. Variations in the sound waves impinging on the microphone create corresponding variations in an electric signal flowing from it. Most hearing aids manufactured at present achieve this transformation by using an electret condenser microphone.

The microphone itself is housed inside the hearing aid case. The location of the microphone may be detected by looking for a small opening in the case. It is important to identify this sound inlet, because it should not be obstructed when the instrument is worn nor occluded by debris.

Some hearing aids have microphones that are *directional.* A directional microphone receives signals from two locations; it has both a front-facing and a rear-facing opening. In such a microphone, sounds occurring from the rear are attenuated, thereby giving emphasis to sounds occurring in front of the hearing aid user.

Amplifier. As the electric current from the microphone passes through the amplifier, its magnitude is increased. This is accomplished through various stages of complex circuitry. In all hearing aids, the amplifier is contained within the case of the hearing aid. It is an extremely small component.

Receiver (Earphone). The part of a hearing aid that corresponds to a loudspeaker usually is referred to as a receiver. The function of the receiver is to convert the amplified electric energy back into acoustic energy. Through magnetic action, the electric current from the amplifier causes physical movement of the diaphragm of the receiver. This movement disturbs the adjacent air molecules, thereby creating sound waves again. Now, however, the converted sound waves are of much greater magnitude than those that originated at the diaphragm of the microphone.

An air conduction receiver may be housed internally inside the hearing aid, or it may be a separate part connected to the aid by a cord. For both types, the amplified sound eventually will be directed into the child's ear canal. For a small number of hearing aid users, such a fitting is not advisable due to draining ears or a malformed or absent ear canal. These children use a *bone conduction oscillator* for a hearing aid receiver. An oscillator is a small, boxlike device attached to the hearing aid by a cord; it fits onto a headband that holds it against the prominent bone behind the external ear. Mechanical vibrations from the side of the oscillator's case transmit sound to the inner ear through the skull.

Battery. Also contained within the hearing aid case is a small battery, which provides the electric power for the instrument. The battery is a reservoir of stored chemical energy that is converted into electric energy when used in the hearing aid. Three different types of batteries, more accurately termed "cells," are available for use in hearing aids—zinc air, mercury, and silver oxide. Some states have banned batteries containing mercury because it is a hazard to the environment. Zinc air batteries, however, are environmentally safer as well as longer lasting; they are used in most hearing aids today. The adhesive tab on a zinc air battery, which covers tiny holes, is removed when the battery is to be used because air must enter the battery for it to function. Specifications from the manufacturer indicate the size and type of battery recommended for use in a particular aid, as well as the voltage it should supply. Generally, hearing aids require 1.3 to 1.5V.

Hearing Aid Arrangements

Wearable hearing aids are available in four different styles, which are named according to their location on the user. They are pictured in Figure 10–4.

Body-Worn. The term "body worn" refers to a small, rectangular instrument usually worn on the chest. It may be clipped to an article of clothing, such as shirt pocket, or, with young children, it may be inserted into a cloth carrier or harness, which is strapped around the chest.

The microphone, amplifier, and battery on a body-worn aid all are within the case of a hearing aid. A flexible cord leads from the body-worn aid to an external, button-sized receiver. In recent years, there has been a definite decline in the use of body-worn hearing aids. With children, they primarily are reserved for the very young (less than 3 years of age), or for those whose profound losses or other physical disabilities necessitate the use of a more powerful or more durable body aid. In most other instances, children now may be fit appropriately with behind-the-ear instruments.

Behind-the-Ear. In this hearing aid style, all components of the system—microphone, amplifier, receiver, and battery—are contained within a small, slightly curved case. It is designed to fit behind the ear of the wearer.

Eyeglass. Eyeglass hearing aids, although rarely considered for children, also are available. In this style of hearing aid, all components are built within the temple bar of an eyeglass frame. This fitting is not recommended for young children because of its bulk and the problems associated with maintaining two sensory aids concurrently. If a child wears eyeglasses, sometimes it is possible to anchor a behind-the-ear hearing aid to the eyeglass frame through use of an adapter.

In-the-Ear. In this style, all parts of the hearing aid, including the battery, are contained within a plastic shell that fits entirely into the outer ear itself. An *in-the-canal* aid is an even smaller version of this style. Because of tiny controls, lack of flexibility of electroacoustic parameters, and the fact that it is not modified easily

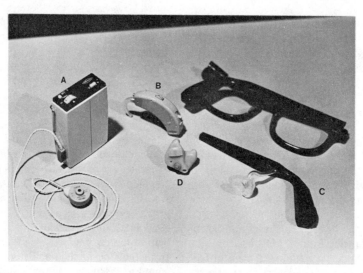

Figure 10–4. Styles of hearing aids. A: Body worn; B: behind-the-ear; C: eyeglass; D: in-the-ear.

as the size of the ear canal changes, in-the-ear aids have not been used widely with children.

As a group, behind-the-ear, eyeglass, and in-the-ear instruments are referred to as *ear-level* hearing aids.

Monaural, Binaural. In a monaural hearing aid arrangement, the output from a single hearing aid is directed into only one ear of the wearer. A *binaural* fitting refers to the use of a complete hearing aid for each ear; ear-level hearing aids provide truer binaural listening than body-worn aids because microphone placement is at each ear. A *pseudobinaural* fitting means that the output of one hearing aid is channeled to both ears. This is accomplished through the use of a Y-cord or V-cord that is connected to a body-worn aid with one plug; then, it divides into two branches so that a cord goes to a receiver in each ear.

CROS, BICROS. "CROS" and "BICROS" are terms used to describe innovative ways in which the components of a hearing aid are arranged on the head and coupled to the ear to provide amplification for those with a unique hearing loss. CROS is an acronym for the *contralateral routing of signal.* A CROS hearing aid is an option for someone with an unaidable unilateral hearing loss and near normal hearing in the better ear. BICROS refers to fitting a conventional hearing aid on one ear and including a second, remote microphone on the other ear, which is unaidable. Neither CROS nor BICROS aids are used often with children.

Hearing Aid Controls

A conventional hearing aid is controlled though dials, switches, and screw adjustments. Figure 10–5 depicts a conventional behind-the-ear instrument to help clarify the descriptions of hearing aid controls in this section. Programmable hearing aids are controlled by a computer chip contained within the hearing aid or, less frequently, in a remote control unit. Various settings for this type of instrument may be programmed by connecting the hearing aid (having a computer chip) via a cable to a programmer or computer. After the settings are stored in the computer chip's memory, the cable is removed. Programming technology may also offer the user a choice of electroacoustic settings to compensate for different listening environments.

On-Off Switch. The switch that turns on the aid may be found in various locations, depending on the design of the aid. It may be incorporated

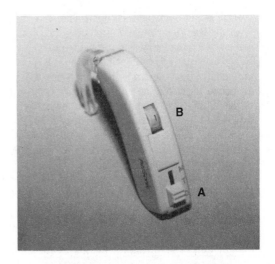

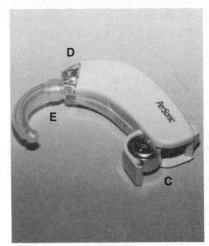

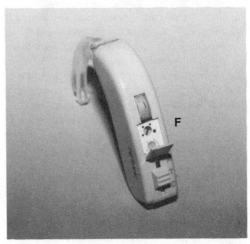

Figure 10–5. View of a conventional behind-the-ear hearing aid. A: Input control; B: gain (volume) control; C: battery compartment; D: microphone port; E: receiver port and earhook; F: panel open to reveal screw setting.

into the swing-out battery compartment, especially in ear-level instruments. Snapping the plastic battery tray completely shut turns on the aid. This switch also may be combined with the rotary volume control, so the first click when this dial is advanced indicates the aid has been turned on, or the aid may have a separate on-off switch with a plus (+) sign indicating when it is functioning. Finally, in some aids this switch may be combined with the input control where O indicates the aid is off and not operating.

Input Control. The input control determines what signal is being transmitted to the amplifier. The choices available for input on a specific hearing aid include: *M*, which means the microphone is picking up airborne signals; *T*, which shows the aid will interact with a telephone or other device emitting a magnetic signal; *MT*, which indicates both the microphone and magnetic inputs are functional; and ⊕ or E, which denotes that the aid may be coupled to an external audio source. Although these latter symbols are advocated by the International Electrotechnical Commission to indicate audio-input entry, some manufacturers may use other markings.

When the control is on *T*, the microphone of the aid is turned off. Instead, an induction coil, commonly referred to as a telecoil, inside the case of the hearing aid receives and transmits a magnetic signal that comes from the telephone handset, which is held in close proximity to the hearing aid. This signal continues through the circuitry of the hearing aid amplifier and receiver. When the telephone switch is in use, the only signal amplified comes from the message emitted over the telephone, and it is not the actual acoustic sound of the voice itself that enters the hearing aid, but rather a magnetic signal that exists simultaneously with it. Other sounds such as room noise and the user's own voice are not amplified, since the microphone of the aid is not functioning. Some telephones come with a receiver that does not have a usable magnetic signal; consequently, a hearing aid telecoil is not compatible with such telephones unless a separate adapter is used with the telephone (see Chapter 13).

Also of interest is the fact that in the *T* position, the hearing aid will pick up magnetic signals emanating from an *induction loop*. An induction loop is created by connecting both ends of a loop of wire to an amplifier whose input is usually a microphone. Sound from the microphone is carried through this loop as electric current, which also produces an electromagnietic field; the elec-

tromagnetic field, in turn, induces current in the telecoil of the hearing aid when in the *T* position. A neckloop is a small induction loop and may be used to couple a hearing aid with various assistive devices. A large induction loop might encircle an entire room to provide an assistive listening system (see Chapter 13). The advantage of an *MT* setting is that, with input from both the microphone and the telecoil, the user may monitor his or her own voice and respond to the voices of others while receiving the signal from the telecoil.

A direct audio input option is available on some instruments. When set for this mode of operation, the hearing aid may be connected directly to an external audio source via an auxiliary cord. In this way, it is possible for a child's personal hearing aid to receive input from assistive devices such as an Frequency Modulation (FM) receiver (see Chapter 12) or a remote microphone. An alternative input setting may exist that allows use of both the hearing aid's microphone and the external audio input source at the same time.

Gain (Volume) Control. This rotary dial on a conventional hearing aid allows the user to adjust the sound of the hearing aid from minimum to maximum amplification. Most often, it is continuously adjustable and operates much like the volume control on a radio. The dial also may be numbered or color-coded to assist the user in finding the desired setting. Some programmable hearing aids have no user-operated gain control; other models regulate this function via a remote control.

Directional-Omnidirectional Switch. On some hearing aids, the use of a directional microphone is optional. A standard omnidirectional microphone may be changed to one with directional capabilities when a selector switch is placed in a certain position.

Tone Control. With the tone control, the relative strength of the high-frequency and low-frequency sounds that are amplified may be changed. A tone control appears either as a selector switch available to the user or as a screw adjustment or programming option that is determined when the aid is dispensed. Usually, when the tone control is set at *S* or *H*, the high frequency range is emphasized by suppressing amplification of low frequencies. On *L*, the opposite occurs; the low frequency sounds are emphasized because high frequencies are suppressed. The position *N* denotes the standard or normal frequency response for that particular instrument. Tone control markings are not standardized and should be verified by consulting performance data from the manufacturer for each model of hearing aid.

Output Control. This screw adjustment or programming choice imposes a limit to the maximum amount of sound the hearing aid will transmit. It sets a ceiling—the hearing aid will not produce a more intense sound than this limiting level no matter how great the input to the microphone. This output limiting may be achieved in the aid's circuitry through either peak clipping or compression; the latter also is referred to as *automatic gain control*.

Earmolds

In body-worn, behind-the-ear, and eyeglass hearing aid arrangements, it is necessary to couple the hearing aid to the user's ear with an individually made earmold. An earmold is a piece of plastic with a channel called the "sound bore" running through the center; the earmold is attached to the hearing aid and inserted into the wearer's ear. Its purpose, of course, is to deliver the amplified sound directly from the receiver into the ear canal. In addition, modifications to the earmold may effect the transmission of sound. For example, a sound bore of constant diameter transmits low frequencies well; however, when the sound bore flares at the end like a horn, and is a certain length, it actually enhances output in the high frequencies.

There are many different types of earmolds. The National Association of Earmold Laboratories uses standard nomenclature to classify them.[20] Only a few are mentioned here. On body-worn hearing aids, the external receiver button snaps onto a solid earmold, which fills the ear; it is termed a "receiver earmold," but also often referred to as a "standard earmold." For behind-the-ear instruments, sound from the internal receiver is directed through a rigid plastic hook or elbow; then, a piece of flexible plastic tubing carries sound from this hook to the earmold, which usually is either a *shell earmold* or a *skeleton earmold*, as seen in Figure 10–6. With in-the-ear aids, a separate earmold is not needed because the casing or shell of the hearing aid itself fulfills this function.

Each earmold is custom-made. An impression is taken of the user's ear to reproduce exactly the contours of the canal and bowl-like portion of the ear flap; this is done by packing these areas with a soft impression material. After this substance has set, it is carefully removed, packaged, and

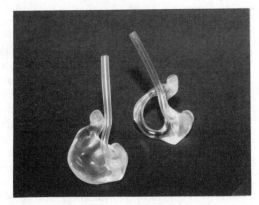

Figure 10–6. Sample styles of earmolds. Left, a shell earmold; right, a skeleton earmold.

mailed to an earmold laboratory with an order describing the type of earmold desired. The laboratory fabricates the actual earmold following these specifications. Materials from which earmolds are made include acrylic, silicone, polyvinyl chloride, and polyethylene. Depending on the material, the result may be either a hard earmold or a soft one. The more pliable earmolds often are used with children because they are less likely to cause injury as a result of any boisterous activity. An earmold must fit comfortably and securely in the ear in order to retain the hearing aid there. In addition, a snug fit ensures that amplified sound from the hearing aid receiver actually will arrive at the eardrum. A properly fitting earmold, which prevents sound from leaking out at the sides of the canal, often is of concern when powerful hearing aids are used on children with severe losses. Special materials or earmold styles may be needed to obtain a mold with a tight enough seal. Conversely, however, for some children with certain audiometric configurations, special earmolds or earmolds with certain modifications are recommended to provide a pathway for amplified sound to escape. This usually is done to alter the output of the hearing aid in some way. The special earmolds are described as *free-field* (open, nonoccluding); the modification frequently made to other earmolds is termed a "vent," which is also used for pressure equalization in the ear.

Since the outer ear grows as the child matures, it is expected that new earmolds will be needed periodically to maintain a proper fit. Children less than 4 years of age may require a new earmold as often as every 3 to 6 months; older youngsters may need to exchange their earmolds yearly until the age of 8 or 9 years.[21]

Electroacoustic Characteristics

A hearing aid is described and compared with other hearing aids according to the way it amplifies sound. Such information about a hearing aid indicates how sound coming from the receiver (output) differs from what entered the microphone (input). These measures of various input- output functions of a hearing aid are referred to as electroacoustic characteristics. The way in which these performance measurements are made and expressed is mandated in the *American National Standard Specification of Hearing Aid Characteristics.*[22] This standard was approved by both the American National Standards Institute (ANSI) and the Acoustical Society of American in 1976; it was revised in 1982 and again in 1987; it is referred to as ANSI S3.22-1987 (ASA 7-1987). The intent of such a standard is to enable measurements of hearing aid performance obtained at different facilities to be compared with one another. It is noteworthy that this standard became law in this country in 1977. This is when the Food and Drug Administration's (FDA) Rules and Regulations Regarding Hearing Aid Devices: Professional and Patient Labeling Conditions for Sale went into effect.[23] As part of this FDA document, it was specified that the performance characteristics of hearing aids be determined in accordance with the existing American national standard. Thus, this standard for hearing aid characteristics became the first to be enforceable. The FDA regulation was later updated to require adherence to the 1987 revision of ANSI S3.22.

Another significant feature of ANSI S3.22-1987 is that it stipulates tolerance limits for each characteristic measured. The reason for having a tolerance limit, or range of acceptable deviation, is to improve quality control. Because of these requirements, each hearing aid of a particular model should perform within the tolerance limits allowed by the standard when measured accurately. Some of the measurements from ANSI S3.22-1987 will be described.

Gain. Gain refers to the amount in decibels by which the hearing aid amplifies or intensifies sound. If a sound of 70 dB sound pressure level (SPL) enters the hearing aid microphone and a sound of 115 dB SPL is measured coming from the receiver, then the gain of this hearing aid, or the additional intensity supplied by the amplifying circuit, is 45 dB. The amount of gain a hearing aid offers varies with the frequency of the entering signal; that is, a hearing aid does not amplify all incoming sounds by the same amount. ANSI S3.22-1987 specifies that the gain present at 1000, 1600, and 2500 Hz, with an input of 60 dB SPL, be averaged. This average is obtained with the gain (volume) control rotated to the full-on position; the resulting gain is referred to as the *high-frequency average full- on gain.* Although it is not required in the standard, manufacturers often repeat this measure with the gain control rotated to a specific setting more nearly simulating use conditions (less than full- on); they report this value as *reference test gain.*

SSPL 90. This term is used to describe the maximum SPL output that a hearing aid is able to produce at its receiver. Previously, it has been referred to as the maximum power output. Procedures of ANSI S3.22-1987 call for the saturation sound pressure level (SSPL) of a hearing aid to be measured with the gain control full-on, and with an input signal of 90 dB SPL applied to the hearing aid microphone. The output for frequencies from 200 to 5000 Hz is recorded. Again, the values at 1000, 1600, and 2500 Hz are averaged, and the resulting number is reported as the *high-frequency-average SSPL 90* for the hearing aid. In addition, the maximum decibel output present for a single frequency is noted and reported, along with the frequency at which it occurred, as the *maximum SSPL 90.* SSPL 90 and, to a lesser extent, gain values are used in determining the relative power of a given hearing aid.

Frequency Response. The frequency response refers to descriptive information about the way in which a hearing aid amplifies various frequencies because it does not increase all frequencies equally. According to ANSI S3.22-1987, a frequency response curve is a graph that illustrates how the output of the aid changes as frequencies progress from 200 to 5000 Hz. It is measured with an input of 60 dB SPL at the microphone and the aid's gain control in reference test position. It is possible, then, to use this graph to determine the *frequency range,* or that band of frequencies from low to high for which the aid provides enough amplification to be potentially useful.

Harmonic Distortion. Distortion is present in an amplifying system when the acoustic parameters of the input sound at the microphone are not reproduced exactly in the output at the receiver. One form of such distortion is harmonic distortion. This occurs when new frequencies that are whole-number multiples of the input frequency appear. ANSI S3.22-1987 states that this should be reported in terms of *percentage of total harmonic distortion*. Total harmonic distortion is measured at 500 and 800 Hz with an input of 70 dB SPL, and at 1600 Hz with an input of 65 dB SPL. The gain control of the aid is in reference test position.

Equivalent Input Noise Level. This measurement pertains to the internal noise present in the hearing aid similar to the *on* noise found in many electrical devices. It is calculated according to a formula given in ANSI S3.22-1987.

Induction Coil (Telecoil). With the input switch on *T* and the gain control full-on, a hearing aid having a telecoil is positioned inside a magnetic field having a strength of 10 mA/m at 1000 Hz. The standard assesses telecoil performance by requiring its output be measured at 1000 Hz.

HEARING AID MAINTENANCE

A maintenance program to ensure continued maximum performance of a hearing aid should be composed of: (1) a daily visual inspection and listening check; and (2) periodic electroacoustic measurement. Through a daily monitoring program, obvious causes of hearing aid malfunction may be identified quickly and sometimes resolved. A few supplies should be assembled to simplify this inspection. The electroacoustic measurements, which require more elaborate equipment, provide information of a different type about the way the hearing aid amplifies sound.

Hearing Aid Maintenance Kit

To implement the first step of this program, it is recommended that several items be obtained and kept, ideally, both in the classroom and in the home of each hearing aid user. These articles will fit into a small utility box; having access to it facilitates the task of caring for a hearing aid. Some suppliers offer a hearing aid maintenance kit already assembled (Appendix A). The suggested contents are listed below and appear in Figure 10–7.

A. Battery Tester (Voltmeter). The battery tester is used to ascertain whether a battery supplies the necessary voltage; consequently, a meter or dial that displays the actual voltage measured is preferred. Often, the battery tester has colored areas to differentiate acceptable batteries (green) from poor ones (red).

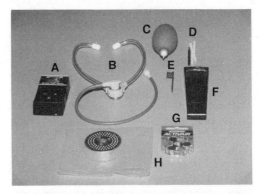

Figure 10–7. Hearing aid maintenance kit. See text for description of contents.

B. Hearing Aid Stethoscope and Adapter. Use of a hearing aid stethoscope enables one to listen only to sounds amplified by the aid because both ears of the listener are occluded. It may be used with any style of hearing aid.

C. Earmold Air Blower. This device is used to remove moisture from earmolds and tubing after they have been cleaned. It is helpful, too, in determining if there is an obstacle to the passage of sound through an earmold.

D. Wax Pick or Pipe Cleaners. These are useful for removing earwax from an earmold sound bore and vent. Pipe cleaners also may be used to dry out the sound bore after an earmold has been washed. These items should not be used with an in-the-ear aid; a wax loop is more appropriate.

E. Small, Soft Brush. This brush helps in clearing dust or lint from hearing aid switches and the opening to the microphone.

F. Small, Lighted Magnifying Glass.

G. Extra Batteries.

H. Plastic Bag and Drying Agent. The chemical silica gel will remove moisture from the air; thus, it keeps dry or dries out the contents of the bag. The hearing aid may be stored in this bag, especially during humid periods. However, zinc air batteries, once the tab is removed, should not be placed in such a bag because this would shorten rather than prolong battery life.

Visual Inspection

Battery. First on any maintenance list should be inspection of the battery. Initially, one should determine that the correct battery is used. Both the desired battery size and the nominal voltage are specified in information supplied with the aid by the manufacturer. Also, the maximum voltage available in each cell may be labeled on the battery package. Battery voltage should be checked with a battery tester. Actually, it is preferable to test battery voltage in the evening when the battery is taken out of the hearing aid. It is possible for batteries temporarily to recover voltage during the night when they are not used. If checked in the morning, misleading information could be obtained because a satisfactory voltage reading might not result in optimal performance. Decreased battery voltage is a significant factor in the unsatisfactory electroacoustic function of hearing aids. Diefendorf and Arthur[24] found battery voltage less than 1.2 V resulted in altered performance of high-gain hearing aids; battery voltage less than 1.1 V was detrimental to moderate-gain aids and mild-gain aids. These general guidelines, however, may vary according to the requirements of specific hearing aids.

One should observe whether the battery and the battery contacts in the aid yield evidence of corrosion. Corrosion on battery contacts may cause a hissing sound in the aid. If minimal corrosion is present, the white powdery substance that forms on the battery contacts may be wiped away with a soft cloth or an alcohol swab. However, care must be taken not to get alcohol on the plastic case of the aid or on the earmold. Sometimes, it may be necessary to rub battery contacts with a pointed eraser to remove all traces of corrosion. Only gentle pressure should be applied, so that any coating covering the battery contacts will not be damaged. A battery that is extensively corroded should not be used. To minimize the possibility of corrosion, the battery should be removed from the aid overnight.

Finally, one should observe if the battery is installed properly in the aid. The plus (+) side of the battery should be aligned with the plus (+) marking usually stamped or engraved in the battery compartment. Instead of this marking, some aids have battery compartments that will only accept placement of a battery in the correct position. If the battery compartment will not close, it is likely that the battery has not been inserted correctly.

Earmold.   The earmold should be examined both alone and coupled to the ear of the child. Note whether the earmold is cracked or chipped because any rough edge will cause discomfort to the wearer. It is vital that the sound bore of the earmold not be occluded with earwax. Such an accumulation in this opening may be removed with a wax pick and then the channel cleaned out with a pipe cleaner. Care must be taken not to push earwax back into the mold, where it is more difficult to remove. When the earmold is inserted into the child's ear, it should fit comfortably; a whistling sound, known as acoustic feedback, should not occur when the aid is in use.

An earmold may be separated from the external receiver of a body-worn aid simply by unsnapping it. To remove an earmold from a behind-the-ear aid, gently slip the tubing from the earhook. The tubing must not be pulled from the earmold itself because it is permanently secured there. With the earmold separated from the aid, it is possible to use the earmold air blower to demonstrate that there is, indeed, a clear passageway through the earmold (and tubing) for amplified sound. Position the bulb at one end of the mold (or tubing), squeeze it, and feel the flow of air at the other end. The earmold may be washed in warm water and mild soap *provided it is detached from the hearing aid*; dry it and use a pipe cleaner and the earmold air blower to remove moisture from the sound bore. Make sure the earmold is completely dry before joining it again to the hearing aid. Moisture will damage the hearing aid. The earmold should be cleaned periodically, but unless the child accumulates an unusual amount of earwax, it should not be necessary to wash the earmold daily. Removing the earmold from an external receiver of a body-worn aid does not present a maintenance problem. However, detaching an earmold from a behind-the-ear aid by slipping the tubing off the earhook eventually will stretch the tubing somewhat. When this connection becomes loose, the amplified sound passing through it can escape and cause acoustic feedback.

Tubing.   Any tubing that forms a loose connection, has yellowed, or is hardened and brittle needs to be replaced by an audiologist or a hearing aid specialist. Check to see that moisture has not collected inside the tubing to block the passage of sound. If moisture problems persist, consider the use of special tubing designed to absorb and exhaust moisture as it accumulates. When the aid is in place on the child, the tubing should not be twisted, thereby obstructing sound.

Receiver.   If the hearing aid is body worn and has an external receiver, look to see if it is cracked or damaged in any way. Often a washer of thin plastic film is placed around the nubbin of the receiver to ensure a tight seal when it is snapped onto the earmold. A receiver-saver also may be used; this is a strip of plastic that forms an additional connection between the receiver and the cord to prevent an accidental separation.

Cord. On a body-worn aid, determine if any sections of the cord appear to be frayed. Connections at the plug receptacles of the receiver and the hearing aid case should be firmly attached.

Settings and Controls. The input switch should be on *M* unless the telecoil (*T,TM*) or direct auditory input is being used with a classroom listening system. The tone and gain control settings should be those recommended for the child.

Hearing Aid Case. If necessary, the case itself should be cleaned with a soft cloth. A brush from the maintenance kit may be used to clean crevices and around controls.

Listening Check

It is important to listen to the hearing aid to obtain information about the function of the switches and controls and to monitor, as much as possible, the quality of sound reproduction. If parents begin this practice when their child's instrument is new, they will establish a reference for future listening checks.

Standard Listening Check. The listener may attach the hearing aid to a hearing aid stethoscope. As seen in Figure 10–8A, the external receiver of a body-worn aid may be snapped onto the stethoscope. Figure 10–8B shows an adapter in use with a behind-the-ear aid that has an internal receiver; the nozzle of a connecting tube is slipped over the aid's earhook, and the other end of the tube is snapped onto the stethoscope. Still another alternative is to place the nozzle end of the tubing extension over the canal portion of an earmold or in-the-ear aid. In this way, one may listen to the combined system of any hearing aid and earmold together or to an in-the-ear aid. This latter method, especially, offers some practical advantages in daily listening checks of behind-the-ear aids by teachers and parents. Because the nozzle may be fastened directly over the end of the earmold, it does not necessitate routinely separating the tubing from the earhook; thus, fewer problems would be likely to develop at this point. In a school program, where several aids are to be checked, the outside of each earmold should be sanitized by wiping it with Cetylcide, or a similar product, before it is inserted into the end of the adapter. Cetylcide is an antibacterial instant earmold cleaner available from a supplier of hearing aid products. It will not harm plastic as alcohol will.

The input switch of the aid should be set on *M*, the aid should be off, and the gain control should be turned down. Because it is difficult to

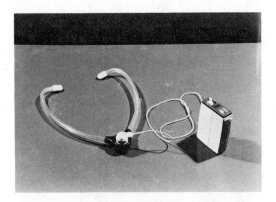

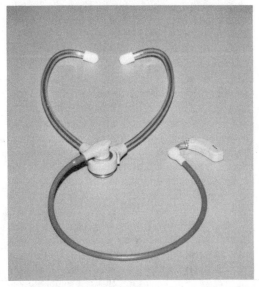

Figure 10–8. A. Attachment of a hearing aid stethoscope directly to the external receiver of a hearing aid. B. Attachment of a hearing aid stethoscope adapter to a behind-the-ear hearing aid.

talk and listen simultaneously, one may want to listen to speech on a tape recorder or radio during this check. While the tester is listening, the aid should be turned on and the gain control rotated slowly back and forth to note if there is a smooth change in intensity, if there is a constant signal, and if the control operates quietly. The various switches should be moved to determine if they are functional. The cord, if the aid has one, should be rolled gently between the fingers in several places; a "break" in the incoming sound would identify a defective cord that should be replaced. Finally, the case should be rotated slightly to ascertain whether this causes interruption of the sound.

Such a listening check will identify faulty controls. Noting a decrease in the quality of sound reproduction is more difficult, especially for an examiner with an untrained ear. Deterioration in the quality of sound may occur gradually over a period of time, and not be readily apparent on a day-to-day listening basis. Another consideration is the intensity of the speech input. When the gain control is set in the position used by the child, the hearing aid normally responds to conversational speech input from about 3 feet away and to the child's own voice at a distance of about 8 inches. When the person making the listening check uses his or her own voice, as so often happens, input to the aid reflects the intensity of the user's own voice, but does not assess how the aid responds to speech at other input levels. Finally, it must be recognized that those with normal hearing may find it uncomfortable to listen to the high output levels of the more powerful hearing aids at gain control settings used by the child. This discomfort precludes careful listening at such a setting. Although distortion of sound may be present for the child, it may not be detected at the lower gain control setting preferred by the adult performing the listening check.

Five-Sound Test.   Ling[25] suggests an approach that uses sounds representing the various octave bands of speech to monitor the frequency response of a hearing aid.. He advocates listening to five speech sounds—*oo, ah, ee, sh,* and *s*—as they are transmitted by the aid. If parents or caregivers do this daily, they will become familiar with how these sounds are reproduced by the child's hearing aid and be able to identify a change with confidence. In the classroom, this test may be given while the child wears the aid to observe any deviation from his or her usual response. The teacher or aide presents the five sounds, one at a time, without visual clues. The child claps after hearing each sound, and, if capable, repeats the sound.

Bone Conduction Hearing Aids.   There is not a satisfactory way to perform an adequate listening check on a bone conduction hearing aid. When the instrument is in actual use, the tension with which the oscillator is held against the head is very important. If the headband does not have sufficient tensile strength, it eventually might be stretched by being placed repeatedly on an adult's head for a listening check. Also, the listener would have to occlude both ears with earplugs or by pressing them shut to hear only through the bone conduction oscillator. It is possible for an audiologist or hearing aid specialist to check the integrity of the aid's controls and switches after substituting an appropriate air conduction receiver. Such persons should provide frequent routine maintenance for these aids. Daily checks

may include testing the battery voltage and inspecting the aid visually.

Acoustic Feedback

"Acoustic feedback" is the term for the high-pitched whistling sound so annoying to those in the company of hearing aid users. Many times the hearing aid user does not hear this sound because of hearing loss. Acoustic feedback occurs whenever there is a clear pathway between the output from a hearing aid receiver and the microphone of the same hearing aid. Ordinarily, this whistling interaction is avoided because the output of the receiver is directed through the earmold into the ear canal and away from the hearing aid microphone. However, if the earmold does not fit snugly in the ear canal, the amplified sound waves may escape around the sides of the mold and be reproduced as feedback when they reach the aid's microphone. This happens most often with a powerful ear-level instrument. The amplified sound also might leak through a crack or pinhole in the tubing or earhook of a behind-the-ear aid or through the sides of tubing if it is too thin.

Preventing acoustic feedback, then, becomes a matter of determining where the sound leakage is occurring by the process of elimination. Once the trouble spot is identified, the cause may be corrected. The following procedures show how to check for the source of feedback in a behind-the-ear aid:

1. Remove the hearing aid, with the earmold attached, from the child.
2. Place your thumb over the earmold sound bore opening, turn the aid on, and rotate the gain control to its maximum. If whistling is heard, quickly turn the aid down and detach the earmold by slipping the tubing from the end of the earhook.
3. Place your thumb over the end of the earhook. Increase the gain control to maximum for only a short time. If the feedback is gone, it must have been present due to damage to the earmold or tubing. If the whistling continues, it must be caused by a leak in the earhook or a problem internal to the aid. Consult an audiologist or hearing aid specialist for replacement of the earhook or repair of the aid.

It may be that feedback occurs when the hearing aid is on the child, but not during this check.

In such cases there are two considerations: (1) this may be an indication of a middle ear problem, and immittance measurements should be obtained to investigate this; or (2) a new earmold may be needed. The latter cause is frequent with growing children. Once the other causes of feedback have been eliminated, a new earmold should be obtained.

Caring for a Hearing Aid

Batteries. Batteries should be stored in a dry location at room temperature in their original protective package; do not place batteries in the refrigerator.[26] Also, do not put zinc air batteries with their tabs removed in a container with a drying agent, as this will shorten battery life. Keep spare batteries in their original "dial" package; this will prevent them from touching metal as they might if carried loosely in a pocket with change and keys, or in a purse. Contact with metal can cause batteries to discharge or short circuit. Wipe the contact surfaces of the battery (top and bottom) before inserting the battery into the aid; try to grasp the battery on the sides only during insertion. A magnetic battery retriever tool is available to assist with this task. Remove the battery from the hearing aid at night; this will prolong its life and decrease the possibility of corrosion. Extra batteries should be kept at school so they may be replaced there.

BATTERY DISPOSAL. Keep used batteries away from children. Zinc air batteries may be disposed of in a routine manner with household waste; mercury and silver oxide batteries may be required by state or local environmental regulations to be collected.[26] Mercury batteries are reclaimed because mercury is a pollutant to the environment. Also, mercury and other batteries (including zinc air) may be recycled to reduce them to their basic elements for use in industry. Some collection programs for used hearing aid batteries exist; please refer to the Appendix.

BATTERY INGESTION. Button batteries, which power ear-level hearing aids as well as other devices, such as calculators and watches, present a potential health hazard because they may be swallowed easily.[27-29] Their popularity and availability have resulted in increasing instances of battery ingestion, especially among children who are attracted to loose or discarded batteries within their reach, or who remove batteries from hearing aids and other products. In 1983, Litovitz[28] reviewed 56 cases of battery ingestion; age could

be determined for 50 cases and, of these ingestions, 78% occurred in children less than 5 years of age. This incidence is typical, in general, of poisonings. Hearing aids were the most common intended use of these batteries. In the majority of cases reviewed, Litovitz found that ingested batteries the size of those used in ear-level hearing aids passed spontaneously through the gastrointestinal system without complications. However, serious injuries may result from caustic chemicals, toxicity, and constant pressure if the battery becomes lodged in the esophagus for any length of time; the small size of ear-level hearing aid batteries makes this unlikely in children 18 months and older. Zinc air batteries pose less of a toxic threat than other batteries, although the possibility of electrolyte leakage does exist. Consequently, it is of paramount importance that parents, caregivers, and teachers be counseled regarding the inherent dangers of button batteries to children. These small batteries may also cause injury if placed in the nose or ears.

Prevention of battery ingestion and other misuses must be stressed at all times. Some hearing aid manufacturers offer the option of a tamper-resistant closure on the battery compartment of a hearing aid; battery manufacturers are printing warning statements on product packages. Clinicians and educators should give the following precautions in verbal and written form to all hearing aid users and those working with children who are hearing aid users:

1. Keep extra batteries and hearing aids not in use out of children's reach.
2. Dispose of batteries properly away from children.
3. Do not dispose of batteries in incinerators or fires because they can rupture and explode.
4. Dispose of any batteries that show signs of leakage.
5. Never change batteries in front of children.
6. Never put batteries in the mouth for any reason, as they are slippery and easy to swallow accidentally. A child may mimic you.
7. Whenever possible, secure the battery drawer from casual access by children (may use tape, a tamper-resistant compartment, or a hearing aid retainer).
8. Always check medications; batteries have been mistaken for tablets.
9. *If a battery is swallowed:*
   a. Find another battery exactly like the one swallowed, or the package from which the battery came, to obtain the identification number.

b. Promptly seek medical advice from a physician.

c. For battery contents and recommended treatment protocol, telephone, collect, the National Button Battery Ingestion Hotline. The number is (202) 625-3333 (voice) or (202) 362-8563 (TT/TDD). This hotline is operated by the National Capital Poison Center at Georgetown University Hospital in Washington, DC.

Cords. Cords can be obtained in several lengths. One of an appropriate size should be used with a child so that it will not have to be wrapped or twisted around the aid to be kept out of the way. A spare cord should be available so that immediate replacement will be possible.

Hearing Aid. Keep the hearing aid away from excessive heat and humidity. For body-worn aids with top-mounted microphones, food guards may be purchased; a food guard is a cover designed to protect the microphone opening from food spills. During especially humid times of the year, place a hearing aid (but not a zinc air battery) overnight in a plastic lock-top bag with a drying agent (silica gel). Avoid dropping the hearing aid. Keep the aid turned off when it is not in use, and never open the case of the hearing aid in an attempt to repair it yourself.

Consult an audiologist or hearing aid specialist promptly if you have any questions or concerns about the function of the hearing aid.

Hearing Aid Retainers. It is often difficult to secure a behind-the-ear aid on a small child, and some dispensers have advocated the use of toupee tape in such situations. However, a retainer for behind-the-ear hearing aids has been developed. It consists of a plastic loop that encircles the external ear flap; this loop contains two plastic clips that fit tightly around the aid. These clips have the possible added advantage of preventing tampering with the aid's gain control and battery compartment, depending on their positions. Other styles of retainers are available for the external air conduction receivers of body-worn aids and auditory trainers, for bone conduction receivers, and for holding aids to the heads of difficult-to-fit children who have absent or deformed ears or misshapened heads. For more information, consult the Appendix under suppliers of accessory items.

Moisture Protection. Nonallergenic latex covers are available for all sizes of behind-the-ear hearing aids to protect them from damage caused by moisture, perspiration, chemicals, and dirt. The covers are applied with a special tool and intended to last until a new battery is needed. They are open at the top to allow sound to enter the hearing aid microphone and air to reach a zinc air battery cell. Manipulation of controls (gain adjustment, *T* switch) through this covering may be difficult for young children and its use would prohibit coupling an FM system via direct auditory input. However, this option may be helpful during some recreational activities. For additional information, consult the Appendix.

Electroacoustic Analysis

An effective hearing aid maintenance program must include monitoring the electroacoustic performance of a hearing aid. While a visual inspection and listening check will contribute to an aid's optimal operation, with the possible exception of the Five-Sound Test, they will not reveal problems in electroacoustic performance unless the aid is grossly malfunctioning.[9,30,31] Electroacoustic measurements may be made with a standard or portable hearing aid analyzer.

Hearing Aid Analyzer. A commercially available hearing aid test system is pictured in Figure 10-9. A test system has the following components.

TEST CHAMBER. Measurements must be performed with the aid in a sound-free environment. This is accomplished by placing the aid in an insulated chamber. Spaces around the sides and the lid of the chamber are filled with sound-absorbent material to minimize standing and reflected sound waves and to reduce the effects of room noise in the test environment. A test point is indicated in the chamber where the hearing aid microphone should be placed.

LOUDSPEAKER. A loudspeaker is situated in the test chamber oriented toward the test point. A sweep of pure tones from 200 to 5000 Hz at a given intensity is directed from the loudspeaker to the microphone of the hearing aid to obtain measures according to ANSI S3.22-1987. A broadband composite signal may also be included in the analyzer to have a stimulus available that reflects the intensity and spectral shape of the long-term value for speech.

REGULATORY SYSTEM. Some system is used to ensure that input from the loudspeaker does not vary from the desired intensity as it enters the hearing aid microphone. A regulating microphone may be positioned inside the chamber at the test point only one-quarter inch from the microphone of the hearing aid. It cooperates with

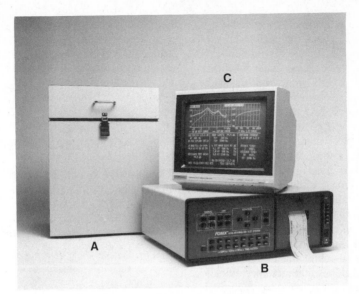

Figure 10–9. Hearing aid analyzer. A. Test chamber. B. Electronics module. C. Monitor. (Courtesy of Frye Electronics.)

a measuring amplifier to regulate the output of the loudspeaker to keep the input to the aid at a constant level across frequencies. Another way in which this uniformity may be achieved is by the use of a predetermined and stored correction curve that compensates for the effects of the test chamber. In this method, one microphone serves both regulatory and measuring functions; a dummy microphone with identical physical dimensions changes places with the real microphone.

2 cc Coupler. Output from the receiver of the hearing aid is sent into a 2 cc coupler. The hearing aid is connected to the 2 cc coupler, which is a stainless steel cylinder containing a cavity with a volume of 2 cc. This size was selected as the standard because it was thought to approximate the space between the tip of an earmold and the eardrum in an adult ear.

Measuring Microphone. A microphone is inserted into the opposite end of the 2 cc coupler to pick- up the amplified signal from the hearing aid receiver. The diaphragm of this microphone forms the bottom boundary of the 2 cc space. Thus, sound leaves the hearing aid receiver, passes through the 2 cc hard-walled cavity, and activates this measuring microphone.

Induction Loop. A hearing aid analyzer will either have an induction loop built-in or provided as an accessory to generate the 10 mA/m magnetic field necessary to measure performance of a hearing aid's telecoil.

Electronics Module. The signal from the measuring microphone is fed into components that analyze this output from the hearing aid. In addition, some type of filter is used so that harmonic distortion measurements may be made—the signal entering the hearing aid must be filtered from the output, so that only sound energy present in its harmonic frequencies may be measured. Data resulting from these various measurements appear visually in a graphic display, which may be recorded permanently in printed form.

Hearing Aid Measurement. Educational programs should take advantage of the availability and ease of operation of hearing aid analyzers. Measurement procedures with them were developed explicitly for the purpose of maintaining quality control and product uniformity. It is in just this way that analyzers may help to meet the needs of rehabilitative programs. Routine electroacoustic monitoring should be used to verify that the amplification characteristics of hearing aids are consistent over time and in agreement with those that the aids had when they originally were selected for the child.

How often a child's aid should be evaluated depends realistically upon the accessibility of the hearing aid analyzer and the number of children it must serve. A recommendation resulting from investigations of hearing aids worn by school children is that aids receive at least an annual electroacoustic evaluation.[4,7] Certainly, any program would be strengthened if it were possible to include such monitoring as often as two to three times per year.[9] Moreover, the need for this monitoring varies with the age of the child. Small children lead more active lives; consequently, it may be beneficial to check the performance of younger children's aids frequently. In addition, such measurements should be made whenever there is a change in a child's aided abilities without apparent reason, or whenever a problem in the aid's electroacoustic performance is suspected on the basis of the daily listening check.

The manufacturer's printed performance specifications for the various instruments worn by children in the school must be on file. Only then may measurements made with the test set be used to determine if an aid is functioning as originally designed. As additional information, it would be ideal to include in each child's records an electroacoustic analysis obtained with the aid adjusted to the use settings recommended when the aid was fit. The aid could be monitored periodically with this information as a reference. The difficulty lies in coordinating this exchange of information between those who fit and dispense the aid and those who monitor its functioning.

Generally, electroacoustic monitoring should consist of determining the major characteristics previously described in this chapter—gain, SSPL, frequency response, harmonic distortion, and telecoil function. A measurement of the internal noise level also may be included. Instruments whose performance deviates significantly from the reference data would be identified as malfunctioning. Limits of acceptable variation, however, must be somewhat arbitrary until the relationship these electroacoustic characteristics have to speech intelligibility and hearing impairment in children is more clearly defined.

Testing Repaired Hearing Aids. Many problems detected with the electroacoustic analysis of children's hearing aids are repairable. Therefore, a hearing aid test set is an asset to a maintenance program in yet another way. Measurements may be made when aids are returned from repair to ascertain if, indeed, they received adequate service before the aids are used.[32]

Testing Loaner Hearing Aids. A hearing aid test set may be used with loaner hearing aids. Because a child's personal hearing aids may be an integral component of the amplification arrangement used in the classroom, the child needs instruments in good working order. Accordingly, some schools supply loaner aids to students whose personal aids are being repaired. With a hearing aid test set, the performance characteristics of a loaner aid may be verified before the aid is issued to the child. If loaner aids do not perform adequately, there is little sense in using

them; their condition will only cause children to reject amplification. Without a doubt, loaner instruments will be needed; resources, however, should be found to ensure that they are kept ready and in good condition.

IMPLEMENTATION OF A HEARING AID MAINTENANCE PROGRAM

Regulations for the Education of All Handicapped Children Act (PL 94-142), which were written in 1977 and reauthorized in 1990 as the Individuals with Disabilities Education Act (PL 101-476), state in Section 121(a)303:

> *Proper Functioning of Hearing Aids:* Each public agency shall insure that the hearing aids worn by deaf and hard of hearing children in school are functioning properly.[33]

Consequently, schools should be engaged in hearing aid maintenance on a routine basis. In addition, members of the Educational Audiology Association have endorsed a policy that supports daily inspections of student amplification.[34] However, Reichman and Healey[35] surveyed residential schools and day schools for children with impaired hearing and reported that 54% did not have daily hearing aid monitoring. Infrequent monitoring in public school programs, also, has been documented by Shepard et al[36] and by Elfenbein et al.[10] Such findings are perplexing when the results of daily hearing aid checks have been most encouraging. Kemker et al[37] showed daily inspections by teachers and aides were preferable to weekly monitoring; battery problems, especially, were greatly reduced. Bendet[38] found a large reduction in the number of defective aids once daily monitoring was implemented by teachers trained in this skill; Potts and Greenwood,[9] also, reduced the incidence of malfunctioning instruments through training teachers to participate.

Schools must expand hearing aid maintenance programs to include student participation.[10,19,39,40] The tools and techniques of simple hearing aid monitoring and troubleshooting may be introduced through demonstration sessions that include the preschool child; then, when school-age, the child may assume responsibility for hearing aid performance, which increases as the child matures. In fact, age-appropriate goals for hearing aid maintenance should become part of an individualized educational plan (IEP) for the child with hearing impairment.[10,41] A training program for students that combines hands-on instruction, criterion-referenced IEP goals, troubleshooting skills, and knowledge of problem-solving resources and personnel at school is advocated by Elfenbein et al.[10]

Finally, parental involvement in hearing aid maintenance should not be overlooked. Diefendorf and Arthur[24] provided parents with more information about hearing loss and amplification along with training in maintenance procedures; as a result, the occurrence of hearing aid malfunctions declined from 30 to 5%.

Involvement of audiologists in educational settings is mandatory; their role in implementing hearing aid maintenance programs, which include in-service training for teachers and instruction for students and parents, emphasizes this fact. In 1993, the American Speech-Language-Hearing Association (ASHA) approved new *Guidelines for Audiology Services in Schools.*[42] These guidelines make recommendations for appropriate cost-effective audiology services in the schools, whether school-based or contracted, and recognize the expanding role of audiologists. Ensuring the proper functioning of hearing aids is one segment of comprehensive services for children with hearing impairments.

There can be no doubt that the need to establish a viable hearing aid maintenance program for children is of the utmost importance. Progress in this area must occur. Teachers, parents, and the children themselves, when they are old enough, must share this responsibility. The immediate result will be more consistent, functional amplification for the child; the additional benefits may be even more far-reaching as children actually experience this improved auditory input in their rehabilitative programs.

APPENDIX

Sources for Materials Helpful in a Hearing Aid Maintenance Program for Children

Suppliers of accessory items

A kit containing the items necessary for hearing aid maintenance may be obtained from: (1) A.G. Bell Association for the Deaf, 3417 Volta Place, N.W., Washington, DC 20007-2778, telephone (202) 337-8767; or (2) HARC Mercantile, P.O. Box 3055, 3130 Portage Road, Kalamazoo, MI

49003-3055, telephone (616) 381-0177. Individual items may be ordered from Hal-Hen Co., 35–53 24th St., Long Island City, NY 11106, telephone, 800-242-5436.

Hearing aid retainers are available from Huggie Aids, LDT, 837 NW 10th St, Oklahoma City, OK 73106, telephone: (405) 232-7848.

Super Seals moisture protectors are manufactured by Just Bekuz Products Co., Castle Rock, CO, telephone (303) 688-5153 for the name of a local distributor.

Recycling programs for batteries

Dispensing audiologists and hearing aid specialists may serve as collection points for used hearing aid batteries, which they contribute to various recycling programs. Also call the Mercury Refining Company, 26 Railroad Avenue, Albany, NY 12205, for information: 1-800- 833-3505.

Audiovisual programs

Hearing Aids: A Daily Check produced by Design Media, San Francisco, CA, 1980. Available as a VHS videocassette from Design Media, 2235 Harrison St., San Francisco, CA 94110, FAX (415) 641-5245. Shows parts of a hearing aid and steps of a daily check. The sounds of common hearing aid malfunctions are duplicated and practical solutions are given.

REFERENCES

1. Gaeth JH, Lounsbury E: Hearing aids and children in elementary schools. *J Speech Hear Dis*, 31 (1966), 283–289.
2. Zink GD: Hearing aids children wear: A longitudinal study of performance. *Volta Rev*, 74 (1972), 41–51.
3. Schell YS: Electro-acoustic evaluation of hearing aids worn by public school children. *Aud Hear Educ*, 2 (1976) 7, 9, 12, 15.
4. Bess FH: Condition of hearing aids worn by children in a public school setting, in Withrow FB, ed: *The Condition of Hearing Aids Worn by Children in a Public School Program*, Report No. (OE)77- 05002. US Dept. of Health, Education and Welfare, Public Health Service, 1977, chap. 2.
5. Coleman RE: *Stability of Children's Hearing Aids in an Acoustic Preschool.* Final Report, Project No. 522466, Grant No. OEG-4-71-0060, US Dept. of Health, Education and Welfare, Office of Education, 1972.
6. Northern JL, McChord W, Fisher, E, et al: *Hearing Services in Residential Schools for the Deaf. Maico Audiological Library Series*, 11 (1972), Report 4.

7. Porter TA: Hearing aids in a residential school. *Am Ann Deaf*, 118 (1973) 31–33.

8. Robinson DO, Sterling GR: Hearing aids and children in school: A follow-up study. *Volta Rev*, 82 (1980), 229–235.

9. Potts PL, Greenwood J: Hearing aid monitoring: Are looking and listening enough? *Lang, Speech, Hear Serv Sch*, 14 (1983), 157–163.

10. Elfenbein JL, Bentler RA, Davis JM, et al: Status of school children's hearing aids relative to monitoring practices. *Ear Hear*, 9 (1988), 212–217.

11. Lass NJ, Tecca JE, Woodford CM: Teachers' knowledge of. exposure to, and attitudes toward hearing aids and hearing aid wearers. *Lang Speech Hear Serv Sch*, 18 (1987), 86–95.

12. Martin FN, Bernstein ME, Daly JA, Cody JP: Classroom teachers' knowledge of hearing disorders and attitudes about mainstreaming hard-of-hearing children. *Lang Speech Hear Serv Sch*, 19 (1988), 83–95.

13. Johnson CE, Stein RL, Lass NJ: Public school nurses' preparedness for a hearing aid monitoring program. *Lang Speech Hear Serv Sch*, 23 (1992), 141–144.

14. Woodford CM: Speech-language pathologists' knowledge and skills regarding hearing aids. Lang Speech Hear Serv Sch, 18 (1987), 312–322.

15. Lass NJ, Woodford CM, Pannbacker MD, Carlin MF, Saniga RD, Schmitt JF, Everly-Myers DS: Speech-language pathologists' knowledge of, exposure to, and attitudes toward hearing aids and hearing aid wearers. *Lang Speech Hear Serv Sch*, 20 (1989), 115–132.

16. Blair JC, Wright K, Pollard G: Parental knowledge and understanding of hearing loss and hearing aids. *Volta Rev*, 83 (1981), 375–382.

17. Fitch JL: Orientation to hearing loss for educational personnel. *Lang Speech Hear Serv Sch*, 13 (1982), 252–259.

18. Ross M: A future challenge: Educating the educators and public about hearing loss. *Semin Hear*, 12 (1991), 402–413.

19. Matkin ND: Wearable amplification: A litany of persisting problems, in Jerger J, ed: *Pediatric Audiology: Current Trends*. (San Diego, CA: College-Hill Press, 1984), 125–145.

20. Staab WJ: *Hearing Aid Handbook* (Phoenix, AZ: WJ Staab, 1978), chap. 4.

21. Northern JL, Downs MP: *Hearing in Children*, ed 4 (Baltimore: Williams & Wilkins, 1991), chap. 2.

22. *American National Standard Specification of Hearing Aid Characteristics*. ANSI S3.22-1987 (ASA 70-1987) (Revision of ANSI S3.22-1982) (New York: Acoustical Society of America, 1987).

23. Rules and Regulations Regarding Hearing Aid Devices: Professional and Patient Labeling and Conditions for Sale, Part IV. Food and Drug Administration, *Fed Reg* 42 (February 15, 1977), 9294–9296.

24. Diefendorf AO, Arthur DA: Monitoring children's hearing aids: Re-examining the problem. *Volta Rev*, 89 (1987), 17–26.

25. Ling D: *Foundations of Spoken Language for Hearing-Impaired Children*. (Washington DC: AG Bell Association, 1989), chap. 3.

26. Duracell USA: An operator's guide to battery care. *Hear Instrum*, 44 (1993), 50.

27. Bebout JM: Hearing aid battery ingestion: Incidence, treatment, and prevention. *Hear J*, 37 (1984), 12–16.

28. Litovitz TI: Button battery ingestions. *JAMA*, 249 (1983), 2495–2500.

29. Rumack BH, Rumack CM: Disk battery ingestion. *JAMA*, 249 (1983), 2509–2511.

30. Busenbark L, Jenison V: Assessing hearing aid function by listening check. *Volta Rev*, 88 (1986), 263–268.

31. Niswander PS: Listening checks on hearing instruments. *Hear Instrum*, 40 (1989) 38, 40, 55.

32. Marston LE: Performance of reconditioned hearing aids. *J Acad Rehabil Audiol*, 18 (1985), 123–127.

33. Education of All Handicapped Children, PL 94-142 Regulations: Implementation of Part B. Office of Education, Dept. of Health, Education and Welfare. *Fed Reg*, 42 (August 23, 1977), 42474–42514.

34. English K: Best practices in educational audiology. *Lang Speech Hear Serv Sch*, 22 (1991), 283–286.

35. Reichman J, Healey WC: Amplification monitoring and maintenance in the schools. *ASHA*, 31 (1989), 43–45.

36. Shepard NT, Davis JM, Gorga MP, Stelmachowicz PG: Characteristics of hearing impaired children in the public schools: Part I—Demographic data. *J Speech Hear Disord*, 46 (1981), 123–129.

37. Kemker FJ, McConnell F, Logan SA, et al: A field study of children's hearing aids in a school environment. *Lang Speech Hear Serv Sch*, 10 (1979), 47–53.

38. Bendet RM: A public school hearing aid maintenance program. *Volta Rev*, 82 (1980), 149–155.

39. Maxon AB, Smaldino J: Hearing aid management for children. *Semin Hear*, 12 (1991), 365–379.

40. Lipscomb M, Von Almen P, Blair JC: Students as active participants in hearing aid maintenance. *Lang Speech Hear Serv Sch*, 23 (1992), 208–213.

41. Allard JB, Golden DC: Educational audiology: A comparison of service delivery systems utilized by Missouri schools. *Lang Speech Hear Serv Sch*, 22 (1991), 5–11.

42. American Speech-Language-Hearing Association: Guidelines for audiology services in the schools. *Asha*, 35 (suppl. 10; 1993), 24–32.

CLASSROOM ACOUSTICS

11

Carl C. Crandell and Joseph J. Smaldino

Sweet is every sound,
Sweeter thy voice, but every sound is sweet.

—Alfred Lord Tennyson, 1809–1892

The accurate perception of speech is essential for academic achievement in the classroom. A number of acoustic, linguistic, or cognitive variables, however, may deleteriously affect perceptual ability in an educational environment. Acoustic variables include the reverberation time of the classroom, the power of the teacher's voice relative to the level of the ambient noise in the room, and the distance from the teacher to the student. Linguistic or cognitive factors consist of the articulatory abilities and dialect of the speaker or listener, knowledge of language patterns, context of the message, memory processes, number of syllables in a word, ability to listen and attend, sex of the speaker, and the word familiarity and vocabulary size of the listener.[1-4] This chapter will examine the *acoustic* variables that can influence speech perception in classroom environments.

REVERBERATION

One of the most important variables that define the acoustic climate of a classroom is the reverberant characteristics of that enclosure.[5,6] Reverberation refers to the prolongation, or persistence, of sound waves within a room as they are reflected off the hard surfaces in the classroom. Operationally, reverberation time (RT) refers to the amount of time it takes for a sound, at a specific frequency, to decay 60 dB (or one millionth of its original intensity) following termination of the signal.[5-9] For example, if a 100 dB sound pressure level (SPL) signal at 1000 Hz took 1 second to decrease to 40 dB SPL, the reverberation time of that enclosure at 1000 Hz would be 1 second. Reverberation time can be expressed via the following formula:[10]

$$RT = 0.05 \text{ V/a} \qquad (1)$$

where V is the volume of the room, a is the total sound absorption in the enclosure, and 0.05

is a constant. Room reverberation increases as a function of the volume of the classroom and is inversely related to the amount of sound absorption in an environment. Consequently, larger classrooms tend to exhibit higher reverberation times than classrooms having smaller dimensions. Interestingly, classrooms with irregular shapes, such as oblong, often exhibit higher reverberation times than classrooms with more traditional quadrilateral dimensions.

Classrooms with bare cement walls, floors, and ceilings tend to exhibit higher reverberation times than classrooms that contain absorptive surfaces, such as carpeting, draperies, and acoustic ceiling tile. A useful index in determining the reverberant characteristics of a classroom is the *absorption coefficient*. Absorption coefficient refers to the ratio of unreflected energy to incident energy present in a room.[11,12] A surface with an absorption coefficient of 1.00 would technically absorb 100% of all refections, whereas a surface structure with an absorption coefficient of 0.00 would reflect all of the incident sound. Absorption coefficients, which are typically indicated from 125 to 4000 Hz, are frequency dependent. Most surface materials in a classroom do not absorb low-frequency sounds as effectively as higher frequencies. Due to these absorption characteristics, classroom reverberation is often shorter at higher frequencies than in lower frequency regions.

Measurement of Reverberation

Reverberation time in a classroom is measured by presenting a high intensity stimulus, such as 1/3 octave bands of noise, into an unoccupied enclosure and measuring the amount of time required for that signal to decay 60 dB. Instruments to measure reverberation time vary from inexpensive, compact, battery units that will allow the audiologist to do rudimentary measures of reverberation to highly technological, computer-based devices that can measure and record numerous aspects of the acoustic decay properties of an environment. Reverberation time can also be approximated using formula (1). Since the primary energy of speech is between 500 and 2000 Hz, reverberation time is often reported as the mean decay time of 500, 1000, and 2000 Hz. Unfortunately, such a measurement paradigm may not adequately describe the reverberant characteristics of a classroom because high reverberation times may exist at additional frequencies. Thus, it is recommended that reverberation time be measured at discrete frequencies from 125 to 4000 Hz whenever possible. Such information could significantly aid the audiologist or acoustic engineer in determining the appropriate degree and type of absorptive materials needed for that environment. The reader is directed to additional sources for further details concerning the measurement of reverberation.[5-9,12]

Effects of Reverberation on Speech Perception

Reverberation compromises speech perception through the masking of direct sound energy by reflected energy.[5,9,12-15] In a reverberant classroom, the reflected signals reaching the child are temporally delayed and overlap with the direct signal, resulting in masking of speech. Figure 11-1 demonstrates the effects of reverberation on speech perception. This spectrogram shows that reverberation typically causes a prolongation of the spectral energy of the vowel phonemes, which tend to mask consonant information (particularly word final consonants). These effects of reverberation are to be expected because vowels are more intense in sound energy than consonants. In highly reverberant environments, words may actually overlap with one another, thus causing reverberant sound energy to replace, or fill in, pauses between words.

In general, speech perception scores decline with increasing reverberation time.[16-21] For example, Moncur and Dirks[20] examined the monosyllabic word recognition ability of adult listeners in four levels of reverberation (RT = 0.0, 0.9, 1.6, and 2.3 seconds). Results from this investigation are presented in Figure 11-2. As can be seen, word recognition scores gradually declined as the reverberation time of the environment increased. Note also that binaural recognition scores were far superior to monaural perceptual abilities in the reverberant listening conditions. This finding has important implications for listeners with unilateral hearing loss. Gelfand and Silman[18] examined consonant perception in a reverberant (RT = 0.8 seconds) and nonreverberant (RT = 0.0

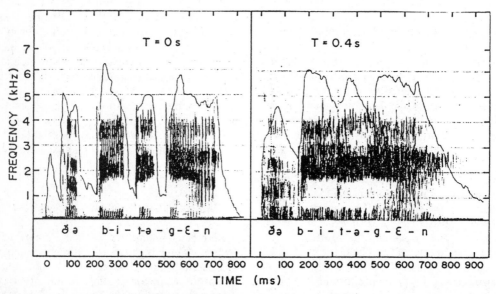

Figure 11-1. A spectrograph of the phrase "The Beet Again" in a nonreverberant (RT = 0.0 seconds) and reverberant (RT = 0.4 seconds). Note that reverberation typically cases a prolongation of the spectral energy of the vowel phonemes, which tend to mask consonant information (particularly word final consonants). (Reprinted with permission from Nabelek and Nabelek.[12])

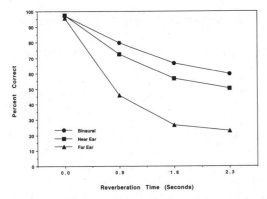

Figure 11–2. Monosyllabic word recognition ability of adult listeners across four levels of reverberation time (RT = 0.0, 0.9, 1.6, and 2.3 seconds) in binaural, near field, and far field listening conditions. Data adapted from Moncur and Dirks.[20]

seconds) listening environment. In the reverberant listening condition, errors for initial and final consonants increased by 5 and 9%, respectively.

Numerous investigators have shown that the speech perception of listeners with sensorineural hearing loss (SNHL) experience more deleterious effects in reverberation than individuals with normal hearing.[13,14,17,22–24] An illustration of this phenomenon is shown in Table 11–1. These data, taken from Finitzo-Hieber and Tillman,[17] represent monosyllabic word recognition at various reverberation times. Subjects included 12 children (ages 8 to 12 years) with normal hearing and 12 children with SNHL. Note that the children with hearing impairment obtained poorer recognition scores at each listening condition. Moreover, differences in perception scores between the two groups increased as the listening environment became more adverse. For example, in a nonreverberant listening condition (RT = 0.0 seconds), the performance difference between the groups was approximately 12%. In a highly reverberant condition (RT = 1.2 seconds), differences in speech perception increased to 32%.

Table 11–1 Mean speech-recognition scores, in percent correct, if children with normal hearing and hearing impairment for monosyllabic words across various reverberation times.

Reverberation Time (seconds)	Groups		
	Normal	Hearing Impaired	Hearing Impaired (Aided)
0.0	94.5	87.5	83.0
0.4	82.8	69.0	74.0
1.2	76.5	61.8	45.0

*Data from Finitzo-Hieber and Tillman.[17]

Data from additional studies have indicated that several populations of children with normal hearing sensitivity experience greater difficulties understanding reverberated speech than adult listeners.[12,25–39] These listeners include children with fluctuating conductive hearing loss, learning disabilities, articulation disorders, central auditory processing deficits, language disorders, minimal degrees of SNHL (pure-tone sensitivity from 15 to 25 dB HL), and unilateral hearing loss. Children for whom English is a second language are also included in this group. Nabelek and Donahue,[38] for example, reported that although native and non-native English-speaking adult listeners (Chinese, Japanese, and Spanish) obtained essentially identical perception scores in a nonreverberant (RT = 0.0 seconds) environment (100% for native English-speaking listeners; 99% for non-native English-speaking listeners), significant differences were noted between the groups (97% for native English-speaking listeners; 88% for non- native English-speaking listeners) when listening to reverberant speech (RT = 0.8 seconds). Boney and Bess[27] demonstrated that children with minimal degrees of SNHL (pure-tone thresholds from 15 to 30 dB HL from 500 to 2000 Hz) experience greater difficulty understanding speech degraded by reverberation than children with normal hearing sensitivity. Specifically, speech perception scores were obtained in nonreverberant (RT = 0.0 seconds) and reverberant environments (RT = 0.8 seconds). Results from this investigation (see Figure 11–3) indicated that the children with minimal hearing loss performed poorer than the control group, particularly in the reverberant listening condition.

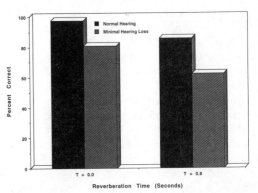

Figure 11–3. Speech perception of children with minimal degrees of sensorineural hearing loss (pure-tone thresholds from 15 to 30 dB from 500 to 2000 Hz) in non-reverberant (RT = 0.0 seconds) and reverberant (RT = 0.8 seconds) listening condition.

Surprisingly, an additional group of normal hearers, who experience more difficulty understanding speech in the classroom than has traditionally been suspected are younger children (13 or less to 15 years of age). Investigators have demonstrated that pediatric listeners require better acoustic environments than adult listeners to achieve equivalent recognition scores.[32,35-37,39] Adult-like performance on speech perception tasks is typically not obtained until the child reaches approximately 13 to 15 years of age. It is thus reasonable to assume that commonly reported classroom reverberation levels have the potential of adversely affecting speech recognition in pediatric listeners. Neuman and Hochberg,[21] for example, reported that 5-year-old children with normal hearing obtained less than 80% correct recognition scores for nonsense syllables at a reverberation time of 0.6 seconds. Finitzo-Hieber and Tillman[17] reported that children, ages 8 to 12 years, obtained recognition scores of only 76.5% at a reverberation time of 1.2 seconds. Certainly, such diminished perceptual ability, as suggested by the investigations just mentioned, would not be appropriate for maximum learning in the classroom setting.

Recommended Criteria for Reverberation Time

Speech perception in adults with normal hearing is not significantly affected until reverberation times exceed approximately 1.0 seconds.[13,14,16,19,34] Listeners with SNHL, however, need considerably shorter reverberation times for maximum speech perception. Sources have recommended that listening environments utilized for the hearing impaired should not surpass 0.4 seconds to provide ideal communicative efficiency.[28,29,40-50]

Unfortunately, acoustic criteria for appropriate reverberation times have not been well established for the diverse populations of children with normal hearing. With these considerations in mind, and until additional research is conducted, a conservative standard for reverberation times in listening environments for children with normal hearing should follow the same acoustic recommendations utilized for listeners with hearing impairment, that is, reverberation time should not exceed 0.4 seconds.

Reverberation Times in Classrooms

Available research suggests that classroom environments are often far too reverberant for maximum communication to occur in pediatric listeners. Specifically, the range of reverberation for unoccupied classroom settings is typically reported to be from 0.4 to 1.2 seconds.[28,29,34,40,41,51-54] McCroskey and Devens[53] reported reverberation levels in classrooms built between 1890 and 1960. Results indicated that the newer classrooms had lower reverberation times (approximately 0.6 seconds) than older classrooms (approximately 1.0 seconds). Nabelek and Pickett[13] reported that reverberation times in medium-sized classrooms ranged from 0.5 to 1.0. Bradley[51] reported that reverberation times in medium-sized classrooms ranged from 0.39 to 1.20 seconds (mean, 0.72 seconds). In 32 classrooms, Crandell and Smaldino[43] reported that mean reverberation times were 0.52 seconds, with a range of 0.35 to 1.20 seconds. The above investigations clearly show that appropriate levels of reverberation (RT = 0.4 seconds) rarely occur in the classroom setting. Indeed, Crandell and Smaldino[43] reported that only 9 of 32 classrooms (28%) exhibited reverberation times less than 0.4 seconds.

NOISE

Noise refers to any undesired auditory disturbance that interferes with what a listener wants to hear.[44] Noise can degrade the perception of speech by distorting, or eliminating, the redundant acoustic and linguistic cues available in the signal.[55-62] Because it is known that the spectral energy of consonant phonemes is less intense than the energy of vowels, noise primarily affects the perception of consonant phonemes, making them less intelligible to the listener. This reduction of consonant perception can significantly influence speech perception because as much as 90% of a listener's speech perception ability is generated from consonant energy.

The effectiveness of any given noise to reduce or eliminate (mask) speech cues depends upon a number of parameters: (1) the long-term spectrum of the noise; (2) the intensity of the noise relative to the intensity of speech; and (3) the intensity fluctuations of the noise over time.[12] Generally, low-frequency noises in a classroom environment are more effective maskers of speech than high-frequency noises because of *upward spread of masking.*[63] The fact that low-frequency noises have a greater effect on speech perception than high-frequency noises is important because the predominant spectra of noise found in classroom environments is low-frequency. It appears that the most effective masking noises are those with a spectra similar to the speech spectrum because they affect all speech frequencies to the same degree.

Measurement of Classroom Noise

The acoustic characteristics of both the signal (the teacher's voice) and the noise (that sound that is masking the signal) vary considerably in the classroom with time. This variability has made it difficult to measure accurately and reliably classroom noise and its effects in a simple manner. In spite of this, single number descriptions of classroom signal and noise characteristics are widespread. One of the most common single number descriptors is the relative SPL of the signal and the noise at specific points in time. The usual way of doing this is to use a *sound level meter*, a device that measures the amplitude of sound. As with reverberation instruments, sound level meters range from compact, inexpensive, battery-operated units to computer-based devices that can measure and record numerous properties of a signal. Sound level meters are classified according to standards set forth in ANSI S1.14.[64] Type I meters meet the most rigorous standards, type II are general purpose, and type III are for hobby use. Most serious measurement of classroom noise would require at least a type II meter. In addition, many sound level meters incorporate weighting filter networks. The A-weighting network is designed to simulate the sensitivity of the average human ear under conditions of low sound loudness (40 phons, to be precise). The B-weighting simulates loud sounds (70 phons), and the C-weighting approximates how the ear would respond to very loud sounds. The convention for classroom measurements is the use of the A-weighting network. Unfortunately, the single number obtained from a sound pressure measurement performed with the A-weighting can be obtained with a number of very different sound spectra. The only really accurate and reliable way to measure spectral intensity would be to do a spectral analysis of the signal and noise, instead of attempting to use a single descriptor.

Noise criteria curves (NCC) can help to determine objectively the suitability of an acoustic spectrum for various human activities.[65] NCCs are a family of frequency and intensity curves based on octave band sound pressure measures across a 20 to 10,000 Hz band and have been related to successful use of an acoustic space for a variety of activities. The value of each NCC is determined by finding the highest NCC the sound pressure intersects. For instance, Figure 11–4 shows NCCs for normal conversational speech (the highest curve intersected is 55, so the NCC = 55) and a typical occupied classroom environment (NCC = 70). This figure strongly suggests that normal conversational speech would be relatively weak in occupied classroom settings. NCCs have also been roughly equated to sound pressure measures made using the A-weighting. An NCC of 25 is considered suitable for a classroom. The computed equivalent sound pressure level using the A-weighting would be approximately 35 dBA. This would then be the target for the long term average spectrum in the classroom and may be the best that can be done without extensive spectral analysis as a function of time. It is recommended, therefore, that whenever possible, ambient noise levels in classrooms or therapy rooms be measured via NCC measures, as this procedure gives the examiner additional information regarding the spectral characteristics of the noise.

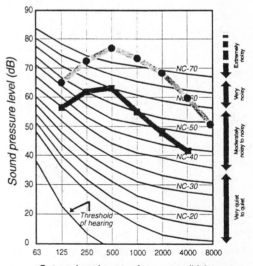

Figure 11–4. Noise criteria curves for an average occupied classroom setting and conversational speech. (Reprinted with permission from Berg[89]).

Sources of Noise
in Classrooms

Ambient noise in the classroom can originate from a number of possible sources.[66] *External noise* sources include construction, traffic, and playground areas. Noise can also originate from within the school building, but outside the actual classroom (*internal noise*). Classrooms adjacent to the cafeteria, gymnasium, or busy hallways often exhibit high internal noise levels. Finally, a significant amount of noise is generated within the classroom itself. *Classroom noise* includes the talking of children, sliding of chairs or tables, shuffling of hard-soled shoes on non-carpeted floors, and school heating or cooling systems. Classroom noise is typically the most detrimental to a child's perceptual ability because the frequency content of the noise is spectrally similar to the spectra of the signal (teacher's voice).

Noise Levels in
Classroom Settings

Ambient noise levels in the classroom have been reported to be high enough to affect deleteriously even adult communication.[28,29,43,48,54,67-78] For example, Sanders[77] measured the occupied and unoccupied noise levels of 47 classrooms in 15 different schools. Mean occupied noise levels ranged from an average of 69 dB(B) in kindergarten classrooms to 52 dB(B) in classrooms for children with hearing impairment. Unoccupied classroom noise levels were approximately 10 dB lower than the occupied classroom settings, ranging from 58 dB(B) for kindergarten classrooms to 42 dB(B) in hearing-impaired classrooms. Nober and Nober[74] reported that the average intensity of four occupied elementary classrooms was 65 dB(A). Bess et al[67] measured ambient noise levels in 19 classrooms for children with hearing impairment. Median unoccupied noise levels were 41 dB(A), 50 dB(B), and 58 dB(C). When the classroom was occupied with students, ambient noise levels increased to 56 dB(A), 60 dB(B), and 63 dB(C). Crandell and Smaldino[43] measured the ambient noise levels of 32 unoccupied classroom settings for children with hearing impairment. Mean unoccupied classroom noise levels were actually higher than previously reported. Specifically, mean unoccupied noise levels were 51 dB(A) (range, 46 to 59 dB) and 67 dB(C) (range, 57 to 74 dB).

Criteria for Classroom
Noise Levels

The noise levels reported in the investigations just discussed are distressing because acoustic recommendations for children with SNHL suggest that ambient noise levels in unoccupied classrooms should not exceed 30 to 35 dB(A) or an NCC of 20 to 25 dB.[28,29,40,48,49] Such a recommendation is based on the assumption that appropriate classroom signal-to-noise (S/N) ratios (see later) are difficult to achieve if classroom noise exceeds these levels. Unfortunately, a review of the aforementioned investigations indicates that this acoustic recommendation is infrequently achieved. McCroskey and Devens[53] demonstrated that only one of nine elementary classrooms actually meet the acoustic recommendations. Crandell and Smaldino[43] reported that none of 32 classrooms met recommended criteria (see Figure 11-5). Overall, it appears that ambient noise levels in the classroom are approximately 10 to 15 dB higher than recommended.

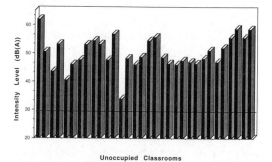

Figure 11–5. The average ambient noise levels, on the A-weighting scale, in 32 classrooms for the hearing impaired. The solid line indicates the recommended acoustic standard [noise level, 30 dB(A)].

Speech Perception in Noise

It is well recognized, however, that the most important consideration for speech perception in the classroom is *not* the absolute ambient noise level, but rather the relationship between the intensity of the signal and the ambient noise at the child's ear. This relationship is referred to as the S/N ratio of the environment. For example, if a speech signal is measured at 65 dB, and a noise is 59 dB, the S/N ratio is +6 dB. For a given noise and speech material, speech perception scores achieve a plateau for favorable S/N ratios and decline for less favorable S/N ratios. Crum,[16] for example, measured word recognition in adult normal hearers at S/N ratios of +12 dB, +6 dB, and 0 dB. Although mean recognition scores were 95% at a S/N ratios of +12 dB, percent correct scores declined to 80% and 46% at S/N ratios of +6 dB and 0 dB, respectively.

In general, the perceptual ability of adult listeners with normal hearing is not significantly affected until the S/N ratio decreases below 0 dB (speech and noise are at equal intensities). To obtain adequate communicative efficiency in noise, adult listeners with SNHL require the S/N ratio to be improved by at least 5 to 10 dB,[79] and by an additional 3 to 6 dB in rooms with moderate levels of reverberation.[80] Stated otherwise, listeners with hearing impairment require considerably better acoustic environments than normal hearers to process and understand speech. As an illustration of the effects of hearing impairment on speech perception, let us examine data from Suter.[59] In this investigation, the author compared speech perception performance in noise for 16 listeners with normal hearing and 32 listeners with various degrees of SNHL. List of monosyllables (Modified Rhyme Test) were presented to the two groups at a level of 60 dB SPL. A multitalker babble served as the competing noise and was adjusted to provide S/N ratios of -6, -3, and 0 dB. Results from this investigation revealed that listeners with hearing impairment performed significantly poorer under all listening conditions. At a S/N ratios of -6 dB, for instance, the listeners with SNHL obtained mean perception scores of 27% correct compared with 63% correct for those with normal hearing.

As with reverberation, research has indicated that the group of children with normal hearing discussed previously also require higher S/N ratios than adult normal hearers to achieve equivalent recognition scores.[25–39] For example, Elliott[36] and Nabelek and Robinson[39] reported that young children require an improvement of approximately 10 dB in S/N ratios to produce equivalent perception scores to those of adults.

Criteria for Classroom Signal-to-Noise Ratios

Acoustic standards suggest that S/N ratios in learning environments for children with hearing impairment should exceed +15 dB.[28,29,40,41,43,44,48,50,54] This recommendation is based on the finding that the speech perception of children with SNHL tends to remain relatively constant at S/N ratios in excess of +15 dB, but deteriorates at less favorable S/N ratios. Moreover, listening effort in children with hearing impairment appears to be minimal at S/N ratios exceeding +10 to +15 dB. At SNRs less than approximately +10 dB, children must utilize so much listening effort that they tend to prefer manual communication and speech reading rather than utilizing auditory input. To date, acoustic standards for S/N ratios are not well defined for "normal hearers." Until such standards are established, the same standards as those advocated for children with hearing impairment should be followed. That is, S/N ratios in learning environments should exceed +15 dB, whereas ambient noise levels should be no more than 30 to 35 dB(A) or an NCC of 20 to 25 dB.

Signal-to-Noise Levels in Classroom Settings

Relatively poor S/N ratios have been reported in many educational settings. The range of S/N ratios for classrooms has been reported to be from +5 dB to -7 dB.[43,54,67–78] Sanders[77] reported that classroom S/N ratios ranged from +5 in elementary classrooms to +1 dB in kindergarten classrooms. Paul[75] reported an average S/N ratio of +3 dB in classrooms. Blair[68] measured classroom S/N ratios in a regular classroom at 0 dB and -7 dB in classrooms for children with SNHL. Finitzo-Hieber[44] reported that classroom S/N ratios ranged from +1 to +4 dB.

In addition to children with hearing impairment, it is reasonable to assume that typical classroom S/N ratios have the capacity of detrimentally affecting speech perception in populations with normal hearing. To support this assumption, let us again examine speech perception data from Finitzo-Hieber and Tillman.[17] In this investigation, the authors also evaluated monosyllabic word perception at different S/N ratios (+12 dB, +6 dB, 0 dB). Results from this investigation are presented in Table 11–2. The most obvious finding from this study is that the children with SNHL obtained poorer perception scores under all listening conditions. However, it is also interesting to examine the data obtained from the children with normal hearing. At an S/N ratio of +12 dB (rarely found in a classroom), the children with normal-hearing sensitivity obtained mean perception scores of 89%. At more

Table 11–2 Mean speech-recognition scores, in percent correct, of children with normal hearing and hearing impairment for monosyllabic words across various signal-to-noise ratios.

Signal-to-Noise Ratio	Groups		
	Normal	Hearing Impaired	Hearing Impaired (Aided)
+ ∞	94.5	87.5	83.0
+ 12	89.2	77.8	70.0
+ 6	79.7	65.7	59.5
0	60.2	42.2	39.0

typical classroom S/N ratios, perceptual abilities were notably poorer. For example, at a S/N ratio of +6 dB, mean perception scores were 80%, and at 0 dB (a common S/N ratio reported in the classroom), mean perception ability decreased to a level of 60%.

In another group of children with normal hearing who exhibit significant perceptual difficulties in noise, Crandell[30] examined the speech perception of children with minimal degrees of SNHL at commonly reported classroom S/N ratios of +6, +3, 0, -3, and -6 dB. The minimally hearing-impaired children exhibited pure-tone averages (0.5 to 2 kHz) from 15 to 25 dB HL. Speech perception was assessed with the Bamford-Koval-Bench Standard Sentence test[81] presented at a level of 65 dB SPL, multitalker babble from the Speech Perception in Noise test[82] was used as the noise competition. Mean sentential recognition scores (in percent correct) as a function of S/N ratio are presented in Figure 11–6. These data suggest that the children with minimal degrees of hearing impairment performed poorer across most listening conditions.

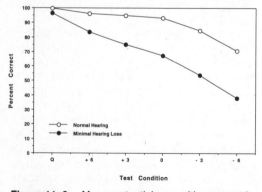

Figure 11–6. Mean sentential recognition scores, in percent correct, as a function of signal-to-noise ratio for children with normal hearing sensitivity (indicated by the open circles) and children with minimal hearing impairment (indicated by the closed circles). (Reprinted with permission from Crandell[30]).

Moreover, note that the performance decrement between the two groups increased as the listening environment became more adverse. For example, at an S/N ratio of +6 dB, both groups obtained recognition scores in excess of 80%. At an S/N ratio of -6 dB, however, the group that was minimally hearing-impaired obtained less than 50% correct recognition compared with approximately 75% recognition ability for those with normal hearing. Interestingly, a similar trend in speech perception was reported by Crandell[31] for non-native English-speaking (Spanish, Chinese, Japanese) children (see Figure 11–7).

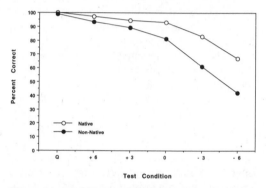

Figure 11–7. Mean sentential recognition scores, in percent correct, as a function of signal-to-noise ratio for native English-speaking children (indicated by the open circles) and non-native English-speaking children (indicated by the closed circles).

Combined Effects of Classroom Noise and Reverberation

In a real-world classroom environment, noise and reverberation are not independent of each other. In fact, in a actual classroom setting, noise and reverberation combine in a synergistic manner to influence speech perception. To explain, the interaction of noise and reverberation adversely affects speech perception greater than the sum of both effects taken independently. If a child experiences a reduction in speech perception of 10% in a noisy listening environment and a reduction of 10% in a reverberant setting, perceptual deficits may actually equate to 30 to 40% in actual listening environments that contain both noise and reverberation. It is reasonable to assume that these synergistic effects occur because when noise and reverberation are combined, reflections fill in the temporal gaps in the noise, making it more steady state in nature. Recall that the most effective maskers are noises with spectra similar to that of the speech spectrum. Although noise and reverberation mask speech differently, there are similarities in how these distortions affect overall speech recognition scores and consonant error patterns. As with noise and reverberation in isolation, individuals with hearing impairment experience considerably greater speech perception difficulties in combinations of noise and reverberation than adults with normal hearing.[12-14,17,19,34,54,62]

Data from several investigations have also suggested that commonly reported levels of classroom noise and reverberation can adversely affect the speech perception of children with normal hearing.[17,28,30,34] In the Finitzo-Hieber and Tillman[17] article, for example, the authors examined the speech recognition of younger children with normal hearing in several conditions of noise and reverberation. Results from this aspect of the investigation are shown in Table 11–3. Note that in typical classroom listening environments, the children with normal hearing generally obtained poor recognition scores. For example, in a relatively good classroom listening environment (S/N ratio = +6 dB; RT = 0.4 seconds), these children were able to recognize only 71% of the stimuli. In a poor, but not a typical classroom environment (S/N ratio = 0 dB; RT = 1.2 seconds) recognition scores were reduced to approximately 30%.

Table 11–3 Mean speech-recognition scores, in percent correct, of children with normal hearing and hearing impairment for monosyllabic words across various signal-to-noise ratios and reverberation times.

Test Condition	Normal Hearing	Hearing Impaired
Reverberation time		
0.0 seconds		
Quiet	94.5	83.0
+12 dB	89.2	70.0
+6 dB	79.7	59.5
0 dB	60.2	39.0
0.4 seconds		
Quiet	92.5	74.0
+12 dB	82.8	60.2
+6 dB	71.3	52.2
0 dB	47.7	27.8
1.2 seconds		
Quiet	76.5	45.0
+12 dB	68.8	41.2
+6 dB	54.2	27.0
0 dB	29.7	11.2

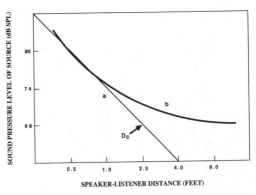

Figure 11–8. The distribution of sound in a classroom, as a function of speaker-listener distance. Adapted from Nabelek and Nabelek.[12]

SPEAKER-LISTENER DISTANCE

In a classroom, the teacher's voice is distributed in several ways that vary as a function of the distance from the source. The distribution of sound in a classroom, as a function of speaker-listener distance, is presented in Figure 11–8. In this figure, Line a represents the SPL of the *direct* sound in the room. Curve b depicts the total sound pressure in the room. The total sound pressure is the sum of the reflected and direct sound energy in the classroom and is often called the *reverberant*, or *indirect sound field*. Point Dc (indicated by the arrow) indicates the critical distance of the room.[83-86] The critical distance refers to that point in a room in which the intensity of the direct sound is equal to the intensity of the reverberant sound. Operationally, critical distance can be defined by the following formula:

$$Dc = (0.20)(VQ/nT)^{-\frac{1}{2}} \quad (2)$$

where V is volume of the room in cubic meters, Q is directivity factor of the source (the human voice is approximately 2.5), n is the number of sources, and RT is reverberation time of the enclosure at 1400 Hz.

Figures 11–9 and 11–10 also demonstrate several of the paths of direct and indirect sound. At distances relatively near to the speaker, the direct sound field (see Fig. 11–9) governs the listening environment. In the direct sound field, sound waves are transmitted from the teacher to the child with minimal interference from room surfaces. Direct sound pressure decreases 6 dB for every doubling of distance from the sound source; a phenomenon known as the *inverse square law*. Due to this linear decease in sound pressure, the direct sound field in a classroom is dominate only at distances close to the teacher.

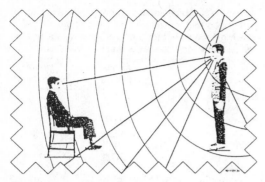

Figure 11–9. Direct sound propagation in a classroom. (Reprinted with permission from Olsen.[48])

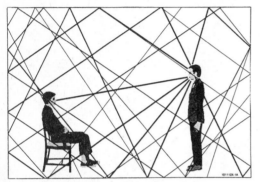

Figure 11–10. Direct and indirect sound propagation in a classroom. The direct sound is indicated by the thickest line, and 1st, 2nd, 3rd, and 4th reflections are denoted by sequentially thinner lines. (Reprinted with permission from Olsen.[48])

For example, in a average-sized classroom (150 m³) with a typical reverberation time of 0.6 seconds, the critical distance would be slightly greater than 3 meters from the teacher. Thus, many of the children in this classroom will be in the indirect sound field.

At increased distances from the speaker, the indirect or reverberant field (see Fig. 11–10) predominates the listening environment. In the indirect sound field (beyond the critical distance), the direct sound from the speaker arrives at the listener first. However, because of the inverse square law, the direct sound is significantly reduced in intensity. In addition to being decreased in intensity, the direct sound is also preceded by numerous reflected sound waves, or reverberation (echoes), which are composed of the original waves that have reflected off hard surfaces within the room (walls, ceiling, and floor). Due to the linear decrease in the intensity of the direct sound, and because the absorptive characteristics of structures in the room absorb some frequen-

cies more than others, the reflected sound reaching the listener will contain a different acoustic content in the frequency, intensity, and temporal domains. Acoustic interaction of this modified spectrum with the direct sound can produce reinforcements and diminutions in the direct sound. These reinforcements and diminutions of the original signal result in an approximately equal distribution of sound energy beyond the critical distance of the room. A uniform distribution of sound energy, however, may not occur in larger listening environments, particularly if the power of the sound source is restricted.

Effects of Distance on Speech Perception

The distance from a student to the teacher can significantly affect speech perception in the classroom.[83-87] If the student is in the direct field (within the critical distance), reflected sound waves have minimal effects on speech perception. In the indirect field (beyond the critical distance), however, reflections can cause difficulties in perception, as there is typically enough of a spectrum or intensity change in the reflected sound to interfere with the perception of the direct sound. Speech perception in a classroom tends to decrease until the critical distance of the room is reached. Beyond the critical distance, perceptual abilities remain essentially constant, particularly in small to moderately sized classrooms. This finding is extremely important, as it suggests that speech perception ability can only be improved by decreasing the distance between a speaker and listener *within* the critical distance of the room. Obviously, increased distance from the teacher deleteriously affects children with hearing impairment greater than children with normal pure-tone sensitivity.

Crandell and Bess[83] examined the effects of distance on the speech recognition of children with normal hearing in a "typical" classroom environment (S/N ratio = +6 dB; RT = 0.45 seconds). Specifically, PB-K monosyllabic words were recorded through the KEMAR manikin at speaker-listener distances often encountered in the classroom (6, 12, and 24 feet). Multibabble was used as the noise competition. Subjects consisted of children 5 to 7 years of age. Results from this investigation are presented in Figure 11–11. As can be noted, there was a systematic decrease in speech-recognition ability as the speaker-listener distance increased. Overall, these results

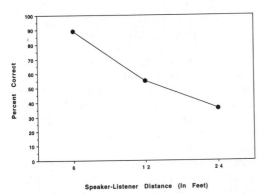

Figure 11–11. Mean sentential recognition scores, in percent correct, as a function of speaker-listener distance for children with normal hearing in a "typical" classroom (signal-to-noise ratio, +6 dB; reverberation time, 0.45 seconds).

suggest that children with normal hearing seated in the middle to rear of a typical classroom have greater difficulty understanding speech than has traditionally been suspected. These findings are understandable by examining the findings of a study by Leavitt and Flexer.[85] In this investigation, the authors utilized the Rapid Speech Transmission Index (RASTI) to estimate speech perception in a classroom. RASTI measurements are based on the hypothesis that noise and reverberation in a room will affect a speech-like signal in ways that can be related to speech perception. Results indicated that in a front row center seat of the classroom, only 83% of the speech energy was available to the listener. Only 55% of the sound energy was available to the listener in the back row center. Clearly, it is reasonable to expect that if only a fraction of the speech signal is available to the listener, poor speech perception would result.

METHODS TO IMPROVE CLASSROOM ACOUSTICS

The perceptual deficits experienced by children with hearing impairment, and with normal hearing, emphasize the necessity of providing appropriate acoustic conditions in listening environments utilized by such populations. Unquestionably, stringent acoustic requirements must be used for rooms occupied by such listeners to ensure that noise and reverberation levels are within recommended criteria. Recall that S/N ratios should exceed +15 dB, unoccupied noise levels should not exceed 30 to 35 dB(A), and reverberation times should not surpass 0.4 seconds.

Reduction of Classroom Noise Levels

Ambient noise levels in a classroom can originate from several possible sources (external, internal, or classroom). The most effective procedure for reducing external noise levels in the classroom is through appropriate planning with architects, contractors, school officials, architectural engineers, audiologists, and teachers for the hearing impaired, *prior* to the design and construction of a building. Unfortunately, consultation among such disciplines prior to building construction is rare. In the absence of such consultation, it is critical that rooms intended for learning, therapy, or instruction be located away from high-noise sources, such as traffic, railroads, construction sites, airports, and furnace or air conditioning units. If relocation of the room or the noise source is not feasible, then acoustic modifications of the room must be considered. Acoustic treatments, such as thick or double concrete construction on the exterior wall, will attenuate extraneous noise sources in the classroom considerably more than having doors or windows on the external wall. Of course, to be effective in noise reduction, all walls must be free of cracks or openings that would allow extraneous noises into the classroom. Architects should attempt to achieve a noise reduction, or a *sound transmission loss* (STL), of at least 45 to 50 dB for external walls. STL refers to the amount of noise that is attenuated as it passes through a particular surface. For instance, if an external noise of 100 dB SPL was reduced to 50 dB SPL in the classroom, the exterior wall of that room would have a STL of 50 dB SPL. A 7-inch concrete wall provides approximately 53 dB attenuation of outside noise, whereas windows and doors provide only 24 dB and 20 dB attenuation, respectively. If windows are located on the external wall, they must be properly installed, heavy weighted or double-paned, and should remain closed. During many acoustic analyses of classrooms, the authors have unfortunately seen exterior windows that remain open the majority of the school day. Landscaping strategies, such as the placement of shrubs, trees (that blossom all year long), or earthen banks around the school building, can also provide interference and absorption of exterior levels of environmental noise. Moreover, solid concrete barriers between the school building and the noise source can reduce noise radiating into the classroom.

Noise can also originate from internal sources. The most cost-effective procedure for reducing internal noise levels in the room is to relocate the classroom to a quieter area of the building. That is, the classroom must not be located next to the gymnasium, bandroom, or other high noise source. At least one acoustically dead space, such as a storage area, should separate classrooms from each other or from high-noise sources in the school building. If relocation of the classroom cannot be accomplished, acoustic treatments such as double wall construction of the interior walls, acoustic ceiling tile or carpeting in hallways outside the classroom, and acoustically treated or well-fitting (preferably with a rubber seal) doorways can attenuate internal noise sources. Doors or interior walls should not contain ventilation ducts that lead into the hallways.

Noise also originates from within the classroom itself. Recall that this type of noise may be particularly damaging to speech perception because its spectrum is often similar to the frequency content of the teacher's voice. The simplest procedure for the reduction of classroom noise is the placement of children away from high noise sources, such as fans, air conditioners, or heating ducts. Often, however, these noise sources produce noise of such intense levels that no location in the classroom is appropriate for adequate communication. Classroom noise sources, such as malfunctioning air conditioning units or heating ducts, need to be replaced or acoustically treated. Heating ducts, for example, can be lined with acoustic materials to reduce airborne and vibratory noise. In addition, acoustic modifications such as the installation of thick carpeting, acoustic paneling on the walls and ceiling, placement of rubber tips on the legs of desks and chairs, the use of acoustically treated furniture, and hanging of thick curtains can also reduce ambient noise generated within the classroom. It is not recommended that children with SNHL, or normal hearing, be placed in openplan classrooms, as it is well recognized that such classrooms are generally considerably noisier than regular classrooms. In addition, instruction should not take place in areas separated from other teaching areas by thin partitions (particularly those that are not permanently fixed to the floor and ceiling), sliding doors, or temporary walls.

Reduction of Classroom Reverberation Times

Reverberation can be reduced by covering the hard reflective surfaces in a room (bare cement walls and ceilings, glass or mirrored areas, and uncarpeted floors) with absorptive materials. Acoustic paneling on the walls and ceiling, carpeting on the floors, the placement of cork bulletin boards on the walls, curtains on the windows, and the positioning of mobile bulletin boards at angles other than parallel to the walls can decrease reverberation levels in an enclosure. It should be noted that many of the aforementioned acoustic modifications can be achieved at little or no cost to the school system. For example, eggshell cartons or pieces of carpet placed on a bare cement wall can, at times, dramatically reduce the reverberation time of that learning environment.

Unfortunately, a review of the literature has demonstrated that classrooms often exhibit minimal degrees of acoustic modifications.[28,30,34,48,67] For example, Bess et al[67] found that 100% of classrooms had acoustic ceiling tile, but only 68% had carpeting and 13% had draperies. No classroom contained any form of acoustical furniture treatment. Crandell and Smaldino[43] reported similar findings: all of the 32 classrooms examined had acoustic ceiling tile, but only 19 (59%) contained carpeting. Moreover, only one of the classrooms had drapes (3%), and none of the rooms had acoustic furniture treatments.

Reduction of Speaker-to-Listener Distance

The deleterious effects of noise and reverberation can also be reduced by ensuring that the child receives the teacher's voice at the most advantageous speaker-listener distance possible. Specifically, the child, particularly the child with SNHL, needs to be in a face to face situation and in the direct sound field, where the interaction of noise and reverberation are less detrimental to speech-recognition skills. Such a placement would also aid the child in utilizing visual as well as auditory cues. To achieve this recommendation, restructuring of classroom activities must be considered. For example, small group instruction should be considered over more traditional room configuration, where the speaker instructs in front of numerous rows of listeners. Such a recommendation has practical limitations, however, because in typical classrooms the critical distance for maximum speech perception is present only at distances relatively close to the teacher. Hence, the simple recommendation of preferential seating is often not enough to ensure an appropriate listening environment for many children. The utilization of a hearing assistance device, such as a personal frequency modulation (FM) amplification system or sound-field FM amplification system, can also decrease speaker-listener distance and significantly augment speech perception in the classroom. A FM sound field system is essentially a room public address system in which speech is picked up via a FM wireless microphone located near the speaker's mouth, where the effects of noise and reverberation are negligible. The signal is then transmitted to a amplifier and delivered to listeners in the room via several strategically placed loudspeakers. The objectives of such a system is: (1) to improve the volume of the teacher's voice approximately 10 dB over the unamplified condition; and (2) provide a uniform direct or a speech reinforcing reflected sound field throughout the classroom. Several investigators have shown that if these objectives are achieved, psycho-educational and psychosocial benefits accrue for children with normal hearing and hearing impairment.[88-94] For instance, Sarff[94] utilized a sound field amplification system in a classroom with children with normal hearing and children with minimal degrees of SNHL. Results indicated that both groups of children, particularly the children with minimal hearing impairment, demonstrated significant improvements in academic achievement when receiving amplified instruction. Moreover, younger children demonstrated greater academic improvements than older children. Crandell[31] reported that sound-field FM amplification devices can significantly improve the speech perception of non-native English-speaking children in a classroom setting (see Chapter 12).

CONCLUSIONS

This chapter has emphasized several of the singular and interactive effects of classroom reverberation, noise, and distance. The acoustic conditions in most classrooms are poorer than what would be recommended for adequate speech perception by children with sensorineural hearing loss and several populations of children with normal hearing. Such findings are alarming, as it is well recognized that inappropriate classroom acoustics can deleteriously affect not only speech perception, but also psycho-educational achievement. Hence, inadequate classroom acoustics may place many populations of children at risk for language, behavioral, literacy, social, and academic difficulties. To reduce this risk, strategies were suggested to improve classroom S/N ratio and reduce reverberation.

ACKNOWLEDGMENT

Portions of the research cited in this chapter were supported by an Advanced Research Project Grant—Texas Higher Eduction Coordinating Board, and by a Department of Education Research Grant (Listening in Classrooms—Utah State University.

REFERENCES

1. Godfrey J. Linguistic structure in clinical and experimental tests of speech recognition, in Elkins E, ed. *ASHA report 14: Speech Recognition by the Hearing Impaired* (Rockville, MD: ASHA, 1984) pp 52–56.
2. Lehiste I. The units of speech perception, in Gilbert J, ed. *Speech and Cortical Functioning* (New York: Academic Press, 1972) pp 187–235.
3. Sanders D. *Management of Hearing Handicap.* (Englewood Cliff: Prentice Hall, 1993).
4. Strange W, Jenkins J: Role of linguistic experience in the perception of speech, in Walk R, Pick H, eds. *Perception and Experience* (New York: Plenum Press, 1978), pp 125–169.
5. Bolt R, MacDonald A: Theory of speech masking by reverberation. *J Acoust Soc Am*, 21 (1949), 577–580.
6. Lochner J, Burger J. The influence of reflections in auditorium acoustics. *J Sound Vibration*, 4 (1964), 426–454.
7. American National Standard Acoustical Terminology. ANSI S1.1-1960, revised 1976.
8. Knudsen V, Harris C: *Acoustical Designing in Architecture.* (New York: American Institute of Physics for the Acoustical Society of America, 1978).
9. Kurtovic H: The influence of reflected sound upon speech intelligibility. *Acoustica*, 33 (1975), 32–39.
10. Sabine W: *Collected Papers on Acoustics.* (New York: Dover, 1964).
11. Lipscomb D: *Noise in Audiology.* (Austin, TX: Pro-Ed, 1975).

12. Nabelek A, Nabelek I: Room acoustics and speech perception in Katz J, ed. *Handbook of Clinical Audiology*, 3. (Baltimore: Williams & Wilkins, 1985).

13. Nabelek A, Pickett J: Monaural and binaural speech perception through hearing aids under noise and reverberation with normal and hearing-impaired listeners. *J Speech Hear Res*, 17 (1974), 724–739.

14. Nabelek A, Pickett J: Reception of consonants in a classroom as affected by monaural and binaural listening, noise, reverberation, and hearing aids. *J Acoust Soc Am*, 56 (1974), 628–639.

15. Houtgast T: The effect of ambient noise on speech intelligibility in classrooms. *Appl Acoustics*, 14 (1981), 15–25.

16. Crum D: The effects of noise, reverberation, and speaker-to-listener distance on speech understanding. Unpublished doctoral dissertation (Northwestern University, Evanston, IL, 1974).

17. Finitzo-Hieber T, Tillman T: Room acoustics effects on monosyllabic word discrimination ability for normal and hearing-impaired children. *J Speech Hear Res*, 21 (1978), 440–458.

18. Gelfand S, Silman S: Effects of small room reverberation upon the recognition of some consonant features. *J Acoust Soc Am*, 66 (1979), 22–29.

19. Irwin R, McAuley S: Relations among temporal acuity, hearing loss, and the perception of speech distorted by noise and reverberation. *J Acoust Soc Am*, 81 (1987), 1557–1565.

20. Moncur J, Dirks D: Binaural and monaural speech intelligibility in reverberation. *J Speech Hear Res*, 10 (1967), 186–195.

21. Neuman A, Hochberg I: Children's perception of speech in reverberation. *J Acoust Soc Am*, 73 (1983), 2145–2149.

22. Crandell C, Henoch M, Dunkerson K:. A review of speech perception and aging: Some implications for aural rehabilitation. *J Acad Rehabil Audiol*, 24 (1992), 121–132.

23. Nabelek A, Robinette L: Reverberation as a parameter in clinical testing. *Audiology*, 17 (1978), 239–259.

24. Plomp, F: Binaural and monaural speech intelligibility of connected discourse in reverberation as a azimuth of a single competing sound source. *Acoutsica*, 34 (1976), 200–211.

25. Bess F. The minimally hearing-impaired child. *Ear Hear*, 6 (1985), 43–47.

26. Bess F, Tharpe A: An introduction to unilateral sensorineural hearing loss in children *Ear Hear*, 7 (1986), 3–13.

27. Boney S, Bess F: Noise and reverberation effects on speech recognition in children with minimal hearing loss. Paper presented at the American Speech, Language, and Hearing Association, San Francisco, November, 1984.

28. Crandell C: Classroom acoustics for normal-hearing children: Implications for rehabilitation. *Educ Aud Mono*, 2 (1991), 18–38.

29. Crandell C: Classroom acoustics for hearing-impaired children. *J Acoust Soc Am*, 92 (1992), 2470.

30. Crandell C: Noise effects on children with minimal sensorineural hearing loss. *Ear Hear*, 14 (1993), 210–217.

31. Crandell, C. The effects of noise on the speech perception of non-native English children. *Lang Speech Hear Schools*, (1994) (in press).

32. Crandell C, Bess F. Developmental Changes in Speech Recognition in Noise and Reverberation. *ASHA*, 29 (1987), 170.

33. Crandell C, McQuain J, Bess, F: Speech recognition of articulation disordered children in noise and reverberation. *ASHA*, 29 (1987), 170.

34. Crandell C, Smaldino J: The importance of room acoustics in Tyler R, Schum, D, eds. *Assistive Devices for the Hearing Impaired*. Baltimore: William and Wilkins, 1994 (in press).

35. Elliott L: Performance of children aged 9 to 17 years on a test of speech intelligibility in noise using sentence material with controlled word predictability. *J Acoust Soc Am*, 66 (1979), 651–653.

36. Elliott L: Effects of noise on perception of speech by children and certain handicapped individuals. *Sound Vibration*, December, (1982), 9–14.

37. Elliott L, Connors S, Kille E, Levin S, Ball K, Katz D: Children's understanding of monosyllabic nouns in quiet and in noise. *J Acoust Soc Am*, 66 (1979), 12–21.

38. Nabelek A, Donahue A. Perception of consonants in reverberation by native and non native listeners. *J Acoust Soc Am*, 75 (1984), 632–634.

39. Nabelek A, Robinson P: Monaural and binaural speech perception in reverberation for listeners of various ages. *J Acoust Soc Am*, 71 (1982), 1242–1248.

40. American Speech, Language, and Hearing Association Standard on Acoustics in Classrooms. (1994) (in press).

41. Bess F, McConnell F: *Audiology, Education and the Hearing-Impaired Child*. (St Louis: CV Mosby, 1981).

42. Borrild K: Classroom acoustics, in Ross M, Giolas T, eds. *Auditory Management of Hearing Impaired Children*, (Baltimore: University Park Press, 1978) pp 145–179.

43. Crandell C, Smaldino J: An update of classroom acoustics for children with hearing impairment. *Volta Rev*, (1994) (in press).

44. Finitzo-Hieber T: Classroom acoustics, in Roeser R, Downs M, eds. *Auditory Disorders in School Children*, ed. 2. (New York: Thieme-Stratton, 1988), pp 221–233.

45. Niemoeller A: Acoustical design of classrooms for the deaf. *Am Ann Deaf*, 113 (1968), 1040–1045.

46. Olsen W: Acoustics and amplification in classrooms for the hearing impaired, in Bess, FH, ed. *Childhood Deafness: Causation, Assessment and Management*. (New York: Grune & Stratton, 1977).

47. Olsen W: The effects of noise and reverberation on speech intelligibility, in Bess FH, Freeman BA, Sinclair JS, eds. *Amplification in Education*. (Washington, DC: Alexander Graham Bell Association for the Deaf, 1981).

48. Olsen W: Classroom acoustics for hearing-impaired children, in Bess, FH ed. *Hearing Impairment in Children*. (Parkton, MD: York Press, 1988).

49. Neimoeller A: Acoustical design of classrooms for the deaf. *Am Ann Deaf*, 113 (1968), 1040–1045.

50. Gengel R: Acceptable signal-to-noise ratios for aided speech discrimination by the hearing impaired. *J Aud Res*, 11 (1971), 219–222.

51. Bradley J: Speech intelligibility studies in classrooms. *J Acoust Soc Am*, 80 (1986), 846–854.

52. Kodaras M: Reverberation times of typical elementary school settings. *Noise Control*, 6 (1960), 17–19.

53. McCroskey F, Devens J: Acoustic characteristics of public school classrooms constructed between 1890 and 1960. *NOISEXPO Proc*, (1975), 101–103.

54. Ross M: Classroom acoustics and speech intelligibility, in Katz J, ed. *Handbook of Clinical Audiology*. (Baltimore: Williams & Wilkins, 1978.)

55. Cooper J, Cutts B: Speech discrimination in noise. *J Speech Hearing Res*, 14 (1971), 332–337.

56. French N, Steinberg J: Factors governing the intelligibility of speech sounds. *J Acoust Soc Am*, 19 (1947), 90–119.

57. Miller G: Effects of noise on people. *J Acoust Soc Am*, 56 (1974), 724–764.

58. Miller G, Nicely P: An analysis of perceptual confusions among some English consonants. *J Acoust Soc Am*, 27 (1955), 338–352.

59. Suter A: The ability of mildly hearing impaired individuals to discriminate speech in noise. *Aerospace Medical Research Laboratory Report No. AMRL-RT-78-4*. (Wright Patterson Air Force Base, Ohio, 1978).

60. Crandell C: Individual differences in speech-recognition ability: Implications for hearing aid selection. *Ear Hear*, 12 (1991), 100–108.

61. Moore B: *An Introduction to the Psychology of Hearing*. (New York: Academic Press, 1991).

62. Plomp R: A signal-to-noise ratio model for the speech reception threshold for the hearing impaired. *J Speech Hear Res*, 29 (1986), 146–154.

63. Danaher E, Pickett J: Some masking effects produced by low frequency vowel formants in persons with sensorineural hearing loss. *J Speech Hear Res*, 18 (1975), 261–271.

64. American National Standards Institute. Specification for Sound Level Meters. ANSI S1.4-1971, New York.

65. Beranek L: *Acoustics*. (New York: McGraw-Hill, 1954).

66. John J, Thomas H: Design and construction of schools for the deaf, in Ewing A, ed. *Educational Guidance and the Deaf Child*. (*Volta Rev*, 59 (1957).

67. Bess F, Sinclair J, Riggs D: Group amplification in schools for the hearing-impaired. *Ear Hear*, 5 (1984), 138–144.

68. Blair J: Effects of amplification, speechreading, and classroom environment on reception of speech. *Volta Rev*, 79 (1977), 443–449.

69. Blair J, Peterson M, Viehweg S. The effects of mild hearing loss on academic performance of young school-age children. *Volta Rev*, 87 (1985), 87

70. Crum D, Matkin N: Room acoustics: the forgotten variable. *Lang, Speech, Hear Serv Sch*, 7 (1976), 106–110.

71. Fourcin A, Joy D, Kennedy M, Knight J, Knowles S, Knox E, Martin M, Mort J, Penton J, Poole D, Powell C, Watson T: Design of educational facilities for deaf children. *Br J Aud*, Suppl 3 (1980).

72. Gleen L, Nerbonne G, and Tolhurst G: Environmental noise in a residential institution for mentally-retarded persons. *Am J Mental Defic*, 82 (1982), 594–597.

73. Markides A: Speech levels and speech-to-noise ratios. *Brit J Aud*, 20 (1986), 115–120.

74. Nober L, Nober, E. Auditory discrimination of learning disabled children in quiet and classroom noise. *J Learn Disord*, 8 (1975), 656–773.

75. Paul R: An investigation of the effectiveness of hearing aid amplification in regular and special classrooms under instructional conditions. Unpublished doctoral dissertation, (Detroit: Wayne State University, 1967).

76. Pearsons K, Bennett R, Fidell S: Speech levels in various noise environments. *EPA 600/1-77-025*. (Washington, DC: Office of Health & Ecological Effects, 1977).

77. Sanders D: Noise conditions in normal school classrooms. *Except Child*, 31 (1965), 344–353.

78. Webster J, Snell K: Noise levels and the speech intelligibility of teachers in classrooms. *J Acad Rehabil Aud*, 16 (1983), 234–255.

79. Moore B, Glasberg B: Relationship between psychophysical abilities and speech perception for subjects with unilateral and bilateral cochlear hearing impairments, in: Schouten M, ed. *Proc. NATO-ARW The Psychophysics of Speech Perception*. (The Netherlands: Martinus Nijhoff, 1987).

80. Hawkins D Yacullo W: Signal-to-noise ratio advantage of binaural hearing aids and directional microphones under different levels of reverberation. *J Speech Hear Disord*, 49 (1984), 278–286.
81. Bench J, Koval A, Bamford J: The BKB (Bamford-Koval-Bench) sentence lists for partially-hearing children. *Br J Aud*, 13 (1979), 108–112.
82. Kalikow DN, Stevens KN, Elliott LL: Development of a test of speech intelligibility in noise using sentence materials with controlled word predictability. *J Acoust Soc Am*, 61 (1977), 1337–1351.
83. Crandell C, Bess F: Speech recognition of children in a "typical" classroom setting. *ASHA*, 29 (1986), 87.
84. Klein W: Articulation loss of consonants as a criterion for speech transmission in a room. *J Audio Eng Soc*, 19 (1971),920–922.
85. Leavitt R, Flexer C: Speech degradation as measured by the Rapid Speech Transmission Index (RASTI). *Ear Hear*, 12 (1991), 115–118.
86. Puetz V: Articulation loss of consonants as a criterion for speech transmission in a room. *J Audio Eng Soc*, 19 (1971), 915–919.

87. Watson T: The use of hearing aids by hearing-impaired children in ordinary schools. *Volta Rev*, 66 741–744, (1964), 787.
88. Anderson K: Speech perception in children. *Educ Aud Mon*, 1 (1991), 15–29.
89. Berg F: *Acoustics and Sound Systems in Schools*. (San Diego: Singular Publishing, 1993).
90. Crandell C, Bess F: Sound-field amplification in the classroom setting. *ASHA*, 29 (1987), 87.
91. Crandell C: Issues in sound field amplification. Paper presented at the Weekend with the Experts Conference, Improving Classroom Acoustics. Orlando, Florida, 1994.
92. Crandell C, Smaldino J: Sound-field amplification in the classroom. *Am J Aud*, 1(4) (1992), 16–18.
93. Smaldino J, Flexer C: Improving listening in the classroom. Paper presented at the 1991 Academy of Rehabilitative Audiology annual meeting, Brakenridge, CO., 1991.
94. Sarff L: An innovative use of free field amplification in regular classrooms, in Roeser R, Downs M, eds. *Auditory Disorders in School Children*. (New York: Thieme-Stratton, 1981), pp 263–272.

CLASSROOM AMPLIFICATION SYSTEMS

12

Carol Flexer

> *The three great elemental sounds in nature are the sound of rain, the sound of wind in a primeval wood, and the sound of outer ocean on a beach.*
>
> —Henry Beston, 1888–1968

A school-based speech-language pathologist recently received recommendations for the use of FM (frequency modulation) technology for the following children:

1. A preschool boy who has a fluctuating hearing loss due to chronic otitis media with effusion (OME)
2. A seventh grade girl with a bilateral, moderately severe, sloping, high-frequency sensorineural hearing loss
3. A third grade boy with normal hearing who was diagnosed with Attention Deficit Disorder (ADD)
4. A first grade girl with a bilateral, severe to profound sensorineural hearing loss
5. A second grade boy with a unilateral hearing loss
6. A tenth grade boy with a bilateral, moderate, sensorineural hearing loss
7. A sixth grade girl with delayed onset, progressive, sensorineural hearing loss
8. A kindergarten girl diagnosed with pervasive developmental delay who is overly sensitive to tactile input— she appears to have normal peripheral hearing sensitivity but she does have attending and auditory processing problems.

In each case, the referring audiologists stated simply, "FM use recommended." The school speech-language pathologist was dismayed. Does the same recommendation for each child mean that the same FM unit is required for each child?

The school system did not have an educational audiologist, so the speech-language pathologist was expected, by the school system, to order and fit the necessary FM equipment.

There are a plethora of FM fitting issues. To begin with, *who* should evaluate and fit the equipment? Would the child do best with a personal FM system or a sound field amplification system?

What are the best output and frequency response characteristics for each FM unit recommended? Why do some of these children even need an FM system? What is the difference between direct input, neckloop, self-contained unit (hearing aid and FM together), and Walkman earphones? When do you use the remote microphone and when should an environmental microphone be activated? How should mainstreamed teachers receive in-service training? Is the school system even responsible for providing FM units for all of the eight children mentioned previously? How do you know if the FM unit is working for a particular child? How do you entice/threaten/motivate an older child to use FM technology? How can we advocate for, obtain, and pay for all of the FM technology that is being recommended? Is FM technology appropriate only for children who are in special education programs?

The purpose of this chapter is to identify, sort through, and solve many questions regarding FM recommendations, management, and use.

DEFINITION OF CLASSROOM AMPLIFICATION SYSTEMS

Historically, the term "auditory training system" has been applied to any amplification system other than a personal hearing aid. Auditory trainers were introduced into programs for children with hearing impairments about 50 years ago. They were high-power-output amplification units that were used primarily for children with severe to profound hearing impairments who were in self-contained schools or classrooms. The reader is referred to Pimentel,[1] Berg,[2] and Bess and McConnell[3] for descriptions of the following auditory trainers: hard-wired, portable desk auditory trainer, loop (induction), loop radio frequency (RF), and infrared systems.

Because of its history, the term "auditory training system" tends to be associated with a rather restricted population of children (those with severe to profound hearing impairments) in rather restricted settings (self-contained, special education programs) who required high-power-output amplification systems. Please note that the term is not negative; it just might not encompass today's diverse population of children. For example, a school-based speech-language pathologist recently received an audiologist's recommendation for an "FM auditory trainer" for a child with a fluctuating hearing loss caused by chronic otitis media, who was in a mainstream classroom. The speech-language pathologist wondered why this child needed the high-power-output unit commonly associated with children with severe hearing impairments in the school's special education program, but he was not familiar with any other kind of "auditory trainer." Because the audiologist's recommendation did not provide a justification for the FM unit, nor did the recommendation state the desired performance characteristics of the FM unit, the speech-language pathologist put an old, high-power output FM unit on the child that had been used in the school's special education program for a child who had a severe to profound sensorineural hearing impairment. That is, this child with a fluctuating, conductive hearing impairment was erroneously fit with a self-contained FM unit (closed earmolds with button receivers, and both environmental microphones on the FM's receiver were activated) that had a 139 dB SPL maximum output. Unfortunately, these types of misunderstandings about auditory trainers are common. Audiologists must justify the need for FM technology for a given child, carefully specify FM performance characteristics, and require a follow-up visit to verify the suitability of the fit.

It seems that currently, the term "classroom amplification system" is more descriptive and not historically self-limiting in use. As this chapter progresses, an argument will be made for the use of the phrase "signal-to-noise (S/N) ratio enhancing technology" as one that seems to be even more descriptive of classroom amplification system effectiveness.

Because of the changing demographics and the current mainstream placement of the vast majority of children with hearing problems, this chapter will focus on the two classroom amplification systems most commonly used: personal and self-contained FM systems, and sound field FM systems.

CURRENT POPULATION OF CHILDREN WITH HEARING PROBLEMS

The use of specific classroom amplification systems is based on the population of children who require the technology. This population has changed over the last few decades.[4] Maternal rubella and Rh incompatibility virtually have been eliminated. Thus, there are fewer than half the number of children with severe to profound hearing impairments today than there were a few decades ago. Conversely, in the last decade, more than 10 times the number of children with mild to moderate hearing impairments have been identified and fit with amplification.

An additional large population of children who often are not clearly identified are those with hearing problems caused by middle ear dysfunction. Indeed, the incidence of children with persistent minimal to mild hearing impairments caused by otitis media may be much higher than school screenings lead us to believe.[5] Hearing screening environments in schools typically have less than ideal levels of ambient noise, causing hearing to be screened at 20 to 35 dB hearing level (HL). When 15 dB HL is used as the criterion for identifying an educationally significant hearing impairment, the numbers of identified kindergarten and first grade children increase dramatically. A study conducted in Putnam County Ohio found that 43% of their primary level students failed a 15 dB HL hearing screen on any given day, and about 75% of their primary level children in classes for children with learning disabilities failed a 15 dB hearing screening.[6] These figures also were found by the Mainstream Amplification Resource Room Study.[7]

The point is that the vast majority of children who will require some type of classroom amplification system will be, or certainly ought to be, in mainstream classrooms and not in a self-contained environment. We cannot manage today's children who experience hearing problems the same way that we managed children at the height of the rubella epidemic in the 1960s. That is, audiological services in school typically have been viewed as *support services* relevant for only a very small population of chidren who are labeled as "deaf."[8] Children who are severely and profoundly hearing impaired certainly require audiological services; however, the need for classroom amplification systems is not limited to these few children. There may be at least 8 million school children who have hearing problems that could be helped by the use of devices that improve the S/N ratio.[9] Audiologists could be even more effective in schools if we expanded our role beyond the special education network into regular education classes.

RATIONALE FOR FM RECOMMENDATIONS AND USE OF A REMOTE MICROPHONE

Typical mainstram classrooms are auditory-verbal environments; instruction is presented through the teacher's spoken communication.[10] The underlying assumption is that children can hear clearly and attend to the teacher's speech. Thus, children in a mainstream classroom, whether or not they have hearing impairments, must be able to hear the teacher in order for learning to occur. If children cannot consistently and clearly hear the teacher, the major premise of the educational system is undermined.

Word/Sound Distinctions

Elliott et al[11] evaluated primary level children with normal hearing and found that the ability to perform fine-grained auditory discrimination tasks (eg, to hear *pa* and *ba* as different syllables) correctly classified 80% of the children in their study either as progressing normally or as having language-learning difficulties. The conclusion is that auditory discrimination is associated with the development of basic academic competencies that are critical for success in school. The young child who cannot *hear* phonemic distinctions is at risk for academic failure. To be able to hear phonemic distinctions, hearing sensitivity for children must be 15 dB HL or better at all frequencies.

Audibility versus Intelligibility

The ability to discriminate individual phonemes, to hear word/sound distinctions, is defined as *intelligibility*. The ability to detect the presence of speech but not identify individual components is called *audibility*. If, because of poor attending skills, a central auditory processing problem, poor classroom acoustics, or a hearing impairment of any degree, a child cannot discriminate *walked* from *walks*, for example, he or she will not learn appropriate semantic distinctions unless deliberate intervention occurs.

Invisible Acoustic Filter Effect of Hearing Impairment

The primacy of hearing in the communicative and educational process tends to be underestimated because hearing loss itself is invisible. The effects of hearing loss are often associated with problems or causes other than hearing impairment.[12] For example, when a child is off-task or cannot keep up with the rapid pace of class discussion, the cause of that child's behavior may be attributed to noncompliant behavior or to attention problems or to slow learning rather than to hearing problems.

One cannot "see" a hearing impairment; therefore, it is easy to confuse the causal hearing loss with the negative consequences of the hearing impairment. To explain, hearing impairment acts like an invisible acoustic filter than interferes with incoming sounds.[13] In addition to a reduction in loudness, sounds are often smeared together, or filtered out entirely. Speech, therefore, might be *audible* by not *intelligible*. A child with a hearing impairment might be able to hear the presence of speech (audibility), but not be able to hear clearly enough to be able to hear one speech sound as distinct from another. Words like *invitation* and *vacation* might sound the same. It is not difficult to imagine what such word confusions could do to a child's vocabulary and conceptual language development.

This acoustic filter effect is the beginning, the cause of an entire chain of negative events. If speech sounds are not heard clearly, then one cannot speak clearly, unless deliberate intervention occurs. The second step in the chain involves reading ability. If one does not have good spoken language skills, then reading, which is a secondary linguistic function, also will suffer. Said another way, we speak because we hear and we read because we speak. If reading skills are below average, an individual will have difficulty performing academically. Limited literacy leads to a reduction in professional options and subsequent opportunities for independent function as an adult. The cause of this entire unfortunate chain of events is the ambiguous, invisible, underestimated, and often untreated acoustic filter effect of hearing impairment. Until the primary problem of hearing impairment is identified and managed, intervention at the secondary levels of spoken language, reading, and academics likely will be ineffective.

The ambiguity of hearing impairment is magnified by the tendency to categorize hearing loss into dichotomous categories of *normally hearing* or *deaf*.[14] Because children who experience minimal, mild, or moderate hearing impairments are not "deaf" (94 to 96% of the population of persons with hearing impairment is functionally *hard-of-hearing* and not *deaf*), their hearing problems are often believed, erroneously, to present an "insignificant" barrier to classroom performance.[15,16]

Any type and degree of hearing impairment can present a significant barrier to the reception of teacher instruction in a typical classroom.

Computer Analogy

One way to explain the negative effects of any type and degree of hearing impairment on language learning and academic performance is to use a computer analogy. Data input precedes data output. A child must have information or data to learn. Information is entered into the brain through the auditory system. If data are entered inaccurately, like having one's fingers on the wrong keys of a computer keyboard or like having a broken keyboard, then the child will have inaccurate, incomplete, and unreliable data to process (see Fig. 12–1). Is it reasonable to expect a child to learn sophisticated spoken communication and to develop academic competencies when the information that reaches the brain is deficient?

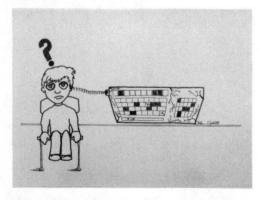

Figure 12–1. Hearing impairment is like having a malfunctioning computer keyboard that enters inaccurate, inconsistent, and incomplete data to the brain. (Illustration by Josh Klynn.)

Using amplification technology such as a hearing aid, a personal FM system, a sound field FM (classroom PA) system, or even a cochlear implant is analogous to having a better keyboard. *The goal in using classroom amplification*

systems is to provide the best, most consistent and reliable keyboard for instructional data entry (see Fig. 12–2a, b). The better a child can detect word/sound distinctions, the better opportunity a child will have for the development of academic competencies.

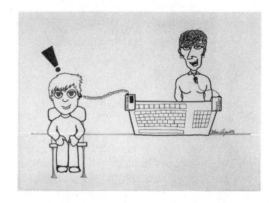

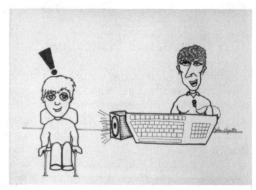

Figure 12–2. Classroom amplification systems, such as a personal FM system (A) and a sound field FM system (B), facilitate data entry by providing a more accessible keyboard. (Illustration by Josh Klynn.)

Once hearing problems are identified and barriers to the clear reception of classroom instruction are removed, analogous to the provision of the best possible keyboard, what happens to all of the previously entered inaccurate and deficient information? Do inaccurate data convert automatically to correct information? Unfortunately, missing data need to be entered and inaccurate data need to be corrected. The longer a child's hearing problem remains unidentified and unmanaged, the more destructive are the negative effects of the acoustic filtering process of that hearing problem.

Managing hearing is the crucial first step in the chain of intervention; providing an accurate and reliable keyboard is the prerequisite step to clear data entry. Once hearing has been accessed, a child has an opportunity to learn spoken language as the basis for developing academic competencies and acquiring knowledge about the world.

Passive Learning/Overhearing/ Distance Hearing

A consequence of hearing impairment and a reason why FM technology needs to be used in a classroom is the concept of distance hearing. Distance hearing is the distance over which speech sounds are intelligible and not merely audible.[13] Hearing problems of any type and degree reduce the distance over which speech sounds are intelligible, even if one is wearing hearing aids. Typically, the greater the hearing loss, the greater the reduction in distance hearing. Reduction in distance hearing has negative consequences for classroom and life performance because distance hearing is necessary for passive learning.[17,18]

A child with a hearing problem, even a minimal one, cannot casually overhear what people are saying. Most children with normal hearing seem to absorb information from their environments; they tend to learn easily information that was not directed to them. Children with hearing problems, however, because of their reduction in distance hearing, need to be taught directly many skills and concepts that other children learn incidentally.

Additional implications of the reduction of distance hearing include lack of redundancy of instructional information and lack of access to social cues. Listening is an active and not a passive process for children with hearing problems, thus, active attention must be directed to appropriate sources at all times. A child's attention will wander often during the school day, causing him or her to miss some of what is being said. Missed information can be offset partially by the use of a remote microphone of a personal or sound field FM system. The remote microphone can be placed close to the speech or sound source, thereby making information available and alleviating some of the strain and effort of constant disciplined attention.

Level of Effort

Children with hearing problems typically expend a high level of effort as they attempt to learn from classroom instruction. For example, a fifth grade girl with a congenital, mild sloping to moderately severe, bilateral, sensorineural hearing impairment and excellent auditory and spoken language skills was earning A's and B's in advanced (mainstreamed) classes. Because she was performing at such a high level, teachers thought that she did not require any support services (such as notetakers, pretutoring of new vocabulary and concepts, captioned instructional materials). She did not use and had never had access to FM technology of any kind. Further questioning revealed, however, that she routinely spent 2 to 4 hours per night doing homework, trying to make up for the redundancy of information that she was being denied access to in the classroom. She was expending such a high level of effort that she needed to nap after school; she also was taking antidepressant medication for anxiety. She had no time for extracurricular activities. Children with hearing impairments typically need to exert a higher level of effort than do children with normal hearing to be competitive in school. However, this girl was expending an unnecessary amount of energy trying to gain instructional information on her own that some basic accommodations could have made available to her in the classroom. Interestingly, when initially asked how she was doing in school, she stated, "Everything is fine!" When asked if she wanted to have any accommodations such as an FM system, she said, "No." She had no idea that classroom learning could be any easier. She had always worked so hard in school; her perceptions were skewed. As Mark Ross has often stated, the problem with hearing loss is that you do not hear so well. Consequently, you hear what you think you hear, and you do not hear what you do not hear. . .and one does not have a perspective about missed information.[12] This young girl finally agreed to experiment with a personal FM system, fit with a neckloop that provided a favorable acoustic signal and was acceptable socially and visually to her. She also accepted the use of captioned video materials and some preview and review sessions with a tutor. Within one semester, she no longer required naps, homework time dropped to about 1 hour per night, she was taken off the medication and she joined a soccer team. She was able to maintain her high level of performance with less expenditure of effort and she had time for a life after school.

Speech-to-Noise Ratio

Unfortunately, children are expected to hear meaningful word/sound distinctions in unfavorable acoustic environments. They must listen to a speaker who is not close and who is moving about the room.

S/N ratio is the relationship between a primary signal, such as the teacher's speech, and background noise. Noise is everything that conflicts with the auditory signal of choice and may include other talkers, heating or cooling systems, classroom or hall noise, playground sounds, computer noise, wind, among others. The more favorable the S/N ratio, the louder the primary auditory signal relative to background sounds, the more intelligible that auditory signal will be for the child, and the better opportunity the child will have to learn the word/sound differences that underlie the development of basic academic competencies. The further the listener is from the desired sound source and the noisier the environment, the poorer the S/N ratio. See chapter 11 on "Classroom Acoustics" in this book for more information.

Persons with normal hearing and listening skills require a consistent S/N ratio of approximately +6 dB for the reception of intelligible speech. Because of internal auditory distortion, persons with any type and degree of hearing problem require a more favorable S/N ratio of about +20 dB. Due to noise, reverberation, and variations in teacher position, the S/N ratio in a typical classroom is unstable and averages out to only about +4 dB and may be 0 dB; less than ideal even for children with normal hearing.[19]

Rapid Speech Transmission Index

The negative effects of a typical classroom environment on the integrity of a speech signal probably have been underestimated. Leavitt and Flexer[20] used the Bruel and Kjaer Rapid Speech Transmission Index (RASTI) to measure the effects of a classroom environment on a speech-like signal. The RASTI signal, an amplitude-modulated broadband noise centered at 500 and 2000 Hz, was transmitted from the RASTI transmitter to the RASTI receiver that was placed at 17 different locations around a typical occupied classroom. The RASTI score is a measure of the integrity of signals as they are propagated across the physical space.[21] A perfect reproduction of the RASTI signal at the receiver has a score of 1.0.

Results showed that sound degradation occurred as the RASTI receiver was moved away from the RASTI transmitter as reflected by a decrease in RASTI scores. In the front row center seat, the most preferred seat, the RASTI score dropped to 0.83. In the back row, the RASTI score was only 0.55, reflecting a loss of 45% of equivalent speech intelligibility in a quiet, occupied classroom. Only at the 6 inch reference position could a perfect RASTI score of 1.0 be obtained. Note that the RASTI score represents only the loss of speech fidelity that might be expected at the student's ear or hearing aid microphone port in a quiet classroom. The additional negative effects of a child's hearing loss, weak auditory or language base, or attention problems are not measured by the RASTI score.

Even in a front-row center seat, the loss of critical speech information is noteworthy for a child who needs accurate data entry to learn. The most sophisticated of hearing aids cannot recreate those components of the speech signal that have been lost in transmission across the physical space of the classroom.

Issue of Acoustic Accessibility

The concept specified by the Rehabilitation Act of 1973 Section 504[22] that will enable audiologists to recommend classroom amplification systems for children in regular classrooms is called "acoustic accessibility." We can advocate, proactively, that a child's hearing problem interferes with that child's opportunity to have access to spoken instruction; therefore, that child is being denied an appropriate education. Recognize that schools typically function on a failure-based model. Classroom amplification systems may be provided for children with hearing problems only after they have failed one to three grades or are significantly behind their same-age peers. Because accommodations typically are not allocated to prevent failure, technology is often provided too late to enable the child to catch-up to grade level.[23]

Perform Speech-in-Noise Sound Field Testing

By adding only two speech tests to the basic audiometric test battery, an audiologist in a school or clinical setting can provide evidence that a child has a hearing problem that interferes with *acoustic accessibility of classroom instruction*. If a child's hearing problem limits acoustic accessibility, then by evoking Section 504 of the

Rehabilitation Act of 1973, we can advocate in a proactive fashion for an appropriate classroom amplification system. That is, we do not have to wait until a child fails and is eligible for special education funding under Individuals with Disabilities Education Act (IDEA),[24] before we can provide services.

To provide functional information about acoustic accessibility, word identification testing should be performed in the sound field in the *unaided* condition, first. If the child wears hearing aids, these same tests also can be performed in the aided condition. Appropriate speech stimuli for the language level of the child should be presented at the average loudness level that speech is received by a child in a favorable classroom environment—45 dB HL. If phonetically balanced (PB) words are presented at 40 dB sensation level (SL) under earphones only, functional information is not provided about accessibility to typical classroom instruction.

In addition, word identification testing in the sound field ought to be conducted at 45 dB HL using a +5 S/N ratio; a favorable noise level in a primary-level classroom.[2] A child might appear to hear very well in the acoustically perfect environment of a sound room but have a great deal of trouble hearing in a typical classroom.

PERSONNEL INVOLVED IN FITTING FM TECHNOLOGY

Role of the Audiologist

As specified by the American Speech-Language-Hearing Association (ASHA) Guidelines for Fitting and Monitoring FM Systems,[25] *the audiologist is the professional who is uniquely and best qualified to select, evaluate, fit, and dispense FM systems.* The necessity of having an audiologist as the "point person" is supported by the American Academy of Audiology, ASHA Codes of Ethics, and by federal regulations. There is a great deal of complexity involved in selecting the appropriate FM options and in fitting and evaluating the equipment. An inappropriate FM fit could be worse for a child than not wearing any amplification technology at all. An audiologist can instruct other personnel in performing daily monitoring checks; however, the audiologist must maintain the supervisory position.

Role of the Speech-Language Pathologist

Speech-language pathologists appropriately can perform daily monitoring of classroom amplification systems after they have received instruction from a licensed/certified audiologist. This monitoring role of the speech-language pathologist relative to FM systems is supported by ASHA's Preferred Practice Patterns for Professions of Speech-Language Pathology and Audiology,[26] ASHA's Scope of Practice: Speech-Language Pathology and Audiology,[27] and ASHA's Code of Ethics.[28] Speech-language pathologists also can (and indeed, should) refer children to an audiologist for an evaluation for FM technology when they encounter children whom they believe would benefit from an improved S/N ratio.

Role of Parents, the Mainstreamed Classroom Teacher, and Other Support Personnel

Parents, mainstreamed classroom teachers, and other personnel who will use the child's FM technology need to receive in-services about the FM equipment. Anyone who is expected to monitor the equipment needs to receive instruction and supervision from an audiologist.

SELF-CONTAINED AND PERSONAL FM SYSTEMS

Description

An FM unit is an assistive listening device that improves the S/N ratio for a child in a classroom by using a remote microphone that can be placed close to the sound source.

FM is a term applied to the radio transmission of signals whereby speech, after being changed into an electrical signal, is frequency modulated onto a carrier wave that is sent from the transmitter to the receiver where it is demodulated and delivered to the listener. A basic FM system consists of two units, a transmitter and receiver, and is like having an individual private radio station that transmits and receives on a single frequency. The FM receiver worn by the child must be set to the same radio frequency as the microphone/transmitter worn by the teacher or the child will not receive the desired signal. Because there are no wires connecting the speaker to the listener, both parties have free mobility. The transmission range can vary with different pieces of equipment from about 30 feet to more than 200 feet.

The speaker (parent, teacher, clinician, or peer) wears the transmitter microphone clipped on his or her clothes at the midline, no further than 6 inches from his or her mouth. Think of the FM microphone as the child's third ear and place that third ear within 6 inches of whatever you want the child to hear. The remote microphone of the FM transmitter improves the S/N ratio by being placed close to the primary sound source. The more favorable the S/N ratio, the more intelligible the speech signal received by the listener. Because sound is degraded as it is propagated across the classroom, the closer the child is to the speaker, either physically or technologically, the better acoustic access the child will have. Whenever a child with a hearing problem is in a classroom, S/N ratio enhancing technology will be necessary to improve intelligibility of the teacher's speech. A hearing aid alone is never enough in a classroom because the teacher physically cannot be consistently close to the child.

Cautions Regarding Use

FM systems can be of enormous benefit to children who have hearing problems in the classroom. Nevertheless, there are some limitations and cautions that ought to be noted. These issues have been emphasized by Ross,[29] and in ASHA's Guidelines for Fitting and Monitoring FM Systems.[25]

1. Many FM systems are purchased without consultation with an audiologist because FMs are available commercially. An audiologist should be the professional who is responsible for fitting, evaluating, and dispensing FM systems.
2. Although there is a committee in progress, the American National Standards Institute (ANSI) has not yet issued a standard for performance measurements of FM systems.
3. Currently, there is little regulatory consumer protection for FM fitting and use because most states do not classify these devices as hearing aids. The Food and Drug Administation may decide differently in the near future.
4. Studies have shown that there are real concerns about specific electroacoustic performance factors. Different FM units and coupling features have shown variability in performance, nonlinearity, lack of stability, and maintenance problems.
5. There are many issues that need to be considered when fitting FM systems on children, including candidacy, a child's many and varied listening/learning domains, effectiveness and flexibility of fit, cost, and psychosocial concerns.

Features of FM Systems

FM systems can be grouped into two general categories, depending on how the signal is delivered to the ear of the listener. A *basic, self-contained FM system* typically delivers the signal via a button receiver/earphone, and the FM receiver contains an environmental microphone or microphones, allowing the FM receiver also to function as a hearing aid (usually a body style hearing aid if the FM receiver is worn on the child's body). A *personal FM system* is similar to a self-contained system except that the child must wear his or her own personal hearing aids to deliver the signal.

The reader is referred to Mark Ross's book, *FM Auditory Training Systems, Characteristics, Selection, & Use,*[29] for additional information.

FM systems can be quite complicated to fit appropriately to a given child because of the many fitting and setting options currently available; there are advantages and disadvantages to each option. Therefore, not only must an audiologist be the professional to select, evaluate, fit, and dispense FM systems, but that audiologist should also in some way be involved in classroom observations and evaluations of FM settings and function. Ideally, there will be an educational audiologist who can manage the FM technology in school.

Self-Contained FM System

Some FM receivers are designed to function both as hearing aids and radio receivers. This self-contained system historically has been referred to as an FM auditory trainer. If the child wears hearing aids, he or she takes them off when wearing a self-contained unit. The signal is delivered to the child's ears typically through button earphones coupled to custom, snap ring earmolds (see Fig. 12–3a). The (hearing aid) environmental

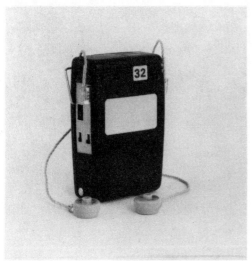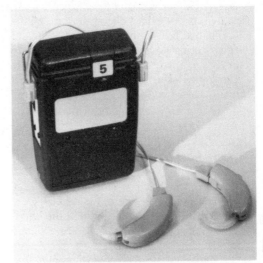

A   B

Figure 12–3. Self-contained FM systems, designed to function both as hearing aids and radio receivers, deliver the signal to the child's ears through button receivers (A) or through receivers housed in behind-the-ear cases (B) which also house the unit's environmental microphones. (Photographs courtesy of Telex Communications.)

microphone or microphones usually are on the FM receiver. Some units have the option of having the environmental microphones and receivers housed in behind-the-ear cases for more effective binaural hearing than body-worn microphones can allow (see Fig. 12–3b).

A bone conduction transducer can be used with some FM receivers. This transducer would be necessary for children who have atresia. A bone conduction transducer could be a viable option for children who have stenotic ear canals or who experience continually draining ears from chronic otitis media.

Most self-contained units have "trimmer screws" or "trim pots" for adjustment of maximum output and frequency response for each ear, as well as for the relationship between FM micro-

phone and environmental microphone sensitivity (see Fig. 12–4).

An audiologist must adjust these trimmer screws appropriately for each child who is fitted with a self-contained unit. Most children who are fitted with self-contained units have severe to profound hearing impairments.

Some audiologists fit self-contained FM units as the primary amplification for infants and young children with severe to profound hearing impairments.[30] The rationale is that FM units can provide superior auditory access, even in home environments.

An audiologist might fit an FM unit instead of a hearing aid for children with more minimal hearing problems as well. However, in this instance, the FM is not intended to function like

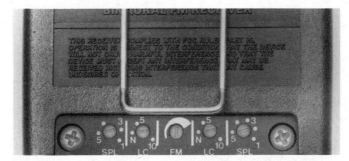

Figure 12–4. Most self-contained FM units have trimmer screws for adjustment of maximum output, frequency response, and for the relationship between FM microphone and environmental microphone sensitivity; these trimmer screws must be adjusted appropriately by an audiologist for each child. (Photograph courtesy of Telex Communications).

a hearing aid but is meant to enhance the S/N ratio in a mainstreamed classroom for children with minimal hearing problems, including unilateral hearing loss, fluctuating hearing impairments, normal peripheral hearing but central auditory processing problems, or attending difficulties. This arrangement will be covered under personal FM systems.

Personal FM Systems

The term "personal FM system" usually refers to an arrangement whereby the FM signal is channeled in some fashion through the child's own hearing aids. For a personal FM system to work, the child's hearing aids must be operating well and must efficiently receive the signal from the FM unit. If the hearing aids are not working, then the FM cannot work either.

The primary coupling options for this arrangement are neckloop, silhouette, and direct-input. Each of these coupling arrangements can alter, often in some unpredictable fashion, the output and frequency response characteristics of the hearing aid.

Neckloop. With a neckloop coupling, the electrical signal from the FM receiver is sent to a wire or loop that is worn loosely around the child's neck and is attached to the FM receiver (see Fig. 12–5a). The neckloop generates an electromagnetic field that is picked up by the T attachment on the child's hearing aid or aids and then amplified. Of course, the hearing aids must be equipped with a strong telecoil appropriately positioned in the hearing aid case. To access the many and diverse listening environments that the child must be in, the hearing aids need to have a three switch setting: M to access the hearing aid's microphone, alone; T to access the hearing aid's telecoil that picks-up the signal from the FM microphone, alone; MT together to pick up both the FM signal and environmental sounds and the child's own voice, all at the same time. Each setting has advantages and disadvantages.

A potential problem with neckloop fittings is that a hearing aid's telecoil rarely has the same maximum output and frequency response characteristics as the microphone; the telecoil typically is weaker and tends to roll off the low-frequency end of the hearing aid's frequency response. In addition, there can often be an increase in internal noise, and signal strength can change with changing head positions. Performance measures need to be obtained.

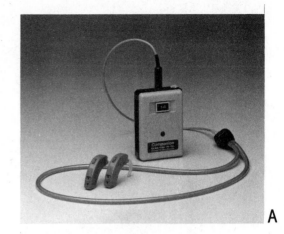

A

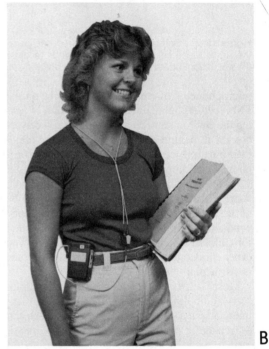

B

Figure 12–5. A neckloop generates an electromagnetic field that is picked up by the T attachment on the child's hearing aids and then amplified (A). (Photograph courtesy of Comtek and Audio Enhancement.) There are no connecting wires between the FM receiver and the person's hearing aids (B). (Photograph courtesy of Telex Communications.)

If an appropriate acoustic fit can be obtained, advantages to a neckloop fitting include:

1. There are no connecting wires between the FM receiver and the child's hearing aid (see Fig. 12–5b)
2. The neckloop can be worn under clothes, which might meet the psychosocial needs of

a particular child, facilitating FM acceptance (a child who refuses to wear an FM receiver with any wires showing may accept a neckloop fit)

3. The FM receiver can be worn in a belt pack or fanny pack provided that the environmental microphone on the FM receiver (if there is one) is turned off. If the environmental microphone is "on" in a fanny pack, think of what that child is hearing. Certainly, clothing and floor noises would mask any intelligible instructional information.

Silhouette.   A T-coil in the hearing aid also is needed for a silhouette coupling because this coupling operates on principles similar to the neckloop. The silhouette is actually a wafer-shaped piece of plastic worn between the head and the hearing aid; the silhouette generates an electromagnetic field. A wire connects the silhouette with the FM receiver. A silhouette has the advantage of minimizing signal variation because the position of the silhouette relative to the hearing aid remains constant with changes in head position. A potential wearer-perceived disadvantage is that there is a visible wire.

Direct Input.   For a direct input connection, the electrical signal from the FM receiver flows through a wire directly into the hearing aid via an audio-shoe or boot (see Fig. 12-6). The hearing aid must be equipped with a special feature that would allow it to accommodate a boot. There are many different shapes of boots; some fit snugly on the hearing aid and some fit so loose

that the signal is disrupted easily. The appropriate boot and cords can be obtained from the hearing aid manufacturer. Note that there can be some change in the output signal with FM coupling.

No Hearing Aids.   Children who do not wear hearing aids and who are fit with FM systems for the single purpose of providing a consistent and favorable S/N ratio, also are described as wearing personal FM systems. That is, *the FM is not intended to function as a hearing aid, but is fit to enhance acoustic accessibility of intelligible speech and to provide instructional redundancy in a classroom environment.* Children who are fit with this intention in mind require a low-power output unit that also has low gain. The gain and output must be specified, known, measured, and controlled by an audiologist.

Coupling arrangements used in this instance may include lightweight Walkman earphones (Fig. 12-7), earbuds, stetoclips, and button earphones attached to special custom earmolds.

Walkman Earphones.   As shown in Figure 12-7, lightweight Walkman type earphones commonly are used to deliver a monophonic signal (same signal to each ear compared with stereophonic). Because they are lightweight, the child still can hear surrounding sounds. Although suitable for short periods of time, many children find the earphones uncomfortable for 6 hours of daily use. Earbuds and stetoclips, because they are not custom fitted, also may become uncomfortable. For long-term continual use, custom earmolds, or a retention earmold with tubing, may be more acceptable to a child. Keep in mind that *any*

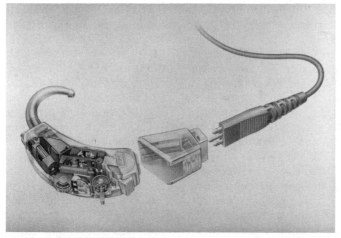

Figure 12-6.   For a direct-input connection, the electrical signal from the FM receiver flows through a wire directly into the hearing aid via an audio shoe or boot. (Photograph courtesy of Phonic Ear.)

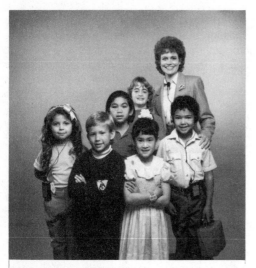

Figure 12–7. When appropriate, a child can be fit with a low-power output FM unit to improve the speech-to-noise ratio in a classroom; the signal can be delivered to a child's ears through lightweight Walkman type earphones. (Photograph courtesy of Phonic Ear.)

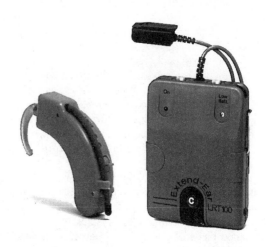

Figure 12–8. Recent technological developments have provided the option of a hearing aid and an FM receiver both housed together in a behind-the-ear hearing aid case. (Photograph courtesy of AVR Sonovation.)

earmold or earpiece potentially changes ear canal resonance.

Telecoil Transducer. An interesting arrangement that has been acceptable to some older children is the use of a telecoil transducer worn with a neckloop. A strong telecoil (no hearing aid components, just a telecoil) is housed in a canal-style case and worn in the ear canal—or one telecoil transducer can be worn in each ear canal for reception of a binaural FM signal. The neckloop is worn under clothing and the FM receiver is carried in a belt pack. The child thus receives an improved S/N ratio with no visible components. As an interesting aside, some actors use this arrangement, unknown to their audiences, to receive cues for their lines.

Behind the Ear FM Receiver. Recent new technological developments have provided the option of a hearing aid and an FM receiver both housed together in a behind-the-ear hearing aid case (see Fig. 12–8). There is no body-worn FM receiver. Of course, the speaker still needs to wear a microphone transmitter. The child can, by moving a switch, have the unit function as a hearing aid only, an FM receiver only, or as both a hearing aid and FM receiver at the same time.

The more options available, the better chance we have of providing an appropriate and consumer-acceptable S/N ratio enhancing device. No single coupling arrangement is automatically superior for all children. The individuality of each child must be considered.

Children Who Could Benefit from FM Use

Anytime a child with a hearing problem is in a classroom or cannot be close to the speaker, an improved S/N ratio will be necessary to facilitate the reception of an intact, consistent, and clear speech signal. It used to be thought that preferential seating was enough. However, information about classroom acoustics (see Chapter 11 in this text) shows that hearing aids alone, no matter how "good" the hearing aid is, cannot substitute for an FM unit in a classroom or in any environment in which the speaker cannot be consistently close to the child.

Fit an FM Unit First on Some Children. There are some instances, such as when a child has a unilateral hearing loss, a fluctuating hearing loss, or a slight permanent hearing impairment, when it might be more effective to fit a mild gain personal FM unit or a sound field FM system instead of, or before, a hearing aid. To explain, a child with the types of hearing problems just mentioned might do fine in a quiet, one-to-one learning situation, but the same child *will* have difficulty in a typical, noisy, distracting classroom. Thus, it makes sense to address the most pressing concern first; classroom listening.

Audiological Management and Monitoring of FM Equipment

There are many audiological management issues to be considered. A child who has a hearing problem and is wearing an FM system should hear the teacher much better when the teacher speaks into the FM microphone. If the child does not hear better with an FM system then without it, check the FM. Is the fit appropriate? Is there interference? Any number of problems could occur. My experience has been that whenever a teacher says that a child does not seem to benefit from an FM system, the FM system has been malfunctioning in some way or has not been fitted or used appropriately. Double check the equipment and teacher use first—do not just remove it. Observe, personally, how the equipment is actually set up and used in the classroom. For example, a mainstreamed kindergarten boy with a moderate conductive hearing loss due to congenital ossicular malformations told his teacher that he heard much better with his hearing aids then he did with his FM unit; the school system was ready to allocate his FM unit to someone else. The child had been fit with a personal FM with a neckloop coupling. His hearing aids had a good telecoil and *M, T,* and *MT* settings. FM performance features were appropriate for the child and the teacher had been taught about equipment use. However, a visit to the classroom revealed that the equipment was not being used as intended. The school had substituted a different FM transmitter for the original one. Unfortunately, the new transmitter was set to a different carrier frequency than the child's receiver. In addition, the teacher had put the child's hearing aids on *T* (they should have been on *MT*), but the receiver was not picking up the teacher's voice anyway (wrong transmission frequency). That is, the child was hearing only static with the FM. Of course he heard better with his hearing aids. When the personal FM was set, adjusted, and used appropriately, this child heard very well and insisted on wearing his FM unit. This teacher obviously had not been performing listening checks on the equipment or she would have discovered that something was wrong. Moreover, this school system did not have an educational audiologist. The director of special education made the decision to change FM transmitters.

Following are some management issues to consider.

Microphones. There are many microphone options. Do we want directional or omnidirectional microphones? Do we want lapel or boom microphones for the transmitter? Do we want to use the FM microphone only, or do we want environmental microphones, too? Do we have environmental microphones at ear level, or are they on the body, or in a pocket, or on the desk, or in a belt pack? How many of them are there? What is the relationship between the FM microphone sensitivity to environmental microphone sensitivity? Think of each active microphone as an "ear" and be sure to identify the location of all ears (See Fig. 12–9).

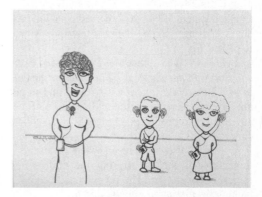

Figure 12–9. Think of each active microphone as an "ear," and know where each ear is located; are all of those ears necessary or are they counterproductive? (Illustration by Josh Klynn.)

The more active microphones, the poorer the S/N ratio. A single directional FM transmitter microphone worn on the head of the speaker (boom microphone) would provide the best S/N ratio. Unfortunately, most children object to not hearing their own speech and the speech of their peers. Thus, microphone use is not a simple matter, nor is it a fixed variable. That is, sometimes the child needs to hear the teacher only, and sometimes the child needs to monitor the environment, monitor his or her own voice, or hear peers.

One solution is to teach the child to control his or her own technology use as mentioned previously—the child switches technology as needed. Another option is to have a teacher (FM) microphone that preempts the child's environmental microphone. Whenever the teacher speaks into the FM microphone, the environmental microphones on the FM receiver automatically are turned off. Some personal FM systems offer this feature.

Another issue about microphone use is that people who are not speaking into the FM microphone will not be heard well, or perhaps not heard at all. So, teachers either will have to pass the FM microphone around to classmates or repeat other's comments.

Capture Effect. The capture effect of FM systems can be a problem for classroom use. As described by Medwetsky,[31] when two or more FM signals are transmitted at the same frequency, the FM receiver responds only to the stronger of the two signals. If the teacher's voice is the strongest signal in the receiver's environment, then the capture effect works in our favor. However, if an outside source such as a CB radio, or a paging system, or the school's radio station produces a stronger signal, then the unwanted signal is picked up.

A child's FM system should be listened to by a person with normal hearing in the environments in which the child functions. An FM unit might not have interference in the audiologist's office, but might be receiving other signals in the child's classroom.

A problem also could result when the teacher's transmitter is turned off, but the child's FM receiver remains on. The receiver is at risk for picking up unwanted sounds due to the capture effect when the strongest signal of the teacher's voice is off.

Daily Monitoring of FM Systems. The one certainty about equipment is that it will malfunction at some point in time. FM breakdowns occur even in normal use situations. Therefore, daily monitoring is essential. A daily visual and listening check should be performed by an audiologist or by someone who has been instructed in the appropriate procedures by an audiologist; speech-language pathologists, parents, and teachers often fill this role. The procedure should be performed by someone with normal hearing in the environment in which the child will be learning. Evans[32] has developed detailed procedures and charts for troubleshooting FM systems.

Spare supplies and equipment should be available to remedy easy-to-fix problems. Examples of supplies include batteries, neckloops, microphones, button receivers, boots, and cords.

Comprehensive Monitoring of FM Systems. Children with hearing impairment who are 3 years and younger should be seen by their audiologist every 3 months for comprehensive evaluation, including FM monitoring. Older children should be seen by their audiologist at least every 6 months. As recommended by ASHA,[25] these assessments may include, but are not limited to: audiologic evaluations, assessments of speech recognition, coupler and real ear performance measurements of hearing aids and FM equipment, consultations with school personnel, observation of FM performance in school settings, and subjective scales of performance benefit.

Performance Measures

There are no validated procedures for measuring and fitting FM systems. Several approaches have been proposed,[33-35] and these have been incorporated into the Guidelines for Fitting and Monitoring FM Systems adopted by the ASHA Legislative Council in November 1993.[25] These guidelines highlight four issues that need to be considered in developing FM measurement strategies:

1. Because the FM microphone is located about 6 inches from the speaker's mouth, *the input level of speech to the FM microphone is more intense than to a hearing aid microphone* that is located about 1 to 2 m from the speaker in a favorable situation. The overall level of speech to an FM microphone is about 80 to 85 dB sound pressure level (SPL) which is about 10 to 20 dB more intense than the typical 60 to 70 dB SPL input to the microphone of a hearing aid. Therefore, if appropriate output measurements are being made to adjust FM systems, then typical input levels should be used. The higher level is particularly important because most FM microphone transmitters use some type of input compression; the gain and output of the FM system could be quite different if lower-level signals are used.

2. *Many FM systems have more than one microphone input possibility.* There could be lapel, lavalier, boom, or conference microphones for the FM transmitter. The FM receiver could have one or two environmental microphones and they could be on the body or at ear level. In addition, the microphones could be omnidirectional or directional. Each input channel in the FM system needs to be evaluated and the microphones need to be positioned appropriately. Input levels would be different for environmental microphones and FM microphones.

3. *Many FM systems have more than one volume control wheel*; some units have one volume control wheel for the FM signal and another one for the environmental microphone

or microphones. On personal FM systems, there will be one volume control wheel for the FM system and one for each personal hearing aid. There also might be a volume control on the FM microphone transmitter. Careful thought needs to be given to the setting and measurement of each volume control wheel.

4. *FM systems are physically arranged on the user in different ways.* Testing procedures need to account for these differences.

Please refer to the Appendix A for the following performance measurements proposed by ASHA:[25]

1. Outline for FM system adjustment using 2 cm³ coupler measurements.
2. Outline for FM system adjustment using probe-microphone measurements.
3. Speech recognition measures with FM systems and personal hearing aid or aids.

SOUND FIELD FM SYSTEMS

Description

Sound field FM systems, an exciting educational tool, allow control of the acoustic environment in a classroom, thereby facilitating acoustic accessibility of teacher instruction for all children in the room. Sound field FM systems are like high-fidelity, wireless, public address systems. By using this technology, an entire classroom can be amplified through the use of two, three, or four wall- or ceiling-mounted loudspeakers. Figure 12–10a, b shows two different sound field units. The teacher wears a wireless FM microphone transmitter, just like the one worn for a personal FM unit, and the radio signal is sent to an amplifier that is connected to the loudspeakers. There are no wires connecting the teacher with the equipment. The radio link allows the teacher to move about freely, unrestricted by wires (see Fig. 12–11a, b).

Features of Sound Field FM Systems

A sound field FM system is one type of assistive listening device. Like a personal FM unit, it improves the S/N ratio by the use of a remote microphone that can be placed close to the desired sound source. Through the loudspeakers,

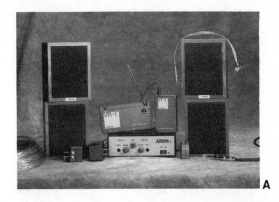

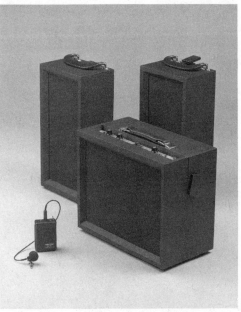

Figure 12–10. Two different sound field FM units (A, B). (Photogaphs courtesy of Lifeline Amplification Systems and Comtek and Audio Enhancments.)

the loudness of the teacher's speech is increased relative to the background noise, allowing all children in the room to benefit from an improved and consistent S/N ratio no matter where they or the teacher are located.

A major difference between a sound field FM unit and a personal FM system is that the personal FM, if fit appropriately, can provide the most favorable S/N ratio; +20 to +30 dB. When wearing a personal FM unit, the speech signal goes directly from the microphone transmitter that is located about 6 inches from the teacher's mouth, into the ear of the child who is wearing the FM receiver. When using a sound field unit, the teacher's speech is transmitted from the

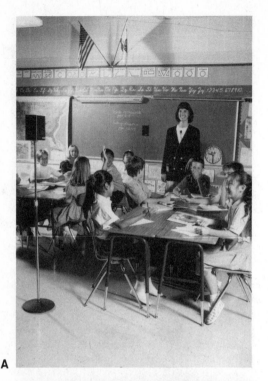

A

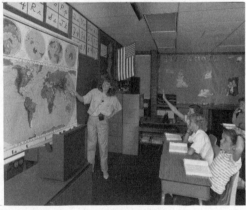

B

Figure 12–11. Two different sound field FM units set up in classrooms (A, B). (Photographs courtesy of Phonic Ear and Comtek and Audio Enhancement.)

microphone worn 6 inches from the mouth to the amplifier/loudspeackers that are located at some distance from the children. The children can be consistently closer to loudspeakers than they can be to the teacher, but not as close as a child could be to the headphones of an FM unit. Sound field FM systems typically improve the classroom S/N ratio by about 10 dB.

Therefore, *sound field FM units are not replacements for personal FM systems because some children require the more favorable S/N ratio provided by a personal FM. Sound field FM*

technology offers audiologists another tool to select from when recommending appropriate classroom amplification systems.

Children Who Might Benefit from Sound Field FM Systems

It could be argued that virtually all children could benefit from sound field FM systems because the improved S/N ratio creates a more favorable learning environment. If children could hear better, clearer, and more consistently, they would have an opportunity to learn more efficiently. Some school systems have as a goal the amplification of every classroom in their districts.[6]

To return to the previous computer analogy, the better and more reliable the keyboard, the more accurate are the entered data. Even adults with normal hearing, language, and auditory processing skills are able to attend better when listening to a well-amplified lecture.

No one disputes the necessity of creating a favorable visual field in a classroom. A school building never would be constructed without lights in every classroom. However, because hearing is invisible and ambiguous, the necessity of creating a favorable auditory field may be questioned by school personnel. Nevertheless, studies continue to show that sound field FM systems facilitate opportunities for improved academic performance.[6,7,36–38]

The following populations seem to be especially in need of sound field S/N ratio-enhancing technology.

1. Children with fluctuating conductive hearing impairments, primarily caused by ear infections or ear wax. Because one fourth to one third of typical kindergarten and first grade children do not hear normally on any given day,[6,7] it seems reasonable to amplify every preschool, kindergarten, and first grade classroom. The ability to hear word/sound distinctions is a primary basis for the development of academic competencies.[11] If young children are at risk for having hearing problems and thus learning phonemic distinctions, why not create an acoustic environment that would enable them to receive intelligible speech consistently and clearly?

2. Children with unilateral hearing impairments also will benefit from a sound field FM system. Some children with unilateral hearing losses may require the more favorable S/N ratio of a personal FM unit, especially if they have major attending problems and language delays.

3. Children with slight permanent hearing impairments (15 to 20 dB HL) might benefit more from sound field FM than from a hearing aid in a classroom environment. Once again, depending on the degree of accompanying attending, learning, and language problems, a personal FM unit might be more suitable.

4. Children who have normal peripheral hearing sensitivity but who are in special education classrooms due to language, learning, attending, or behavioral problems would benefit from the increased instructional redundancy provided by a sound field FM unit. Note that several studies have found that as many as three fourths of the children who are in primary level special education classrooms do not have normal hearing sensitivity, and their hearing problems usually have not been identified nor managed by the school systems.[6,7,37]

5. Children with mild to moderate hearing impairments who wear hearing aids might do as well with a sound field FM unit as they would with a personal FM system.

6. Children who have normal peripheral hearing sensitivity but who have difficulty processing, understanding, or attending to classroom instruction could benefit from sound field FM technology. As stated previously, a child with a more severe central auditory processing problem might need the more favorable S/N ratio provided by a personal FM unit.

7. Children for whom English is a second language benefit from a more intelligible signal provided by the enhanced S/N ratio of a sound field FM system.[36] When one is learning a new language, how much of the acoustic signal needs to be heard to differentiate the new words of the language? *All of the signal*, every sound, every syllable, every word marker; the entire message needs to be intelligible because there is not an internal program in the new language in the child's brain that would enable the child to fill in the blanks.

8. Teachers who use sound field technology report that they also benefit. Many state that they need to use less energy projecting their voices, they have less vocal abuse, and are less tired by the end of the school day. Teachers also report that the unit increases their efficiency as teachers, requiring fewer repetitions, thus allowing for more actual teaching time. One school system noted fewer teacher absences from amplified classrooms.[6]

With more and more schools incorporating principles of inclusion where children who would have been in self-contained placements are in the mainstream classroom, sound field FM systems offer a way of enhancing the classroom learning environment for the benefit of *all* children. It is a win-win situation.

Audiological Equipment Selection Considerations

There are many issues to consider prior to recommending sound field FM equipment.

1. *Should an audiologist recommend a personal FM system or a sound field FM system for a given child?*

Once we determine that a child has a hearing problem that interferes with acoustic accessibility, the next step involves recommending, fitting, and using some type of S/N ratio-enhancing technology. One thing is certain, we cannot manage hearing by not managing hearing. For example, a school system admitted that a kindergarten child with a persistent mild to moderate hearing impairment from chronic otitis media had enormous problems with hearing classroom instructions. They went on to state that they had no money for any S/N ratio-enhancing technology to manage her hearing in the classroom and wanted to know what else they could do that would not cost any money. In other words, they wanted to know how to manage hearing without providing any way for the child to hear better. This child was in a mainstreamed classroom environment where the entire instructional basis is auditory, yet they knowingly would deny her acoustic accessibility to primary instructional information! What they wanted to do was illogical, unreasonable, and illegal. Even though this child had *not yet* failed enough to be eligible for special education funds and intervention through IDEA,[24] she did qualify for assistance under Section 504 of the Rehabilitation Act of 1973[22] that mandates acoustic accessibility. Please recognize that the recommendation of preferential seating does not control the background noise and reverberation in the classroom nor does it stabilize teacher or pupil position, nor does it provide for an even and consistent S/N ratio. The recommendation of preferential seating serves the purpose of having the school system think that they are doing something to manage hearing without really doing anything to manage hearing.

The point is, as audiologists, we must not equivocate on our recommendation for S/N ratio-enhancing technology. If a child cannot hear clearly in a classroom, his or her opportunities for academic success are sabotaged. As audiologists and speech-language pathologists, we can attempt to help the school system obtain funding (see later). However, we cannot back down on our recommendation and deny the importance of S/N ratio-enhancing technology simply because the acquisition of that technology is inconvenient for the school system.

Once we establish that S/N ratio-enhancing technology is important for a particular child, we need to make an initial decision regarding the specific technology to recommend. We do know that children with more severe hearing impairments and with more severe auditory processing and attending problems benefit more from the superior S/N ratio provided by an appropriately fit personal FM system. In addition, a child with a permanent hearing impairment will require S/N ratio-enhancing technology throughout his or her school career, including post secondary education. It is unlikely that every classroom will be amplified for this child, so a personal FM system would be a more parsimonious recommendation because it could be brought by the child to each class.

2. *What factors need to be considered for selection of a sound field unit?*

There are several companies that manufacture sound field FM equipment and some people assemble their own equipment from component parts sold by companies such as Radio Shack. More companies are getting into the business as time goes on. The cost of current units varies from about $650 to $2000, depending on the quality of the equipment, the number of loudspeakers, service contracts, ease of installation, durability, special features such as extra microphones, and flexibility. Refer to Berg[2] for an in-depth discussion of sound field FM components. A high-quality, permanently installed public address and sound system, such as that used in a theater, can cost thousands of dollars. Selection issues to evaluate include:

a. What is the carrier frequency of the radio signal? Manufacturers use different frequency bands, some of which are very crowded, and thus are subject to interference. For example, much of the equipment that is assembled from component parts purchased from outlets such as Radio Shack, use the same transmission/carrier frequency bands as AT&T.

b. Consider the number of available discrete channels within the frequency band used by the manufacturer. Does it meet your needs? Some sound field FM systems have only two to four discrete channels available. This means that only two to four units could be used in a building without potentially interfering with one another. Conversely, the more discrete channels that a frequency band is divided into, the poorer the S/N ratio might be. Too few bands limit the number of units that can be used in a building, while too many bands per carrier frequency might cause interference and an unfavorable S/N ratio within the equipment itself.

c. How many loudspeakers should be ordered for a particular classroom? More research is required on this issue, but to have an even and consistent S/N ratio throughout a typical classroom, it appears that at least three loudspeakers are required. Larger classrooms may require four or more loudspeakers, whereas a smaller resource room or therapy room may need only one or two loudspeakers.

d. How should loudspeakers be positioned around the classroom? Unfortunately, there are no data-based guidelines for speaker placement. Some manufacturers recommend placement of loudspeakers at the children's ear level on speaker stands. Others recommend placement three quarters of the way up a wall or mounted in the ceiling. Many schools position loudspeakers on available shelves or cabinets, safely out of the way of curious hands. Placement near the ceiling can cause additional reverberation, whereas placement too low can cause feedback when the teacher's microphone comes in-line with a loudspeaker. Some recommend placing the loudspeakers near the four corners of the room to bathe the room in an even sound. Others say to amplify the primary teaching/learning centers in a classroom. Some placement strategies include: making sound level measurements,[37] obtaining RASTI scores, and just listening to the sound of the unit, called "ear cuing." Speech heard through a sound field system should be easily and uniformly audible from and at all locations throughout the classroom. In addition, speech should be comfortably intelligible and nonstressful. Note that an empty classroom might sound different from an occupied classroom. That is, we typically install a unit in an empty room. Then, when the children arrive with their sound absorbent bodies and their noise-generating properties, the sound field unit might need to be readjusted.

e. What is the durability, quality, and service availability of the system? How robust is the equipment? Equipment that is fickle or that breaks down easily is of no value to anyone. How easily and quickly can equipment be repaired? Are loaner units and parts available? How supportive is the manufacturer?

f. What is the portability, flexibility, and ease of installation of the equipment? Some units are meant to be permanently installed, whereas others need to be moved to other rooms or within a room as seating arrangements and teaching styles change. How easy is it to move the loudspeakers and connecting speaker wires?

g. What is the overall fidelity of the equipment? Room acoustics shape the signal. It appears that a high-frequency emphasis enhances the intelligibility of speech and enables children to detect word/sound differences better.[37] Does the equipment crackle? Is there interference? Does the signal sound like it is on the verge of feedback when set to a comfortable listening level?

A sound field FM system is meant to be a valuable teaching tool that facilitates classroom instruction, thereby enhancing learning. If equipment malfunctions in any way or interferes with teaching, teachers likely will turn off the unit rather than fix the problem.

3. *How can we entice school systems to try sound field FM technology?*

a. Audiologists and speech-language pathologists need to recognize that most school personnel have limited information about the relationship of hearing and hearing problems to academic performance.[12] Thus, discussions and recommendations of S/N ratio-enhancing technology need to be preceded by discussions about hearing and the acoustic filter effect of hearing loss as presented in the first part of this chapter.

b. Most people have no idea about the value of sound field FM systems until they actually hear and experience the equipment for themselves. Equipment demonstrations and allowing opportunities for trial periods are necessary strategies.

c. Administrative support is critical for successful equipment utilization. Building principals, directors of special education, school superintendents, and the school board all need to be informed and supportive. Without their support, classroom amplification projects could fail.

d. Provide in-service education to teachers before the equipment is installed in their rooms. Teachers need to have an opportunity to become enthusiastic about this new teaching tool and to volunteer to use it. Equipment that is forced on a frightened, skeptical, or timid teacher probably will not be used. Training needs to cover the importance of hearing, the acoustic filter effect of hearing loss, the rationale for classroom amplification, and strategies for equipment use.

e. Assure teachers that they will have a trial period and that equipment will be removed if they do not find it helpful. Almost all teachers find sound field FM technology to be an invaluable teaching tool once they have an opportunity to experience its effectiveness in their own classroom.

f. Do everything possible to assure that the first sound field FM unit that is installed in a school district or in a school building is a successful experience. That is, the equipment has to work efficiently and effectively and the teacher must be a willing participant. If that first unit is a dismal experience, then the school system will not be receptive to additional units. Spend additional time in the classroom with that first teacher. Provide support, suggestions for operation, and encouragement. If that first teacher promotes sound field equipment use, then other children in that district likely will have opportunities to benefit from additional units. On the other hand, if that first teacher spreads the word that sound field classroom amplification systems are distracting, too much work, or not helpful, then other teachers tend to become resistant.

g. A critical variable is the presence of a support/contact person within or easily available to the school district to install the equipment, to present training, and to monitor equipment function and use. Classroom amplification systems represent a significant change for school systems both in operation and philosophy, and that change requires a facilitator. Without a facilitator/

support person, equipment might not be used or may be used inefficiently.

OBTAINING FUNDING FOR FM TECHNOLOGY

A major issue relative to FM equipment use is money. Who is going to pay for this technology? A personal FM unit costs from $500 to $1200 for a transmitter and receiver. For some units, coupling options (earphones, neckloops, direct-input cords, and boots), battery chargers, and patch cords all are extra. Sound field FM units can cost from $650 to $2000.

One point to emphasize when advocating for S/N ratio-enhancing technology for a student is that acoustic accessibility is not a luxury—it is a necessity. Hearing is a first-order event for children in mainstreamed classrooms. If a child cannot clearly and consistently hear classroom instruction, the entire premise of the educational system is undermined. Few families or schools have money for devices that are perceived as frills. However, when hearing takes its proper place at the head of the line relative to academic opportunities, then recommendations for S/N ratio-enhancing technology are taken seriously.

Client Pays and Controls Equipment Use

Some families choose to purchase FM equipment themselves, especially personal FM systems. If a family owns the technology, they control its maintenance and use. They can perform listening checks and trouble-shooting procedures themselves each day and know that malfunctions will be recognized immediately. They can use the unit on weekends and holidays. They can expedite repairs because they do not need to get the unit to the proper department in the school and then wait for a purchase order.

Most important, families can purchase an FM unit in a timely fashion. Some school systems are organized to act promptly. However, many schools require meetings for individual education plan development or revisions, and for budget reallocation. Some schools might need a legal proceeding to show that the FM unit is necessary for a child. Delays from one semester to over 1 year could result. Time is not on our

side. The longer a child is forced to function with the unnecessary barrier of acoustic inaccessibility, the further behind the child will get.

Community Agencies Pay

Local civic groups (like the Lion's club or Quota club), Parent-Teacher Associations, Foundations, and individuals have donated personal and sound field FM equipment to school systems or to individual families. Unless the donor wishes to remain anonymous, the local newspaper can be invited to record the "passing over of the microphone." The donor's name also can be engraved on a plaque that is placed in the school or on the equipment.[39]

School Pays and Controls Equipment Use

There are three primary federal laws that mandate audiological services for children in schools: Education for All Handicapped Children Act of 1975 (Public Law 94-142)[40] Education of the Handicapped Act Amendments of 1986 (Public Law 99-457 that reauthorized and expanded Public Law 94-142);[41] and the Rehabilitation Act of 1973, Section 504.[22] In 1990, Public Law 99-457 was amended by Congress. Its name was changed to IDEA.[24]

All of these laws require that children with disabilities have access to a Free Appropriate Public Education. Please refer to Chapter 1 in this book and to Flexer[42] for detailed information about federal laws. Note that federal law supports the full spectrum of audiological services required for hearing management of children of all ages and with all degrees of hearing problems.

SOME FINAL COMMON SENSE TIPS ABOUT FM USE

Following are several points common to both types of FM equipment that could facilitate use and function.

Try the Equipment

People must experience FM equipment for themselves; they cannot speculate about function.

When asked if they want an FM unit or if they believe that an FM system could be important to them, if they have not tried it already, teachers and students will almost always decline usage saying they do not really need it—they are doing just fine right now without any special technology.[43,44] Often, the direct approach is the best one. Try saying, listen to this equipment. Try on this unit.

Be Mindful of Appropriate Microphone Placement

Teachers have been known to place the FM microphone on necklaces, on waistbands, way off to the side on their clothing, or on a flimsy collar that turns inside-out with the microphone weight. Inservice presentations to teachers need to stress that microphone placement dramatically affects the output speech spectrum. Specifically, high frequencies are weaker in off-axis positions. A headset, boom microphone probably provides the best, most complete and consistent signal. If a lapel microphone is worn, it should be placed midline on the chest about 6 inches from the mouth.

Check the Batteries First

Not surprisingly, when any malfunction occurs, check the batteries first. Weak battery charge can cause interference, static, and intermittent signals.

Audiologists Should Write Clear Recommendations for FM Equipment

At the beginning of this chapter, eight examples were given about children who received recommendations for FM technology. Unfortunately, even though they were very different children, they all received the same recommendation, "FM use recommended."

As stated earlier, the audiologist is the professional who is uniquely qualified to select, fit, and dispense FM systems. If the school is purchasing the systems, the audiologist needs to carefully specify:

1. The rationale for an FM recommendation
2. The type of S/N ratio technology most appropriate, self-contained or personal FM system, or sound field FM unit

3. The frequency response and output characteristics of the equipment
4. The coupling arrangement chosen
5. Examples of specific FM units that would meet specifications could be provided
6. That the child must return to the audiologist with the FM unit (if the unit is a self-contained or personal FM system) for a performance evaluation
7. That inservicing needs to be provided to all who will use the equipment
8. That classroom observations need to occur for both personal and sound field FM technology.

SUMMARY

The purpose of this chapter has been to identify, discuss, and solve many issues regarding recommendations, management, and use of classroom amplification systems.

Hearing is a first-order event in a mainstream classroom. If a child cannot clearly hear spoken instruction, the entire premise of the educational system is undermined. Due to poor acoustic conditions and a variety of hearing and attending problems, there are millions of children who are being denied an appropriate education due to the lack of acoustic accessibility.

Classroom amplification systems can enhance significantly the classroom learning environment by improving the S/N ratio. The better and more consistent the S/N ratio, the more intelligible will be the teacher's spoken instruction.

Audiologists and speech-language pathologists are uniquely positioned to make critical differences for children. We must not underestimate the power of hearing. Our advocacy for a child could mean the difference between success or failure in school.

REFERENCES

1. Pimentel RG: Classroom amplification systems for the partially hearing student, in Roeser R, Downs M, eds: *Auditory Disorders in School Children*, ed 2 (New York: Thieme Medical Publishers, 1988), chap 12.
2. Berg FS: *Acoustics & Sound Systems in Schools* (San Diego: Singular Publishing Group, 1993).
3. Bess FH, McConnell FE: *Audiology, Education, and the Hearing-Impaired Child* (St. Louis: C.V. Mosby, 1981).
4. Upfold LJ: Children with hearing aids in the 1980's: etiologies and severity of impairment. *Ear Hear,* 9 (1988), 75–80.

5. Anderson KL: Hearing conservation in the public schools revisited. *Semin Hear,* 12 (1991), 340–364.

6. Flexer C: Turn on sound: An odyssey of sound-field amplification. *Educ Audiol Assoc Newslet,* 5 (1989), 6–7.

7. Ray H, Sarff LS, Glassford FE: Soundfield amplification: an innovative educational intervention for mainstreamed learning disabled students. *Directive Teacher,* 6 (1984), 18–20.

8. Blair JC: Services needed, in Berg FS, Blair JC, Viehweg SH, Wilson-Vlotman A, eds: *Educational Audiology for the Hard of Hearing Child* (New York: Grune & Stratton, 1986), chap 2.

9. Berg FS: Characteristics of the target population, in Berg FS, Blair JC, Viehweg SH, Wilson-Vlotman A, eds: *Educational Audiology for the Hard of Hearing Child* (New York: Grune & Stratton, 1986), chap 1.

10. Simon CS: *Communication Skills and Classroom Success* (San Diego: College Hill Press, 1985).

11. Elliott LL, Hammer MA, Scholl ME: Fine grained auditory discrimination in normal children and children with language-learning problems. *J Speech Hear Res,* 32 (1989), 112–119.

12. Ross M: A future challenge: Educating the educators and public about hearing loss. *Semin Hear,* 12 (1991), 402–413.

13. Ling D: *Foundations of Spoken Language for Hearing Impaired Children* (Washington, DC: The Alexander Graham Bell Association for the Deaf, 1989).

14. Ross M, Calvert DR: Semantics of deafness revisited: total communication and the use and misuse of residual hearing. *Audiology,* 9 (1984), 127–145.

15. Bess FH: The minimally hearing-impaired child. *Ear Hear,* 6 (1985), 43–47.

16. Davis J, ed: *Our Forgotten Children: Hard-of-Hearing Pupils in the Schools* (Bethesda MD: Self Help for Hard of Hearing People, 1990).

17. Ramsdell DA: The psychology of the hard-of-hearing and deafened adult, in Davis H, Silverman SR, eds: *Hearing and Deafness,* ed 4 (New York: Holt, Rinehart and Winston, 1978), chap 8.

18. Ross M, Brackett D, Maxon A: *Assessment and Management of Mainstreamed Hearing-Impaired Children* (Austin TX: Pro-Ed, 1991).

19. Berg FS: *Facilitating Classroom Listening: A Handbook for Teachers of Normal and Hard of Hearing Students* (Boston: College-Hill Press/Little Brown, 1987).

20. Leavitt RJ, Flexer C: Speech degradation as measured by the rapid speech transmission index (RASTI). *Ear Hear,* 12 (1991), 115–118.

21. Houtgast T, Steeneken HJM: The MTF concept in room acoustics and its use for estimating speech intelligibility in auditoria. *J Acoust Soc Am,* 77 (1985), 1069–1077.

22. Rehabilitation Act of 1973. (P.L. 93-112, September 26, 1973). *United States Statutes at Large,* 87, 355–394.

23. Blair JC: Educational audiology and methods for bringing about change in schools. *Semin Hear,* 12 (1991), 318–328.

24. Education of the Handicapped Act Amendments of 1990. (P.L. 101-476, October 30, 1990), *United States Statutes at Large,* 104, 1103–1151.

25. American Speech-Language-Hearing Association: Guidelines for fitting and monitoring FM systems. *ASHA,* 36 Suppl 12 (1994 March).

26. American Speech-Language-Hearing Association: Preferred practice patterns for the professions of speech-language pathology and audiology. *ASHA,* 35 Suppl, 11 (1993 March).

27. American Speech-Language-Hearing Association: Scope of practice, speech-language pathology and audiology. *ASHA,* 32 Suppl 2 (1990 April).

28. American Speech-Language-Hearing Association: Code of ethics. *ASHA,* 34 Suppl 9 (1992 March).

29. Ross M, ed: *FM Auditory Training Systems: Characteristics, Selection & Use* (Timonium, MD: York Press, 1992).

30. Madell JR: FM systems for children birth to age five, in Ross M, ed: *FM Auditory Training Systems: Characteristics, Selection, & Use* (Timonium, MD: York Press, 1992), chap 7.

31. Medwetsky L: Maximizing the potential benefits from FM system technology. *ASHA Special Interests Division 9 Newsletter,* 3 (1993), 4–6.

32. Evans CH: Troubleshooting FM systems, in Ross M, ed: *FM Auditory Training Systems: Characteristics, Selection, & Use* (Timonium, MD: York Press, 1992), chap 6.

33. Hawkins D: Assessment of FM systems with probe tube microphone system. *Ear Hear,* 8 (1987), 301–303.

34. Lewis D, Feigin J, Karasek A, Stelmachowicz P: Evaluation and assessment of FM systems. *Ear Hear,* 12 (1991), 268–280.

35. Seewald RC, Moodie KS: Electroacoustic considerations, in Ross M, ed: *FM Auditory Training Systems: Characteristics, Selection, & Use* (Timonium, MD: York Press, 1992), chap 4.

36. Crandell C, Smaldino J: Sound-field amplification in the classroom. *Am J Audiol,* 1 (1992), 16–18.

37. Flexer C, Millin J, Brown L: Children with developmental disabilities: the effects of sound field amplification on word identification. *Lang, Speech Hear Serv Sch,* 21 (1990), 177–182.

38. Zabel H, Tabor M: Effects of soundfield amplification on spelling performance of elementary school children. *Educ Audiol Monogr,* 3 (1993), 5–9.

39. Sexton JE: Team management of the child with hearing loss. *Semin Hear,* 12 (1991), 329–339.

40. Education for All Handicapped Children Act of 1975. (P.L. 94-142, November 29, 1975), *United States Statutes at Large*, 89, 773-796.

41. Education for the Handicapped Act Amendments of 1986. (P.L. 99-457, October 8, 1986), *United States Statutes at Large*, 100, 1145-1177.

42. Flexer C: *Facilitating Hearing and Listening in Young Children* (San Diego: Singular Publishing Group, 1994).

43. Flexer C, Wray D, Black T, Millin J: Amplification devices: Evaluating classroom effectiveness for moderately hearing impaired college students. *Volta Rev*, 89 (1987), 347-357.

44. Allen L: Promoting the usefulness of classroom amplification. *Educ Audiol Monogr*, 3 (1993), 32-34.

APPENDIX

Inserts 1, 2, and 3 showing performance measures for FM systems. Reprinted with permission of the American Speech-Language-Hearing Association.

Insert 1

Outline for FM System Adjustment Using 2 cm³ Coupler Measurements

1. Verify through coupler measurements and/or probe-microphone measurements that the client's hearing aid is functioning properly and has been fit appropriately for the hearing loss.
2. Obtain 2 cm³ measurements on the client's personal hearing aid.
   a. Obtain an SSPL90 curve using a 90 dB SPL swept pure tone with the hearing aid VCW full-on.
   b. Adjust the hearing aid VCW to the use position. Using a 65 dB SPL input, obtain an output (not gain) curve in the 2 cm³ coupler.
3. Set up the FM system for 2 cm³ coupler measurements (See Figure 1-A).
   a. Place the FM microphone in the calibrated test position.
   b. With the FM receiver outside the test box, set the receiver for FM-only reception. Attach the button or behind-the-ear (BTE) receiver to the HA-2 2 cm³ coupler. Maintain a minimum distance of 2 ft between the FM transmitter and receiver.
   c. If a personal FM system is used, connect the FM receiver to the personal hearing aid (also located outside the test box) via the coupling method that the client will use (direct audio input, neck loop, or silhouette). If a neck loop is used, the hearing aid should be placed on the client (or other person of similar size, if possible, if the client is not available) and the earhook connected to the HA-2 2 cm³ coupler (or individual earmold connected to the HA-1 2 cm³ coupler) which is held next to the client's ear (See Figure 1-B).
4. Adjust the FM system SSPL90 to match the personal hearing aid SSPL90.
   a. Turn the FM receiver VCW full-on (also turn the personal hearing aid VCW full-on if a personal FM system is being evaluated) and obtain an SSPL90 curve with a 90 dB SPL pure-tone sweep.

   b. Adjust the FM systems SSPL90 control until the SSPL90 curve most closely matches that of the personal hearing aid (#2 above).
5. Adjust the FM system output and frequency response to match the personal hearing aid.
   a. Using an 80 dB SPL input delivered to the FM microphone in the test box, adjust the FM receiver VCW and tone control(s) until the 2 cm³ coupler output (not gain) most closely matches the output obtained with the personal hearing aid (#2b above).
   b. With a personal FM system, leave the hearing aid VCW and tone control(s) at the user setting and adjust only the FM receiver VCW and tone control(s) to obtain the closest match to the personal hearing aid alone response (#2b above).
6. Measure the maximum output and frequency response of the environmental microphone(s) if a self-contained FM system is being used.
   a. Turn the FM VCW to full-on, measure the SSPL90, and adjust as necessary. If the SSPL90 control is changed, measure the FM-only SSPL90 again and determine if readjustment is needed.
   b. Measure the output using a 65 dB SPL input. If only one VCW exists on the FM receiver and it controls both the level of the FM signal and the environmental microphone(s), then a decision must be made as to where the single setting will be. If separate VCWs are present for the FM signal and environmental microphone(s), then the environmental microphone VCW can be adjusted to an appropriate level relative to the FM signal (see Lewis et al., 1991, and Lewis, 1993, for more discussion of this issue). If matching desired output values for the FM-only mode and environmental microphone mode leads to different control settings, priority should be given to matching the FM-only targets.
7. Measure harmonic distortion to verify acceptable values.
8. Perform a complete listening check to assure acceptable clarity and low distortion.

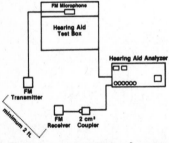

FIGURE 1-A. Physical arrangement for 2 cm³ coupler measurements FM systems when measuring FM transmission mode only. The FM receiver may be attached to the HA-2 2 cm³ coupler via an external button receiver, BTE receiver, or via a personal hearing aid if direct audio input or a silhouette inductor is utilized. (Adapted from Thibodeau, 1992).

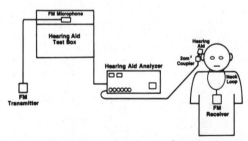

FIGURE 1-B. Physical arrangement for 2 cm³ coupler measurements of the FM system connected to a personal hearing aid via a neck loop. The hearing aid is set to the "T" position and the environmental microphone(s), if present, on the FM system are deactivated if possible.

Insert 2

Outline for FM System Adjustment Using Probe-Microphone Measurements

1. Determine a set of target real-ear maximum output and frequency response values through either
   a. using existing real-ear measurements obtained from an appropriately fit personal hearing aid
   OR
   b. a published amplification selection scheme, e.g. DSL (Seewald et al., 1991)

2. Prepare the test environment for probe-microphone measurements.
   a. The placement of the FM microphone in the sound field will depend on the specific probe-microphone system. See Figure 2-A for a possible arrangement if the probe system uses an off-line (or stored) equalization method. During equalization, the reference microphone is placed at the location of the FM microphone. During the measurements the reference microphone is disabled. If the system uses a controlling microphone for on-line equalization, it can be located near the FM microphone, as shown in Figure 2-B. (Note: In this latter arrangement, if the reference microphone is near the ear, then feedback may be a problem in higher gain instruments.)
   b. Place the probe tube in the ear canal at an appropriate location, connect the FM system (set to FM only) to the client via the coupling method that will be used.

3. Adjust the FM system maximum output to the desired position.
   a. Set the maximum output control to the minimum position.
   b. Set the FM VCW to the highest level before feedback (and the client's hearing aid VCW to the highest possible use position if it is a personal FM system). Obtain a measure of the Real Ear Saturation Response (RESR) by introducing a 90 dB SPL swept tonal signal and measuring the output in the ear canal. (NOTE: Extreme care should be exercised in making this measurement so as to prevent excessive output and/or discomfort; the output control should be set to the minimum position for the first measurement.) An alterna-

tive to directly measuring the RESR has been outlined by Sullivan (1987) and described further by Hawkins (1992, 1993).
   c. Adjust the output control until the RESR most closely matches the personal hearing aid RESR or the desired RESR targets.

4. Adjust the FM system real-ear output and frequency response for the FM signal to match the personal hearing aid values or the desired real-ear values.
   a. Using an 80 dB SPL signal delivered to the FM microphone, adjust the FM receiver VCW and tone control(s) until the desired real-ear values are most closely matched.
   b. With a personal FM system, leave the hearing aid VCW and tone control(s) at the user setting and adjust only the FM receiver VCW and tone control(s) to obtain the closest match.

5. Measure the real-ear maximum output and frequency response of the environmental microphone(s) if a self-contained FM system is being used.
   a. Turn off the FM microphone and place the user in the sound field as for probe-microphone measurements with a personal hearing aid.
   b. Adjust the FM VCW to just below feedback, measure the RESR, and adjust as necessary. If the SSPL90 control is changed, measure the FM-only RESR again and determine if readjustment is needed.
   c. Measure the real-ear output using a 65 dB SPL signal. If matching desired output values for the FM-only mode and environmental microphone mode leads to different control settings, priority should be given to matching the FM-only targets.

6. Remove the FM system from the user and measure harmonic distortion in a 2 cm^3 coupler to verify acceptable values.

7. Perform a complete listening check to assure acceptable clarity and low distortion.

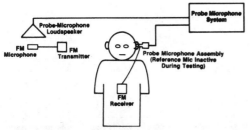

FIGURE 2-A. Physical arrangement for probe-microphone evaluation of FM system for the FM-only mode when the probe-microphone system uses an off-line (or stored) equalization method. During the equalization procedure the reference microphone is active and located next to the FM microphone. During the actual probe measurements the reference microphone is disabled.

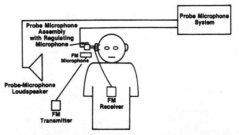

FIGURE 2-B. Physical arrangement for probe-microphone evaluation of FM system for the FM-only mode when the probe-microphone system uses a controlling microphone for on-line equalization.

Insert 3

Speech Recognition Measures With FM Systems and Personal Hearing Aid(s)

1. Select a speech recognition test that is appropriate for the age and language of the client.

2. Place the hearing aid(s) on the client and set up the arrangement shown in Figure 3-A.
   a. Speech is at 55 dB HL (68 dB SPL) and noise at 50 dB HL (63 dB SPL), producing a S/N ratio of +5 dB. The loudspeakers are located at plus and minus 45 degree azimuths.
   b. Obtain a speech recognition score.

3. Place the FM receiver set to FM-only on the client and set up the arrangement shown in Figure 3-B.
   a. Speech is 70 dB HL (83 dB SPL) and noise is 50 dB HL (63 dB SPL), producing a S/N ratio of +20 dB at the FM microphone. The loudspeakers are located at plus and minus 45 degrees azimuth. With directional microphones, point the microphone at the loudspeaker producing the speech signal.
   b. Obtain a speech recognition score.

4. If a speech recognition measure is desired for FM system with environmental microphone(s) active, set up the arrangement shown in Figure 3-C.
   a. Speech is 55 dB HL (68 dB SPL) at the client's location and noise is 50 dB HL (63 dB SPL), producing a S/N ratio of +5 dB at the environmental microphone(s).
   b. The FM microphone is positioned in front of the speech loudspeaker at a location designed to produce 83 dB SPL speech input to the FM microphone.
   c. The environmental microphone(s) on the FM system are activated.
   d. Obtain a speech recognition score.

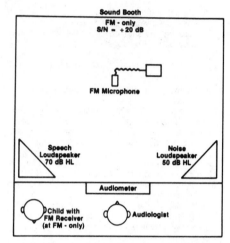

FIGURE 3-B. Physical arrangement in sound booth for speech recognition testing of FM system set to FM-only for comparison purposes to hearing aid(s) only. (Modified from Lewis et al., 1991)

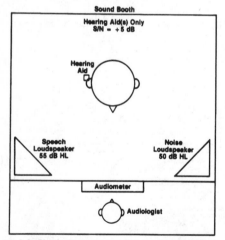

FIGURE 3-A. Physical arrangement in sound booth for speech recognition testing of hearing aid(s) only for comparison purposes to FM system. (Modified from Lewis et al., 1991)

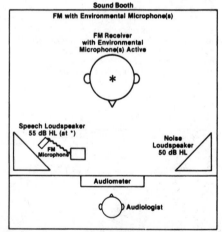

FIGURE 3-C. Physical arrangement in sound booth for speech recognition testing of FM system with environmental microphone(s) active. (See Lewis et al., 1991, for potential difficulties in high-frequency input to the FM microphone using this arrangement.)

13

ASSISTIVE DEVICES FOR STUDENTS WITH HEARING IMPAIRMENTS

Carolyn H. Musket

> *"The time has come,' the Walrus said,*
> *To talk of many things: ...."*
>
> —Lewis Carroll, *Through The Looking Glass*, 1871

An *assistive device* is any device, other than a personal hearing aid, designed to improve the ability of those who do not hear well to communicate or to be aware of auditory signals in the environment. An assistive device may be used alone or may supplement hearing aid use in specific situations. For example, some assistive devices are used to transmit speech efficiently when large distances exist between the speaker and the listener or when the presence of ambient noise in the setting hinders communication. Other devices improve use of the telephone or television. Finally, there are devices that alert a person to environmental events by transforming an auditory signal into a visual or tactile stimulus.[1,2] The purpose of this chapter is twofold: (1) to provide an overview of the help available to the student with hearing impairment through the use of assistive devices; and (2) to consider the role of the school with regard to assistive devices.

OVERVIEW OF ASSISTIVE DEVICES

Assistive Devices for the Telephone

Telephones and Hearing Aid Compatibility. Some hearing aids include a telecoil, also known as an induction coil, to help the wearer use the telephone. Telecoils usually are found in behind-the-ear instruments; it is more difficult to incorporate them effectively into smaller in-the-ear hearing aids because of space restrictions. When the input switch of the hearing aid is on T (telecoil), the hearing aid will amplify only the telephone signal. However, for this to occur, the telephone receiver must generate a magnetic field sufficient to induce current flow in the hearing aid telecoil. Surrounding noise in the area is not amplified because the hearing aid microphone (M) is not activated.

Problems arise because not all telephone handsets are capable of producing a suitable magnetic field and, therefore, are not compatible or usable with hearing aids having a T switch. This situation was somewhat improved with enactment of the Telecommunications for the Disabled Act of 1982 (PL 97-410)[3] and the adoption of implementing regulations by the Federal Communications Commission (FCC). This act stipulated that essential telephones must be compatible with hearing aids and mandated that technical standards be established specifying the magnetic field strength necessary for such compatibility. The term "essential telephones" included all coin-operated telephones; all telephones provided for emergency use, such as those in rodeside areas, elevators, and police and fire department call boxes; and other telephones frequently needed by those using hearing aids. According to PL 97-410, new telephones provided in business and public buildings for use by the public, such as hotel house phones and airport paging phones, must be hearing aid compatible; new telephones installed in hotels and motels must be compatible until 10% of the rooms meet this requirement. Several years later, the FCC expanded the definition of essential telephones to include credit-card telephones and telephones found in common areas of the workplace. Moreover, PL 97-410 required that packages containing telephones be labeled to provide information about their compatibility with hearing aids.

Universal compatibility was furthered in 1988 when Congress passed the Hearing Aid Compatibility Act (PL 100-394),[4] which stated that all corded telephones manufactured or imported in this country must be hearing aid compatible by 1989; cordless models, by 1991. PL 100-394 originally required that all workplaces and hospitals make all existing telephones hearing aid compatible; however, in 1993 the FCC suspended requirements to retrofit all telephones because of the costs involved and this delay is still in effect at the time of this writing.[5]

Amplified Replacement Handsets. Amplified replacement handsets are easily installed on modular telephones by inserting the existing detachable handset cord into a plug receptacle in the end of the amplified handset. Of course, they cannot be used with telephones having the dialing mechanism in the handset. These replacement receivers have built-in amplification with a volume control wheel in the handset that may be rotated to increase the intensity of the signal. If the handset is hearing aid compatible, the magnetic signal, also, will be increased. One model has a touch bar in the middle of the handle that is lightly depressed at one end to increase loud-

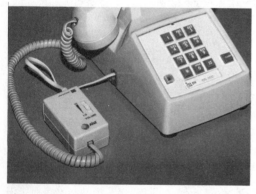

Figure 13-1. An in-line amplifier connected to the telephone.

ness and at the other end to decrease loudness. The volume of this latter type of handset returns to normal when the receiver is replaced on the cradle of the telephone base; this is an advantage if the telephone also will be used by those with normal hearing. Amplified replacement handsets are available in several colors and in styles that are either round (G-type) or square (K-type) at each end. However, such handsets are not interchangeable with all telephones; the suitability of a particular amplified replacement handset for a certain telephone must be verified. For the older style nonmodular telephone, which has cords wired directly into the handset and base, an amplified handset may be obtained with an attached

cord ending in four connecting spade clips to be attached inside the base of the telephone.

In-Line Amplifiers. In-line amplifiers are convenient to use provided the telephone is modular and does not have the dial in the handset. An in-line amplifier may be plugged into the base of a modular telephone after removing the existing handset cord; this cord is then connected to the amplifier (Fig. 13-1). Either a rotary dial or a sliding switch on the amplifier increases the intensity of the telephone signal. An in-line amplifier should have its own power source—either a battery or AC transformer—because the electronic telephones so prevalent today do not provide the necessary power for these add-on devices to operate.[6]

Portable Amplifiers and Adapters. A portable amplifier or adapter may be carried with the user and placed over the receiver end of a telephone handset when the need arises; the unit is held tightly in place by an elastic strap. A rotary dial or sliding switch controls the intensity, and power is supplied by a battery.

Various models of these portable devices perform different functions. One type contains a microphone so it amplifies the acoustic signal and, therefore, may be used with any telephone; it also provides a magnetic field. Less useful is a model that amplifies the accompanying magnetic field and converts it into an acoustic signal because it may be used only with hearing aid compatible telephone handsets. Another model may be used only with hearing aids having a telecoil; it transforms an acoustic signal into the strong magnetic field necessary for the telecoil to operate. Such an adapter is helpful because it allows incompatible telephones to be used with hearing aids. An example of this latter type, the Rastronics TA-80, is unique because a silhouette inductor may be plugged into it; this allows the user to hear binaurally through the telecoils of two hearing aids by holding the receiver (with the adapter attached) to one aided ear and placing the silhouette alongside the second hearing aid.

Amplified Telephones. Amplification has been built into some modular telephones and is controlled through a rotary dial or sliding switch located on the base. Such telephones may have special features. Some amplified telephones, for example, provide greater gain in the high-frequency range and are available as either a standard single-line phone or a two-line business model. The Williams Sound TeleTalker offers dual adjustments for both gain and frequency response and requires the use of an alternate current (AC) power transformer; in addition, the user may couple a hearing aid's direct auditory input cord or inductive coupler (neckloop or silhouette) to this phone. The preselected amplification of the TeleTalker reverts to normal operating levels whenever the handset is returned to the base; it may be activated again by depressing a single button. Often these special telephones have large push button number pads and adjustable ringer volume controls.

Text Telephones. A text telephone (TT), also known as a telecommunication device for the deaf (TDD), offers visual access to telephone communication for those who cannot understand an amplified voice over the telephone or for those who are speech impaired. A TT typically has a keyboard for touch-typing; an illuminated light emitting diode (LED) screen to display the message; acoustic couplers; and either a rechargeable battery or AC transformer to supply power (Fig. 13-2). Some TTs have a printer to provide a hardcopy record of the conversation. More elaborate models have an array of options, which may include a voice synthesizer to announce a TT call, automatic answering, and memory for storing messages. A typical TT is a little larger than a standard telephone; compact models are available small enough to be carried in a purse or briefcase; payphone versions exist. When using this device, a telephone handset is placed in the cups of an acoustic coupler on the TT. The user types a message that is converted into tones and conveyed over the telephone line to another TT, which transforms the message back into visual form. Other models allow the TT to be connected directly to the telephone line by means of a modular plug. In this arrangement, both the sender and receiver of the message must have a TT; they communicate by sending a visual, typed message over a telephone connection.

In some settings, TTs and personal computers may be modified to communicate with each other.

TTs in the United States use the Baudot code, which operates at 45.45 baud; this is a comparatively slow transmission and receiving rate, but suitable for manual typing.[7] However, personal computers use the ASCII code (American Standard Code for Information Interchange), which allows much faster data exchange rates. Consequently, special provisions must be made for communication to occur between a TT and a personal computer. It is possible to obtain a TT that has the added capability of using ASCII at a maximum speed of 300 baud.[7] In addition, modems and software are available that allow personal computers using ASCII to communicate with TTs using Baudot.

Telephone Relay Service. Telephone calls may occur between TTs and standard voice telephones through use of a third-party relay service. Title IV of the Americans with Disabilities Act of 1990 (PL 101-336)[8] stipulated that telephone companies must provide local and long distance 24-hour relay services nationwide by July, 1993. Consequently, a TT user now may place a call to a relay operator or communication assistant (CA) at a central location and provide the name and number of the person to call; the CA calls the voice telephone party; when the connection is established, the CA reads to the person called what the TT user types, and types the reply back to the TT user. Calls from voice telephones to TTs follow the same procedure. Persons with intelligible speech and impaired hearing may expedite the process by using the voice carryover (VCO) option; once the telephone connection is made, the caller speaks directly to the person called and reads only the reply typed by the CA to the TT.

Touch-Tone Text Receivers. Another telecommunication device uses tonal signals from the telephone. A portable touch-tone text receiver may be placed over the telephone handset and secured with a strap. When a connection is made with a push-button telephone, tones that result from depressing the buttons of this phone cause letters, numbers, and symbols to appear on the screen of the touch-tone text receiver. This arrangement allows a person who speaks, but has a severe hearing impairment, to talk over the telephone and receive a visual reply without the aid of a telephone relay service; only one device is needed.

ASSISTIVE DEVICES FOR TELEVISION

Assistive devices, using either auditory or visual approaches, are available to improve television

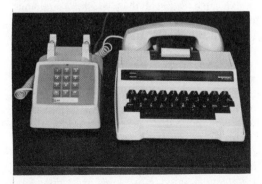

Figure 13–2. A text telephone (or TDD) coupled for use with the telephone.

Case study 13–1.   Amy T., age 9 years, had a moderately severe, bilateral sensorineural hearing loss above 500 Hz and wore binaural behind-the-ear hearing aids most of the time. She was mainstreamed and enrolled in a regular third grade classroom. Amy enjoyed watching TV, but sat very close to the TV set at home and did not wear her hearing aids. Mrs. T. brought Amy to our Assistive Devices Center to investigate help when viewing TV. This mother and daughter were shown a closed captioned version of the previous day's *Sesame Street* program, which had been recorded in anticipation of their appointment. In addition, Amy was fitted with an infrared receiver coupled via a silhouette inductor to her hearing aid set on *T* (telecoil). A wireless system was chosen because of other small children in the family; the cost was within the family's budget. Amy watched and listened from across the room. "Gee, Mom," she volunteered, "I never knew that fellow's name before!"

Amy's parents purchased a closed caption decoder and an infrared TV listening system. Later, the grandparents presented the family with a videocassette recorder so Amy could enjoy closed captioned movies available on videotapes. Moreover, Mrs. T. moved the infrared system to another room in the evenings to use as a personal communicator, with a microphone input, when she tutored Amy in her lessons. Next, Amy started taking the infrared system to school whenever use of TV or a tape recorder was scheduled for the class. Her teacher used the system when announcing the weekly spelling test words.

In fact, Amy's use of an infrared listening system with her personal hearing aids demonstrated to both family and teachers that improved performance was possible in certain situations. At the last meeting of her school's Admission, Review, and Dismissal Committee, the decision was made to provide a personal FM system for Amy to use daily in the classroom. Surely, Amy's use of assistive devices is a success story.

(TV) viewing for those with hearing impairments; some devices are also suitable for systems that reproduce recorded music and for the radio. Those devices involving audition are based on the concept of presenting an amplified audio signal much closer to the ear of the listener with hearing impairment, thereby overcoming the problems associated with distance, room reverberation, and noise. Most personal listening systems, discussed later in this chapter, may also be adapted for use with television, as is demonstrated by case study 13–1.

Hardwire.   A simple hardwire arrangement involves plugging a headset into the earphone jack of a television set; however, this may disconnect the TV loudspeaker for others unless a second jack provides the option of hearing simultaneously via both loudspeaker and earphones. Not all television sets have this output jack. Therefore, it is also possible to position a small microphone with an adhesive clip by the TV loudspeaker to capture sound; a long cord from this microphone leads to a battery-powered amplifier, which allows the user to select additional volume. Various couplers may be used with the amplifier—monaural or binaural earbuds or button receivers; a headset; and a neckloop or silhouette inductor or a direct auditory input cable to be used with hearing aids. Although many variations of the preceding description are possible, a feature all have in common is that components are connected by wires.

Frequency Modulation Broadcast.   The battery-powered transmitter of a frequency modula-

(FM) radio system may be coupled to a television set either directly through a cable inserted into an earphone jack or acoustically with a microphone placed near the loudspeaker. The audio portion of a TV program then becomes an FM radio signal which is broadcast to a battery-powered receiver worn by the viewer; various couplers including earbuds, a headset, and neckloop or silhouette inductor or direct auditory input to a hearing aid, may be chosen by the user. Instead of a personal receiver, some manufacturers offer small, remote loudspeakers that may be located next to the listener with hearing impairment. FM systems are wireless between the TV and the viewer.

Infrared Light.   An infrared (IR) system also is wireless from the TV set to the viewer (Fig. 13–3). An IR transmitter, AC powered, is situated near the TV and connected to either a microphone (to pick up sound from the loudspeaker) or to a cable leading to the television's audio output jack. This transmitter contains several LEDs that send invisible beams of IR light to a battery-powered receiver used by the viewer. The style of the receiver varies according to the manufacturer; it may be worn suspended under-the-chin (stethophone), as a headset, or clipped to a pocket. All receivers contain a small, IR-sensitive receiving diode that must be exposed to the IR beams from the transmitter to operate. Some receivers may interface with a hearing aid having a telecoil or direct auditory input capability.

Induction Loop.   An area induction loop may be used when viewing television. Again, a

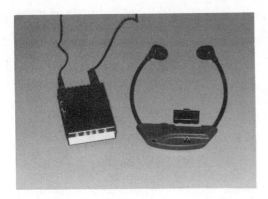

Figure 13–3. A television infrared listening system having a transmitter (left) and stethophone receiver and battery (right).

microphone placed near the TV loudspeaker serves as input to an AC-powered amplifier; the electrical signal from this amplifier is sent throughout a closed wire loop antenna that encircles the listening area. The loop may extend around the room or enclose only the chair of the viewer. To receive the electromagnetic signal emanating from the loop, the listener needs either a hearing aid with an induction coil (telecoil) or a personal receiver containing an induction coil, which may be used with earphones.

Television-Band Radio. A simple, yet effective, way to amplify TV sound for those with impaired hearing is with a portable or table top radio that has very high frequency channels 2 to 13 for the audio portion of TV programs. TV sound is transmitted in FM bands outside the range of most FM radios, but special radios with this feature are available. The radio may be located beside the viewer, tuned to the station also selected for the TV, and adjusted to a comfortable volume. An earphone, headset, or inductive coupler may be plugged into an output jack. A limitation of this device is that it cannot be tuned to UHF or cable channels and must be readjusted every time the TV channel is changed.

Closed-Captioned Television. Visual information about TV programs may be supplied through closed captioning. With a decoder, the audio portion of a TV program appears as captions on the screen, much like subtitles for a foreign film. Thus, a viewer with impaired hearing may read dialogue and narration to supplement what is heard; for the deaf, captions replace the sound track. These captions appear as white letters against a black background; their size varies

according to the size of the screen. Closed-captions are transmitted on line 21 of the TV broadcast signal, which has been reserved by the FCC for this purpose.[9] Closed captions may be seen *only* with a decoder. When the decoding function is turned on, the captions appear; when the decoder is off, only the picture is seen. A closed-caption decoder may be purchased separately and connected to the television. However, the Television Decoder Circuitry Act of 1990 (PL 101-431)[10] required that TV sets, with screens 13 inches or larger, manufactured or imported into this country after July 1993, contain built-in decoders for displaying captions. Internal circuitry to decode closed captions may also be found in some videocassette recorders.

The National Captioning Institute (NCI) was established by the United States Congress in 1979 to provide closed captioning services for TV broadcasts.[9] NCI, along with some other companies, continues to caption all types of TV programs. Prerecorded shows are captioned in advance of the broadcast. News programs and live events, such as sports, are captioned as they occur through *real-time captioning*; these captions are created on a computerized stenotype machine.[11] Both broadcast and cable networks offer closed captioned programs; most of broadcast networks' prime time programming is closed captioned. Program listings in the newspapers and magazine guides identify a closed captioned program through use of the initials CC.

Closed caption decoders also may be used with videocassette recorders. A large number of movies are closed captioned in their videocassette versions and are identified as such on the packages. Some music videos, too, have closed captions.

Studies have shown that students with hearing impairments who read at the third-grade level and above significantly increase their comprehension of televised programs when closed captions are added.[12,13] Captioned TV has the potential to not only increase comprehension of a program, but also to improve reading and language skills when used over a period of time. Children with hearing losses, like all children, find televised material highly interesting. Certainly, closed captioned television gives these students access to spoken language and a means of enriching vocabulary never before available. It is an effective tool, also, for non-English-speaking students learning English.

Alerting Devices

As a part of daily activities, one must respond appropriately to a variety of nonspeech auditory signals. The ring of the telephone, the chime of a doorbell, and the buzz of an alarm clock are essential cues for independent living (see case study 13-2). Moreover, one's actual safety depends on being able to hear the sound of a fire alarm or smoke detector. These auditory signals may not be heard by those with impaired hearing. Consequently, there is a wide array of devices and systems that offer help in this area.[14] Primarily, these assistive devices must detect a special sound and announce its occurrence by converting it into a stimulus that will be perceived in various places. The number of options and possible combinations makes this a complex topic. First, sounds may be detected through: (1) a monitoring microphone; (2) a direct electrical connection; or (3) inductive coupling. Second, the occurrence of a sound may be converted into: (1) a more suitable auditory signal (louder or lower in pitch); (2) a visual signal (flashing light); or (3) a vibrotactile signal (pager or bed shaker, for example). Finally, these devices may signal the existence of a sound: (1) near the original sound; or (2) in a remote location. To add still further possibilities, there are single-purpose devices as well as systems designed for total facility monitoring. The following list of common solutions for certain situations should help acquaint the reader with the type of help available to improve the detection of alerting and warning sounds.

Telephone Ring. Portable telephone ring amplifiers may be plugged into any modular telephone outlet. These amplifiers change the actual ring into a warble tone or low-pitched sound more likely to be heard by those with high frequency hearing losses. Other units are available that feature a strobe light or make it possible for a household lamp to become a flashing signaler in any room. A vibrotactile receiver, worn on the body, can be activated by the ring of the telephone through use of a transmitter connected to the telephone line.

Doorbells. Doorbell chimes may be replaced with extra volume bells or buzzers. Visual signaling systems may be installed with an existing doorbell or connected to a pushbutton provided to be placed at the door. The doorbell, also, may trigger a wearable vibrotactile receiver.

Door Knocks. A device containing a strobe light may be attached to a dormitory or bedroom door; it will flash in response to a knock at the

---

Case history 13-2. Mrs. H. telephoned the Assistive Devices Center to inquire about alarm clocks modified for use by those with impaired hearing; her son needed one. She was told such clocks were available with either a flashing visual or vibrotactile signal; in standard or travel size; and as a single function clock or combined with an alert for the ring of the telephone. She was amazed—and so were we; her son was 23 years old. Why did this mother wait until now to learn about this assistive device? Why did not her son contact us? How can our educational system help those with impaired hearing learn about assistive devices to enable them to make telephone calls and to awaken each morning—to enable them to have communication access and independence?

---

door. It may be obtained in a model that works in conjunction with a vibrotactile receiver.

Wake-up Alarms. Bedside alarm clocks are manufactured with outlets for connection to either a visual or vibrotactile alerting device (Fig. 13-4). Smaller, travel-sized models have battery-powered vibrators contained within the clock. Still another electrical device is sensitive to the sound of any regular alarm clock placed atop it and will cause a lamp or bed shaker plugged into it to be activated whenever the alarm sounds.

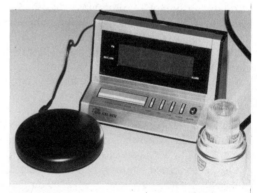

Figure 13-4. An alarm clock that may be used with a vibrotactile alarm (left) or a strobe light (right).

Smoke Detectors. One type of device activates a strobe light or bed shaker when its microphone senses the occurrence of the sustained, intense sound of a smoke alarm. In other systems, the smoke detector and transmitter are combined in one unit that activates a visual or vibrotacticle alert.

Computer Prompts.   The audible prompt of a personal computer may be replaced by a flashing colored screen or blinking words to relay an attention-getting visual signal.

Multipurpose Systems.   Monitoring of several different auditory signals may be accomplished through the use of a single multipurpose system. A central controlling unit will recognize input from various sensing transmitters and give a response unique to each. Thus, in a visually based system, a light may flash a distinctive coded pattern to differentiate the doorbell from the telephone. For a vibrotactile system, each remote sensor transmitter may be identified by a specific light and symbol on the receiver.

Hardwire Assistive Listening Devices

Personal assistive listening devices (ALDs) improve interpersonal communication in difficult listening situations. In most instances, they offer the user a way to overcome problems occurring because of speaker distance, reverberation, and noise in the listening environment. ALDs may be used alone or in conjunction with hearing aids. Hardwire devices for stationary, one-to-one use are less flexible, but inexpensive, when compared to the classroom auditory trainers described in Chapter 12. A hardwire ALD has the basic components of an amplification system: a microphone, which may be contained within the unit or connected to it by a cord; an amplifier; and a receiver, which is usually a single earphone or headset. In the most useful hardwire ALD configuration, the microphone may be extended with a cord some distance from the amplifier/receiver. Thus, it is possible for the person speaking to hold this remote microphone 6 inches from the mouth, or clip it to a lapel, making the message spoken much more intense than any surrounding noise. The listener, a comfortable conversational distance away, is tethered to the talker with cords, but profits from the enhanced speech-to-noise ratio that this system allows. An unaided listener may require only a small amount of amplification and wear an earphone or headset. An aided listener may combine the ALD and a hearing aid through direct auditory input, if the aid has this option, or by induction with a neckloop or silhouette inductor if the aid has a telecoil. Such a listening arrangement has been found to be helpful in restaurants and automobiles, for example, by those who wear hearing aids. Hardwire ALDs are flexible; the remote microphone may be placed near the loudspeaker of a television set, radio, or stereo as well.

Several manufacturers produce hardwire ALDs. It is also possible to assemble a simple system from components readily available at electronics stores. One needs a tie clip or hand-held microphone, a low-gain miniamplifier-speaker, and a monaural, lightweight headset. Sudler and Flexer[15] reported on the success they encountered when using the latter inexpensive ALD during speech-language therapy. They noted improved articulation and self-monitoring skills in high school students with hearing impairments. Children with normal hearing also had better self-monitoring of speech with the system, and were more motivated when using the device. Flexer[16] and Flexer and Savage[17] recommend consideration of a personal low-gain hardwire ALD with other groups of children as well: (1) children with articulation errors and a continuing history of fluctuating hearing loss; (2) infants and toddlers with Down syndrome; and (3) preschoolers with language delay.[16,17] It is important to stress that this equipment should provide only minimal amplification and be used with supervision and a program of monitoring when recommended for children with normal or near-normal hearing.[18]

Large Area Assistive Listening Systems

Assistive listening systems for the benefit of those with impaired hearing may be found in large assembly areas, such as auditoriums, convention centers, stadiums, cinemas, theaters, and houses of worship. Recent growth in the availability of such assistance is due to several factors, which include new applications of technology and governmental regulations.

Frequency Modulation Broadcast.   FM sound systems may be installed in large assembly areas in addition to the classroom use presented in Chapter 12. A base station transmitter is connected to a facility's existing public address system; low-gain FM receivers compatible with the transmitting frequency of the base station are available on site for loan to those with hearing losses. Provision may be made for these receivers to interface with hearing aids having a telecoil or direct auditory input. The potential exists for radio wave interference should nearby, or more powerful, transmitters share the same frequency.[19] However, FM systems are economical for large areas and free of electrical interference; they allow mobility among users. These advantages have encouraged the use of FM listening systems in assembly areas. For example, American Multi-

Cinema, the second largest theater chain in the United States, announced they will install more than 2000 FM listening systems in 1993.[20]

Infrared Light. IR sound systems are confined to large *indoor* areas because bright sunlight is a source of interference. Panels containing a large array of LEDs are connected to a public address system or a movie's soundtrack, for example, and positioned strategically above the assembly area; they transmit information by radiating invisible IR light waves over the entire audience. IR receivers, described in a previous section of this chapter, are available for use by those with impaired hearing in attendance. IR light cannot penetrate walls; consequently, this technology is often chosen for adjoining rooms or settings where security of the information transmitted is of prime importance. Persons who use IR receivers at home usually may take these same receivers to use at facilities equipped with an IR sound system; the same transmitting carrier frequency is used by the major manufacturers of hearing assistance IR systems.[21] IR listening systems have been installed in theaters on Broadway as well as in many other theaters throughout the country.

Induction Loop. Because an induction loop is simply a loop of wire, it may encircle a listening area of any size; the two ends of the wire are attached to the output of a power amplifier whose input is a microphone or other signal source. The current passing through the wire creates an electromagnetic field that reflects the strength and frequency of the input signal. It is possible for this electromagnetic field, through magnetic induction, to generate voltage proportional to the current in the loop in another coil of wire (such as a telecoil) within its range. Thus, to benefit from this arrangement, those with hearing loss need either a hearing aid with a telecoil or a special receiver equipped with a telecoil; the latter may be pocket-sized with earphones attached or a wand held to the ear like a telephone handset.

High-powered amplifiers are needed for a large area loop; if only a smaller section of an assembly area is looped, then listeners using it must sit in a designated place, which some view as a disadvantage. Induction loop systems are susceptible to electromagnetic interference from electrical wiring, florescent lighting, transformers, electric motors, and similar sources. Moreover, the strength of the signal varies according to location within the loop, being stronger near the perimeter and weaker in the center. An electromagnetic field will pass through walls; thus, spillover to receivers in adjacent rooms is possible. Oval Window Audio has developed a three dimensional (3-D) induction loop embedded in a special mat designed to be placed under a floor covering such as carpet.[22] Major advantages of the 3-D system are reported to be greater uniformity of the signal and minimal spillover. Induction loops have been used in this country to offer hearing assistance since the 1950s.[23] In some settings, this is the most suitable option.

Rehabilitation Act of 1973. An important influence on the use of large area assistive listening systems originated with Title V of the Rehabilitation Act of 1973 (PL 93-112). Section 502 of this act created an independent federal agency, the Architectural and Transportation Barriers Compliance Board (ATBCB) to enforce the Architectural Barriers Act of 1968.[24] This 1968 law prohibited architectural barriers in federally funded buildings to ensure accessibility to people with disabilities. The elimination of communication barriers in assembly areas is included in the "Minimum Guidelines and Requirements for Accessible Design" adopted by the ATBCB in 1982.[25] These regulations define an assembly area as a room or space accommodating 50 or more persons. Such areas with audio amplification systems are required to have a listening system to assist a reasonable number of people, but no fewer than two, with severe hearing loss. Audio loops and radio frequency systems, which include light wave systems, are listed as acceptable. For assembly areas without amplification systems, a permanently installed or portable listening system is mandated. Many states also have similar architectural barrier laws.

Americans with Disabilities Act of 1990. Communication access was extended to the private sector through implementation of the Americans with Disabilities Act (ADA) (PL 101-336). Title III, Public Accommodations, of the ADA prohibits discrimination on the basis of disability by private entities in places of public accommodation and commercial facilities.[26] The term "public accommodation" in this law refers to 12 categories of facilities; among these are the large assembly areas found in places of exhibition (museums), entertainment (theaters, stadiums, concert halls), and public gathering (auditoriums, convention centers). Private membership clubs and religious organizations are exempt. According to this regulation, a public accommodation must provide auxiliary aids to remove communication barriers for those with hearing loss unless doing so would result in an undue burden or a fundamental alteration in the nature of the goods or services being provided. Among the auxiliary aids listed by the ADA are assistive listening systems. Permanently installed assistive listening systems are required for existing or new assembly areas that seat at least 50 persons or have audio amplification systems. If the assistive listening system is permanently installed to serve fixed seats, as with an induction loop, then such seats must be within a distance of 50 feet from the stage or playing area. In addition, receivers must be provided equal to 4% of the total number of seats.

ROLE OF THE SCHOOL WITH REGARD TO ASSISTIVE DEVICES

To Provide Information.   It is important that those who are in daily contact with students having hearing impairments and their families be knowledgeable about the vast resources available to help those with hearing loss achieve communication access. Teachers, audiologists, speech-language pathologists, counselors, nurses, and administrators may contribute by providing information and referrals regarding assistive devices to students and families. A school library might add books and videotapes that demonstrate assistive devices to its collection.[27] A program concerning assistive devices may be scheduled for meetings of parent groups affiliated with the school. A school-based assistive device fair, similar to a health fair or book fair, has been reported by the organization of parents of children with hearing impairment at Camelot Elementary School in Fairfax County, Virginia, to be "one of the most popular and productive programs ever sponsored."[28] Vendors were invited to display their products at this fair and to give a brief product presentation. Then, those in attendance visited the various exhibits to view demonstrations, ask questions, and obtain literature.

Because assistive devices contribute to communication access in everyday living, information about these important technological options should be included in a student's comprehensive education. One resource is Deyo's teacher guide and student workbook, *On My Own,*[29] which introduces children ages 10 to 16 to alerting devices, closed captioned TV, and personal and large area listening systems. Schools should have some devices available to demonstrate and to help children gain familiarity with them. The school should ensure that children understand the basic technology of various assistive devices as well as the coupling options for devices to hearing aids. Children should be prepared to know which assistive devices might best meet their needs in certain situations.

To Provide Training in the Use of Assistive Devices.   Although some assistive devices are relatively uncomplicated, others require a period of training to be used most effectively. Consequently, in addition to supplying information about assistive devices, educators should help students with hearing impairments learn to use this technology.[30] Such efforts have been made in the area of telephone communication. Both Castle[31] and Erber[32] have developed and written about equipment options and instructional programs to facilitate telephone use. The materials these authors make available may be modified for various age groups. Another teaching aid is a training system that allows practice with TTs (Fig. 13-5). This device, powered by AC, is outfitted with telephone handsets to connect either two or four TTs so children may communicate via this mode without the necessity of an actual telephone line. Because these handsets have magnetic leakage, this training system also may be used to demonstrate the advantages of a telecoil in a hearing aid. The teacher may simulate a telephone conversation by talking to a child using the training system's handsets. Then, the child can learn: (1) to activate the telecoil of his or her hearing aid by moving the input switch to *T*; and (2) to position the telephone handset so the proper orientation is achieved with the telecoil for best listening results. Another training device has circuitry that duplicates the noise conditions existing on real telephone lines; it may be used to connect either two standard telephones or one telephone and a cassette recorder. Such equipment is vital to help children with hearing aids learn to use telecoils and to communicate over the telephone. Understanding the operation of a telecoil should not be underestimated. It will enable children to utilize this feature to optimal advantage in the

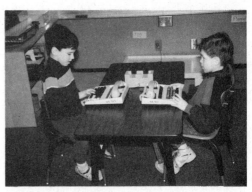

Figure 13-5. Children using a training system connecting two text telephones (TDDs).

future with the telephone and as a means of coupling hearing aids and assistive listening devices.

Because assistive devices can be used in the home, sessions may be organized at school to provide parents with hands-on demonstrations. Once parents become familiar with these devices, they will encourage their children in this area.

Finally, school systems should schedule periodic in-service instruction to keep teachers and other staff members up-to-date regarding technological advances in the area of assistive devices. Everyone must be knowledgeable if communication access in daily life is to become a reality.

REFERENCES

1. Vaughn GR, Lightfoot RK: Assistive listening devices and systems for adults who are hearing impaired, in Hull RH, ed: *Aural Rehabilitation* ed 2 (San Diego, CA: Singular Publishing Group, Inc, 1992), chap 14.
2. Compton C: Assistive technology for deaf and hard-of-hearing people, in Alpiner JG and McCarthy PA, eds: *Rehabilitative Audiology: Children and Adults* ed 2 (Baltimore, MD: Williams & Wilkins, 1993), chap 16.
3. *Telecommunications for the Disabled Act of 1982.* P. L. 97-410 (96 Stat. 2043).
4. *Hearing Aid Compatibility Act of 1988.* P. L. 100-394 (102 Stat. 976).
5. Cherow E, Thompson M, eds: *Audiology Update,* 12, No. 3 (1993), 10.
6. Slager RD: Romancing the phone: the adventure continues. *Seminars in Hearing,* 10 (1989) 42–55.
7. Harkins JE: Visual devices for deaf and hard of hearing people: state-of-the-art. *GRI Monograph Series* (Washington, DC: Gallaudet Research Institute, Series A, No 3, 1991), sec. II.
8. Title IV, Telecommunications, *Americans with Disabilities Act of 1990,* P. L. 101-336 (104 Stat. 327).
9. DuBow S, Geer S, Strauss KP: *Legal Rights: The Guide for Deaf and Hard of Hearing People* ed 4 (Washington, DC: Gallaudet University Press, 1992), chap. 11.
10. *Television Decoder Circuitry Act of 1990,* P. L. 101-431 (104 Stat. 960).
11. Harkins JE: Visual devices for deaf and hard of hearing people: state-of-art. *GRI Monograph Series* (Washington, DC: Gallaudet Research Institute, Series A, No 3, 1991), sec. III.
12. Braverman B: Television captioning strategies: A systematic research and development approach. *Amer Annals of the Deaf* 126 (1981), 1031–1036.
13. National Captioning Institute: Hearing impaired children's comprehension of closed captioned television programs, research report 83-5 (Falls Church, VA: National Captioning Institute, 1983).
14. Jensema CJ: Specialized audio, visual, and tactile alerting devices for deaf and hard of hearing people. *GRI Occasional Paper Series* (Washington, DC: Gallaudet Research Institute, No. 90-2, 1990).
15. Sudler WH, Flexer C: Low cost assistive listening device. *Lang, Speech, Hearing Serv Schools,* 17 (1986), 342–344.
16. Flexer C: *Facilitating Hearing and Listening in Young Children* (San Diego, CA: Singular Publishing Group, Inc., 1994), chap. 5.
17. Flexer C, Savage H: Using an ALD in speech-language assessment and training. *The Hearing Journal,* 45 (1992), 28–35.
18. American Speech-Language-Hearing Association: Amplification as a remediation technique for children with normal peripheral hearing. *ASHA,* 33, Suppl. 3 (1991), 22–24.
19. Boothroyd A: The FM wireless link: an invisible microphone cable, in Ross M, ed: *FM Auditory Training Systems* (Timonium, MD: York Press, Inc., 1992), chap 1.
20. News announcement, *Hearing Instruments,* 43 (1992), 6.
21. Lieske M: Infrared systems, in Ross M, ed: *Communication Access for Persons with Hearing Loss* (Baltimore, MD: York Press, Inc., 1994), chap. 3.
22. Hendricks P, Lederman N: Development of a three-dimensional induction assistive listening system. *Hearing Instruments,* 42 (1991), 37.
23. Williams GI: The five technologies of large space hearing assistance systems. *Assistive Listening Devices and Systems* (Rockville, MD: ASHA, 1985), chap 4.
24. DuBow S, Geer S, Strauss KP: *Legal Rights: The Guide for Deaf and Hard of Hearing People* ed. 4 (Washington, DC: Gallaudet University Press, 1992), chap. 3.
25. Architectural and Transportation Barriers Compliance Board (ATBCB): Minimum guidelines and requirements for accessible design: final rule. *Federal Register,* 47 (August 4, 1982), 33862.
26. Department of Justice: Nondiscrimination on the basis of disability by public accommodations and in commercial facilities: final rule. *Federal Register,* 56 (July 26, 1991), 35544.
27. Compton CL: *Assistive Devices: Doorways to Independence* (videotape and book), (Washington, DC: Gallaudet University, 1989).
28. Fellendorf GW: *Current Developments in Assistive Devices for Hearing Impaired Persons in the United States* (Washington, DC: Gallaudet Research Institute, 1982), 36.
29. Deyo D: *On My Own, Student Workbook and Teacher Guide* (Washington, DC: Pre-College Programs, Gallaudet University, 1984).
30. Fellendorf GW, Castle DS, Ravich R, Gammel C: Institutional panel on trends and issues, in Fellendorf GW, ed: *Develop and Deliver II: The Proceedings of the Second International Forum on Assistive Listening Devices and Systems for Hearing Impaired Persons* (Washington, DC: Fellendorf Associates, Inc, 1985), 85–97.
31. Castle D: *Telephone Training for Hearing-Impaired Persons: Amplified Telephones, TDD's, Codes* ed 2 (Rochester, NY: NTID/RIT Press, 1984).
32. Erber NP: *Telephone Communication and Hearing Impairment* (San Diego, CA: College Hill Press, 1985).

COCHLEAR IMPLANTS AND TACTILE DEVICES FOR STUDENTS WITH PROFOUND DEAFNESS

Ross J. Roeser

> *The universe is full of magical things, patiently waiting for our wits to grow sharper.*
>
> —Eden Philpotts, 1862–1960

Conventional amplification through personal hearing aids provides significant benefit to the majority of children and adults with hearing loss. With conventional hearing aids, acoustic signals are amplified to an intensity great enough to make them audible to the impaired ear. In the preschool and school-age child, the added acoustic stimulation should help to improve the reception of speech and, as a consequence, foster the development of speech and language skills.

A basic tenet of audiological management for children with hearing impairment is to provide amplification as soon as possible to promote communication skills (see Chapter 10 and 12). Although the vast majority of children and adults with hearing impairment benefit significantly from conventional amplification, it is clear that there are some who do not. Specifically, those with profound deafness typically receive so little additional information from the amplified signal that they will not wear a hearing aid when given the choice. Case study 14–1 describes a child with profound deafness who does not benefit from amplification.

PROFOUND DEAFNESS DEFINED

As described in Chapter 2, degree of hearing loss is defined by a shift of threshold sensitivity from 0 dB hearing level (HL) (ANSI, 1989). The classifications are usually based on the average of the thresholds in the frequencies 500, 1000, and 2000 Hz. Although the classification systems vary somewhat, each typically contains five major categories: minimal or slight, mild, moderate, severe, and profound. These classification systems provide a general way to describe the effects of hearing loss on speech communication. In children,

predictions can be made regarding the development of speech and language based on the degree of hearing loss present (adapted from Boothroyd).[1]

Minimal or Slight. Children with minimal or slight (15–25 dB HL) hearing loss may experience speech and language delay (see Chapter 9). Hearing aids are not typically used with these children, but classroom amplification and special training is recommended (see Chapter 12).

Mild. Children with mild (26–40 dB HL) hearing loss will experience minimal delay in speech and language development. Hearing aids, special training, and classroom amplification are sometimes used, depending on the individual child.

Moderate. Children with moderate (41–60 dB HL) hearing loss will experience speech and language delay, but speech and language development will not be prevented. Hearing aids and modest intervention will allow these children to develop almost normally.

Severe. Children with severe (61–90 dB HL) hearing loss require intervention to *prevent* significant delays in the speech and language development. With appropriately fit hearing aids, frequency modulation (FM) systems in the classroom, proper early intervention and special training, hearing can become the principal avenue for speech and language development; most children with severe hearing loss can develop almost normally.

Profound. Children with profound (91+ dB HL) hearing loss will require intense intervention for speech and language to develop, and even then development will be slow and difficult. Hearing will not be the primary avenue for learning, but will be *a complement to lipreading*. Within the profound deafness category, there are three subcategories.

Case study 14-1. K.S. has no significant clinical history, except for a series of ear infections beginning about 1 year of age. At 1 year, 7 months of age, K.S. contracted meningitis. Following hospital discharge, her parents noted a lack of awareness to sound and had K.S. evaluated by an audiologist. Despite her visual attentiveness, behavioral testing over two sessions revealed a lack of response to auditory stimuli, except for low frequencies presented at the limits of the audiometer; immittance testing revealed no apparent middle ear disease. Auditory brainstem response testing indicated no response at audiometric limits, confirming a severe to profound sensorineural hearing loss.

K.S. was fit with high-gain binaural amplification, and she and her family were placed in a parent education program for children with hearing impairment. Formal hearing aid evaluation showe d that K.S. demonstrated benefit from her hearing aids; low-frequency unaided thresholds improved from 95–100 dB HL to the 55–60 dB range with her instruments. Initially, both parents reported more awareness to environmental sounds and speech when K.S. was wearing her hearing aids, and felt that she was benefiting from them. At 3 years of age, K.S. was placed in a preschool program for children with hearing impairments, which she attended daily. Her teachers felt that K.S. had excellent learning potential, but her limited speech was unintelligible, and she was significantly delayed in her language skills on formal tests. None of her teachers felt that she was benefiting from hearing aid use, as was evident from her performance on listening tasks. She consistently was unable to perform auditory tasks whether aided or unaided. On occasion, routine daily checks of her hearing aids would reveal that one or both instruments were not functioning, and she did not indicate that she knew the difference.

At 14 years of age, K.S. finished grade school and entered into a high school program for students with hearing impairment. Many of the students used sign language. Although K.S. had some intelligible speech, she no longer wore her hearing aids voluntarily, and reacted when attempts were made by her parents to encourage their use. At 18 years of age, after being graduated from high school, she discontinued the use of her hearing aids altogether. Sign language became her only means of communication.

1. *Those with considerable residual hearing.* Children in this subcategory will have hearing loss from 90 to 100 dB HL and have hearing above 1000 Hz at 105 dB HL. Information about intonation and vowel articulation and some information about consonant articulation will be provided through hearing. With high quality, high gain amplification and intense intervention, children in this category will develop like children with severe hearing loss.[2]

2. *Those with little residual hearing.* Children in this subcategory will have hearing loss from 100 to 110 dB HL and hearing above 1000 Hz at 110 dB HL or more. With high-gain amplification, hearing is only able to provide information regarding intensity, duration, rhythm, and maybe intonation and vowel cues. There are remarkable children who fall into this category and develop oral language skills, but they are rare. However, most children in this subcategory fall into subcategory 3 described below.

3. *Those with no residual hearing.* Children in this subcategory will have average thresholds in the 110+ dB HL range. Hearing, even with high gain amplification, will provide minimal benefit; these children will learn speech and language skills only through vision. Children (or

adults) in this subcategory will need special consideration. Two devices that are available for those who do not receive benefit from conventional amplification are cochlear implants and tactile devices.

COCHLEAR IMPLANTS AND TACTILE DEVICES

Cochlear implants are like hearing aids in that they attempt to process acoustic signals so that they are audible and have meaning. However, cochlear implants differ from hearing aids in that they use more sophisticated technology and deliver an electrical signal, rather than an acoustic signal, to the ear through an electrode array having several channels, which has been surgically implanted in the cochlea. Because surgery is needed, the technique requires the expertise of a specially trained otolaryngologist for implanting the electrode, and it is expensive. First year costs, including the hardware, hospitalization, surgery, and rehabilitation, range between $35,000 and $40,000. The high cost of cochlear implants severely limits their availability to many persons with profound deafness. Third party coverage is available for the cochlear implant device, hospitalization and surgery; Medicare covers these costs in some states. However, coverage for the critically important postoperative rehabilitation and device adjustment can be difficult to secure; some insurance policies specifically exclude any type of therapy, education, or rehabilitation.[3] As a result, there are many schoolchildren using cochlear implants in the classroom who are in need of special training.

With tactile stimulation, acoustic signals are changed into vibratory or electric patterns, which are delivered to the skin. The goal of a tactile communication system is to extract relevant information from the acoustic signal and to present it to the individual in a tactile mode as a means of supplementing the auditory reception of the acoustic signal—with the successful reception of speech as the ultimate challenge. Surgery is not required for tactile stimulation, and the typical cost of a tactile aid ranges from about $900 to $2500. Several types of cochlear implants and a number of tactile aids are now available commercially and are being used in the educational setting.

What is the need for cochlear implants or tactile instruments? Who are candidates? How do they work? What devices are available? Are they safe? Are they effective? What differences are there between the two devices? What intervention strategies should be used with those receiving the devices? These, as well as other issues, are addressed in this chapter.

THE NEED FOR COCHLEAR IMPLANTS OR TACTILE AIDS

The need for cochlear implants or tactile aids depends on the prevalence of severe to profound deafness, and an estimate of those among this population who might benefit from their use. Following approval of the single channel cochlear implant by the Food and Drug Administration (FDA) in 1984, sensationalism by the news media resulted in claims that the device represented the solution for deafness for millions of people.[4] This claim, quite obviously, was an overstatement. An early attempt to delimit the eligible population for cochlear implants was undertaken by Carhart.[5] He estimated that, in 1974, there were between 70,000 and 80,000 children and adults in the United States who were potential candidates for cochlear implants. A more recent estimate was provided by The American Speech-

Language-Hearing Association (ASHA) Ad Hoc Committee on Cochlear Implants.[6] The ASHA committee used data reported by The National Center for Health Statistics and indicated that there were between 131,000 and 294,000 individuals 3 years of age and older nationwide who would be candidates for cochlear implants.

These estimates represent the population of all individuals with profound deafness 3 years of age and older in the United States. Clearly then, the number of eligible school-age children is less than these figures. Ries[7] reviewed data from the 1982 Annual Survey of Hearing Impaired Children and Youth and reports that 51,962 school children with hearing loss were identified in 6000 schools. Among this population, there were 35,735 children with no additional handicapping conditions that potentially could eliminate the child from cochlear implant candidacy; and of the 35,735, there were 16,607 with hearing loss in the profound (91 dB International Standards Organization or above) range. To account for error, Kachmer recommended increasing the estimates by one third, giving a range from 16,607 to 22,087. If one eliminates the 20 to 55% of this population who would not be stimulated due to insufficient nerve fibers,[6] the result would be from 9170 to 17,670 school age children nationwide who are eligible for cochlear implants.

With regard to tactile aids, except for rare sensory disorders of the skin, there are no clear physiological contraindications. Also, a favorable aspect of tactile aid use is that a trial period can be carried out with little difficulty because the instrument is not permanently implanted in the body through surgery. Thus, tactile aids have a potentially wider application and can be used with less trauma than cochlear implants. As many as 367,000 individuals with profound deafness 3 years of age and older, and an even greater number of children (if those under 3 years of age are included) may benefit from tactile instruments.

SAFETY, EFFECTIVENESS, AND LABELING—THE ROLE OF THE FOOD AND DRUG ADMINISTRATION

FDA Medical Device amendments of 1976 initiated regulations to guide the medical devices industry. In essence, these amendments set up guidelines to be followed by medical device manufacturers before the devices are offered to the public for use and sale. In 1982, the Center for Devices and Radiological Health (CDRH) was established to protect public health in the fields of medical devices and radiological health. One purpose of the CDRH program is to assure the safety, effectiveness, and proper labeling of medical devices. Medical devices that are not "substantially equivalent" to devices that were on the market prior to May 28, 1976, must now be approved by the FDA before they can be sold in the United States. The term "substantially equivalent" implies that the device has the same function or composition, or both.

The procedures that are required to gain FDA approval of a medical device are complex and need not be detailed here. However, there are two steps in the process. First, manufacturers must submit an investigational device exemption (IDE), which outlines procedures to collect data on safety and effectiveness. Once the IDE is approved, a limited number of investigators are selected to use the device under controlled conditions. After completion of the IDE stage, a premarket approval application (PMA) is filed, describing the device in detail and the data that were collected on safety and effectiveness. The PMA also contains information on labeling. IDEs and PMAs are reviewed by a panel of experts who act as consultants to the FDA to determine whether the claims made by the manufacturer are supported by the data collected.

Cochlear implants must follow the FDA process. However, tactile aids are exempt from FDA approval because of their substantial equivalence; they were on the market prior to May 28, 1976.

Once approved by the FDA, the public can be assured that devices are safe and effective *for the claims that are made about them*. An adult who is a candidate for a cochlear implant, or parents of children who are candidates, should read the claims carefully before deciding to have an implant. The claims will enable the user to determine the expected benefits.

The FDA approved the first PMA for cochlear implants for adults in 1984 and later approved the device for children 2 years of age and older in 1985. The initial device approved was the 3M/House single-channel cochlear implant. However, since 1984–1985, a number of other cochlear implants have been approved or are under consideration by the FDA (Table 14–1). It is clear that in the future clinicians and educators will be faced with providing for the (re)habilitative and educational needs of an expanding population of chldren and adults with profound deafness wearing cochlear implants.

COCHLEAR IMPLANTS

In the past few years the literature on cochlear implants has exploded with reports describing cochlear implants and their use with children and adults. Because it is impossible to cover this vast literature in this chapter, the material will be limited to how implants work and the devices that are currently available, candidacy, risks, benefits, comparison between cochlear implant systems and cochlear implants in children.

Figure 14–1 is a schematic showing one type of cochlear implant system; most systems use the basic techniques shown here. During surgery, an electrode array is placed through the round window of the cochlea into the scala tympani, and an internal receiver or stimulator is secured in the temporal bone above and behind the ear. As sound is picked up by the microphone (1), it is converted into an electric signal and delivered to a speech processor (3), where selected acoustic characteristics are coded. The primary function of the processor is to prepare and code the incoming acoustic information for delivery to the electrode array. The electric code from the speech processor is delivered to a transmitter coil (5), and is electromagnetically induced across the skin to an internal receiver/stimulator (6). The internal receiver/stimulator converts the code to electric signals, and they are delivered to the electrode or electrodes placed in the cochlea (7). As the electric signals stimulate the structures in the inner ear and cranial nerve VIII, the signals are recognized as sounds, and a sensation of hearing occurs (8).

Most systems work essentially in this way, although one has direct input to the internal coil, meaning that it is hardwired using a percutaneous plug (see Table 14–1). It should be noted that not all channels are always used with the systems having multiple channels. Instead, only the channels that are found to be functional through testing are activated. Moreover, some implants have been placed in cochleas obliterated by bony growth. In these cases, less than a full array of electrodes is placed in the cochlea. Interestingly, many patients with partially inserted electrodes do very well with their implants, and data from adults indicate that less than a full array of electrodes does not appear to affect speech perception performance.[8]

Table 14–1 lists four devices that currently have either IDE or PMA approval by the FDA. The following describes specific features of each device.

Table 14–1 Comparison of Four Cochlear Implant Systems Available in the United States

Manufacturer	Name of Device	Cost of Device to Hospital	FDA Status	No. Elec-trodes	No. Chan-nels	Electric Nave-form	Coupling to Internal Transmitter/ Electrode	No. Patients Implanted Chil-dren	Adults
3M (see text)	House	N/A	PMA approved for adults IDE approved for children	1	1	Analog	Transcutaneous (induction coil)	280*	680*
Cochlear Corp. 61 Iverness Dr. Suite 200 Englewood, CO 80112 303-790-9010	Nucleus Mini-22	$14,695	PMA approved for children and adults	22	Varies	Pulsatile	Transcutaneous (induction coil)	2800 (4/1/94)	3700 (4/1/94)
MiniMed Technologies 12744 San Fernando Road P.O. Box 9219 Sylmar, CA 91391 818-362-5958	Clarion	$13,995	IDE for adults only	16	8	Pulsatile or analog	Transcutaneous (induction coil)	N/A	78 (4/1/94)
Smith & Newphew Richards 2925 Appling Rd. Bartlett, TN 34134 901-373-0200	Ineraid Coch-lear Implant System†	$13,000	IDE for adults only	6	4	Analog	Percutaneous Pedestal (direct)	N/A	200 (4/1/94)

*Estimate based on available data.
†Prior to 1989, this device was named Symbion.

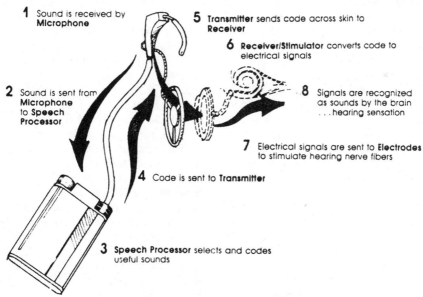

1 Sound is received by **Microphone**

2 Sound is sent from **Microphone** to **Speech Processor**

3 Speech Processor selects and codes useful sounds

4 Code is sent to **Transmitter**

5 **Transmitter** sends code across skin to **Receiver**

6 **Receiver/Stimulator** converts code to electrical signals

7 Electrical signals are sent to **Electrodes** to stimulate hearing nerve fibers

8 Signals are recognized as sounds by the brain . . . hearing sensation

Figure 14–1. Illustration of how cochlear implants produce sound sensations (see text for detailed explanation). (Courtesy of Cochlear Corporation.)

3M House. The 3M House cochlear implant was developed under the direction of Dr. William F. House. In 1972, Dr. House was the first surgeon in the United States to implant a wearable signal processor. The device was approved by the FDA for adults in November 1984 and for children in 1985.

The 3M House device is a single channel instrument. As a result, it cannot deliver separate information to the different parts of the cochlea. Although this instrument represented a major breakthrough at the time, clinical studies began showing that as a group, patients performed better with multiple-channel instruments and single-channel instruments are no longer routinely implanted in the United States.

3M sold the technology for the House device in August 1989 and a decision was made to discontinue with the FDA PMA process. During the course of studies with the 3M device, the best estimate is that 280 children and 680 adults were implanted. Interestingly, at the time of this writing about 200 patients have had the single-channel electrode removed from their cochlea and have been reimplanted with a multichannel electrode array; clinical reports from these patients indicate that they are performing quite well. For example, Chute et al[9] report on a child who received a multichannel cochlear implant after the internal coil of her single-channel implant failed. The explantation/reimplantation process did not impair the child's auditory perceptions from the cochlear implant. In fact, after about 6 months with the new device, her performance was equal to the single channel device and after a year her performance was superior with the multichannel device.

Cochlear Corporation, Nucleus Mini-22. The nucleus device is named the Mini-22 system. The work that led to the development of the Mini-22 was performed at the University of Melbourne in Australia in the late 1970s. The initiation of clinical trials in the United States began in 1986, shortly after the FDA approved clinical trials for adults for the 3M device. Currently, the Mini-22 is the only device still being implanted and having PMA approval by the FDA for both children and adults. Consequently, more patients have been implanted with this system than any other device. As of April 1, 1994, 2800 children and 3700 adults are using this system in the United States.

The distinctive features of the Mini-22 system are:

1. It has an array of 22 evenly spaced platinum band electrodes. The electrodes are mounted on a flexible silicon rubber structure that allows them to be inserted into the spiral-shaped cochlea. Although each electrode is capable of receiving separate input and providing stimulation, there is a scientific debate about the actual number of functional channels that can be stimulated simultaneously. However, this system does allow for the greatest number of possible stimulation sites in the inner ear.
2. The device has a single manufacturer. Other devices have changed manufacturers. This factor is important in that resources must

be made available to support the devices implanted, as well as to continue development.

MiniMed Technologies, Clarion. The Clarion device was developed through collaborative efforts at the University of California at San Francisco, the Research Triangle Institute (in North Carolina), and MiniMed Technologies (Sylmar, California). At present, this device is under IDE status from the FDA for adults only.

Distinctive features of the Clarion device are:

1. It consist of 16 stimulus contacts (electrodes) arranged in staggered pairs (channels). The electrode array is contained in a silicon rubber carrier molded in a coil to fit within the snail-shaped cochlea. Because of the unique preshaped form of the electrode array, a special tool is used to insert it into the cochlea during surgery.
2. It is the only system that permits more than one type of speech coding; that is, the user can select between pulsatile or analog electric wave forms (see Table 14–1). This versatility allows patients to choose the electric code that offers the most advantageous sound reception in different environments. Although the exact advantage of having this option has yet to be clearly documented, there are theoretical advantages.

As of 4/1/94, 78 adults have been implanted with this device.

Smith & Nephew Richards, Ineraid Cochlear Implant System. The initial work that led to the Ineraid device was performed at the University of Utah in the 1970s. The system was first designed to provide electric stimulation directly to the cortex of the brain. However, because of technical problems, the emphasis was shifted to inner ear stimulation. Originally, Symbion obtained a license to manufacture and distribute the system under an IDE and the device was called the Symbion Device. However, in August 1989 Smith & Nephew Richards, Inc. purchased the system and the device was renamed Ineraid. The Ineraid is currently under IDE status from the FDA for adults only.

Distinctive features of the Ineraid Cochlear Implant System include:

1. It has eight electrodes. Six of the electrodes are inserted into the cochlea and the other two are used as reference/ground. The external signal processor has four channels.
2. It is the only system that uses a percutaneous (through the skin) pedestal to connect (interface) the external hardware to the internal hardware. As described earlier

and shown in Figure 14–1, other systems use an external coil (transmitter) and internal coil (receiver) and transmit information through the skin using magnetic induction. As of April 1, 1994, 200 adults have been implanted with the Ineraid Cochlear Implant System.

Selection of Implants

Adults who are candidates, and parents of children who are candidates, for cochlear implants should seek advice from audiologists and otolaryngologists about the technical advances that are being made with the various devices that are available before selecting the device to be implanted. Factors that should be considered in selecting a cochlear implant include:

The technical capabilities of the system.

The availability of service. That is, how many centers will provide support for the system.

The time required for repair.

The availability of a loaner external signal processor in the event that the unit malfunctions.

The manufacturer's research and development capabilities; resources must be available and there must be a commitment from the manufacturer to continue supporting the device.

Candidacy

The FDA has established separate candidacy requirements for children and adults for cochlear implants. For children, candidacy requires the following:

1. Aged 2 to 17 years.
2. Bilateral profound sensorineural deafness (electrophysiological assessment must corroborate behavioral evaluation for younger children).
3. Little or no benefit from a hearing (or tactile) aid as demonstrated by failure to improve on age-appropriate closed-set word identification tasks (a minimum of a 6 month trial with appropriate amplification and rehabilitation is recommended to ascertain the potential for aided benefit).
4. Families and (if possible) candidates should be well motivated and possess appropriate expectations.

For adults the FDA candidacy requirements are as follows:

1. Profound sensorineural deafness.

2. Little or no benefit from a hearing aid.
3. Postlingually deafened.
4. Eighteen years of age or older.
5. Psychologically and motivationally suitable.

For both children and adults contraindications include:

1. Deafness due to lesions of the acoustic nerve or central auditory pathway.
2. Active middle ear infections.
3. Cochlear ossification that prevents electrode insertion as determined through preoperative high-resolution computed tomography (CT) scans.
4. Absence of cochlear development as determined through preoperative high-resolution CT scans.
5. Tympanic membrane perforations.

Case study 14–1, presented earlier in this chapter, describes a child who would have been an ideal candidate for a cochlear implant at an early age. As indicated in this case history, despite the fact that this child was receiving some benefit by formal hearing aid evaluation, she demonstrated little or no advantage with the use of high-gain instruments in her everyday listening environment. This is one primary reason accepted by clinicians for considering any individual with profound deafness for either a cochlear implant or a tactile instrument.

Although all of the above procedures have some value in determining candidacy, results from the audiological evaluation, and past experience with hearing aids—more than any of the other single presurgical considerations—are the primary considerations used to determine candidacy. Patients who receive cochlear implants must have profound deafness and not be able to benefit from conventional amplification.

Owens and Telleen[10] reinforce the need for conclusive documentation of hearing aid performance prior to cochlear implant surgery. They studied the performance of two profoundly deaf patients with hearing aids compared to three patients with single-channel cochlear implants on audiometric and speechreading procedures. Those using the cochlear implants showed wide variations in their responses, but results from the two patients using conventional amplification were consistently superior to those of the subjects with implants. This report reinforces the requirement that experience with a suitable hearing aid is mandatory before a cochlear implant should be considered. Tests of auditory speech perception and speechreading with a suitable hearing aid are necessary as part of the preimplant testing.

The requirement that children be at least 2 years of age is needed not as the result of technical surgical considerations, but to establish firmly the presence of deafness and the lack of benefit from traditional amplification. Such a time period is required when deafness is established at birth. Even though the age of 2 years has been set as a minimum criterion for cochlear implant candidacy, there are those who believe that this is too young. They argue that audiometric testing on children age 2 years and younger is much too variable to ensure that profound bilateral deafness is present with 100% accuracy. Although auditory brainstem evoked response (ABR) audiometry is available, the maximum stimulation levels are limited and low-frequency hearing can be present when ABR responses are absent.

Behavioral audiometry using observation techniques can be used, but responses are influenced by the maturational level of the child and the observers' experience and response criteria (see Chapter 2). In addition, especially for the child with acquired deafness, at 2 years of age the benefits of hearing aid use cannot always be firmly established. Sufficient time is needed with appropriately fit amplification before the decision is made to implant a young child. Based on these concerns many believe that specifying a minimum age for a cochlear implant is not appropriate. Unfortunately, this minimum age becomes the accepted standard for all children to receive an implant. Instead, each child must be considered individually and candidacy be determined only when profound deafness and the inability to benefit from appropriately fit amplification are firmly established.

Intelligence testing for children who meet the hearing loss criteria is critical. Due to the questions that still surround cochlear implants in children, candidates must present with no other complicating factors, such as low intelligence; it would not be clear whether any lack of progress in an implanted child with below-normal intelligence was a result of the cochlear implant or the child's intellectual level. Due to the inherent difficulties in establishing intellectual function in children with deafness, each child's age, motor performance, and communication level and skills must be considered in selecting the most appropriate measures. Children with autism and significant learning disabilities should be eliminated from candidacy.[6]

A unique criterion, evidence of strong family support, is a key ingredient for success with children. The obligations and responsibilities associated with cochlear implants are considerable and critical to the child's overall success. The family must be aware of the requirements through preimplant counseling, and then be able and agreeable to meet the increasing needs following surgery. Table 14–2 provides examples of how family support can be documented overtly.

Table 14–2   Evidence of Strong Family Support*

Accept child's hearing loss
Keep appointments
Are Knowledgeable about child's hearing aids
Communicate well with child
Have appropriate expectations
Display high interest and motivation levels
Spend ample time with child
Use same language at home and school
Have concern for child's educational and physical development

*Reprinted with permission from Northern et al.[11]

Risks

Proponents of the cochlear implant believe that the benefits provided by the implant far outweigh any potential risks, even though it is recognized that most users will not be able to discriminate open set speech. The risks involved with cochlear implants are low, but their existence must be recognized. With any surgical procedure, consideration must be given to the low-incidence risks associated with general anesthesia and with possible infection. Besides these general considerations, there are several others that are specific to the cochlear implant. Initially, concern was raised about the possibility of bone growth in the cochlea, because animal studies have shown that electric stimulation of the cochlea will cause this condition to occur, which results in disruption of hair cell function.[11] However, clinical experience has demonstrated that many patients have used cochlear implants for years without significant changes in electric threshold sensitivity. This finding would suggest that there are no obvious adverse affects of cochlear implant use for these time periods, but does not address the important question of lifetime use for periods of 70 to 80 years for the infant wearing a cochlear implant. However, the question remains as to the possible effects on the discrimination ability or recognition of more complex sounds over extended use.

Downs[13] expressed concern for children being considered for cochlear implants who are at risk for recurring otitis media; during the infection stage, there is a potential for bacterial invasion of the cochlea. To help identify children who might be affected, she gives high-risk categories for otitis media pronicity. Despite this logical cautionary stance, studies have failed to document a higher incidence of otitis media or secondary complications in patients receiving cochlear implants.[14] As a result, otitis media does not appear to be a major complicating factor at present.

A particular concern with children is head growth. At birth, the cochlea has reached adult size.

However, the temporal bone that houses the components of the cochlear implant continues to grow and enlarge as the infant develops. As a result, allowances need to be made with infants, so that the intracochlear electrode will not be extracted from the cochlea. O'Donoghue et al[15] found that maximum head growth occurs in the first 2 years of life and recommended prolonging surgery until after this age. In addition, these investigators recommended that a stretching allowance of 1 to 3 cm be made for the intracochlear electrode array in young children to account for head growth.

Device malfunctions have occurred in some patients. In fact, several years ago one manufacturer voluntarily called a moratorium on implanting a device due to a failure of the internal coil in several patients. When device malfunctions occur, reimplantation is necessary, and reports have indicated auditory sensations are possible from the reimplanted electrode array.[16]

Other possible complications include tinnitus, dizziness, and facial muscle twitching; facial muscle twitching is most likely with extracochlear devices. Although these potential complications exist, their occurrence is reportedly rare because they have been found in only a few patients.[17]

Benefits

As stated earlier in this chapter, once the FDA approves a device, manufacturers can then label the device and advertize the benefits that can be expected from using the device. However, the claims made must be based on the data that were collected during the PMA. Quite obviously, the expected benefits from cochlear implants are different for children and adults, and separate claims are available for the two populations. For children

who receive cochlear implants (specifically the Nucleus 22 channel device), the expected benefits are as follows:

1. Implant patients are able to detect medium to loud environmental sounds, including speech, at comfortable loudness levels.
2. Some (34 to 52%) children can identify environmental sounds chosen from a closed-set of alternatives, at comfortable loudness levels.
3. Many (more than 52%) children can identify the timing and rhythm of speech as well as identify words from a closed-set of alternatives without lipreading.
4. Some (34 to 52%) children demonstrate enhancement of their lipreading abilities.
5. For many (more than 52%) children, speech production is improved after training and experience with the device.
6. A few (5 to 34%) children demonstrate the ability to recognize speech without lipreading.
7. Children who are born deaf or become deaf shortly thereafter may derive less benefit than children who acquire deafness later in life.

Despite careful screening of implant recipients, significant variability exists in speech perception performance. Some recipients perform remarkably well, being able to discriminate open-set sentences and talk over the telephone, whereas others do not. Neural survival in the cochlea, correct fitting of the device, and speech processor coding strategy are possible factors. In children, personality, cognitive ability, and the availability and quality of rehabilitation and educational support are also variables. Studies have shown that educational setting and mode of communication are additional factors influencing cochlear implant use.[18,19]

Age at onset of deafness is a critical factor for young children. Compared to children with congenital or prelingual deafness, better performance is seen for children having cochlear implants who are postlingually deafened. As a group, children with congenital and prelingual deafness are very slow to acquire auditory skills, sometimes requiring 1 to 2 years before measurable speech perception performance is noted.[20] In contrast, postlingually deafened children perform similar to adults with acquired deafness, readily adapting to the device and demonstrating benefit almost immediately.

Comparison Between Cochlear Implant Systems

A significant design consideration is whether to use single or multiple channels. It is logical to conclude that a multiple-channel system will provide superior performance because of the additional information that can be coded for processing in the cochlea.

Gantz and Tyler[21] were among the first to provide objective evidence that multiple-channel cochlear implants are superior to single-channel implants. They evaluated the performance of 10 adults who were implanted with three different devices: seven with a single-channel system and three with systems having up to 20 channels. All three of the implant systems enhanced speech-reading ability and improved performance on tests using speech and nonspeech stimuli. However, superior performance was found for the three patients who were fit with the multichannel devices, especially on open-set speech tests. Since this early report, a number of other investigations have documented the superiority of multichannel cochlear implants over single channel devices.[22]

Do different multichannel devices or coding strategies provide different amounts of benefit? In addition to comparing single to multichannel implants, Waltzman et al,[21] compared the performance of 60 adults with two different multichannel implants, 30 with the 22 electrode Nucleus prosthesis and 30 subjects with the 8 electrode Ineraid prosthesis. Overall, no significant differences were found between the Ineraid and Nucleus prostheses when the same coding strategies were used. However, when the coding strategy was changed (from wearable speech processor using F_0, F_2, and F_3 to minispeech processor using multipeak processing) significant improvements in performance were observed for the Nucleus device after a 3-month period. This study provides preliminary evidence that improvements in coding strategies can significantly improve speech perception performance.

Although it is clear that better performance is observed with multichannel stimulation than single-channel stimulation, a significant issue is the number of channels necessary to achieve maximum performance. Haskell and Jordan[23] examined this very complex issue by evaluating the results from 30 adult subjects with different numbers of channels activated using the Nucleus 22 electrode prosthesis and the same number of subjects using the Ineraid 4 electrode prosthesis. No clear relationship was observed between the number of active electrode pairs and performance on speech perception tests. There was a relationship between coding strategy and the number of active electrodes, but large intersubject variability was found. At the present time, a clear answer to the question of how many electrodes is best is not available.

Cochlear Implants in Children

The most controversial issue surrounding cochlear implants is their use in children. On the one hand, there are major consequences of severe to profound deafness, especially for children with congenital losses. Language learning and speaking will be significantly impaired when profound deafness exists and the child is made to rely on speechreading alone. For most children with profound deafness, total communication is the only means of providing language. Vocabulary development and reading skills will be affected—compared to a vocabulary of 5000 to 26,000 words for the normal 5-year-old child, a child with deafness will have a speaking vocabulary of about 200 words. One study reported that 50% of children having hearing losses greater than 85 dB HL had no reading comprehension at all.[24] Severe to profound deafness impacts on all aspects of educational and psychosocial development and will greatly influence socioeconomic status. In addition, some cochlear implant recipients receive extraordinary benefit from their instruments, even to the point of being able to discriminate openset sentences.

On the other hand, there are uncertainties about the potential benefits from cochlear implants. At present, it is not possible to predict those who will benefit from cochlear implants. Degree of neural survival in the impaired ear is probably the single most physiological important factor to predict success of cochlear implant use. However, there are no preoperative procedures available to measure neural survival in the cochlea.[19] In addition, costs (monetary, psychological, time, effort, etc) are high. These factors must receive serious consideration in the decision to implant a child.

Those who favor implanting children argue that the device provides valuable timing and intensity cues for contact with the sound environment and assists in speechreading. It is their contention that the information processed by the cochlear implant will provide significant benefit in speech and language development. They argue that even if irreversible damage occurs in the implanted ear, the other ear is available for implantation if improved technology leads to a better system. Failing to provide a cochlear implant will deprive the child of the potential benefits during the critical years for speech and language development. Few would argue with these principles, but the fact remains that the exact benefits a child will derive from a cochlear implant cannot be determined prior to surgery.

Until conclusive data are made available documenting the advantages that can be gained from cochlear implants in children, this issue will continue to be controversial. Several studies comparing performance with cochlear implants and alternative devices (hearing aids and tactile aids) have been reported and are described later in this chapter. Generally, the results from these studies have supported cochlear implants *for some children*. However, there continues to be a wide range in performance, from those who derive only limited sound detection skills to those with open-set word understanding ability. A critical need is the ability to identify those children who will benefit significantly from cochlear implants and those who will derive only limited benefit.

TACTILE AIDS

Acoustic signals that are presented at a sufficiently high-enough intensity can be perceived by the skin (through the tactile mode), rather than the ear (through the auditory mode), by individuals with profoundly deafness. Nober[25,26] was among the first to caution clinicians that at high intensities acoustic signals presented by air and bone conduction can be felt rather than heard by the profoundly deaf individual. For air conduction stimuli, he demonstrated that low-frequency pure-tone thresholds obtained from the ears and hands of 94 profoundly deaf subjects were almost identical once the intensity reached levels of 75 to 105 dB HL at 125 to 1000 Hz, respectively.[25] For bone conduction, the levels were between 25 and 55 dB HL. This finding helps to explain why the individual with profound deafness obtains minimal benefit from conventional amplification; the high-intensity acoustic stimuli delivered through the hearing aid provides tactile, rather than acoustic stimulation.

Providing tactile stimulation through hearing aids has adverse consequences. Whereas the individual with some residual hearing should be able to obtain spectral and temporal cues through the amplification provided by a hearing aid, the individual with profound deafness who relies on tactile sensations will receive only rudimentary awareness and possibly temporal cues from the low frequencies delivered to the ear canal by the hearing aid.[27] Additional detail regarding this concept is provided in Figure 14–2. In this figure a comparison is made between the frequency sensitivity of the ear (see Chapter 2, Fig. 2–2) and the skin measured at the forearm and fingertips. Two important points are made in this figure. The first is that the frequency response of the skin and tactile sensitivity vary with the body location. In this figure, the fingertip is shown to be more sensitive and has a greater frequency range than the forearm. It is known that the fingers and lips are among the most sensitive locations for tactile stimulation,[28] but (as will be discussed in a later section of this chapter) neither location is ideally suitable for tactile stimulation using a communication aid.

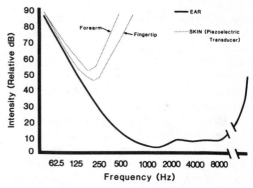

Figure 14–2. Frequency response of the skin measured at the forearm and fingertip compared to the normal frequency response of the human ear.

Figure 14–2 also points out that compared to the broadband frequency response of the ear, the skin is limited to only low frequencies. The frequency response of the ear is between 20 and 20,000 Hz, with the optimal frequency response between 300 and 3000 Hz. However, the skin is limited to frequencies of 10 to 500 Hz, with the optimal frequency response at 220 to 240 Hz. The reduced frequency response of the skin only to low-frequency stimulation is a major limiting factor when hearing aid amplification is used, because hearing aids typically do not amplify frequencies below 400 to 500 Hz. This most likely is the primary reason why the majority of individuals with profound deafness obtain little benefit from hearing aid use, and as many as 23%

of the school-age population with profound deafness choose not to wear hearing aids.[29] The goal of a tactile aid is to improve communication by changing acoustic signals into vibratory or electric signals and delivering them to the skin in the most efficient way possible, maximizing the physiological capabilities of the skin.

Educators of students with profound deafness have for years been using tactile stimulation informally. For example, having a student touch the therapist's larynx during phonation is one approach used to teach voicing. A unique approach to teach musical rhythm is to have students hold large balloons between their hands in the presence of music presented through a phonograph or tape recorder at a high intensity, allowing them to feel the low frequencies. Or, placing a loudspeaker on the chest of the student and playing music or speech will provide a form of tactile stimulation. Although these techniques have been used for quite some time, they provide a limited, but still effective, form of tactile stimulation.

Systematic work on tactile aids dates back more than 70 years.[30,31] Over this span of years, researchers, clinicians, and educators have invested extensive amounts of energy in searching for the ideal way to stimulate the skin to achieve maximum communication. In recent years a number of devices with varying characteristics have been developed and evaluated. Kirman[32,33] and Sherrick[28] both provide excellent historic reviews of this early work and major issues that are in this area.

A number of commercially available wearable tactile devices have been developed. Table 14–3 lists the various devices, provides information on their operating characteristics, indicates whether they are currently commercially available, and the approximate costs for those that are commercially available. Issues concerning tactile aids have centered around the type of stimulation, location of stimulation, and single versus multiple channels.

Table 14–3 Commercially Available Tactile Instruments*

Name of Device	Company	Type of Stimulation	Channels	List Price
Tactaid II+	Audiological Engineering**	Vibrotactile	2	$955
Tactaid 7	Audiological Engineering**	Vibrotactile	7	$2955
Trill	AVR Sonovation***	Vibrotactile	2	$895

*U.S. manufacturers only.
**35 Medford Street, Somerville, MA 02143.
***1450 Park Court, Chanhassen, MN 55317.

Type of Stimulation

Tactile aids can use two types of stimulation: (1) vibrotactile, in which acoustic signals are presented as vibrations to the skin using mechanical transducers; and (2) electrotactile (or electrocutaneous), in which acoustic signals are presented to the skin as electric currents. The use of the vibrotactile approach has been preferred over the electrotactile approach due to the availability of vibrators for experimental use, and also the inherent difficulties experienced with applying an electric current to the skin. Many early investigators used standard audiometric bone conduction vibrators, causing serious limitations due to their poor frequency response and high power requirements. Recently, specially constructed vibrators have been developed to match the impedance characteristics of the skin. This development is the most significant factor that has allowed efficient, wearable vibrotactile aids to be introduced.

Location of Stimulation

Unlike cochlear implants, which are designed to stimulate only structures within the cochlea, with tactile instruments a decision must be made concerning the location on the body to provide stimulation. The majority of studies have used the hands, arms, abdomen, jaw, thorax, forehead, or thighs as stimulation sites. As a sensor for vibrations, the fingers of the hand have structural and functional characteristics indicating they are among the more sensitive body parts.

Only a limited number of comparative studies with tactile aids using different body parts in clinical trials are available. Early studies failed to show an apparent advantage of one body location over the other. For example, Englemann and Rosov[34] trained their subjects using the forearms and fingertips. When the transducers were relocated to the thighs of their subjects, transfer was reported to be immediate. Also, Yeni-Komshian and Goldstein[35] transferred tactile patterns from the right hand to the left and from the fingers to the palm of the same hand and found no performance differences. Findings from these studies support the interpretation that tactile performance is a function of pattern recognition, more than increased sensitivity of a particular body part or neurological adaptation.

Geldard and Sherrick[36] reported data indicating that the fingertips of the hand are superior for recognizing vibratory patterns compared to

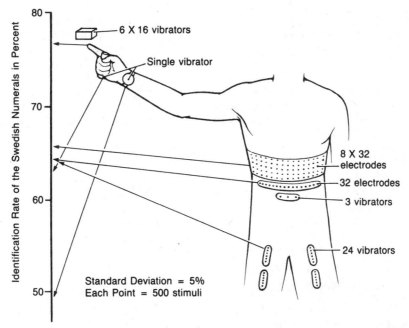

Figure 14–3. Identification rate of Swedish numbers as a function of the stimulating place, the stimulating method, and the number of stimulators. (From data presented by Spens.[37])

the arm, thigh, and thorax. Additional data supporting the superiority of the fingertips for tactile recognition comes from Spens.[37] He used a variety of different tactile arrays on seven different body locations of one subject (himself); the task was number identification. Results from this study are shown in Figure 14–3. As displayed in this figure, performance ranged from a low of 46% for a single vibrator placed on the wrist to a high of 77% for a 6 × 16 vibrator array placed on the index finger. From these results, as well as those of Geldard and Sherrick,[36] it is clear that for maximum discrimination the fingertips should be used. One problem with using the fingertips is their accessibility; using them for tactile stimulation would affect manual dexterity and, perhaps, be a serious drawback.

Although the data are beginning to favor the fingertips as the ideal location for tactile stimulation, commercial devices are not yet available to use the apparent superiority of this location. The clinician choosing to use tactile stimulation must explore various body locations (abdomen, sternum, forearm, thighs) in choosing which location is best for a given patient. One clinical method to select location of stimulation is to obtain sound field awareness thresholds for warbled pure tones and speech in making the initial placement decision. The location on which the best thresholds are obtained is used for the

initial stimulation site. After using this location for several days, alternate sites are selected for comparison until a preferred site is found. In some cases, there does not appear to be a clear superiority of one body location over another.

Single Versus Multichannel Tactile Aids

Simple one-channel to extremely complex multichannel devices with up to 288 different points of stimulation have been developed and tested under different conditions.[38] With single-channel devices, the available information is limited to simple awareness of environmental sounds and temporal cues (stress patterns and prosody). For speech, the single-channel device is severely limited and is capable of displaying only rudimentary fundamental frequency (F_0) information. However, single-channel devices, as limited as they are, have proven to be beneficial in supplementing speechreading.[39]

Currently, there are no direct comparisons available using single- and multiple-channel instruments, so it is not known which is actually superior.[28] With the advent of wearable tactile aids, it is now possible to field test performance with single-channel and multi-channel tactile aids, and it is expected that data on this type of comparison will be forthcoming in the near future.

COMPARISON OF HEARING AIDS, COCHLEAR IMPLANTS, AND TACTILE INSTRUMENTS

The goals of hearing aids, cochlear implants and tactile aids are essentially the same: (1) to provide wearers with increased auditory contact with their environment, including awareness of their own voice; (2) improve their ability to speechread; and (3) ultimately to provide the ability to discriminate connected discourse. Although the goals are the same, inherent limitations exist for each device. How are they the same and how do they differ?

Functional Differences Between Hearing Aids, Cochlear Implants, and Tactile Instruments

Functional differences between hearing aids, cochlear implants, and tactile aids are compared on seven factors in Table 14–4. Hearing aids and cochlear implants are recommended for daily use. After orienting a child to the instruments audiologists encourage parents and classroom teachers to monitor hearing aid and cochlear implant use to ensure maximum wearing time. However, with tactile aids, the question of daily usage pattern remains. Tactile instruments provide maximum benefit in face to face conversation, where the signal-to-noise ratio is favorable and the use of visual cues is maximized. Tactile instruments can also provide alerting signals to inform the wearer of the presence of warning or functional acoustic signals. However, whether the wearable tactile systems available provide tactile information in a sophisticated enough manner to be useful in a normal, everyday environment, where background noise is prevalent, has not been fully demonstrated.

Some preliminary evidence exists to indicate that tactile aids are of limited use in situations other than face to face interactions. Friel-Patti and Roeser[40] documented highly significant improvements in the communication skills of four children with profound deaf children who were fit with a three-channel vibrotactile aid and placed in individual, triweekly language intervention sessions. As part of the study, the four children were also monitored in the classroom, and careful monitoring of their behavior in this environment failed to show significant carryover into general classroom activities.[41] Most likely, the lack of carryover was a result of hardware limitations, because the noise rejection system in the aid used in the study was limited. However, refined noise rejection systems may expand the use of tactile instruments to a variety of listening situations.

Comparison of trial period, initial costs, risks, safety, and long-term sequela in Table 14–4 should need no further expansion. However, the issue of effectiveness is complex. With hearing instruments, as discussed earlier in this chapter, effectiveness depends on the type of loss and the amount of residual hearing. Patients with conductive loss receive maximum benefit from hearing aid usage. In fact, for most patients with conductive loss, threshold sensitivity can be brought within the range of normal limits and normal speech understanding is expected. With sensorineural hearing loss, the major factors determining effectiveness are the degree and configuration of the loss. Those with mild or mild to moderate losses generally obtain more benefit than those in the severe range.

For cochlear implants, the number of residual neural populations in the cochlea and cranial nerve VIII and the coding techniques used by the implant system to process the electric signal are the primary factors determining effectiveness of

Table 14–4 Primary Differences Between Hearing Aids, Cochlear Implants, and Tactile Aids

Factor	Hearing Aid(s)	Cochlear Implants	Tactile Aids
Daily usage	Yes	Probably	?
Trial period	Yes	No	Yes
Initial cost	$550–1200	$10,000–20,000	$450–3000
Risk	None	Yes	None
Safety	Safe	?	Safe
Long-term sequela	Minimal	?	None
Effectiveness	Depends on type of loss and amount of residual hearing	Depends on residual neural population and coding/processing technique	Depends on skin's ability to process sound and processing technique

cochlear implants. Exactly why some patients are able to function at extremely high levels of accuracy, even to the point of communicating over the telephone, remains a mystery. Could this behavior be accounted for by their ability to synthesize the limited information delivered through the system? Or is the system delivering a superior signal for these patients? This question cannot be readily resolved, because there are currently no noninvasive techniques to determine the number or integrity of neural populations in the cochlea.

With tactile aids, as discussed previously, the skin's limited ability to process sound is a major limiting factor. The ear has: (1) a dynamic range of 130 dB and (2) a frequency response between 20 and 20,000 Hz, with an optimal frequency range from 30 to 3000 Hz. On the other hand, the tactile system has (1) a dynamic range of only 30 to 35 dB and (2) a frequency range of only 10 to 400 or 500 Hz, with an optimal frequency range at 220 to 240 Hz.[42] These limitations inflict serious restrictions on the ability of the skin to process sound, and dictate the maximum benefits and use that can be expected.

Sound Awareness/Detection

Sound awareness is the ability to detect the presence of auditory stimuli in the environment. Detection of sound is important in providing alerting signals, and must be present if discriminations are to be made. However, simple detection of sound does not imply that the acoustic signals detected can be discriminated. Regardless, sound awareness is an important behavioral measure, and it is based on highly objective information in a cooperative patient. How do sound awareness thresholds compare for cochlear implants and tactile aids? Table 14–5 shows

published data comparing awareness thresholds for the two systems when the instruments were set at their typical volume settings. The data for cochlear implants were taken from a summary of findings from a large number of children,[43] and the data for tactile aids were from four children fit with a three-channel vibrotactile aid.[46] As indicated by this comparison, awareness thresholds from the two devices are similar, being within 0 to 4 dB for the frequencies 500 to 4000 Hz. Speech awareness thresholds were slightly better for the tactile aid than the cochlear implant: 47 dB compared to 55 dB, respectively. Overall, these data indicate essentially the same performance is possible when using tactile aids compared to cochlear implants when sound awareness is measured.

Comparable findings for sound awareness with cochlear implants and tactile aids are not surprising because the amplitude of the stimulating signal—whether it is an electric signal delivered to the cochlea or tactile signal delivered to the skin—is determined by the volume setting of the amplifier. The higher the volume setting, the greater the gain of the amplifier, the more sensitive the system, and the lower the intensity at which the wearer will respond. In fact, it would be possible to increase the volume setting of either a cochlear implant or a tactile aid and to reduce significantly the levels at which the patient will be aware of sound. However, the negative effect of increasing the sensitivity of an amplifier is that there will be increasing difficulty with background noise as the sensitivity is increased; that is, the background sounds will increasingly disrupt the processing of the primary signal as the sensitivity is increased. The application of microprocessing techniques, such as automatic noise suppression circuits, should significantly improve sound detection thresholds for both cochlear implants and tactile aids in the presence of background noise.

Table 14–5 Comparison of Mean Aided Awareness Thresholds for Cochlear Implants and Tactile Aids (dB SPL)*

	Warbled Pure Tones (Hz)						Speech Awareness Thresholds
	250	500	1000	2000	3000	4000	
Cochlear implants at 24 mo†	59	56	57	57	59	64	55
Tactile aid‡	68	58	60	61	59	63	47

*Data were obtained at user-level volume settings
†From Thielemeir et al.[43]
‡Thresholds converted from HL to SPL. From Friel-Patti and Roeser.[40]

Research Studies

Geers and Moog[39] were among the first to study the differences between hearing aids, tactile instruments, and cochlear implants. They observed performance in two large groups of children with profound deafness wearing hearing aids: 10 children wore single-channel vibrotactile instruments, and two children with single-channel cochlear implants. Included in their analysis was a comparison of their findings to results reported for 54 children implanted with a single-channel device. Performance was compared on a number of audiological tests, and measures of speech production and language development were obtained. Children were placed in one of four categories based on their test performance: category 1, no pattern perception; category 2, pattern perception; category 3, some word recognition; and category 4, consistent word recognition. Their results indicated that single-channel devices provide only pattern information (category 2) not spectral information. For children in category 2 who had learned to categorize words according to stress pattern, and had learned to monitor their vocalizations through hearing aids, the single-channel devices appeared to provide little advantage. Based on their findings, Geers and Moog[39] concluded that, in most cases, single-channel vibrotactile aids and single-channel cochlear implants provide similar information with no apparent advantage to either device. These authors encourage the development of multichannel tactile aids and cochlear implants.

Evidence supporting superior performance of multichannel cochlear implants over tactile devices is provided by Skinner et al.[44] They report data from adults with postlingual deafness on tests using sound only, vision plus sound, vision only, and speech tracking. Although sound field warble tone thresholds were similar for both devices, scores from the multichannel cochlear implant far surpassed those with the one or two channel vibrotactile device. Miyamoto et al[45] reported similar findings with 42 children ages 4 to 12 years wearing a two-channel tactile device and two cochlear implant systems. Performance was better with both cochlear implant systems than the two channel vibrotactile device.

Predicted performance from cochlear implants and tactile instruments on a number of different tasks by retrospective analysis of available research studies is shown in Table 14–6. This table compares expected performance between the two devices on eight different auditory func-

Table 14–6   Comparison of Cochlear Implant and Tactile Aid Expected Performance

Task	Cochlear Implant	Tactile Aid
Discriminate loud and soft sounds	Yes	Yes
Discriminate continous and interrupted sounds	Yes	Yes
Discriminate long and short sounds	Yes	Yes
Differentiate no. of sounds	Yes	Yes
Differentiate no. of syllables in words	Yes	Yes
Differentiate no. of syllables in sentences	Yes	Yes
Differentiate different types of sounds in the environment; eg, door knock vs speech	Yes	No
Discriminate open-set speech	Maybe	No

Sources: Thielemeir et al,[43] Proctor and Goldstein,[46] Goldstein and Proctor.[20]

tions. As shown by this comparison, there does not appear to be a difference between the two devices in expected performance for six factors. However, for two factors, the ability to discriminate between environmental sounds and discrimination of open-set speech, cochlear implants are clearly superior. These two factors make it clear that cochlear implants are superior to tactile instruments.

One additional factor is patient acceptance. When given the option of using either of the instruments, all subjects show a preference for the cochlear implant. This factor is probably the best indicator that the advanced cochlear implants provide a superior signal for the reception of speech and better performance than even the most advanced tactile devices.

Miyamoto et al[48] encourage incorporating vibrotactile aids into cochlear implant programs, allowing patients to experience tactile stimulation prior to receiving the implant. They report this technique to be highly favorable. Through this approach, basic stress differentiation and temporal concepts can be taught, and the ability of the subject to incorporate these cues into speech identification can be assessed. Since the procedure can be incorporated into the initial phases of cochlear implant rehabilitation, they can be demonstrated prior to surgery and greatly enhance the probability of success. It appears that this use of tactile devices is effective.

Training Strategies with Cochlear Implants and Tactile Devices

Comprehensive training is required for members of implant teams who are responsible for providing rehabilitation (basic guidance) of patients with cochlear implants. Audiologists, speech-language pathologists, or teachers who are not part of an implant team and are faced with a patient having an implant, will need some guidance for rehabilitation strategies. Since cochlear implants and tactile aids have similar operating characteristics, with some exceptions therapeutic strategies for the two devices can be interchanged.

Tye-Murray and Kelsay[49] describe an effective five-component training program for parents of children with cochlear implants, which is briefly described as follows.

Introduction to cochlear implant use. During the introduction to cochlear implant use a schedule is developed for when the child will wear the cochlear implant. At first, the device is worn for 1 or 2 hours several times during the day, with the goal of full time use after 2 months. During regularly scheduled device adjustment sessions, any concerns are addressed, the need for auditory stimulation is stressed, and suggestions for providing auditory stimulation at home are given. Parents are also taught informal speech perception training activities so they can integrate them into their daily routines and a diary is completed and returned to the cochlear implant center at regular intervals.

Assessment of parents' communication behavior. This step uses the Communication Index for Parents (CIP) to evaluate how well parents can verbally repair communication breakdowns. During the CIP parents communicate 20 different instructions while sitting at a table across from his or her child, without using sign. If the child does not understand the instruction, it is repeated, restructured, or different information is repeated. After 1 minute, the parent can use signs. The CIP is audiovideotaped for later scoring and the material is used during the parent seminar.

Parent seminar. This session occurs about 10 months after implant connection. By this time, the parents have had an ample opportunity to feel comfortable with the device, a routine has been established, and sound awareness and some discrimination of words has occurred. Parents are instructed in methods to converse with their child, learn to initiate conversation, how to practice good speaking behaviors, how to engage the child in conversation, and how to repair communication breakdown. Videotapes are used as examples and role playing and modeling are used to reinforce didactic materials. Formal instruction is provided, but ample opportunity for parents to practice concepts, share experiences, and critique themselves is given.

Home-training program. The home training program consists of completing a workbook and computerized activities; it is carried out for 8 weeks after the parent seminar. A lesson in the workbook is completed at the end of each week, mailed to the implant center where it is reviewed and returned to the parents with comments. The material in the workbook reinforces the material covered during the parent seminar. The computer is placed in the home and teaches parents repair strategies.

Parent library. The library contains a wealth of written materials and videotapes on all aspects of hearing impairment (auditory training, speech-reading training, sign language, educational options, etc), which are made available for parents to take home.

Although this program was developed specifically for children with cochlear implants, it could be adapted for children with tactile devices or hearing aids. As with most auditory training programs, formal auditory training with cochlear implants and tactile instruments progresses in a hierarchy from simple to complex as follows:

1. Presence or absence of sound.
2. Onset or cessation of sound.
3. One versus two sounds.
4. Long versus short sounds.
5. Fast versus slow sounds.
6. Continuous versus interrupted sounds.
7. Gross word discrimination.
8. Voiced versus voiceless phonemes.
9. Telephone training.
9. Recognition of environmental sounds.
10. Speech-tracking.

Clinicians can use a number of techniques from auditory training manuals, or devise their own to work on each of these areas.

Speech tracking is a procedure that was first described by DeFilippo and Scott[50] as an objective measure of speechreading. Subsequent to their introduction, the technique has been used to train and measure speechreading performance by a number of clinicians and investigators, and it can be used with older children and adults. In the procedure, a talker—reading from a text, a novel, or short story—presents short segments to a receiver who then attempts to repeat the text back verbatim. Performance is measured by the number of correct words per minute that the speechreader with hearing loss is able to repeat back; that is, tracking is performed over 10-minute intervals, and the measure of performance is the mean number of words correctly repeated by the subject per minute. As a guide, subjects with normal hearing average about 100 to 120 words per minute when this type of sender-receiver exchange is used.

Robbins et al[51] point out a number of limitations with speech-tracking. Included are: (1) possible bias of the sender; (2) lack of standardization; (3) the receiver must have a basic knowledge of the English language (which limits its application to postlingually deafened subjects); and (4) learning. Despite these limitations, Robbins et al conclude that speech-tracking is an excellent strategy for teaching speechreading. Its use is especially applicable for patients with implants and tactile aids. The clinician must realize that tracking is a time consuming technique, requiring about 40 minutes to complete three 10-minute sessions, which is about all the average patient will be capable of completing because of the concentration required. A good therapy strategy is to have implant or aid users track with their spouses or others with whom they regularly communicate, and keep a record of their performance. This way, the patient can work on speechreading skills outside of the therapy sessions, and others can become involved in the therapy process.

Regular telephone communication is possible for some cochlear implant users. Dorman et al[52] found that about one third of 80 cochlear implant patients responding to a survey reported being able to understand a telephone conversation with a familiar speaker and a familiar topic. Those with high scores on speech intelligibility tests used the telephone more than those with lower scores. Even when speech perception is not possible, older children and adults can communicate through coded messages learned through telephone training. This technique is even possible with tactile instruments.

Telephone training involves teaching wearers to use coded signals to make emergency and simple informational communications over the telephone with the assistance of their device. Training begins by having the patient practice listening (or feeling with a tactile aid) for a dial tone. After its presence is established, the telephone number is dialed and the patient listens or feels for the ring or, if the telephone is in use,

the busy signal. Practice is given with the three signals (dial tone, ring, and busy signal) until the patient can differentiate them. A code can be set up with family and close friends using one through four syllable phrases. For example:

No . . . . One syllable
Yes, Yes . . . . Two syllables
Please, repeat . . . . Three syllables
I don't know that . . . . Four syllables

In this way, the individual wearing an implant or tactile instrument could ask a series of questions and have them answered using this system. This type of communication is limited to family members and close friends of prelingually deaf implant or tactile instrument users because their speech is often difficult or impossible to understand by others. For the adult with postlingual deafness and good speech, the telephone code could be used in a variety of situations by beginning the conversation with instructions to the listener that the caller is deaf, by using an implant or aid, and by giving instructions on how to use the code. In emergency situations the ability to use telephone code may be vitally important.

SUMMARY

This chapter reviews the techniques that are available for the people with profound deafness. Hearing instruments, tactile instruments, and cochlear implants can be provided so that even students with the most severe hearing loss can achieve their maximum educational potential.

ACKNOWLEDGMENTS

Portions of this work were supported by National Institutes of Heal grant no. 1 RO1 NS 15982-01A1.

REFERENCES

1. Boothroyd A: Tactile aids: Development issues and current status, in Owens E, Kessler DK, eds: *Cochlear Implants in Young Deaf Children* (Boston: College Hill Press, 1989), pp 101–136.
2. Ling D, Milne M: The development of speech in hearing-impaired children, in Bess F, Freeman B, Sinclair J, eds: *Amplification in Education* (Washington, DC: Alexander Graham Bell Association for the Deaf, 1981), pp 98–108.
3. Moora C: Financing a cochlear implant current and future considerations. *SHHH J*, 15 (1994), 26–28.

4. Sonnesschein MA: Cochlear implant update. *SHHH J*, 7 (1986), 16–19.

5. Carhart R: Sensorineural hearing loss: an overview, in Merzenich MM, Schindler RA, Sooy FA, eds: *Proceedings of the First International Conference on Electrical Stimulation of the Acoustical Nerve as a Treatment for Profound Sensorineural Deafness in Man* (San Francisco: University of California, 1974).

6. ASHA Ad Hoc Committee in Cochlear Implants. *ASHA*, 28 (1985), 29–52.

7. Ries PW: *Hearing Abilities of Persons by Sociodemographic and Health Characteristics: United States*, Series 10. No. 140 (Washington, DC: National Center for Statistics, 1982).

8. Kileny, PR, Zimmerman-Phillips, Zwolen TA, Kemink, JL: Effects of channel number and place of stimulation on performance with Cochlear Corporation multichannel implant. *Am J Otal*, 13 (1992), 117–123.

9. Chute PM, Hellman SA, Parisier SC, Tartter VC, Economou MA: Auditory perception changes after reimplantation in a child cochlear implant user. *Ear Hear*, 13 (1992) 195–199.

10. Owens E, Telleen DD: Speech perception with hearing aids and cochlear implants. *Arch Otolaryngol*, 107 (1981), 160–163.

11. Northern J, Black FO, Brimacombe JA, et al: Selection of children for cochlear implantation. *Semin Hear*, 7 (1986), 341–446.

12. Sutton D: Cochlear pathology: hazards of long-term implants. *Arch Otolaryngol*, 110 (1984), 164–166.

13. Downs MP: Implanting electrodes? *ASHA*, 23 (1981), 567–568.

14. House, WF, Luxford WF, Courtney B: Otitis media in children following the cochlear implant. *Ear Hear*, 6 (1985), 24S–27S.

15. O'Donoghue GM, Jackler RA, Jenkins WM, Schlinder RA: The problem of head growth. *Otolaryngol—Head Neck Surg*, 94 (1986), 78–81.

16. Luxford WM, House WF: Cochlear implants in children: medical and surgical considerations. *Ear Hear*, 6 (1985), 20S–24S.

17. Tyler RS, Davis JM, Lansing CR: Cochlear implants in young children. *ASHA*, 29 (1987), 41–49.

18. Somers MN: Speech perception abilities in children with cochlear implants or hearing aids. *Am J Otol*, 12 (1991), 174S–182S.

19. Fryauf-Bertschy H: Pediatric cochlear implantation: an update. *ASHA*, 35 (1993), 13–16.

20. Miyamoto RT, Osberger MJ, Robbins AM, Myers WA, Kessler K, Pope ML: Longitudinal evaluation of communication skills of children with single- or multichannel cochlear implants. *Am J Otol*, 13 (1992), 215–222.

21. Gantz BJ, Tyler RS: Cochlear implant comparisons. *Am J Otolaryngol* (1985), 92–98.

22. Waltzman SB, Cohen NL, Fisher S: An experimental comparison of cochlear implant systems. *Semin Hear*, 13 (1992), 195–207.

23. Haskell, GB, Jordan, HN: Cochlear implant performance as a function of electrode number. *Semin Hear*, 13 (1992), 239–253.

24. Berliner KS, Eisenberg LS: Methods and issues in the cochlear implantation of children: an overview. *Ear Hear*, 6 (1985), 6S–13S.

25. Nober EH: Pseudoauditory bone conduction thresholds. *J Speech Hear Res*, 29 (1964), 469–476.

26. Nober EH: Vibrotactile sensitivity of deaf children to high intensity sound. *Laryngoscope*, 1967), 2128–2146.

27. Sweetow RW: Amplification and the development of listening skills in deaf children. *Audiology, An Audio J Cont Educ*, 4 (1979).

28. Sherrick CE: Basic and applied research on tactile aids for deaf people: progress and prospects. *J Acoust Soc Am*, 75 (1984), 1325–1342.

29. Karchmer MA, Kirwin L: *The Use of Hearing Aids by Hearing Impaired Students in the United States*. Series No. 2, (Washington, DC: Office of Demographic Studies, 1977).

30. Gault, RH: Progress in experiments on tactual interpretation of oral speech. *Soc Psychol*, 14 (1924), 155–159.

31. Gault RH: Touch as a substitute for hearing in the interpretation and control of speech. *Arch Otolaryngol*, 3 (1926), 121–135.

32. Kirman JH: Tactile communication of speech. A review and analysis. *Psychol Bull*, 80 (1973), 54–74.

33. Kirman JH: Current developments in tactile communication of speech, in Schiff E, Foulke E, eds: *Tactual Perception: A Sourcebook* (Cambridge, UK: Cambridge University Press, 1982), 234–262.

34. Englemann S, Rosov R: Tactual hearing experiments with deaf and hearing subjects. *Except Child*, 41 (1975), 243–253.

35. Yeni-Komshian GH, Goldstein MH: Identification of speech sounds displayed on a vibrotactile vocoder. *J Acoust Soc Am*, 62 (1977), 194–198.

36. Geldard FH, Sherrick CE: The cutaneous saltatory area and its presumed neural basis. *Percept Psycholphy*, 33 (1983), 299–304.

37. Spens KE: *Experiences of Tactile "Hearing" Aid*. Paper presented at the International Congress on the Education of the Deaf (Tokyo, Japan, 1985).

38. Sparks DW, Kuhl P, Edmonds AE, Gray GP: Investigating the MESA (Multipoint Electrotactile Speech Aid): The transmission of segmental features of speech. *J Acoust Soc Am*, 65 (1979), 810–815.

39. Geers AE, Moog JS: *Long-term Benefits from Single-Channel Cochlear Implants*. A paper presented at the Annual Meeting of The American Speech-Language-Hearing Association (Detroit, MI, 1986).

40. Friel-Patti S, Roeser RJ: Evaluating changes in the communication skills of deaf children using vibrotactile stimulation. *Ear Hear*, 4 (1984), 31–40.
41. Roeser RJ, Friel-Patti S, Scott B, et al: *Evaluating a Vibrotactile Aid with Profoundly Deaf Subjects*. A miniseminar presented at the Annual Meeting of The American Speech-Language Hearing Association (Cincinnati, OH, 1983).
42. Roeser RJ: Tactile aids for the profoundly deaf. *Semin Hear*, 6 (1985), 279–298.
43. Thielemeir MA, Tonokawa LL, Peterson B, Eisenberg LS: Audiological results in children with a cochlear implant. *Ear Hear*, 6 (1985), 27S–35S.
44. Skinner MW, Holden LK, Holden TA, Dowell RC, Seligman PM, Brimacombe JA, Beiter AL: Performance of postlinguistically deaf adults with the wearable speech processor (WSP III) and mini speech processor (MSP) of the nucleus multi-electrode cochlear implant. *Ear Hear*, 12 (1991), 3–18.
45. Miyamoto RT, Myres WA, Pope ML, Carotta CC: Cochlear implants for deaf children. *Laryngoscope*, 96 (1986), 990–996.
46. Proctor A, Goldstein MH: Development of lexical comprehension in a profoundly deaf child using wearable, vibrotactile communication aid. *Lang Speech Hear Serv Sch*, 14 (1983), 138–149.
47. Goldstein MH, Proctor A: Tactile aids for profoundly deaf children. *J Acoustic Soc Am*, 77 (1985), 258–265.
48. Miyamoto RT, Myres WA, Punch JL: Tactile aids in the evaluation procedure for cochlear implant candidacy. *Hear Instrum*, 38 (1987), 33–37.
49. Tye-Murray N, Kelsay DM: A communication training program for parents of cochlear implant users. *Volta Rev*, 95 (1993), 21–31.
50. DeFilippo CL, Scott BL: A method for training and evaluating the reception of ongoing speech. *J Acoust Soc Am*, 63 (1978), 1186–1191.
51. Robbins AM, Osberger MJ, Miyamoto RT, et al: Speech-tracking performance in single-channel cochlear implant subjects. *J speech Hear Res*, 28 (1985), 565–578.
52. Dorman M, Dankowski K, McCandless G, Smith L: Consonant recognition as a function of the number of channels of stimulation by patients who use the Symbion Cochlear Implant. *Ear Hear*, 10 (1989) 288–291.

15

TECHNIQUES AND CONCEPTS IN AUDITORY TRAINING AND SPEECHREADING

Helen A. McCaffrey

> *Education does not mean teaching people to know what they do not know; it means teaching them to behave as they do not behave.*
>
> —John Ruskin, 1819–1900

The person who has a hearing impairment must overcome the challenge of perceiving spoken language through a degraded auditory signal that is enhanced by visual information contributed by speechreading. When the person with a hearing loss is a child, the perceptual challenge impacts on language acquisition and academic performance. Intervention targets skill and strategy development as well as perception, as shown in Case study 15–1. The ultimate goal in intervention is the child's successful use of the acoustic and visual cues in spoken language to acquire language, to gain academic skills, and to communicate successfully throughout the life span.

An underlying assumption of this chapter is the primacy of the auditory signal in human communication. Visual cues in spoken language enhance auditory perception. Audition is more adaptive than vision for processing information.[1] Auditory information travels over distance and across obstacles; visual information does not. In localizing sound one need not direct the ear to the source; with vision, however, one must see the source and time is lost in reception when movement for visual access is required.

CHARACTERISTICS OF THE SPEECH SIGNAL

To implement the most effective intervention, the clinician or educator must have a fundamental knowledge of the acoustic and visual characteristics of spoken language, and the role that these play in perception. A full description of acoustic and visual characteristics is beyond the scope of this chapter. The reader is encouraged to refer to the many excellent texts that are available.[2,3] Some fundamental concepts, useful for implementing a perceptual training program, are provided here.

Acoustic Characteristics

The sounds of spoken language can be described along three acoustic dimensions: intensity, frequency, and time. The average conversational speech intensity measured from a distance of about 1 m is 65 dB sound pressure level (SPL), ranging from faint speech at 45 dB SPL to a shout at 85 dB SPL.[4] The vowel /ɔ/ has the greatest intensity among English speech sounds. The fricative consonant /θ/ has the weakest.

The frequency spectrum of speech ranges from 50 to 10,000 Hz, with greatest energy appearing from 100 to 600 Hz, or the region where suprasegmentals and vowels lie.[5] The voice fundamental, or F0, carries suprasegmental information, or rhythm, intonation, and stress. Vowels are differentiated by the location of peaks in the frequency spectrum known as formants. Formant peaks differentiate vowel height, or degree that the tongue is raised, and vowel place, the location in the mouth where the tongue is raised. Vowel height is signaled by the the first formant peak (F1), along with the voice fundamental. Vowel place is signaled by the second and third formants, F2 and F3, which are higher in frequency than F0 and F1, but are lower in intensity. The predominant energy of consonants is weaker in intensity than vowels, and appears at higher frequency ranges. The primary cues of consonant manner of production appear at and below 1000 Hz. The primary cues of consonant place of production appear in the region between 2000 and 4000 Hz.

Case study 15–1. Stephen was a 6-year-old boy with a severe-to-profound bilateral sensorineural hearing loss (Fig. 15–1). Stephen was first fit with hearing aids at age 18 months and enrolled in a parent-infant program. At the time of therapy, Stephen was mainstreamed in a first grade classroom. His support services included the use of a frequency modulation (FM) system, individual speech/language therapy, tutoring with an itinerant teacher of the hearing impaired, and private therapy. Stephen uses oral communication. Among his language and speech goals were comprehension and expressive use of complex sentences, including passives and relative and subordinate clauses, comprehension and use of new vocabulary from the classroom, expressive use of negative contractions and the /s/-/z/ morphemes, reduced stopping of fricatives, and reduced neutralization of the vowels /æ/, /I/, and /ɛ/. Auditory skills assessed revealed that he had difficulty remembering more than three critical elements and the details of a short story. In addition, Stephen's teacher and parents have observed that he did not consistently cue the teacher when he did not understand what was being said in the classroom.

Stephen's auditory goals were shaped by his speech and language goals as well as the results of auditory skills testing. Stephen's auditory memory improved with practice listening to and identifying lists of words with increasing number of elements. Nevertheless, greater effort was directed toward improving comprehension of sentences made more complex by added phrase structures. Elaboration of the phrase structure served to increase critical elements within the sentence.

Simple stories were presented during the therapy sessions. Stephen answered questions about these stories and retold them. Questions were directed toward exposing Stephen to story grammars (Who is in the story? Where was the boy? Was there a problem?) in preparation for his second grade language arts curriculum. In the classroom Stephen had showed some difficulty reading "short vowels" during phonics lessons. These were essentially the same vowels that were neutralized in his speech productions. Stephen and the clinician read stories to each other from primers that were loaded with words containing short vowels.

Most auditory work proceeded at the comprehension level with connected discourse, with some exceptions appearing for the purpose of highlighting a target. For example, Stephen demonstrated auditory awareness and discrimination of fricatives, all vowels, and negative contractions when these were presented in syllables or single words. However, these elements were difficult for him to perceive in running speech and as a consequence he did not establish rules for the use of these speech sounds or morphemes in receptive or expressive language. Stephen practiced auditory identification and production of these targets in syllables, words, and phrases, and rules for their use were explicitly presented (Is there more than one boy? What do you add at the end of the word?). Since these elements tend to be less audible in running speech, Stephen also practiced identification via lipreading as well.

Stephen's reticence to cue the teacher when he did not understand came from two sources. First, Stephen did not always know when he did not understand. Second, he needed skills to notify the teacher. The clinician embedded vocabulary that Stephen did not know throughout her conversations with Stephen, and he practiced finding these words and asking for an explanation. The clinician and Stephen talked about different ways to clue the speaker if the person were a teacher talking to a class, an adult talking to him individually, or a teamate on the soccer field.

The temporal characteristics of a speech segment may be described as (1) the duration of a segmental aspect or (2) the transition, or change over time, from one aspect to another. For example, the voice/voiceless distinction among consonants can be characterized by a difference in the time of onset of voicing (duration of silence) in the case of an initial plosive or in the duration of the preceding vowel in the case of a final stop. Semivowels contrast with diphthongs by differences in the speed of formant transitions within the segments.

A description of the acoustic characteristics of speech does not necessarily specify for the clinician those characteristics that will serve as cues for speech recognition. Ling[10] reminds us that one should be concerned less with average overall intensity levels of speech in various frequency bands than with the levels of crucial speech components within these bands. Despite the predominance of speech energy from 100 to 600 Hz, the sounds most important for speech recognition do not lie in this frequency region. The more crucial segments are the consonants, which lie in higher frequency regions of lower intensity.

Each speech sound possesses a variety of acoustic cues that can lead to its identification.[7]

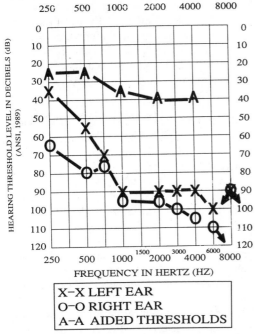

X–X LEFT EAR
O–O RIGHT EAR
A–A AIDED THRESHOLDS

Figure 15–1. Case study 15–1. Six-year-old boy with a severe to profound bilateral sensorineural hearing loss.

Table 15–1   Hearing Levels at Which Identification of Speech Characteristics Drop to 50% Probability*

Speech Feature/Characteristic	Hearing Level
Consonant place	75 dB
Initial consonant continuance	85 dB
Initial consonant voicing	90 dB
Vowel place	100 dB
Talker sex	105 dB
Syllabic pattern	115 dB
Vowel height	In excess of 115 dB

*Adapted from Boothroyd.[10]

Furthermore, the acoustic characteristics of a speech sound vary from one context to another. Speech sounds influence the acoustic characteristics of adjacent sounds by way of coarticulation. It benefits the child to practice perception of a sound in a variety of contexts to take advantage of facilitative context effects. Trading relationships exist among perceptual cues so that when an acoustic cue is not available to the listener for identification of a speech segment, then others will take prominence.[8] If a frequency cue is not available to a listener with hearing impairment, then intensity or temporal information might be used to identify the speech sound. There is evidence that listeners who are hearing impaired prioritize cues in identifying speech segments differently than listeners with normal hearing when certain cues are not audible.[9]

Sensorineural hearing loss affects the audibility of suprasegmentals and speech segments by reducing the sensation level of the conversational speech spectrum and filtering frequency components of speech. Sensorineural hearing loss tends to have greater effect on high frequency speech components than low-frequency speech. The result is greater ease of perception of speech features that are of the strongest intensity and lowest frequency or coded temporally. These include syllable number, the suprasegmentals, vowel height, consonant manner, and for some listeners, consonant voicing. Table 15–1, adapted from Boothroyd,[10] lists hearing threshold levels at which the probability of identification of various speech features drops to 50%.

The data in Table 15–1 can be used to determine which speech features are most likely to be audible to a child when selecting stimuli for auditory training. Stimuli are selected from analyses of (1) the aided or implant audiogram, (2) the speech processing algorithm of the hearing aid or cochlear implant, and (3) auditory confusions on identification or imitation tasks. Analysis of speech information that is furnished by the cochlear implant or hearing aids should not eliminate cues for training but should instead guide the clinician in organizing stimuli from the easiest perception to the most difficult.

In summary, speech sounds may be described by intensity, frequency, and temporal aspects. As a rule, the high frequency characteristics of speech sounds are lower in intensity than mid- or low-frequencies, and are less likely to be audible to the listener with hearing impairment. Each speech sound possesses a variety of acoustic characteristics that may serve as cues to the identification of a sound. A listener does not utilize all cues each time a segment is identified. The listener with hearing impairment may utilize cues differently than one with normal hearing.

Visual Characteristics

A complementary picture emerges when one considers the visual characteristics of speech. Visual speech cues enhance or disambiguate the auditory signal. Features that are potentially the least audible, such as consonant place of articulation, tend to be visible. Other speech features, however, are characterized by low visibility or ambiguous visual cues.

Suprasegmental aspects are not coded visually. Vowels and diphthongs may be differentiated visually by lip shape and jaw height, but tongue position is generally not visible. Adjacent vowels are easily confused visually. Among consonants, few acoustic manner features are coded visually. Some manner features such as frication and plosion can be contrasted visually by duration of position, but these are difficult to resolve in connected speech. Voicing contrasts cannot be visually differentiated within the spoken signal.

Consequently, some 60% of the spoken code is visually uninterpretable.[11] Approximately 50% of English phonemes and words are so reduced in contrastiveness that they are identical. Identical visual speech segments are called "visemes."[12] The low visibility of speech sound features reduces their contrastiveness, resulting in an inventory of visible speech features that are different from acoustic features. Woodward[14] and Woodward and Barber[15] identified four visually constrastive areas among speech sounds as a function of place of articulation: the bilabials, rounded labials, labiodentals, and nonlabials.

Low visibility and ambiguity of visual cues in spoken language require the perceiver to exploit additional sources of information in spoken language for comprehension. Fortunately, human communication is highly redundant. Information that leads to the comprehension of a spoken message is available simultaneously across several channels. These include structural, or syntactic and phonotatic constraints, contextual, or semantic and experiential constraints, and situational, or pragmatic constraints. The speechreader fills in the visual gaps by sizing up the communicative context, identifying the topic of conversation, and ruling out phrases or words that do not belong in the message, thus improving the chances of comprehension.

Acoustic and visual cues in speech combine to provide an intelligible message. For the listener with normal hearing, the acoustic signal is ordinarily sufficient for speech recognition, provided that there is little interference from noise, distance, or reverberation. The listener with hearing loss will miss crucial auditory information and rely on information from other sources to supplement audition, including visual cues in spoken language. Ambiguity and low visibility of visual cues, however, render sole reliance on vision to be a difficult route to comprehension.

The simultaneous information provided by context facilitates comprehension. Consequently, the clinician who designs a program for training the use of vision for comprehension must address not merely *lipreading*, or perception of spoken language via lip and mouth movements, but the more wholistic process of *speechreading*. Speechreading incorporates information appearing on the lips, in a speaker's facial expressions and body language, and the situational and linguistic context.

DEVELOPMENT PERCEPTION AND COMPREHENSION

Humans are innately predisposed to decode spoken language. For infants with normal hearing, many auditory behaviors are "hard-wired" into the perceptual system from birth.[15] Newborns demonstrate an awareness to sound.[16] They show a listening preference for speech in general and for their own mothers' voices in particular.[17,18] From the first moments of life, audition provides a bridge between the infant and his environment.

During the first year of life, auditory behavior is increasingly selective, constraining recognition to cues that are linguistically important in the mother language. As early as 1 month of age, infants discriminate among speech sounds, including sounds not present in their "mother" tongue.[19] This ability declines around 12 months of age when most infants discriminate solely speech sounds that are native to their language.[20] The infant learns what to pay attention to and what to ignore. This perceptual process develops simultaneously with cognitive skill in categorization, the acquisition of receptive language, and the emergence of the child's first words.[21]

From early on, infants are aware of visual aspects of spoken language and show some ability to use these to enhance auditory perception. Studies of visual perceptual development have focused on the child's response to congruence between visual and auditory presentations of spoken language. Infants as young as 18 to 20 weeks old demonstrate differential response to incongruencies between visual and auditory presentations of a spoken vowel.[22] Children as young as 18 months old recognize incongruence when shown a picture of an object with the silent videotape of a face producing the label of an object different from the picture presented.[29]

Despite the infant's demonstrated ability to discriminate individual speech sound contrasts presented in the experimental context, it is not likely that he or she segments individual speech sounds from the continuous stream of spoken language directed to him or her by the caregivers.

Evidence from studies of infant and toddler language comprehension suggest that the acquisition process is founded on developing skill in segmenting spoken language into meaningful units. Conscious segmentation of continuous speech into individual sounds does not appear until late preschool age when phonemic awareness emerges and the process of literacy acquisition begins.

Peters[30] proposes four strategies that the child applies in breaking down language input into meaningful units: (1) pay attention to perceptually salient stimuli; (2) discriminate stimuli along salient dimensions; (3) remember stimuli; and (4) classify stimuli according to the result of the discrimination. Peters' algorithm requires sufficient repetitiveness and predictability of the input so that many opportunities are present for attention and discrimination. There should be a consequence to the child's response so that he can receive feedback as to the correctness of his behavior, allowing classification and storage into memory.

The child first applies Peters' strategies to chunks of speech that can be as large as the daily routines of dressing or feeding. Daily routines occur with regularity and tend not to vary in linguistic content, providing predictability. Routines also provide communication turns for the child's participation, requiring appropriate, discriminated response.[25] Caregivers give saliency to spoken language by using *motherese*—varying pitch, simplifying the lexical content, reducing utterance length, paraphrasing, repeating, and providing contextual support.[26] As a result, motherese is easier to segment and process for discrimination and comprehension.

Repetitiveness and predictability are essential aspects of learning experiences in a perceptual training program. Saliency of input can be achieved by applying the principles of motherese. The clinician scaffolds the child's participation by providing opportunities for turn-taking and verification of response during the training session.

The child's family and school, however, look not for perceptual development, but for the establishment of *comprehension*. The clinician working with a child with hearing impairment must pay attention to perception, yet cannot lose sight of the fact that the ultimate goal, and the predominantly observable behavior in therapy, must be language comprehension. Among the first words comprehended by young children with normal hearing are simple labels and action nouns.[27] Comprehension appears to be strategy based, at least in its early stages as language is developing.[28] Children use comprehension strategies to figure out meaning on the basis of situational cues and past experience, strategies similar to those used by speechreaders young and old alike. The evidence that children use strategies suggests that comprehension is a cognitive process as well as linguistic, and subject to general notions about learners and skill development.

Ultimately children with normal hearing comprehend spoken language automatically, with little reliance on context or personal experience. This ability appears with the onset of school age. The school-age child is expected to acquire knowledge and academic skills through comprehension of instructional language that is presented at each grade level with increasing abstraction and departure from direct experience. Table 15–2 lists auditory skills targeted in a typical elementary level language arts program for children.[30] By the time a child is in the fourth grade he is expected to function independently in the use of receptive language (listening and reading) and expressive language (speaking and writing) to acquire knowledge and think critically.[31]

The child with hearing loss operates from several levels of skill development, and each influences the clinician's plan as well as the child's response. These include: (1) the skill level of the perceptual task to be trained; (2) the level of expertise with language form, content, or use in

Table 15–2 Listening Skills in the Elementary Language Arts Curriculum*

I. Basic listening
  A. Sound/object association
  B. Sound/letter association
  C. Ryhming sounds
  D. Following directions
  E. Auditory memory
  F. Listening for specifics: for letter sounds, color words, names, etc.
  G. Listening to identify categories
II. Critical listening/listening for information
  A. Getting the main idea
  B. Recalling facts, major details
  C. Listening to answer *who, when, where,* or *what*
  D. Recalling the sequence of events
  E. Differentiating major from minor details
  F. Making inferences
  G. Drawing conclusions
  H. Determining cause and effect
  I. Giving explanations
  J. Interpretation of mood or tone
  K. Stating personal reactions to auditory information

*Adapted from Maxwell.[30]

which the perceptual task is embedded; and (3) the child's competency with the response required. The language levels of school children with hearing loss are often significantly lower than their peers with normal hearing, even among those children who participate in mainstream classes.[32,33] Consequently the child with hearing loss may utilize comprehension strategies more typical of younger children. The clinician thus has two tasks with regard to intervention. The first, when planning perceptual training tasks, is to accommodate the level of comprehension strategies used by a particular child. The second is to foster more sophisticated strategies that might give the child greater access to the instructional language in his classroom.

PERCEPTUAL TRAINING

Auditory Training

Discrete Skill and Auditory Learning. Auditory training programs for children can be assorted into two general types: discrete skill or language based.[33] Erber's[34] skill objectives in Table 15–3 are fundamental to both discrete skill and language based auditory training curricula. Discrete skill programs tend to train specific auditory skills in a context separate from learning experiences that target the development of other communicative behaviors. The clinician

Table 15–3   Erber's[34] Hierarchy of Auditory Skills

Skill Level	Description	Response Type
Detection	Awareness of the presence or absence of sound	"On" vs "off"
Discrimination	Perception of differences between sounds	"Same" vs "different"
Identification	Labeling or naming what has been heard	Imitating, pointing to, naming, writing the label
Comprehension	Understanding the meaning of an auditory message	Answering questions, paraphrasing, maintaining a conversation

applying a discrete skill program will select stimuli based on audibility and the perceptual task. In contrast, the stimuli in a language based approach are encased within an interactive language development program.

The clinician applying a language based approach will use audibility and perceptual skill criteria similar to a discrete skill approach but will also select stimuli that teach specific linguistic principles.[35,36] Auditory skills are positioned within the more pervasive context of targeting objectives according to what would be expected according to normal language development. Ling[37] applied the term "auditory learning" to describe the language based process. He observed that real-life experiences develop listening skills more effectively than isolated tasks. Learning to listen occurs when children extract meaning from everyday acoustic events. Language based approaches integrate auditory learning experiences into activities that target language development and communication in general. The auditory-verbal approach is the most widely applied auditory learning approach in the United States today. Pollack's[38] auditory-verbal skill hierarchy is seen in Table 15–4.

The most efficacious approach to developing auditory skills judiciously applies the best of discrete skill and auditory learning methods. There are times that the child benefits from the separation of auditory tasks from other language or communication tasks to introduce a skill or to allow for practice of a skill toward developing automaticity. Discrete skill training also permits easier observation of auditory performance in isolation from other language behaviors and can be introduced throughout the auditory learning program as a check on progress. One must also keep in mind that integrating auditory learning into the more general language intervention program requires careful planning to avoid burdening the child with too many new skills to be attained in a single experience.

Discrete skill training sessions tend to be more structured than language based auditory learning experiences. Simser[39] describes an effective auditory training program as one that moves in and out of structured tasks, to the extent that structure does not overpower conversational interaction. Patterson[33] points out that auditory training programs tend to vary in the amount of structured adult-directed activities so that in the real clinical setting there may be no clear dividing line between discrete skill training or language based approaches, but rather a continuum of sorts. Erber[34] describes a continuum of structure among auditory training programs:

1. Structured practice on specific tasks
2. A moderately structured approach that first elicits identification within a closed set and

Table 15–4   Pollack's[38] Auditory-Verbal Curriculum

Level	Objectives	Performance Criteria
I	Change the learning environment Develop auditory awareness, vocalization, and use of sound for contact Conduct baseline evaluation	Move to level II when hearing aids are worn daily and sound awareness is established
II	Develop auditory attention and vocalization	Child shows a consistent behavior to sound.
III	Develop auditory localization and distance hearing Teach appropriate response to sound Increase vocalizations	Child is aware when sound stops Child may turn to name Child looks for the source of sounds. Move to level IV when orienting response appears
IV	Develop vocal play	Child attempts to imitate pitch, rhythm, volume, or some vowel sounds
V	Begin to develop auditory discrimination Develop auditory feedback and feedforward through babbling	Babbling increases in frequency and type Quieting may occur in presence of sound, indicating listening
VI	Develop auditory discrimination and short term memory Use sounds in babbling for the formation of functional words	Recalls a word associated with a situation ("bye-bye") Recalls a sound associated with an object ("moo" for cow) Spontaneously makes some sounds associated with objects
VII	Develop auditory processing Develop first nouns and action labels	Steady increases in vocabulary Outside the instructional context, child uses some of the words he knows
VIII	Develop the auditory processing of patterns Increase auditory memory Increase vocabulary Begin understanding and expressing word combinations	This level should be reached by the third or fourth birthday in an auditory-verbal program Begin formal evaluation for documentation of progress
IX	Prepare for school entry Discriminate against background noise Associate speech sounds with written symbols Hold conversations, tell stories and answer questions Learn school readiness concepts, following directions	Continue formal evaluation procedures for school programming
X	Coordinate auditory activities with academic content	Coordinate evaluation with school program

follows with a related comprehension task

3. Natural conversational approach

Tye-Murray[40] recommends short, intense sessions of formal training, 10 to 15 minutes per day, similar in practice to Ling's[6,41] recommendations for phonetic level speech drill. Formal objectives are then pursued throughout the day in the natural context.

Dimensions of Skill Acquisition. Auditory skills hierarchies tend to be similar with regard to the fundamental process of leading from detection to full comprehension of a message. Curricula vary in focus on the dimensions along which auditory skill is acquired. Auditory skills are multidimensional, shaped by three influences: (1) development, (2) stimulus characteristics, and (3) constraints on the child's reponse. Pollack's[38] curriculum in Table 15–4 represents an approach that is strongly shaped by developmental aspects. The child's language and cognitive development dictate the content and learning experiences in an auditory skills program.

The curricula abstracted in Tables 15–5 and 15–6 incorporate the dimensions of stimulus characteristics and responses constraints into auditory skill heirarchies.[42,43] One stimulus aspect is the listening environment. Auditory skills may be practiced under conditions of varying level and type of interfering noise or distance between listener and signal source. The linguistic unit of perception is another stimulus characteristic that influences auditory skill. Linguistic unit refers to the structures that are processed. These comprise a continuum proceeding from individual speech sounds, to syllables, to words, to phrase units or critical elements within the sentence, to whole sentences, and finally to connected discourse.

Movement along this continuum is bidirectional. The larger the unit to be processed, the more information available for comprehension. The information actually used by a child, however, is constrained by attention, memory, the match between the child's developmental language

Table 15–5 Objectives from the Auditory Skills Curriculum[42]

Curriculum Area	Performance Objective
Discrimination	Demonstrates selective attention to sound
	Discriminates nonverbal sounds
	Discriminates speech on the basis of suprasegmental features
	Discriminates linguistic messages with contextual cues
	Discriminates words on the basis of segmental features
Memory-Sequencing	Recalls and sequences critical elements in a message
	Demonstrates auditory/cognitive skills within a structured listening set
	Demonstrates auditory/cognitive skills in a conversation
Auditory Feedback	Demonstrates preverbal behavior
	Imitates vocal production
	Modifies vocal production
Figure-Ground	Demonstrates auditory skills at varying distances in quiet
	Demonstrates auditory skills at varying distances in noise
	Demonstrates auditory skills in the presence of a verbal distraction

Table 15–6 Objectives from the Developmental Approach to Successful Listening[43]

Skill Area	Subskills
Sound awareness	Responds to loud environmental and speech sounds
	Indicates when a sound stops
	Discriminates and identifies environmental sounds
Phonetic listening	Discriminates vocal duration
	Discriminates vocal intensity
	Discriminates rate of speech
	Discriminates vocal pitch
	Discriminates and identifies vowels
	Discriminates and identifies consonants
Auditory comprehension	Identifies name
	Derives meaning from vocal characteristics
	Discriminates common expressions
	Follows directions from one through four critical elements in a closed set
	Critically listens: identifies true/false statements, follows a sequence, learns new vocabulary from context
	Listens for information
	Follows directions in an open set

level and that of the stimulus, and the child's ability to segment, or chunk, meaningful units from connected discourse. The clinician may restrict the length and complexity of the stimulus to match these constraints. The clinician may further restict the stimulus to a lower level of input to highlight or isolate a linguistic unit for processing. For example, the child who exhibits confusions among speech sounds may benefit from some syllable level drill contrasting the sounds that need differentiation. In addition, practice in auditory chunking may help move the child toward larger units of processing.

A number of constraints function to limit the range of possible responses to auditory input, and thus provide predictability to the auditory task. The set of possible responses may be limited by restricting the number of items or pictures from which a child might choose in an auditory task. Keying the child in to the topic of conversation can also limit the range of responses. *Closed* sets refer to those responses that are constrained in the auditory learning session. *Open* sets refer to those responses that have no constraints, or have constraints that are not applied by the child. Some children will benefit from experiences geared toward leaning to recognize response constraints, such as identifying the topic of conversation from hearing sets of related words, or connected discourse, or looking at a picture of a communicative setting and talking about what is typically said (see Case study 15–2).

The real acquisition of auditory skills does not necessarily follow an iterated hierarchical path.

There will be plateaus in learning. Multiple skills develop simultaneously. Auditory learning can even appear to regress. Attention to the dimensions along which auditory skills are attained permit an understanding of the varied routes that children will take within an auditory skills heirarchy. As a child attempts to process more complex and less predictable input along each dimension, he may need to return to lower skill levels. Access to a variety of curricula that address different dimensions of auditory skill permit the clinician to match learning experiences to the individual needs of the child.

A final word must be said about a related area of learning that appears within many auditory skills hierarchies, the establishment of the

Case study 15–2.   Anthony was an 8-year-old boy with a profound bilateral sensorineural hearing loss (Fig. 15–2). He was first fit with hearing aids at age 31 months and was enrolled in an auditory-oral preschool. When Anthony entered therapy, he had received a cochlear implant and had been wearing the device for 3 months. He was mainstreamed in a second grade classroom. His support services included individual speech/language therapy, tutoring with an itinerant teacher of the hearing impaired, and private therapy.

Prior to implantation, Anthony received intensive auditory therapy and had developed a number of auditory skills. Nevertheless, Anthony's aided hearing levels barely reached the conversational speech spectrum, and he relied heavily on lipreading for ordinary communication. When Anthony entered therapy, he demonstrated the following auditory capabilities in a closed set: word identification by syllable number, sentence identification by length, and vowel discrimination on the basis of the second formant. Anthony also demonstrated emerging recognition of common sentences or expressions (How old are you? It's time for PE). Anthony also expressed a desire to use the telephone with his implant.

Auditory goals incorporated language and speech goals in the same manner as seen with Stephen in Case study 15–1. Specifically, auditory goals included:

1. Recognition and comprehension of open-set speech material
   a. Common sentences or expressions
   b. Sentences within a given topic
   c. Unrelated sentences with clue words
   d. Unrelated sentences without clue words
2. Participation in interactive telephone practice following the goals listed
3. Process three and four critical elements with known vocabulary, two to three critical elements with less familiar vocabulary

Therapy was directed toward bridging open and closed set identification skills. Anthony easily identified what he heard when the choices were explicitly available, either in picture or written form. Anthony practiced identifying sentences or answering questions after listening to an auditory message and looking at pictures that were related to what was said, but did not contain all the information. He listened to sentences describing events while looking at pictures that illustrated these events and then sequenced the pictures. Later, foils were included among the pictures that could logically be sequenced, but were not contained in the message. Still later, the simultaneous presentations of pictures and message was changed to presentation of the message first followed by pictures.

Anthony progressed to message identification with the message topic first announced by the speaker. Conversations were practiced at this stage. Anthony and the clinician would select a topic (''Let's talk about the Cowboys game today.'') and the conversation would continue in an auditory-only mode. In the beginning, there would be some discussion about what might be said to give Anthony an opportunity to practice anticipatory strategies. Anthony made a list of anticipatory and repair strategies that he could refer to during the session, and these were modified as Anthony determined what was most effective for him. Anthony needed to be able to determine the topic of a conversation on his own in order to develop open set auditory skill. He practiced listening to groups of related words, short descriptions, and definitions and identifying what the speaker was talking about.

Telephone practice proceeded at a slow and careful pace. When Anthony was successful with an auditory task during the therapy session, he completed the same kind of task with the message delivered over the telephone. Anthony also explored the components of a telephone conversation, including how to recognize that a speaker was ready to change a topic or to end a conversation. He wrote conversations and rehearsed them on the telephone with his clinician.

Six months after Anthony's implant was first hooked up, he achieved a word discrimination score of 68% to monosyllables presented in a closed set at 50 dB HL. Anthony's error responses were analyzed to catalogue his auditory confusions. These formed the basis of syllable level drill to give Anthony practice in identifying these speech sounds. Anthony created variations to make the drill more interesting, moving to different locations in the therapy room and introducing different kinds of background noise.

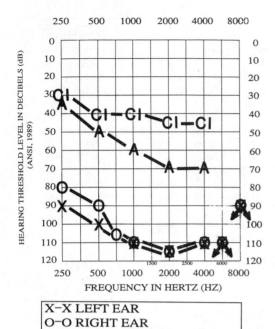

X–X LEFT EAR
O–O RIGHT EAR
A–A AIDED THRESHOLDS
CI·CI COCH IMPLANT THRESH

Figure 15–2. Case study 15–2. Eight-year-old boy with a profound bilateral sensorineural hearing loss.

phonology, or the speech sound system, in the child's native language. Speech abilities in children with hearing loss are fundamentally influenced by residual hearing and auditory skill acquisition, which establishes auditory feedforward and auditory feedback.[44] Auditory feedforward allows the child to set an acoustic target for the production of a speech sound. This is not easily achieved without the auditory experience and practice that establishes a phonology both motorically and auditorially. Auditory feedback allows for continual monitoring of speech production and ongoing adjustments as needed to maintain accuracy. The child who does not have an established phonology auditorially will utilize other sources for feedback, such as kinesthesia and tactile information. These appear to be less effective than auditory information. The inclusion of speech production tasks within the auditory learning program appears to facilitate both speech production and auditory skills development more effectively than auditory training alone.[45]

Hearing Age. Several factors influence performance in an auditory training program. The extent to which a child succeeds at auditory learning depends largely on the degree of the hearing loss. This influences rate of learning as much as the final product. Nevertheless, the wide range

of individual variation in performance within a given degree of hearing loss prevents the clinician from forming a prognosis based on hearing level alone.

The age at which auditory training is initiated also influences progress. Certainly, the ideal is to provide amplification or a cochlear implant and training during the optimal language learning period.[46] Some authors apply the notion of "hearing age" to establish expectations for performance based on the length of time that a child has been fit with amplification or has been stimulated by an implant.[47,48]

The application of hearing age to predictions of auditory behavior is most straightforward when the child is fit with amplification or receives a cochlear implant at an early age and the discrepancy between chronological and hearing age is minimal. As the gap between chronological and hearing age widens, motoric, cognitive, and experiential levels that are present in the older child must be taken into account, as well as the effects of starting intervention beyond the optimal period for learning language. The effect of starting intervention outside the optimal period may slow progress, but maturity in other skills areas may actually positively influence performance. Some discrete skills may emerge at an earlier level simply due to the cognitive demands of a discrete skills program. For example, the metalinguistic task of "same-different" judgments in Erber's hierarchy of discrete skills may be more cognitively appropriate for the older child who has an established language base, even if that language base is a manually coded system. Similarly, imitative skills that might be used in an identification task may appear earlier in an older child, simply because of better motoric control or more generalized imitative behavior, providing the child more expert knowledge as the task demands than the younger child.

Although the ideal age for implementation of an auditory learning program is during the optimal language learning preschool years, children with hearing loss do begin auditory learning during the school years. This may occur for three reasons: (1) the child has not been identified until school age, (2) the child moves from a program that has not emphasized auditory skills to one that does, or (3) the child receives a cochlear implant and now possesses auditory potential that was previously not available for training.

In the case of children who have only recently been identified, there will be two types: (1) those who do not present unaided hearing levels sufficient for processing spoken language and enter the school program with no formal language system, and (2) those who have unaided residual hearing capable of processing some spoken language and enter school with an established, albeit probably deficient, language system. In the first case, perceptual training might take on a highly structured discrete form. These children will not have an established auditory base and progress may be slow and proceed in small steps. In the second case, the child may already have an established auditory function, and the task of the clinician is to orient the child to hearing aids and newly available auditory cues so that the child may continue with language based auditory learning. Focused practice with syllables and words incorporating speech features that were previously inaudible may be helpful.

Children who have attended programs for children with hearing impairment and first begin auditory training at school age due to transfer from one program to another or an improvement in auditory potential are likely to have a language base of some sort. Auditory skill development may be mapped onto existing language, and a language-based approach included in the training program. Although the child may posses the potential for auditory processing, he may either be unaware of his abilities or have learned to doubt them. The training program initially might look like that for children who have not been identified until school age, with small, discrete, first steps so that the child's awareness and confidence are established.

Among children with profound loss, those who are implanted often follow a different time course in performance than those with hearing aids, although the approach to training and the sequence of auditory skill development are similar. Detection skills may be more quickly established among those children with implants. There is a greater probability of vicarious auditory learning, more sensitivity to high frequency sounds, and greater facility with informal, language-based activities.[49]

Speechreading Training

In establishing a speechreading training program for a child with hearing loss, one must first determine how speechreading will function for him. Among children with usable residual hearing, speechreading is likely to function as an enhancement to audition and will be used when the auditory signal is less than optimal—in noise,

in reverberant environments, or if hearing levels fluctuate. For other children, speechreading takes on a larger role in speech perception, particularly if hearing aids or cochlear implantation fail to achieve functional audition. A child might also be considered for speechreading training if an oral interpreter is to be used in the classroom.[50] The clinician must keep in mind that children with profound hearing losses can and do demonstrate functional residual hearing, so that the determination of the relative importance of speechreading in an intervention program should not be made on the basis of the audiogram alone.

Speechreading training programs are designed in general to develop two types of skill: analytic or synthetic. Analytic skill programs train the recognition of each sound or word in a training stimulus. Synthetic approaches require that the speechreader recognize the general idea of a message.[51,52] Analytic and synthetic speechreading skills use different information processing strategies. Analytic skills use "bottom-up" strategies; synthetic skills employ "top-down" strategies.[53] A bottom-up approach emphasizes the units of processing and their recognition. A top-down approach emphasizes thought and language. Accordingly, training stimuli in an analytic approach tend to be syllables or single words. Stimuli in a synthetic approach tend to be units of spoken language that are sufficiently large so that meaning is present—phrases, sentences, or longer stretches of conversation.

Evidence for speechreading learning exists for both analytic and synthetic training approaches.[54,55] Not surprisingly, the strongest evidence for either approach is obtained when the materials used to test learning utilize the same skills that are being trained.[56] There is, however, little evidence of generalization from one training approach to the other.[57]

Linguistic/sensory processing is probably a continual interaction between top-down and bottom-up information processing, requiring that speechreaders use analytic as well as synthetic skills. A combined approach to speechreading training is probably the more fruitful clinical method. Parasnis and Samar[58] propose an interactive training program that focuses first on context and semantic content to comprehend a message and then drawing the speechreader's attention to phonemic detail.

Individual differences in speechreading ability are considerable.[59] The presence of substantial individual differences in speechreading ability may indicate a need for a variety of training approaches to training speechreading skill.[57] However, the variables that separate poor from expert speechreaders and that might dictate the design of a training program have not been clearly defined by research.[60] Good speechreaders do tend to have better language skills, lending support to the establishment of training programs that target language development as well as speechreading skill, similar to language based auditory training.[61] Research and clinical evidence also demonstrate that the most efficient speechreaders integrate visual and auditory information,[62] lending support to the application of speechreading training in association with a clearly defined auditory skill development program.

Sensory Modality

The question arises whether the input signal in a perceptual training program should be delivered bimodally, so that both vision and audition are used, or whether the modality should be unisensory. Most auditory training programs assign some learning time to perception of the auditory signal alone. In a discrete skill approach, this may be the only time during training that the student receives an auditory-only signal. Language based approaches may vary in the use of a unisensory modality. A hallmark of the auditory-verbal approach is unisensory training. A significant proportion of an auditory-verbal learning session focuses exclusively on the processing of auditory information without speechreading. Children are encouraged to use audition as a principal means of speech perception.

The child with hearing impairment is likely to have learned to process speech input visually prior to receiving amplification or a cochlear implant. This can occur among children who are identified as early as 8 to 10 months old due to the substantial cognitive development that takes place during infancy. When the child is fit with hearing aids or receives a cochlear implant, he must reorganize existing visual schemas, adapting these to include audition. Perceptual reorganization can be facilitated by providing the child with intense scaffolded experience and practice with auditory processing.

If a child is constantly oriented to look at the speaker's face he selects visual information. Similarly, when directed to listen, the child is programmed to process auditory information. There is evidence that a unisensory approach facilitates integrated processing of auditory and visual speech information more effectively than multisensory training, as obtained in rates of identification of syllable patterns presented bimodally in the experimental context.[63]

When considering the choice of sensory modality in speechreading training, it is helpful to recall that speechreading is seldom sufficient for achieving comprehension without the support of auditory information. The choice of sensory modality in speechreading training is also affected by role that speechreading will play in the child's comprehension of spoken language. For the child who will use speechreading information to complement the information provided by the auditory signal, bimodal presentation of auditory and visual speech information has clinical validity for speechreading training. For the child who will rely heavily on speechreading information for comprehension, some practice with the visual signal alone may be useful, although among adult learners, there is little evidence that exclusively unisensory visual training achieves significantly greater gains than combined modality training.[64] An approach with greater face validity than unisensory visual training might be to replicate the conditions under which the auditory signal is degraded, such as in conditions of competing noise, distance, or reverberation.

Perceptual Training in an Interactive Context

The comprehension of spoken language is interactive, necessitating attention to strategies used by the talker as well as the communicative demands of the perceiver. The child who succeeds in comprehending spoken language is likely to have internalized communication strategies for avoiding and repairing the breakdowns that can occur in everyday communication. A perceptual training program that is designed with communicative interaction in mind will more easily facilitate the development of these strategies than a simple stimulus-response paradigm that targets similar auditory skills, but fails to program for generalization to the give-and-take of conversation. Yoshinaga-Itano[53] includes in her speechreading program goals that increase the child's sense of responsibility toward communication: (1) increase ability to evaluate his own skills in a variety of communicative situations; (2) increase ability to generate strategies to improve communication; and (3) increase tolerance for frustrating communication situations.

Kaplan et al[65] divide communication strategies into two types: anticipatory and repair. Anticipatory strategies are applied before a message occurs to minimize potential problems. Repair strategies address a breakdown after it has occurred. Anticipatory strategies include anticipation of the vocabulary, topic, and dialogue that may take place in a particular situation, and preparation for the auditory environment with plans for modifications. Repair strategies include requests for repetitions, paraphrasing, saying or spelling key words, gestures or writing, or asking questions about the message.

Erber[34] incorporates clinician-initiated adaptive strategies in the traditional stimulus-response perceptual training paradigm. Adaptive strategies influence the input presented by the clinician based on the child's response to a perceptual task. If the child is successful, the clinician maintains the task, introduces new semantic content or more complex linguistic form, or moves to a higher level of perceptual demand. If the child is not successful, a task analysis reveals the nature of the unsuccessful response and the clinician applies strategies to facilitate success. Breakdowns may be behavioral, linguistic, perceptual, or based in the child's knowledge about the topic.

Tracking procedures provide yet another avenue of training involving interaction and repair strategies. Tracking was first described and Defillipo and Scott.[66] Text is read to the child and she repeats what she hears or speechreads. The clinician utilizes adaptive procedures to correct the child's response until her repetition is verbatim of the read text. The perceiver can also utilize cues to direct the sender as to the adaptive procedures that might be applied, thus making the listener a more active and responsible participant in the comprehension task.

Tracking procedures allow for simultaneous training and evaluation. Performance is typically measured by the number of words of text that are repeated correctly over a period of time, giving the clinician a continuous measure of the child's success throughout the training period. Tye-Murray and Tyler[67] warn against the use of tracking assessment as anything other than a measure of a single individual's performance over time, citing difficulty in finding controlled texts and variability that appears from presentation to presentation. Mathhies and Carney[68] also point out the variability that can result from using different adaptive procedures from session to session and recommend a standardization of these. Nevertheless, tracking can be a useful tool for

practice with connected discourse and assessment of how the child processes textual materials that might be presented in the classroom. Tracking procedures also provide a structured activity for the child to practice repair strategies.

Tye-Murray[69] points out three challenges to incorporating communication strategies training in a program designed for children: (1) presenting these strategies in a way that children will understand them; (2) choosing strategies that are appropriate for children's conversation; and (3) developing materials and procedures that are interesting to children. Skits and role playing provide an avenue for illustrating the need for and use of conversational strategies.[70,71] Furthermore, children with hearing impairment may need training to use the structure of conversation. Practice of conversational routines, or scenarios, is one way to establish conversational function and makes use of routinized language from which linguistic rules may be derived.[72]

STRATEGIES FOR PERCEPTUAL TRAINING

The suggestions below are not intended to be a cookbook for developing a perceptual training program from start to finish. A cookbook approach would fail to meet the varied needs of schoolchildren with hearing loss, as is shown in Case study 15–3. Furthermore, discussion of the rich topic of assessment of auditory and speechreading skills, beyond the scope of this chapter, is necessary for a complete description of program implementation. Instead, the following translates the preceding chapter into practical hints for auditory training and speechreading.

1. *Determine the nature of the perceptual training program.* How will audition and speechreading be used by this child? Will audition be a primary mode of speech reception? Will some training in the use of speechreading cues be beneficial? What should be the balance between discrete skill training and auditory learning?

2. *Specify the learning objectives.* Consider perceptual skill to be the learning objective with language form and content as stimuli for the intervention. With schoolchildren, academic content also comprise the stimuli. The clinician may retreat to an earlier-appearing auditory skill if new language or academic content are being acquired.

3. *Plan for exposure time.* The development of listening skills demands enormous amounts of input before similar output from the child is

Case study 15-3.   Tina was an 11-year-old girl who was seen for a consultation at the request of her parents and school. She had a congenital bilateral profound sensorineural hearing loss of unknown etiology (Fig. 15-3). She was first fit with hearing aids at age 20 months and was enrolled in a total communication preschool. Tina received a cochlear implant at age 9 years. At the time of consultation, Tina had been wearing her implant for 18 months. Tina is partially mainstreamed in a third grade classroom with an educational interpreter. She receives instruction in language arts and reading in a self-contained classroom with other children with hearing loss. Tina also received individual therapy with a speech-language pathologist at her school in two 15 minute sessions per week. Tina's school program used a manually coded English sign system.

The school and parents expressed disappointment at Tina's progress in the production and comprehension of spoken language since the cochlear implantation. They asked for suggestions for improving Tina's skills. In addition, Tina's parents wanted to know if signs should be removed from her daily communication to facilitate the establishment of oral skills.

Formal language measures, observation of Tina in school and in the clinic, and school and parent interviews showed Tina to be functioning within 2 years of her chronological age in the form, content, and use of language. Speech use was greatly reduced relative to language. Tina rarely used her voice when she signed. Nevertheless, Tina's speech-language pathologist reported an increase in her phonetic inventory since receiving the cochlear implant. Generalization to the phonological level was limited.

Observation of Tina in the classroom revealed that most of the language input she received was sign language input, and much of this was not accompanied by spoken language. When Tina was in the mainstream setting, she made good use of her educational interpreter to follow classroom instruction, but the signal she was attending to was primarily signed with few lipreading cues accompanying the signal. In Tina's class with other children with hearing loss, instruction presented by the teacher occurred without voice some 40 to 60% of the time that was observed. In both settings, Tina was rarely encouraged to accompany her signed communications with spoken language.

Assessment of auditory skills showed that Tina had an awareness of sound, recognized some environmental sounds, and differentiated human from environmental sounds. Speechreading assessment revealed that Tina had little recognition of common words through the combined modalities of speechreading and listening, despite the fact that she understood the words when they were signed. The observation of the clinician was that Tina was not aware of information available through speechreading and listening.

Tina received her implant relatively late in life. The timing of Tina's implantation suggested that auditory learning would be slow and her skills may not progress to the same level as a child with similar capacities who receives an implant during the optimal language learning years. In addition, Tina had established a visual language system that was English based, but did not have the underlying auditory phonology that exists in spoken English. The presence of an already established visual language system and the absence of functional use of audition or speechreading suggested that auditory language learning should be mapped onto existing signed structures, and removal from a signing environment was not recommended.

Looking at Pollack's[50] curriculum in Table 15-4, we see that Tina is at level I, sound awareness. The objectives in Level I include changing the learning environment, developing auditory awareness, and developing use of voice. The prognosis that auditory learning would be slow and recommendation that signs remain in Tina's communication system did not indicate that changes were not recommended in the learning environment. Despite the fact that the school program was managing a child with a different level of auditory potential once Tina was implanted, expectations and interactions did not change. Unless Tina had opportunity throughout the day to listen to, speechread, and produce spoken language, then prognosis for improvement beyond the level of rudimentary auditory awareness was poor.

The perceptual program for this child did not follow a model of direct instruction, but instead followed a model of consultation with the family and school to modify the learning environment and assist personnel in developing techniques that had not previously been incorporated into the curriculum. In addition, the school program increased Tina's time with the speech-language pathologist for discrete skill training. The school also provided for increased participation of the speech-language pathologist in the classroom for children who are mainstreamed and hearing impaired classroom to assist in the incorporation of added techniques with this child. Tina's auditory skills improved to the level of closed set discrimination and there was an increase in Tina's vocalizations. In addition, other children in the program showed improvements in auditory skills as a result of the incorporation of auditory techniques in the instructional program.

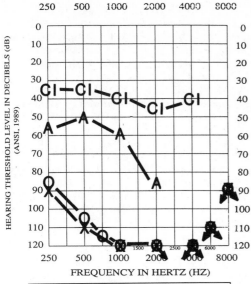

X–X LEFT EAR
O–O RIGHT EAR
A–A AIDED THRESHOLDS
CI·CI COCH IMPLANT THRESH

Figure 15–3. Eleven-year-old girl with a congenital bilateral profound sensorineural hearing loss of unknown etiology.

observed. An exposure, or stimulation, period is often necessary even for higher levels of listening skills. The inclusion of an exposure phase in training requires simultaneous targeting of future and current objectives so that exposure and stimulation are provided on an on-going basis.

4. *Consider the guidelines found in milieu language teaching*[73]

a. Follow the child's interest.

b. Provide multiple, naturally ocurring examples.

c. Explicitly prompt the child's production or response.

d. Embed the teaching episode in ongoing interactions.

e. Program for generalization by using multiple encounters in multiple conversational contexts.

f. Use familiar vocabulary.

5. *Use linguistic prefacing.* Before an activity is presented, describe it to the child so that the child first attends to spoken language. Repeat this language throughout the activity.

6. *For each learning objective, provide a variety of response alternatives and learning experiences.* These will accommodate the various comprehension strategies that might be applied

by the novice learner. If necessary, target the development of mature comprehension strategies.

7. *Provide negative examples.* Disequilibrium precedes the formation of new knowledge structures. Activities that do not produce expected results allow for disequilibrium. The child develops the expectation that there will be a certain amount of unpredictability in what he hears.

8. *Learning is active and interactive.* The child should do something with what he hears.

9. *Integrate content and process.* Integrate the process of listening while teaching content of academic subject areas.

10. *Plan auditory learning experiences along the dimensions of linguistic level, linguistic unit, and response constraint.* Target auditory skill development according to the child's performance within these levels. Add on rather than check-off skills.[74]

11. *Once mastery of a skill has occurred, provide opportunities for reinforcement and generalization.*

12. *Proceed at an appropriate pace.* Goals and activities should be distributed among a variety of levels of skill mastery.

13. *Listening is an internal process that cannot be measured directly.* Include some tasks in a stimulus-response framework, so that training will elicit a specific response to each activity and performance can be monitored.[75] This should not be confused with testing. It may be necessary to teach the response and give the child experience with the correct response before performance is observed.

14. *Prepare the child to take responsibility for successful communication.* Allow for breakdowns in the therapy session, and guide the child in the repair and prevention of these.

15. *Identify influences on performance and account for these in expectations of performance.*

Child characteristics such as degree of hearing loss or age at identification that might slow the attainment of learning objectives should not rule out the application of an auditory training program. Instead, realistic expectations for the rate of learning and final level should be considered as training ensues.

REFERENCES

1. Lindblom B, MacNeilage P, Studdert-Kennedy M: Self-organizing processes and the explanation of phonological universals, in Butterworth B, Comrie B, Dahl O, (eds., *Explanations of Linguistic Universals* (Mouton: The Hague, 1983), pp. 181–203).

2. Kent RD, Read C: *The Acoustic Analysis of Speech.* (San Diego, CA: Singular, 1992).

3. Pickett JM: *The Sounds of Speech Communication* (Baltimore: University Park Press, 1980).

4. Fletcher H: *Speech and Hearing in Communication* (Princeton: D. Van Nostrand, 1953).

5. Denes P, Pinson E: *The Speech Chain* (Garden City, NJ: Anchor Press, 1973).

6. Ling D: *Foundations of Spoken Language for Hearing-Impaired Children.* (Washington, DC: A.G. Bell Association, 1989).

7. Lisker L: *Rapid vs Rabid: A Catalogue of Acoustic Features That May Cue the Distinction. Status Report on Speech Research, SR-54.* (New Haven: Haskins Laboratories, 1978), pp 127–132.

8. Diehl RL, Walsh MA: An auditory basis for the stimulus-length effect in the perception of stops and glides. *J Acoust Am*, 85 (1989), 2154–2164.

9. Fry DB: The role and primacy of the auditory channel in speech and language development, in Ross M, Giolas TG, eds.*Auditory Management of Hearing-Impaired Children.* (Baltimore: University Park Press, 1978), pp 15–43.

10. Boothroyd A: Auditory perception of speech contrasts by subjects with sensorineural hearing loss. *J Speech Hear Res*, 27 (1984), 134–144.

11. Berg KW: Visemes and homophenous words. *Teacher Deaf*, 70 (1972), 396–399.

12. Fisher CG: Confusions among visually perceived consonants. *J Speech Hear Res*, 11 (1968), 796–800.

13. Woodward MF: Linguistic methodology in lip reading research. *John Tracy Clin Res Papers IV*, (1957).

14. Woodward MF, Barber CG: Phoneme perception in lipreading. *J Speech Hear Res*, 3 (1960), 212–222.

15. Kuhl PK: Psychoacoustics and speech perception: internal standards, perceptual anchors, and prototypes, in Werner, LA, Rubel EW, eds. *Developmental Psychoacoustics* (Washington, DC: American Psychological Association, 1992), pp 293–332.

16. Schneider BA, Trehub SE: Sources of developmental change in auditory sensitivity, in Werner LA, Rubel EW, eds. *Developmental Psychoacoustics* (Washington, DC: American Psychological Association, 1992), pp 3–46.

17. Fernald A: The perceptual and affective salience of mothers' speech to infants, in Feagans L, Garvey C, Golinkoff R, eds. *The Origins and Growth of Communication* (New Brunswick, NJ: Alkex Press, 1985), pp 285–306.

18. DeCasper A: Newborn preference for maternal voice: an indication of early attachment. Paper presented at the meeting of the Southeastern Conference on Human Development, Alexandria, VA. (1980).

19. Aslin RN, Pisoni DB, Jusczyk PW: Auditory development and speech perception in infancy. *Research on speech perception, Technical Report No. 4* (Bloomington, IN: Indiana University Infant Perception Laboratory, 1982), pp 132–143.

20. Werker JF, Tees RC: Cross-language speech reception: evidence for perceptual reorganization during the first year of life. *Infant Behav Devel*, 7 (1984], 49–63.

21. Moeller MP, Carney AE: Assessment and intervention with preschool hearing-impaired children, in Alpiner JG, McCarthy PA, eds: *Rehabilitative Audiology: Children and Adults* (Baltimore: Williams & Wilkins, 1993), pp 106–135.

22. Kuhl P, Meltzoff A: The intermodal representation of speech in infants. *Infant Behav Dev*, 7 (1984),361–381.

23. Dodd B: The acquisition of lip-reading skills by normally hearing children in Dodd B, Campbell, R, eds: *Hearing by Eye.* (London: Erlbaum, 1987).

24. Peters AM: *The Units of Language Acquisition.* (London: Cambridge University Press, 1983).

25. Ninio A, Bruner J: The achievement and antecedents of labelling. *J Child Lang*, 5 (1978), 1–15.

26. Newport EL, Gleitman LR, Gleitman H: Mother, I'd rather do it myself: Some effects and non-effects of maternal speech style, in Snow CE, Ferguson CA, eds: *Talking to Children: Language Input and Acquisition.* (New York: Cambridge University Press, 1977).

27. Benedict H: Early lexical development: comprehension and production. *J Child Lang*, 6 (1979), 619–635.

28. Milosky LM: Children listening: the role of world knowledge in language comprehension, in Chapman RS, ed: *Processes in Language Acquisition and Disorders* (Baltimore: Mosby Year Book, 1992), pp 20–44.

29. Sternberg R: *Intelligence Applied.* (New York: Harcourt, Brace & Jovanovich, 1986).

30. Maxwell MJ: *Listening Games for Elementary Grades.* (Washington, DC: Acropolis Books, 1981).

31. Laughton J, Hasenstab MS: Assessment and intervention with school-age hearing-impaired children, in Alpiner JG, McCarthy PA, eds: *Rehabilitative Audiology: Children and Adults* (Baltimore: Williams & Wilkins, 1993), pp 136–175).

32. Osberger, MD, ed: *Language and Learning Skills of Hearing-Impaired Students. ASHA Monogr*, 80 (1986).

33. Davis JM: Performance of young hearing-impaired children on a test of basic concepts. *J Speech Hear Res*, 17 (1974), 342–351.

34. Paterson M: Maximizing the use of residual hearing with school-aged hearing-impaired students—a perspective, *Volta Rev Monog* 88 (1986), 93–106.

34. Erber NP: *Auditory Training* (Washington, DC: A.G. Bell Association, 1982).

35. Kretschmer RR, Kretschmer L: *Language Development and Intervention with the Hearing*

Impaired. (Baltimore: University Park Press, 1978).

36. Estabrooks W: Still listening...auditory-verbal therapy for "older" children. *Volta Rev,* 95 (1993), 231–252.

37. Ling, D: Devices and procedures for auditory learning. *Volta Rev Monogr,* 88 (1986), 19–28.

38. Pollack D: *Educational Audiology for the Limited-Hearing Infant and Preschooler, 2nd ed.* (Springfield, IL: Charles C Thomas, 1985).

39. Simser J: Auditory-verbal intervention: Infants and toddlers. *Volta Rev,* 95 (1993), 217–230.

40. Tye-Murray N: Aural rehabilitation and patient management, in Tyler R, ed: *Cochlear Implants: Audiological Foundations* (San Diego: Singular, 1993), pp 87–144

41. Ling D: *Speech and the Hearing-Impaired Child: Theory and Practice.* (Washington, DC: A.G. Bell Association, 1976).

42. *Auditory skills curriculum.* (N. Hollywood, CA: Foreworks, 1979).

43. Stout GG, Windle J: *The Developmental Approach to Successful Listening.* (Englewood, CO: Resource Point, 1986).

44. Tye-Murray N: Articulatory organizational strategies and the roles of audition. *Volta Rev,* 94 (1992), 243–259.

45. Novelli-Olmsted T, Ling D: Speech production and speech discrimination by hearing-impaired children. *Volta Rev,* 86 (1984), 72–80.

46. Brackett D: Rehabilitation/education strategies for children with cochlear implants, in *Clinical Bulletin,* (Englewood, CO: Cochlear Corporation, 1991).

47. Pollack D: *Educational Audiology for the Limited-Hearing Infant and Preschooler,* 1st ed (Springfield, IL: Charles C Thomas, 1970).

48. Northcott W: *Curriculum Guide: Hearing Impaired Children—Birth to Three Years—and Their Children* (Washington, DC: A.G. Bell Association, 1972).

49. Tye-Murray N, ed: *Cochlear Implants and Children: A Handbook for Parents, Teachers, Speech and Hearing Professionals.* Washington, DC: A.G. Bell Association, 1992).

50. Castle D, Gonzales K, eds: *Oral Interpreting Selections from Papers.* (Washington, DC: A.G. Bell Association, 1988).

51. Nitchie EB: *New Lessons in Lip Reading.* (Philadelphia: J.B. Lippincott, 1950).

52. Kinzie CE, Kinzie R: *Lipreading for the Deafened Adult.* (Chicago: John C. Winston, 1931).

53. Yoshinaga-Itano C: Speechreading instruction for children. *Volta Rev Monogr,* 90 (1988), 241–259.

54. Lesner S, Sandridge S, Kricos P: Training influences on visual consonant and sentence recognition. *Ear Hear,* 8 (1987), 283–287.

55. Gagné, J-P, Dinon D, Parsons J: An evaluation of CAST: a computer-aided speech-reading train-

ing program. *J Speech Hearing Res* 34 (1991), 213–221.

56. Blamey PJ, Alcántara JI: Research in auditory training. *J Acad Rehabil Audiol Monogr,* 27 (1994), 161–191.

57. Gagné J-P: Visual and audiovisual speech perception training: Basic and applied research needs. *J Acad Rehabil Audiol Monogr* 27 (1994), 133–159.

58. Parasnis I, Samar V: Visual perception of verbal information by deaf people, in Sims DG, Walter GG, Whitehead RL, eds: *Deafness and Communication: Assessment and Training* (Baltimore: Williams & Wilkins, 1982), pp 53–71.

59. Erber N: Auditory, visual, and auditory-visual recognition of consonants by children with normal and impaired hearing. *J Speech Hear Res,* 14 (1972), 496–512.

60. Jeffers J, Barley M: *Speechreading (Lipreading).* (Springfield, IL: Charles C Thomas, 1971).

61. Berger KW: *Speechreading: Principles and Methods* (Kent,OH: Herald Publishing, 1972).

62. Binnie CA, Montgomery AA, Jackson, PL: Auditory and visual contributions to the perception of consonants. *J Speech Hear Res,* 17 (1974), 619–630.

63. Ling D, Leckie D, Pollack D, Simser J, Smith A: Syllable reception by hearing-impaired children trained from infancy in auditory-oral programs. *Volta Rev,* 83 (1981), 451–457.

64. Walden BE, Grant KW: Research needs in rehabilitative audiology, in Alpiner JG, McCarty PA, eds: *Rehabilitative Audiology: Children and Adults* 2nd ed (Baltimore: Williams & Wilkins, 1993), pp 501–528.

65. Kaplan HF, Bally S, Garretson C: *Speechreading: A Way to Improve Understanding,* (2nd ed (Washington, DC: Gallaudet University Press, 1985).

66. De Filippo CL, Scott BL: A method for training and evaluating the reception of ongoing speech. *J Acoust Soc Am,* 63 (1978), 1186–1192.

67. Tye-Murray N, Tyler R: A critique of continuous discourse tracking as a test procedure. *J Speech Hear Disord,* 53 (1988), 226–231.

68. Matthies ML, Carney EA: A modified speech tracking procedure as a communicative performance measure. *J Speech Hear Res,* 31 (1988), 394–404.

69. Tye-Murray N: Communication strategies training. *J Acad Rehabil Audiol Monogr,* 27 (1994), 193–207.

70. Elfenbein J: Coping with communication breakdown: a program of strategy development for children who have hearing losses. *Am J Audiol* 1 (1992), 25–29.

71. Trychin S, Bonvillian B: *Actions Speak Louder: Tips for Putting on Skits Related to Hearing Loss* (Bethesda, MD: Self Help for Hard of Hearing Press, 1992).

72. Stone P: *Blueprint for Developing Conversational Competence: A Planning Instructional Model with Detailed Scenarios* (Washington, DC: A.G. Bell Association, 1988).

73. Kaiser AP, Yoder PJ, Keetz A: Evaluating milieu teaching, in Warren SF, Reichle J, eds: *Causes and Effects in Communication and Language Intervention* (Baltimore: Brookes, 1992) pp 9–47.

74. Network of Educators of Children with Cochlear Implants (in preparation). *Children with Cochlear Implants: An Inservice Curriculum* (in preparation).

75. Pollack D: Reflections of a pioneer. *Volta Rev*, 95 (1993), 197–204.

16

REMEDIATION OF CHILDREN WITH AUDITORY LANGUAGE DISORDERS

M. Suzanne Hasenstab and Joan Laughton

All we know is still infinitely less than all that still remains unknown.

—William Harvey, 1578–1657

Many remediation programs have been designed to develop auditory skills in children with auditory-based deficits. However, most of these approaches are applied without meaningful language contexts or adequate cognitive bases. Therefore, the result is a limited transfer of targeted skills to the domains of communication and academics. The purpose of this chapter is to provide information to help professionals integrate their knowledge and resources to meet the needs of school-age children with auditory-based language and learning deficits. We make no effort to resolve theoretical differences with respect to the role or impact of central auditory processing on disorders of language (linguistic-cognitive), speech (auditory-phonological), or selective areas of attention. The discussion here stems from a broad perspective of auditory processing and emphasizes commonalities across various diagnostic categories of auditory disruption, for example, learning disabilities, attention deficit disorder, or auditory processing deficits. The goals of this chapter are: (1) to provide a focus based on the language and learning demands placed on children in school; and (2) to suggest assistive strategies to help children circumvent their auditory deficits in the school context.

AUDITORY LEARNING

Information that children use for learning and communication comes from experiences within their environment. Sensory modalities are the "avenues" through which experiences reach cognitive and linguistic processing areas of the brain. Children with intact input modalities are able to analyze incoming information from all stimulated modalities efficiently and effectively.

They are able to integrate this information and create a perceptual balance. Thus, they are able to benefit from the experience. If, however, a modality, such as hearing, is deficient in some way, information cannot be analyzed appropriately. Problems will occur in the affected sensory avenue and the total perceptual balance of the experience will be altered.

Hearing is the only sensory modality that permits the direct appreciation of the parameters of spoken language. It is also requisite for auditory learning. Auditory learning is the result of receiving, processing, representing, symbolizing, comprehending, interpreting, storing, and recalling auditory information. It is dependent on a child's ability to analyze and make appropriate decisions about auditory information. Auditory learning is critical to spoken communication and to success in school.

Problems in auditory learning are the result of auditory deficits that cannot be attributed solely to peripheral hearing loss. Auditory learning deficits are not hearing sensitivity problems. By definition, children with auditory learning problems have normal hearing sensitivity but they are unable to analyze auditory information adequately. This does not negate the possibility, however, that a child with hearing impairment could also have an auditory learning problem that is concurrent with a conductive or sensorineural hearing loss. If a peripheral hearing loss is present, the overlay of an auditory learning deficit will present as a problem in utilizing auditory information that is more extensive than the peripheral hearing loss alone would warrant. Therefore, even with appropriate amplification, the child is unable to utilize existing residual hearing effectively in the development and use of spoken language or for the purposes of learning in the school setting. Since an auditory learning deficit places children at risk for problems in both spoken language acquisition and learning, we will refer to these children as students with auditory language learning deficits (ALLD).

CHARACTERISTICS OF STUDENTS WITH AUDITORY LANGUAGE LEARING DEFICITS

The ability to analyze auditory experiences is necessary for the meaningful interpretation of auditory signals, especially those that code spoken language. As mentioned, an auditory language learning deficit impedes the development and use of spoken language and affects success in academic areas of reading, writing, mathematics, and spelling. Children with ALLD also present difficulties in auditory tasks that require attention, discrimination, organization, representation, recognition, symbolization, comprehension, storage, and retrieval of auditory information. In addition, they frequently manifest behaviors that interfere with successful adjustment and function in the classroom. For example, children with ALLD are often described as restless, forgetful, impatient, or socially inappropriate. Characteristics observed in students with ALLD are presented in Table 16-1.

Characteristics used to describe students with ALLD may seem diverse, but they are bound by a common theme: restricted function of the auditory modality for the effective development of spoken language and the purpose of learning. Not all children with ALLD present all of these characteristics. ALLD is a disorder that compromises children in their auditory learning capabilities, but it does not have a homogeneous effect with respect to obvious characteristics. Individual problem profiles vary across children and the complexity of difficulty falls along a continuum so that students with ALLD are not always alike in their abilities or in their patterns of strengths and weaknesses. A profile of a child with ALLD is illustrated in Case study 16-1.

AUDITORY LEARNING PROBLEMS: CHARACTERISTIC VERSUS DEFICIT

The characteristics used to describe children with ALLD are also attributed to other disorders, most notably attention deficit hyperactivity

Table 16-1 Characteristics of Children with Auditory Language/Learning Deficits

Normal auditory threshold sensitivity with or without normal auditory discrimination

or

Presence of a peripheral hearing loss that cannot account solely for the auditory problems experienced by the child

Problems in speech sound discrimination

Delays in speech acquisition

Delays and/or deficits in either/both receptive and expressive language

Problems in academic areas (reading, mathematics, spelling, content subjects)

Problems focusing on a task

Problems completing a task

Problems ignoring auditory or visual distractions

Problems in following directions

Problems in immediate recall of information

Problems in retrieving of previously learned information

Problems in transferring learning from one context to another

Problems in generalizing information

Problems in organizing general information

Problems in organizing sequential patterns

Difficulty understanding spoken language in the presence of background noise

Difficulty in responding quickly to an auditory stimulus (question or directive)

Difficulty in rapidly processing auditory information

Difficulty monitoring own voice

Difficulty localizing sound

Difficulty prioritizing sounds (selective attention)

Difficulty maintaining attention to an auditory signal (sustained attention)

Difficulty tolerating loud sounds

Limited flexibility in problem solving strategies

Limited ability to use language in problem solving

disorder (ADHD) and learning disabilities (LD). Children with ALLD, ADHD, and LD frequently share common characteristics, such as, apparent inattention, distractibility, excessive or nonpurposeful activity, difficulty in focusing on and completing tasks, listening and auditory processing problems, and difficulty in learning to read. Differentiating the source of the problem is often complicated when conditions share characteristics or symptoms. In the case of ADHD or LD, an auditory learning problem may be seen as merely a set of symptoms of the disorder rather than a deficit per se. The variation in perspective, symptom vs deficit, can complicate remediation for students with auditory-based difficulties associated with attentional deficits or learning disabilities.

There has been a tendency to implement a separate auditory skills curriculum as an intervention approach for these children. However, we suggest that the integration of visual approaches

Case study 16–1.   RJ is a 7-year-old boy enrolled in a second grade class who has been experiencing problems in school. He shows overall delay in academic subjects in comparison to expected norms for second grade children. He also presents deficits in specific areas of reading (vocabulary, word recognition strategies, comprehension), mathematics (word problems), and spelling (letter reversals). RJ's ability to grasp information and complete assignments was reported to be highly inconsistent from one day to another. He was described by his teacher as inattentive, easily distracted, and often confused by verbal directions and questions.

RJ's history indicates that he has had frequent episodes of otitis media with effusion (OME) that began before his first birthday. Although the occurrences have lessened over the past 2 years, he is still prone to OME. RJ's history is also positive for delay in the development of spoken language. He did not use consistent productions for words until age 2 years. Minor misarticulations are still evident in connected discourse, although RJ can accurately imitate all speech phonemes from a model production.

An audiological evaluation indicated that RJ had normal hearing sensitivity and normal tympanograms at the time of testing. Further testing to determine the presence of auditory processing problems indicated that RJ has difficulty sequencing auditory information and making figure-ground decisions. He also demonstrated a slower response time than would be expected for a child his age, especially for more complex tasks.

Psycho-educational testing results verified problems in academic areas. RJ's scholastic performance averages a delay of about 1.5 grade levels. He demonstrated poor flexibility in problem-solving strategies and used a trial and error approach almost exclusively. His repertoire of task analyses was likewise limited. For example, approaches to sequential tasks were neither efficient nor effective.

and other organizational techniques may be more beneficial in fostering auditory learning and problem-solving strategies. Addressing auditory learning problems as truly a deficit and not just symptomatic of another problem can ameliorate difficulties across the academic curriculum, within various communication contexts, and in the classroom setting.

ACADEMIC PERFORMANCE AND STUDENTS WITH AUDITORY LANGUAGE LEARNING DEFICITS

Poor achievement in academic areas is one of the most frequently cited problems ascribed to students with ALLD. Although much is written about the reading disabilities of children with ALLD, less attention is given to other academic areas. Mathematics, for example, is seldom recognized as a deficit area because many children with ALLD perform well on computation and number operation problems. Spelling, on the other hand, is viewed as an area of potential difficulty, but the usual avenue of remediation assumes that more drill equals better skill. This section discusses problems encountered by students with ALLD in mathematics and spelling and suggests strategies and techniques to assist these students achieve success in these important aspects of school curriculum.

Mathematics

Mathematics is an extremely broad area of academic learning that permeates the scholastic curriculum throughout the school years. Formal reading instruction and spelling lessons usually end with the passage from elementary grades to middle school and are replaced by the language arts curriculum called "English." Mathematics, however, expands to more sophisticated arithmetic, algebra, geometry, and other higher mathematical forms throughout the secondary school curriculum. Success in the quantitative areas becomes a criterion for acceptable scores on various standardized achievement tests, such as the Scholastic Aptitude Test, and a requisite for study at colleges and universities. Principles of early, basic mathematics, such as counting, adding, or subtracting may pose little or no difficulty to young children in the primary school years. However, the introduction of applied problems in the context of written word formats presents a very different situation. Many students have difficulty solving word problems in mathematics. Children with ALLD have particular difficulty solving these problems even when their computation skills are adequate. High school students with ALLD may have abilities to solve word problems that are no more advanced than those of fifth graders.[1] Students with ALLD are often unable to select relevant information and determine the appropriate operational processes to derive a correct answer. They also have difficulty evaluating the correctness of their problem-solving strategy. Word problems with extraneous information are especially difficult. The challenge of separating necessary information from unrelated information is usually overwhelming for these students.

Difficulty with mathematical word problems reflects the language and learning deficits of these children. Word problems are mathematical situations that are set in a language format. Word problems have a semantic component that constitutes meaning specific to mathematics. The meaning in mathematical language does not necessarily mirror meaning in social language. The vocabulary of mathematics, for example, codes concepts and references that are not directly equivalent to word meanings in interpersonal language. The meaning in mathematical language is conveyed through the syntactic component: the word, phrase, and sentence structure, that is unique to mathematical word problems. Again, the organization of mathematical syntax is often different from the familiar formats of social language. For example, the question "How much longer will it take Dan to reach home than Reggie?" is not one that is usually found in daily conversation. To solve a word problem, a student must accurately interpret both the semantic and syntactic aspects of the word problem language. Word problems with simple vocabulary and less complex syntax are the easiest to solve, yet a glance at problems on standardized tests or in mathematical textbooks will readily show that this fact is typically disregarded.[2]

The language of mathematics varies dramatically from interpersonal language in another important way. A small number of select words are used to convey complex concepts and meanings in a context that carries minimal linguistic redundancy or interpretive cues. Word problems contain indirect questions, unnecessary data, and implied information without clarification and explanation found in interactive spoken language or other types of written text. Precise comprehension of the language used in a word problem is expected without the aid of nonverbal support cues, topic introduction, content explanation, or contextual and referential support.[3]

The complexity and difficulty of mathematical word problems places unreasonable demands on the language competency and learning abilities of students with ALLD. These students will inevitably require special instruction in mathematical word problem-solving strategies. These children need to be taught to focus on solving word problems in a systematic way. Students with ALLD require more time to process and internalize information and skills than their non-ALLD peers; therefore, they will require frequent opportunities for practice in mathematical word problem solving. These children need more than drill and practice in computation and number operations. Assistive techniques, such as simplifying the language of the problem, highlighting key words in the problem statement, writing the problem in a math sentence or formula, using structured questions, drawing pictures, manipulating objects, writing a word problem to match a computation problem, and reducing the problem to more manageable units, have all been helpful approaches in guiding the student to select the correct information and appropriate strategies to solve mathematical word problems.

Remedial instruction to develop necessary strategies in solving word problems must begin in the early primary grades when children are first learning to add and subtract. Early instruction forms a foundation for the development of appropriate processes in attacking the challenges of applied mathematics through word problems. Introducing the word problem formats early in the curriculum, through simple and basic one step problems, provides a gradual exposure to written mathematical structures and helps eliminate the intimidation that many ALLD students feel when faced with these problems in multiple sentence and paragraph form. Simultaneous exposure to computation and the format and language of word problems allows children to integrate mathematical operations and understand the relationship of calculation to application. In addition, the use of manipulatives and drawings that are commonly part of early mathematical operations teaching, is concrete and gives the ALLD student a hands-on advantage in making connections between computation and word problems. Early success afforded by controlled exposure and ample opportunities to practice solving word problems also helps develop both skill and confidence necessary when traditional or formal problems appear in a standard mathematical curriculum.

Language is the basis for difficulties that ALLD students have with mathmematical word problems. Therefore, early exposure to word problems should contain few words and should relate to drawings or manipulatives used in teaching. Gradually the number of words should be increased but extraneous information should still be omitted. The objective is to increase the language in word problems from words to phrases to sentences and eventually to paragraphs. As word problems become more sophisticated, they will also become more complex through the addition of extraneous information that is not necessary to solving the problem.

Other linguistic variables will also require attention. For example, word problems require increased problem-solving time when the unknown is presented first, as:

Mary and Paul bought balloons from a man in the park. How may balloons did the children by all together if Mary bought 6 and Paul bought 2?

$$\text{\_\_\_\_} = 6 + 2 \quad \text{or} \quad X = 6 + 2$$

One strategy that is helpful for children is to first cross out all of the unnecessary information and then rewrite an abbreviated form of the problem listing the known information first and the unknown entity last, as:

I do not need—cross out this sentence:
Mary and Paul bought balloons from a man in the park.
I know:
Mary bought 6 balloons
Paul bought 2 balloons
I need to find out:
How many balloons all together
I will:
Add 6 + 2

Students with ALLD will benefit from direct explanation regarding phrase formats that cue the type of operation needed to solve the word problem. Thus, "How many more...?" always means that subtraction is the correct strategy for solving the problem, while "How many... altogether?" indicates that addition is required. The type of verb used in the word problem presentation likewise should be targeted as an important clue to solving the problem. In single-step word problems verbs will generally refer to gain or loss. A "gain" verb (got, bought, received, found) codes addition, but a "loss" verb (gave away, lost, ate) indicates subtraction.[4]

In addition to solving problems, activities that encourage children to make up their own word problem to reflect a mathematical calculation problem requires children to select language (words and structure) with the appropriate meaning to express real world mathematical experiences. The ultimate scholastic test of a student's mastery of mathematics in elementary school is his or her ability to comprehend, interpret, and solve word problems. The ability to create a word problem indicates that the student with ALLD understands the language, purpose, and format of word problems.

Summary. Mathematics is governed by concepts, vocabulary, phrases, and sentence formats that create a language of mathematics that must be learned. Unfortunately, mathematics is often approached from a direction of skill development, such as memorization of number facts, rather than from a perspective of a learning process based in a language genre. Mathematics is also pragmatic and applicable, therefore, evidence of the internalization of mathematical language and principles is reflected in a child's ability to apply and understand both in real-life situations.

Spelling

Spelling is considered to be primarily an auditory task because of how it has been traditionally taught. In reality, however, spelling is a visual task; it constitutes written orthography. This dichotomy can prove to be confusing to students with ALLD. Spelling words are presented visually in spelling texts; spelling practice usually requires a writing task using the assigned words; and children are graded on the correctness of their spelling in creative written language activities. Nevertheless, spelling tests require children to hear a word, interpret the correct phoneme-letter exchange, and write the visual form of the word on paper. Even in an oral spelling test the requirement is to say the letters not the sounds that make up the word. For example, the correct response to "Spell the word 'cat'" is c-a-t (letter names), not kuh-ae-tuh (speech sounds). Students with ALLD will not automatically recognize or understand these sound-letter exchanges. Spelling is a visual phenomenon taught in an auditory format; therefore, emphasis should be placed on guiding the student to see as well as hear spelling patterns in words.

Spelling problems are pervasive among students with ALLD because these children are often unable to recode spoken language phonemes into corresponding written language orthography. They also have problems in sequentially ordering letters correctly. Thus, reversals or element shifts occur in their spelling patterns. Students with ALLD require modifications of typical spelling instruction. Spelling remediation procedures can be helpful in assisting these children develop the ability to spell more accurately. Several strategies for teaching spelling have been found to be effective.

Traditional presentation of spelling units usually begins with the introduction of a list of 10 or more target words to be learned. The words are presented to the children at the beginning of the week and are then practiced through daily lessons designed to help the students learn to spell the assigned words. The procedure culminates with an orally dictated spelling test at the end of the week. A smaller target list presented daily, most optimally three words, reduces overload in spelling instruction. The presentation of the spelling minilist should be accompanied by relevant practice and followed by purposeful and meaningful review rather than drill for rote memory of word spellings. Positive practice and reinforcement are important to spelling mastery.

In addition to presenting spelling lists that may be too long for students with ALLD to master, spelling texts often introduce various spellings of a sound in one lesson. Although all of the words may have the same sound target, the orthography is very different. For example, the spellings for the long *a* sound are *a-e*, *ai*, *eigh*, and *ei*. Concentration on three examples of only one spelling convention in a miniword list will allow children to focus on the spelling rule and note regularities in the sound/spelling pattern. Integration of other spelling variations over time is made easier if each can be learned as an organized pattern.

Reduced word lists and consistency in spelling patterns (sound/spelling families) can be combined with organized study approaches to provide structured practice in learning spelling words. Specific study steps are helpful for students with ALLD and can be used in small group or peer instruction and as independent practice. Structured procedures reduce haphazard study and encourage a uniform way to approach new words. These strategies also emphasize visual steps and memory practice that are important in spelling. Structured study procedures which are helpful with children having severe spelling deficits typically consist of the steps summarized in Table 16–2.

Spelling quizzes or tests should provide an opportunity for improving spelling as well as assessing learning of target words in the spelling

Table 16–2 General Steps in a Structured Study Procedure for Spelling Words

Look at the word and say it
Copy the word in writing (or use letter tiles)
Say the word
Write the word saying each letter as it is written
Say the word
Check spelling accuracy with the model
Write the word from memory
Check spelling accuracy with the model
Practice and review the word for 5 consecutive days
Repeat these steps until mastery is reached

unit. However, words on spelling tests are often marked incorrect with little or no feedback to the student as to the nature of the error. Unless specific attention is directed to misspellings, most children with ALLD will simply accept that they have spelled yet another word incorrectly and fail to learn from their mistake. Error imitation or modeling the child's error and then providing a correct spelling form is another procedure to assist ALLD students. This approach is especially helpful with words that are spelled nonphonetically. The student's spelling error is rewritten by the teacher/aid/peer and then presented in the correct form. The child is then helped to compare his misspelling with the correct spelling. This procedure provides clear and accurate feedback to the student in a very concrete manner, whereas merely marking a spelling word wrong fails to give the student with ALLD any information about the spelling error. Error imitation permits observation of the misspelling and a comparative model for correction. It is also a helpful strategy to use in a language arts program when students are required to produce creative written assignments.

Computer-assisted instruction (CAI) is helpful in providing practice opportunity for learning to spell accurately. Computer lessons capitalize on students' motivation for this medium for learning. CAI lessons can be individualized to meet student needs and abilities. Classroom computers can also be programmed to provide immediate feedback, reward for correct responses, and control instructional pace. However, students should not merely be assigned to complete drill or practice tasks on the computer as a substitute for direct teacher instruction and other meaningful spelling experiences. Computer activities should be integrated into the scheme of spelling instruction, not constitute the entire learning process. Spell checks for word processing software can also be an effective learning procedure for ALLD students.

Peer tutoring is another approach that can provide one on one instruction that is often so beneficial to students with ALLD. Daily peer tutoring provides intensive individualized practice that is usually not feasible in the busy day of most teachers. This format for learning can also be enjoyable to both students when used in a game format. Peer instruction is a valuable means of providing direct and individualized assistance.

Spelling activities, especially for younger children, may include motor activities such as tracing letters of written words or letter tiles. Writing words on paper, the blackboard, overhead projector, or computer are also helpful motoric activities. Motor activities, however, should be more than just repetitive copy tasks.

Learning to spell accurately is more than rote memorization of letter patterns in words. Spelling requires the ability to relate phonology (sounds) to orthography (letters), the facility to order letters in a correct sequence, and the knowledge of when to apply a given spelling rule. Spelling is not just a skill, but it is viewed as the most skill-based of all the instructional areas in elementary school. The ability to spell correctly is relevant to reading and writing and should be viewed as an integral part of the written language process.

In most cases spelling instruction follows the strict procedures outlined by the spelling textbook and little creative activity accompanies teaching. Lessons are usually structured over the course of the 5-day school week with a test administered on the fifth day. Activities demand little teacher guidance or require only cursory teaching. The lack of instructional requirements combined with the emphasis on drill for memorization frequently relegates spelling to a seatwork assignment or independent study activity. Such focus will do little to assist the student with ALLD achieve spelling success; rather, spelling instruction for these children should be based on the remediation components summarized in Table 16–3.

Table 16–3 Remediation Components for Teaching Spelling

A daily instructional list limited to three words
Concentration on consistent sound/spelling patterns
Teaching to mastery (independent spelling of the word without a model)
Opportunity for self-check for accuracy
Clear feedback
Error analysis

WRITTEN LANGUAGE

We have opted not to address reading and writing directly in the context of this chapter, although deficits in reading and writing constitute a legitimate concern for children with ALLD. There is a substantial volume of useful information currently available to clinicians that addresses reading and writing problems and strategies to offset them. Reading and writing are approached here as written language, which is integral to school success. Competence in reading and writing is codependent and interactive with achievement in mathematics, spelling, and content subjects (for example, science and social studies). Using this perspective, three topics are discussed that concern written language. Word knowledge is presented because it is an ongoing process that permeates all aspects of school achievement. Phonics was selected because of continued debate on its value as a word decoding technique and as a primary reading approach. Finally, an intervention perspective, called the whole language approach to learning, is briefly explained with illustrations as to how it can benefit students with ALLD.

Vocabulary Development and Word Knowledge

The majority of children with ALLD have limitations in their receptive and expressive vocabularies for both spoken and written language. Overall, these children lack exposure to an extensive corpus of words. Limits in vocabulary restrict a child's flexibility in any language activity. A constrained lexicon has implications for reading and academic content areas, as well as for understanding and expressing spoken conversation. Students with ALLD have difficulty in listening, which affects development of spoken language vocabulary and limits the number of new words they internalize. Reading vocabulary and the variety of words students with ALLD use in writing activities are also restricted because these students have problems using word recognition techniques and understanding contextual meaning in written language format. Also, because of their limitations in reading performance, children with ALLD select books that present limited vocabulary, thus reducing their opportunities to meet new words.

Vocabulary development is usually associated with word recognition, such as the ability of a child to match a picture or object to a word presented in speech or written form. However, vocabulary development is more than recognizing words. It also involves knowledge of word meanings. There are three important dimensions of vocabulary and word knowledge. The first dimension is the number of words in a child's lexicon. The number of word meanings a child has for a given word is the second aspect. The third factor is the flexibility a child is able to exercise in fitting word meaning to context. Children with ALLD usually present limitations in all three areas.

Traditional methods of vocabulary development are not explicit enough for students with ALLD. Often new words are presented in vocabulary lists with only superficial instruction to explain meaning, as in reading lessons or in the introduction of a content area topic. However, a single definition or explanation of a word in isolation of other related words does not necessarily provide an exemplar for the meaning of a word. Most words, especially common words that children are exposed to, have multiple uses so that the function or meaning of the word changes with context. It is important to present and discuss new words or new meanings for words so that children can establish a framework for understanding the purpose of the word in the text or lesson to be taught. Constructing a basis for understanding the topic of a passage or conversation and building new meanings on prior knowledge are necessary for accurate comprehension.

Children acquire new words and expanded meanings for words they already know in many different situations. Most children learn different applications for words through listening and are able to transfer this spoken language word knowledge to reading and writing. However, due to their limited capabilities in effective listening, students with ALLD do not have this advantage and are frequently unable to generalize meaning from one context to another. These students require more in-depth and frequent exposures to new words and new meanings for words than their peers, but in actual practice, ALLD children are given less opportunity to expand their vocabularies and meaning bases.

An integral component in word knowledge is the ability to define words. Knowing the definition of a word reflects understanding of word meanings. This ability develops and expands over time. For example, a young child might be able to match a picture or object to a like picture or object but be unable to label it or the child might

be able to label an object but be unable to define it. General levels in the expanded development of definitions given by children are summarized in Table 16–4. These levels can serve as indications of sophistication children possess in their ability to define words and as guidelines to fostering further expansion in explaining word meanings.

Table 16–4 Levels in Teaching Word Definitions

Matching an object or picture to a like object or picture

Indicating an object or picture in response to a word label

Indicating an action by movement in response to a word prompt

Labeling or naming an object or picture

Defining an object by function or purpose (A bike is to ride.)

Defining an object by characteristic parts (A bike has wheels and pedals and handlebars.)

Defining an object by attributes or appearance (The sun is round and kinda yellow and it's hot.)

Defining an object or action by explanation (You know, running is like when you are going down the street real slow, and then you start going very fast with your feet.)

Defining an object, action, or descriptor by general category (A cat is an animal, actually a mammal.)

Defining an object, action, or descriptor by example (The color crimson is red, but deep like cranberry sauce.)

Defining an object, action, or descriptor by a synonym (To comprehend means to understand.)

One skill area that is considered advantageous to the development of vocabulary and word knowledge, and is included in reading and language arts curricula, is use of a dictionary. This is certainly a useful ability, but it does have limitations in teaching word meanings. Dictionary definitions are general word meanings that are out of context. They are often abstract or restricted and references to multiple meanings offer little guidance for applying the word to a specific situation. Activities, such as assigning students a list of words to locate in the dictionary, copy and memorize the definitions, and regurgitate the word meanings on a quiz or workbook exercise, will do little to enrich a child's word knowledge. Memorizing dictionary definitions does not transfer to understanding the meaning of a word in conversation or text. Simply learning a word by its dictionary definition fails to develop any conceptual basis for comprehension; therefore, the word is easily forgotten or used only in a specific context.

Other approaches to the development of definition are more effective. Words learned in a semantic set or network, such as words for feelings or names of animals found in the jungle, are more easily internalized. The common characteristics of a semantic network assist children in their organization of words into meaningful categories. Using new words in storytelling or story writing activities helps children develop definitions that reflect context. Discussing and comparing new meanings to ways that a word has been previously used helps students see functions of words in different contexts and builds on previous learnings. Strategies such as these will provide the necessary exposure and experiences that children with ALLD need to develop their lexicon and expand their knowledge of word meanings.

Vocabulary decrements tend to increase over time so that as children with ALLD proceed through the elementary grades the gap in their word knowledge becomes greater when compared to their peers. Children with ALLD require specific remedial instruction in the development of vocabulary and word meanings. This intervention is critical to spoken and written language comprehension and to expression used in conversation and writing. It is also crucial to success in academic areas and recreational reading and writing activities.

Summary. An adequate lexicon and knowledge of a variety of word meanings is critical to school success. Word knowledge is necessary for proficiency in reading and writing and for achievement in academic content areas as well.[5] Children's vocabularies (number of words and corpus of word meanings) are expected to grow in immense proportions during the school years. However, students with ALLD will require extensive experiences with, examples of, and applications for new vocabulary words and their various meanings. ALLD students are not able to internalize novel concepts, meanings, and words rapidly; thus the value of incidental learning is lost to them. Systematic and formal remedial instruction must become part of the learning process for these children.

Phonics

Perception of individual phonemes is not necessary for a listener to identify a word. In fact, every phoneme, when combined with other phonemes, is altered within each syllable or word context. Remedial interventions that depend on a strict analysis of individual phonemes for discrimination or recognition of speech stimuli or phonics techniques for written word recognition in reading, will not be the best strategies for students with ALLD. Many children are simply unable to master successfully the repertoire of phonics skills that are needed to recode printed letters into their corresponding sounds and synthesize the sounds into a meaningful spoken word.

Phonics is an integral part of most reading systems used in schools today. The phonics approach to reading is based on the premise that once a word is "sounded out" and correctly pronounced, that is, decoded from its printed form, the word will be part of a child's spoken language vocabulary and, therefore, readily recognized and understood. Unfortunately, this is not always true. A child's mastery of phonemic recognition will not guarantee success in word recognition. Children may use phonics skills but not be able to comprehend what they read. For example, a student may successfully articulate each letter of a word, but be unable to "blend" them correctly. Even if individual sounds can be meshed into a word, there is no assurance that the word will be recognized. Word recognition, likewise, will not ensure word understanding in either spoken language or reading. Reading comprehension depends on meaning of words in the context of other words, not recognition or meaning of individual words, but too often there is overattention to developing decoding skills to the exclusion of meaning.

The nature of phonics is based on three requirements. First, there is a system of rules representing the verbal pronunciation of printed words. Second, use of phonics to recode words requires knowing when these rules apply in letter/sound transfer. Finally, knowledge of exceptions to the rules, including how and where the exceptions apply, is also necessary. In light of these points, use of phonic skills may be seen as only one possible method of determining word pronunciation. The American English sound system is extremely complex. It is difficult to learn and remember all of the rules and exceptions of sound/letter transfer that are requirements for using phonics to decode or recode words not immediately recognized.

Children may be able to hear speech sounds (phonemes) and discriminate between them but be unable to grasp the notion that a symbol (letter) represents that sound. Children may also be unable to blend sounds into a word pattern even if they are able to determine the sound/symbol relationship. Finally, even if a word is accurately decoded, there is no certainty that it will be either familiar to the child or part of his or her lexicon.

Summary. Phonics has been a topic of debate since the 1920s, enjoying various degrees of support. Currently, it is in vogue as evidenced by a television marketing program directed to parents and presented as a way to ensure reading success for their children whether they are preschoolers or school-age students. This over reliance on teaching phonics stems from a correlational, rather than causal relationship between successful reading and the knowledge of phonics. However, the use of phonics as a primary approach to reading for children with ALLD must be seriously questioned. It is, at best, a method of determining the pronunciation of a word. However, it does not automatically result in comprehension of any word meaning let alone the contextual meaning in the reading passage. The phonics approach to reading assumes that once a word is decoded from its printed form and correctly pronounced it will be both recognized and understood by the reader. Unfortunately, this is not always true. Phonics, however, continues to receive enormous acclaim and credit as the ultimate method of teaching children to read.

WHOLE LANGUAGE APPROACHES

The perspective that underlies whole language approaches to learning has positive implications for beneficial intervention with ALLD students. It is based on the premise that language is the basis for listening, speaking, reading, and writing and that learning in each area strengthens abilities in all others. In a whole language approach, school-age children enhance their listening and speaking abilities and learn to read and write by participating in interactive situations that require using language in natural, real-life ways. The goal of a whole language approach to learning is to make language both personal and social so that children develop a strong motivation to involve themselves in all aspects of both written and spoken communication.[6] Students learn the purposes and functions of language as well as form and structure. For example, a child may want to write a letter. Letter writing rules are then learned by actually writing a purposeful letter. The emphasis is not on drill for skill mastery, but on relevant and meaningful practice.

Students with ALLD need many opportunities for language experiences, especially reading and writing, yet school instruction may actually provide fewer situations conducive to language learning for these children than for children without this disability. Too often, valuable time is devoted to workbook exercises and drill on skill development rather than to meaningful and relevant reading and writing experiences. Exposure to language-enriching instruction is frequently withheld until children "master" certain skills that are considered to be prerequisite to literacy. A whole language approach places language, including literacy, as the central focus of learning; thus, children learn through authentic language experiences from the earliest stages of academic development.

In selecting instructional materials used in any whole language approach, all printed formats are acceptable. This can be a powerful incentive for students and also makes reading and writing applicable to real life. It is as valuable, or even more so, to read the directions on a can of tomato soup as it is to read an unmeaningful story in a second grade reader.

Another benefit of a whole language approach is that students see themselves as active in the process as language learners, as readers, and as writers. Use of various language formats assists accomplishment and provides control. Reading and writing are useful, functional avenues for interacting, accomplishing tasks, and acquiring what is needed or desired.

Summary. The whole language perspective offers an intervention approach that is conducive to the language and learning needs of students with ALLD. It fosters the use of language in real life experiences that children encounter every day. Learning is applicable, practical, and functional. Mathematics and content subjects are easily phased into this approach. Content subject areas can provide the core topic for learning units, for example, postal services. Concepts, vocabulary, and reading and writing activities as well as mathematical principles, such as money, addition, and subtraction can all be integrated into a holistic learning experience. Because spelling is necessary to writing, it naturally becomes an integral part of instruction. Thus, all components of the elementary school curriculum can interface in a linguistically based and learning-focused environment.

AUDITORY CAPABILITIES

Intact auditory capabilities are necessary for effective listening, and effective listening is necessary for school success. School success entails both adequate academic performance and appropriate classroom behavior. Children with ALLD have limited or fragmented auditory capabilities; therefore, they have difficulty in all aspects of listening. It then follows that their school success is seriously at risk. As discussed earlier in this chapter, problems in listening are primary characteristics in the profiles of children with ALLD. This section presents a taxonomy of auditory analyses and decisions that underlie auditory capabilities and explains how they relate to listening, language, and learning.

Auditory Awareness

Auditory awareness is also called acuity, sensitivity, or detection and is the first requisite to listening. Auditory awareness is the ability to hear a sound. It requires the listener to determine if a sound exists. Listeners are aware of many sounds occurring at any given moment in any given situation. Children with ALLD usually have normal auditory awareness. If, however, they do present a peripheral hearing loss, it is not sufficient to account for the linguistic or academic difficulties experienced by the child.

Intervention for problems in auditory sensitivity usually involve amplification and aural (re)habilitation. These interventions can also be helpful to children with ALLD. For example, classroom sound field amplification, such as that used in the Mainstream Amplification Resource Room project, can provide an improved auditory signal for students and result in better listening and academic performance.[7]

Auditory Attention

Auditory attention requires a listener to prioritize a sound and follow the growing pattern of auditory information over a relevant time period. Attention to sound is mandatory for information to be processed, used, and stored. The decision to attend or not attend to an auditory stimulus results in listening or in abandoning focus. There are three aspects of auditory attention that warrant discussion: localization, selective attention, and sustained attention.

Localization is the ability to determine the source of a particular sound. Once a child is aware of a sound, and if the sound is salient, there is motivation to search for the source of that sound. Localization links awareness or detection of a sound to more complex analyses and decisions about the auditory stimulus. Localization is the initial step in auditory attention and is fundamental to all other attending behavior.

Many students with ALLD cannot or are slow in locating the source of a sound, especially in a noisy classroom. Visual cues, such as, pointing to or touching the important sound source, show the student where to localize. Verbal cues given by the teacher help students determine the source of the important auditory event. For example, leader statements, such as "OK children, look at me. Time to listen and watch. Time for reading group" or "Now, listen to the message on the intercom" are explicit indications of direction and sound source. When the important sound source changes, as when the teacher asks a question and a child in the class then answers, the ALLD student will also benefit from cues toward location of the new sound source. Explaining the source of an extraneous sound likewise provides information as to direction, for example, "Listen, who hears someone knocking on the door?" or "What do you hear?"

Selective attention is the ability to separate and prioritize the target auditory stimulus over all others that may be occurring at the same time. In the classroom, the target sound is usually the teacher's voice. Sometimes the figure-ground relationship is captivating, such as a novel sound or one with sudden increased intensity. Other times the selection must be a deliberate focus by the listener. The auditory system is constantly presented with auditory experiences. To process and use auditory information efficiently and effectively, some priority must be established. If not, listening cannot occur.

Children with ALLD have problems prioritizing sound and selecting the most important auditory information in a listening context (usually the teacher's voice). This situation is exacerbated if there are competing auditory stimuli in the listening environment. Efforts must be made to control potential auditory distractions during verbal instruction and directives. Children's focus must be captured before information is given. Verbal, visual, or physical cues are all effective. Often cues as simple as saying the child's name or asking "Are you ready?" will help the child focus or get ready to listen.

Frequency Modulation (FM) systems have also been used effectively with children with ALLD. These devices reduce figure-ground interferences and enhance reception of the teacher's input.

They should be used carefully and only in learning situations that require control of the signal-to-noise ratio. Many school administrators may associate FM systems with hearing impairment and are unaware that such devices can also benefit children with ALLD. Cost is a concern in most school systems and so it may be difficult to justify purchase of an FM system, especially if school personnel are naive as to their potential benefit.

Sustained attention is the ability to maintain focus on the target auditory experience for as long as necessary. Time is the essential factor in sustained attention. The length of time required to focus depends on the stimulus or task. The duration of sustained attention is often referred to as "attention span." Sustained attention is the decision to eliminate interfering stimuli to devote full attention to the target auditory stimulus for whatever time is required.

Saliency plays an important role in sustained attention. If a child is motivated by either internal or external factors, it is easier for him or her to maintain focus. Control of distractions is also critical to sustained attention. If a child is constantly pulled off task by competing auditory or visual occurrences, extended focus cannot occur. Extended focus can be encouraged by requiring periodic feedback from the student. Asking the child to repeat directions, questions, or pertinent comments helps ensure attention and, in addition, encourages more responsibility from the student in a listening task.

Auditory Determinations

Auditory determinations are attempts to establish a description of the incoming sound. They are analyses about the nature of the auditory stimulus. These analyses and the resulting decisions depend on a child's ability to compare the auditory event to identical or similar previous experiences. Thus, auditory determinations are closely related to cognitive operations of representation and recognition and are necessary to determine how a sound should be processed. Auditory determinations also help distinguish between new information and previously existing knowledge. There are four steps in determining the descriptive parameters of auditory information: general description, acoustic differentiation, prosodic distinction, and segmental discrimination. Each step in the determination process analyzes the auditory stimulus in finer detail.

General description of an auditory signal is the ability to analyze the overall nature of the auditory experience. The formation of a general description of a sound is pivotal in auditory learning and in utilizing auditory information in linguistic forms. Determining the parameters of the incoming stimulus has a two-way effect. It influences the attention decisions as to whether the event warrants continued focus, and it also determines how the sound, for example, speech or music, should be further analyzed and processed. A general description of an auditory stimulus is established through "questions" such as, "Is the sound internal or external to my body?" "Is the stimulus familiar or novel?" "Is it meaningful or nonmeaningful to me?" "Is it spoken language or an environmental sound?" "Is it verbal or vocal?" This general analysis of an auditory experience affects new learning as well as previously acquired knowledge, including the auditory aspects of cognitive concepts and meaning (semantics) in spoken language.

If children cannot effectively make this initial descriptive determination about a sound, they will be unable to attach any relevancy to the experience. Thus, even if attention has been established and listening occurs, failure to define the basic descriptive parameters of the auditory event will result in abandoning attention. For example, if a child cannot determine familiarity with the topic or content of a discussion presented by the teacher, he or she will cease to attend and will not make any further analyses about the auditory experience.

Problems associated with children's limitations in determining basic descriptions of auditory events can be offset by explaining the nature of a sound. For example, "I have a tape for you. The man on the tape tells the story of *Peter and the Wolf.* Remember, I read the story to you yesterday. It will be the same story." Once the general description of the auditory experiences is determined, the listener has the foundation to make more refined analyses regarding the nature of the auditory signal.

Acoustic differentiation or auditory discrimination is more than noting similarities and differences between phonemes; it is the ability to determine similarities and differences within auditory patterns. Acoustic differentiation is discrimination based on perceptual variables of length, complexity, structure, temporal relationships, frequency, and intensity. Acoustic differentiation analyses are necessary for both linguistic and nonlinguistic auditory stimuli. For example, all of the perceptual variables pertain to music. These perceptual variables likewise govern the unspoken meaning in language. The unspoken information is not coded by the meaning of the words in the message, but by the acoustic aspects of the signal. Acoustic perceptual variables can actually change the literal meaning of words in a sentence. For example, the mere shift in stress from word to word in the question "Do you expect me to do that?" creates subtle changes in its precise meaning. In actuality, it is the combination of meaning coded by words and meaning coded by auditory perceptual variables that contributes to the total meaning of a message. Acoustic differentiation is necessary for understanding the cues and requirements for coding language intent and purpose, discourse rules of conversation, and topic negotiations. This analysis is also critical to the understanding of subtle variations in meaning.

Children with ALLD are often insensitive to the perceptual variables of auditory experiences. They do not use these cues in their own spoken language expression and they do not understand or respond appropriately to the application of acoustic cues in the speech of others. Students with ALLD are frequently described as being literal in their interpretation of language. They understand a message only through the direct meaning of the words in the sentence. For example, they fail to grasp subtle meanings in humor or sarcasm. This difficulty is the result of their inability to recognize the nuances carried by auditory perceptual variables.

Problems in acoustic differentiation are very difficult to remediate. Skill development often seems successful because children can be taught to discriminate the differences between long vs short, loud vs soft, high pitch vs low pitch, etc, but they do not readily generalize these learnings to the complex context of spoken language. The best approach to accommodate problems in acoustic differentiation in children with ALLD is to provide them with direct, literal messages and avoid the possibility of misinterpretation and failure to understand important information.

Prosodic distinction or suprasegmental discrimination is an extension of acoustic differentiation. It is the ability to note variations in sound patterns. Pattern variations in spoken language are coded by syllable and word emphasis, and intonation changes in phrases and sentences that are cued by pitch, stress, and pause variations. Prosodic distinction in English is based on syllable, word, and phrase stress, tone, or pitch changes, intonation contours or rhythmic patterns in sentences or across an utterance, and timing factors such as pauses and rate changes.

There is a close developmental relationship between prosodic distinction and the acquisition of pragmatics, syntax, and phonology. Children who are unable to make prosodic distinctions may be unable to understand the differences between statements and questions. In addition, they may incorrectly interpret subtle meaning cues that are coded by variations such as word stress in a sentence. Again, the best approach in the school setting is to present instructional information, directions, explanations, and other pertinent and necessary messages in a clear, direct format and minimize the possibilities of misunderstandings by children with ALLD.

Segmental discrimination is the ability to "hear" differences between phonemes and phoneme patterns. The language components of phonology and morphology are dependent on this ability. Segmental discrimination receives extensive attention in the literature, in testing procedures, and in intervention programs. It is what most clinicians refer to as auditory discrimination. Segmental discrimination is viewed as important because it is closely associated with word pronunciation, which in turn affects speech and certain word recognition or sound/letter approaches in reading and spelling. However, segmental discrimination is only one step in the discrimination/determination analysis of an auditory stimulus. Caution must be exercised in adopting drill approaches that are designed to develop children's "discrimination skills," but address only the differences between syllables or phonemes. It is important to remember that the ability to determine the differences between phonemes and even phoneme patterns in syllables does not guarantee comprehension of spoken language or success in auditory learning. The value of segmental discrimination is that it provides a refined analysis in a child's attempt to determine a description of an auditory experience. Complete and successful auditory discrimination permits a child to determine the nature of a sound and the critical variables that make that sound a unique stimulus.

Auditory Organization

If auditory information is to be used for spoken communication and learning, it must be properly organized. Information without proper organization is useless. Once auditory determination decisions are made, the sound information must be patterned according to criteria established by previously experienced auditory events and rules of spoken language. There are three components of auditory organization: short-term store, sequencing, and synthesis.

Short-term store is an organization requisite and a function of the auditory system in response to the temporal characteristics of the auditory signal. Short-term store is necessary because auditory information occurs as a pattern over time. A sound exists and then it is gone. Therefore, if a child is to make any connection between discrete auditory stimuli, whether they are individual phonemes in a word or individual sentences in discourse, there must be some accommodation for temporarily holding the information until a relevant pattern can be established. Short-term store is the ability to retain auditory information so that the pattern boundaries of an auditory experience can be defined. Short-term store influences and is influenced by knowledge of meaning units and rules of syntax.

Short-term store is often labeled as "auditory memory" and equated with short-term memory or immediate recall of an auditory stimulus. However, short term store is not a memory process per se. Memory processes are cognitive operations and entail storage of information or experience that has already been organized according to sensory parameters. Short-term store, in contrast, is a critical step in organizing the sensory parameters of an auditory event.

It is usual for children with ALLD to present difficulties in auditory organization. They are often ignorant of auditory cues and linguistic rules that dictate meaning unit boundaries. The efficiency of short term store decisions will reflect a child's knowledge of meaning units combined with his or her understanding of syntactic rules. For example, the words *a*, *big*, *red*, and *balloon* can constitute a meaning unit according to the syntactic rules that govern nouns and their modifying adjectives. Spoken and written language instruction directed toward grouping and organization of meaning units assists students with ALLD in developing organizational strategies that are necessary to language comprehension and learning.

Auditory sequencing is the second phase of auditory organization and is the ability to order auditory information into relevant patterns. It determines the relative positions of elements within meaning unit boundaries and is necessary to interpret word, phrase, sentence, and discourse patterns. Auditory sequencing underlies and reflects structural rules of syntax and phonology. Correct auditory sequencing analyses are also required in for the organization of nonlinguistic information into a meaningful or relevant pattern, as in music.

Sequencing problems are common in students with ALLD and are observed in both linguistic and nonlinguistic tasks. Difficulty in the immediate recall of sequential information is extremely common in these children and is frequently cited as a characteristic problem in their classroom performance. Sequencing problems may also show modality cross-over and affect success in tasks that require visual or motor sequencing.

Sequencing problems of students with ALLD can be reduced in several ways. Providing positional cues in spoken instructions, for example, will help the child organize the order in which the steps occur. Stating directions such as, "First, get your math book out of your desk. Second, open your book to page 21. Third, put a check mark next to problems 1,3, and 5. Problems 1, 3, and 5 are your homework math problems." Written directions will be less likely misunderstood if they are listed and written with order cues rather than presented in sentence or paragraph form.

The directions may seem overly detailed, but this degree of specificity and organization is often necessary to ensure that the student with ALLD organizes and understands information. All activities designed to extend children's auditory or visual sequencing ability should begin with only two elements. Each picture or step should have a specific position cue. Additional steps should be gradually added as the child becomes successful in the ordering task. It is also important to require only minimal inference by the child. Auditory or visual information may seem obvious, but the typical student with ALLD does not grasp implied information and cannot fill in the necessary gaps to sequence correctly. Sequencing activities should be cohesive at first and slowly increase increments of implied information.

Auditory synthesis is the ability to blend or merge information into a total cohesive presentation so that cognitive processes can take place. Auditory synthesis allows the listener to determine the completeness of the auditory experience, from beginning to end. It is preparation for integration with sensory information from other contributing sensory modalities that pertain to a given experience. Once synthesis is complete, the auditory stimulus can be processed by cognitive and linguistic operations.

AUDITORY COMPONENTS OF COGNITIVE AND LINGUISTIC PROCESSES

In the interest of simplicity, the cognitive processes of representation and recognition, and the linguistic processes that include parallel operations of symbolization and comprehension, are discussed. Both cognition and language involve memory (long- and short-term storage) and retrieval. Auditory components of cognitive and linguistic processes depend on operational auditory capabilities, that is, accurate analyses and decisions regarding incoming auditory information. The auditory aspects of cognitive processes dictate the integration, conceptualization, and schema formation of the auditory facets of objects, actions, and events that occur in the environment. The linguistic processes ensure interpretation and understanding of the spoken language code.

Auditory Representation

Auditory representation is the ability to conceptualize a sound as it corresponds to an object, action, or event in the environment. For example, the auditory representation of a fire engine is the sound of the siren. Auditory representation is a prerequisite to enable children to use auditory information for learning or communication. Auditory representation is a child's reference to the reality of acoustic events; it is the internal model for sounds as they exist in the child's environment.

Without representation each experience a child has would be completely novel and unrelated for the child. Thus, the child would be unable to categorize information into generic sets or generalize and transfer learning from one experience to another. Each auditory experience is compared to existing auditory images. If a match can be made, the event will be familiar. If no prior reference exists, the experience is considered novel and serves as the beginning of a new concept formation. Learning expands and develops as new experiences are formatted in representation and as existing auditory information imaged in representation is refined, expanded, modified, or changed through repeated exposures to the reciprocal auditory event over time.

Auditory representation interfaces with determination analyses and provides the reference base for description and discrimination decisions. This is an example of the interrelationship between auditory capabilities and cognitive processes. If auditory determination capabilities function appropriately, continued and repeated exposures to an auditory experience will result in accurate representation. However, if auditory decisions are fragmented, incorrect, or inconsistent across exposures, representation will not reflect reality. In addition, several different representations of the same auditory event can occur. For example, the synthesized auditory signal may be analyzed incorrectly and appear to vary across multiple experiences.

Auditory Recognition

Auditory recognition is the ability to match an auditory experience to one that has occurred previously. Representation occurs when the child matches an experience to the existing model or reference. Once a sound has been represented, a reference for recognition has been established. However, one exposure to an auditory event is usually not enough for its subsequent recognition. Just as repeated exposures and correct analyses provide accurate representation, increased opportunities with auditory experiences ensure recognition. In general, the more complex the auditory stimulus, the more experiential repetition is needed to allow recognition.

Auditory recognition is also interrelated with determination analyses and decisions. For example, if the general description analysis determines that an auditory signal is a novel experience, that is, it is not recognized, it will be processed as "new data." The refined determinations provided by acoustic differentiation, prosodic distinctions, and segmental discrimination (if the signal is speech) will aid recognition by creating a more complete image in representation. If the auditory experience is only partially familiar, more information will be necessary to expand the form existing in representation. If the event is already represented and can be recognized, it can be used in some way.

The auditory aspects of representation and recognition are critical to learning. If auditory capabilities fail to deliver an accurately synthesized analysis of an acoustic experience, learning accuracy, efficiency, and effectiveness are greatly compromised. Children with ALLD are at risk for cognitive misrepresentation and problems in recognition of auditory stimuli as well as for deficits in representing and recognizing multimodality experiences that contain significant auditory characteristics. Multiple, realistic, and consistent exposures to auditory occurrences are necessary for students with ALLD. Only then can their cognitive processes be honed sufficiently to process auditory information adequately.

Auditory Symbolization

Representation and recognition are necessary for all sounds, but the sounds of spoken language require two additional processes to be utilized: symbolization and comprehension. Auditory symbolization is necessary for both reception and expression of spoken language because words in themselves are arbitrary, that is, phonemic sound patterns have meaning only in that they symbolize a referent. Symbolization is similar to representation but it is not an iconic form. A symbol is an arbitrary element of a code so the child must be able to match the symbol to its referent. For example, the spoken word *table* is a symbol for the object as it exists in reality.

Accurate analyses by auditory capabilities are as important for symbolization as they are for representation. A correct match to the symbol image is necessary for effective linguistic processing. If a comparison cannot be made, interpretation of the code is not possible.

Auditory Comprehension

In spoken language the auditory information, that is, the linguistic code, must be both recognized and comprehended. Auditory comprehension is similar to recognition but is a process that, in conjunction with symbolization, permits interpretation and understanding of the spoken language code. It is the ability to translate the acoustic information of the spoken language code into meaning. Auditory comprehension enables the child to decode the auditory linguistic symbols into meaning.

Long-Term Storage

Learning relies on a system that stores knowledge that can be retrieved and applied as demands require. "Memory" is the term most often applied to that process. It is the system that houses information (including auditory data) once it has been analyzed and processed by cognitive and, if necessary, linguistic operations. In a simplistic scheme, memory can be viewed as a catalogued information bank that holds data until it is needed. In reality, however, memory has been an area of interest and research for many years, yet we still do not fully understand either its forms or its functions.

Children tend to remember real life events best. Memory for information and facts that are based on participation and experience are stored more effectively than those that are merely presented and discussed. Long term memory can be enhanced by gradual movement through academic units, frequent review of previously learned material, and integrating new concepts, ideas, and facts with knowledge that is already well established. It appears that memory provides an organized information storage that can also be readily transferred to related learnings and that categories and classifications of information are necessary if memory stores are to be accessed and used.

Retrieval and Recall of Information

Knowledge storage is of limited value if it cannot be tapped in some way. Knowledge cannot be used if it cannot be retrieved from memory stores. Memory access is possible only when key triggers activate the retrieval process.

Information recall is a problem that is frequently observed in students with ALLD. Even facts and information that seem well established one day will not necessarily be remembered in the next lesson. The exact reason for problems in information recall is often difficult or impossible to determine. Information may not be analyzed correctly and thus may never reach memory. Another possibility is that the information was stored improperly and therefore cannot be accessed. A third cause may be an actual inability to retrieve information from memory.

CLASSROOM SURVIVAL

Instructional Practices

Teaching approaches and instructional practices have a direct impact on the quality and quantity of learning that takes place in any classroom. The teaching-learning relationship should be an interactive dyad, but in many classrooms it is not achieved. Children who are capable learners are usually able to learn in any instructional environment. They are self-motivated and can internalize information effectively with little guidance. Less than optimal instructional practice may inhibit even the best students' learning, but generally when a child is free from learning deficits, he or she learns regardless of instructional limitations. Students with ALLD, however, do not fare as well. Even commonly accepted or traditional teaching approaches may not be conducive to their learning requirements.

One of the most frequently used instructional practices in contemporary classrooms is the large group, teacher-lecture format. Many students with ALLD experience difficulty in classrooms where large group or undifferentiated instruction is the usual format for teaching. Unfortunately, this teaching mode is the rule rather than the exception, especially beyond the primary grades. However, even in the early school years, content areas, such as science and social studies, are taught by large group instruction. When this format is used, children must understand information that is being presented or they must be capable of requesting clarification if they do not understand. This may seem easy enough; however, students with ALLD may not even be able to relate sufficiently to a discussion to realize what it is that they do not understand. The ability to request clarification depends on a child's ability to have some idea of what they know and do not know about a topic.

Students with ALLD are often passive learners. They seldom ask questions in class, even when they need clarification. They rarely volunteer to answer questions or comment on topics. In many cases there are linguistic and knowledge gaps between the child's functioning level and the level of the information presented in a lesson. When this occurs, the student is unable to participate in the learning process. Students with ALLD have successful learning experiences only when they are oriented to previously acquired information about a topic, and then guided and directed to relate that knowledge to new ideas and concepts.

Students with ALLD require concrete manipulation or strong visual illustrations of new concepts, vocabulary, or word meanings. Learning is best accomplished in an associative context that capitalizes on the connections between reality and its symbols and abstractions.

Following Directions

Two indispensable aspects of teaching and learning are giving and following directions. Within any given school day, directives guide the procedures for seatwork assignments, learning tasks, and classroom routines. Directions entail a dual responsibility. The teacher must provide a clear, direct, coherent instructional message and the student must attend to, understand, and perform as the directive prescribes. One nearly uniform characteristic of children with ALLD is the inability to follow directions. Common problems in following direction include: retaining only partial information contained in the directions, substituting information for the actual content, and confusing the order of steps in multistep commands. Many of the difficulties that students with ALLD experience with spoken directions in the classroom can be reduced by the teacher's attention to how oral directions are presented. The considerations presented in Table 16–5 will assist students' comprehension of verbal instructions.

Table 16–5 Suggestions to Help Students Follow Oral Directions

Auditory and visual distractions should be eliminated

The child's complete attention should be secured before any information/directives are given

Instructions should be given in clear and well-articulated voice

Sentences should be direct, simple, short, and precise

Visual cues should be given to support auditory information (notes on the board, overhead projector, or written handout)

Passive Learning Styles

As mentioned earlier in this section, many children with ALLD are described as passive learners. Passive learners are disengaged from the learning process. They do not monitor the lesson or themselves to determine what they already know and what is new information. They cannot or do not determine their problems; they do not ask questions; they do not request assistance or clarification. They seldom appear to be frustrated or confused. In contrast, an active learner realizes that a difficulty exists and will demonstrate signs of confusion or ask for help.

Passive learning behaviors may form a coping strategy that permits the student to pass through the school day without drawing undue attention to his or her problems and thus eliminate what the child considers to be unnecessary stress. It is common for children with ALLD to show interactive and assertive learning behaviors in kindergarten, first, or second grade, but then to withdraw from the learning situation as they pass through later elementary years. Middle school and high school students with ALLD present minimal task oriented interaction with teachers or peers in the academic classroom. In addition, teachers ask less of them in the instructional setting. Students seem to learn by the time they enter the intermediate grades that if they are quiet, well-behaved, and accommodating, teachers will leave them alone. Unfortunately, this is predominantly the case.

Problem-Solving Strategies

Learning style is closely associated with the problem solving strategies that children use in daily living and in the educational setting. Problem-solving strategies allow a learner to approach a task and select the best method of successfully mastering it. Effective problem-solving strategies prevent learners from being overwhelmed by novel, complex, or elaborate information. Students with ALLD frequently have a restricted repertoire of problem solving strategies. They are also inflexible in applying the strategies they have developed and in selecting the most efficient strategy for a given situation. For example, they often work too quickly and fail to analyze, evaluate, and plan appropriately to complete a task. Their approach may be impulsive, using trial and error attempts rather than forethought and prediction to select the best strategy.

Problem-solving strategies can be taught by guiding children step by step through activities or tasks. Breaking a task into its component parts tells the student where to begin and what to look for. It also provides a direction to pursue in solving the problem or completing the task. Instruction to help develop effective problem-solving strategies should begin in the primary grades so that children can establish appropriate routes of learning early in their school career. Problem-solving strategies can be presented in both a utilitarian and game format so that children can recognize the value of such techniques as well as find the learning experience enjoyable. Teaching effective problem-solving strategies can also be integrated with practice in following directions.

Attention to Tasks

In addition to problems related to localization, selective attention, and sustained attention in listening situations, students with ALLD also have difficulty attending to tasks, such as seatwork assignments or independent study. They are often easily distracted by visual stimuli in the classroom, such as other children moving about as well as auditory occurrences that are normally present in the instructional setting. Auditory distractions can be reduced through the use of sound-attenuating earmuffs or earplugs. These assistive devices modify classroom noise and can help students concentrate on assignments. If earmuffs and ear plugs are an option for any student in the mainstream classroom, ALLD students may be less inhibited to use them. Sound barriers to reduce excess noise by placement of furniture or display boards can also be used to the benefit of the student with ALLD.

Finding the Best Place to Sit

Classroom logistics can have either a negative or positive effect on learning for the student with ALLD. Various seating arrangements are possible, but the objective should be to place the student with ALLD in a location that affords the best conditions for listening and visual monitoring. Children with ALLD should also be seated away from areas of noise, such as doors, heating or air conditioning vents, windows facing noisy outdoor areas, and pencil sharpeners. Seating selections may also depend on teaching style and classroom arrangement. Position placement, for example, in desk groupings, should permit adequate visual contact with the teacher as well as optimal auditory input. It should not be assumed that the best seating location is in the front row of the classroom. This placement may actually inhibit the student's auditory functioning. It may be necessary to try several different seating options before both student and teacher feel comfortable.

Coping and Survival Strategies

Coping strategies are behavioral responses to one's condition or state and the context at the time. All individuals devise ways of reducing stress and techniques for surviving day to day problems. Some coping strategies are positive, healthy, and successfully temper life's frustrations. Other strategies provide immediate reduction of negative effects but create long-term problems. There are also strategies that are negative and inefficient in both the immediate situation and the long term context. Students with ALLD develop and use coping strategies in the form of behaviors and attitudes to accommodate or reduce the negative effects of their language-learning deficit, especially in the school setting. Unfortunately, many coping devices utilized by children with ALLD are not beneficial to them.

Passive learning behaviors were discussed as one example of a coping strategy that students with ALLD, especially older students, use. This low profile stance toward school may alleviate the immediate stress of having to respond in class, but it also eliminates a student's opportunity to secure information, explanation, or clarification. Another coping strategy is redefining the purpose or value of school. Case study 16–2 presents a child who capitalizes on her appearance and personality in lieu of academic abilities to win the favor of teachers and peers.

Case study 16–2. TC is an 11-year-old girl who has demonstrated characteristics and performance of a child with ALLD since she entered kindergarten. Formal testing verified the presence of both language and learning problems and she has received special education services through the school system's learning disabilities program since first grade.

TC is an extremely attractive child with an arresting personality. She is very assertive socially and actively cultivates friendships with other children. She is well-behaved in school and is liked by her teachers and peers.

One of TC's coping strategies is to openly joke about her academic problems in school. For example, "Of course I can't do math, I am a blond you know!" She has developed an "I don't really care" attitude toward the scholastic component of education, yet has thrived on the social opportunities school provides for her. Although TC's fifth grade classroom may be an arena of success for bright, non-ALLD children, for TC it is a stage to show off cleverly assembled wardrobe options or a new hairdo. TC's coping strategies have done little to improve her academic performance, but they do provide her with an avenue of acceptance among her peers.

Another common coping strategy is to become aggressive, either verbally, physically, or both, to control a situation. Children who use this device may appear to be destructive, but their objective is purposefully to redirect attention away from a challenging or difficult task or activity.

REMEDIATION PERSPECTIVES

Remediation for children with ALLD is often a compromise between the optimal ideal considered necessary to develop a child's auditory learning potential and the reality of services that exist. Remediation must include a broad spectrum of intervention strategies and activities. Intervention options for remediation include more than 10 to 15 minutes of listening exercises that are presented two or three times per week. Children with ALLD must be placed in an environment that nurtures and facilitates auditory learning. A context conducive to auditory learning constantly and consistently provides both structured and informal opportunities for developing auditory capabilities that are necessary for communication and school success.

Interventions for children with ALLD should not only focus on discrete skill development, yet many remediation programs and strategies are based on practice and drill to perfect individual skills. Auditory capabilities are interactive and interdependent. Areas of difficulty presented by students with ALLD have an underlying theme and are all related. Intervention emphasis should be directed toward auditory function and integration because it is interference in this process that underlies the problem. Auditory capabilities are related to language and cognition. An auditory language/learning deficit is manifested in communication and cognitive performance as well as academic areas of reading, language arts, content areas, and mathematics. It is not logical to believe that one aspect can be separated from the others. Therefore the idea of remediation of discrete skills in specific areas is not plausible as a sole successful intervention strategy.

It is important to remember that there are persisting effects of ALLD as well as immediate problems experienced by affected children. Although many students benefit from early identification and remediation, many others are not so fortunate. Even with sensitivity toward the impact of ALLD and appropriate intervention, it is unlikely that the disorder will dissipate completely with time. In addition, there will be increases in listening expectations and demands as children progress through school. As students with ALLD reach high school or even progress into post-secondary education, auditory requirements continue to tax their capabilities. Although students with ALLD may have developed positive and helpful coping and problem-solving strategies that assisted them in elementary school, they face new demands of the high school curriculum, such as the study of a foreign language. The linguistic and auditory requirements of learning a second language may present an unattainable challenge for the high school student with ALLD. Students with ALLD will have extreme difficulty mastering a second language even with additional, special support and tutoring services available to high school students to assist with foreign language learning. The auditory requirements of learning a foreign language coupled with the metalinguistic ability to analyze language increase dramatically with second language learning. Case study 16-3 presents an example of a student who had progressed successfully in academic areas in spite of significant ALLD until he attempted to master a language other than English.

Although the focus of this chapter has been the primary through elementary school-age student with ALLD, the impact of this disability on social interaction may become as significant as the effect on spoken language, written language, and academic achievement when a student moves into middle or high school. Peer interaction and development of independence from the family is further marred by ALLD during the adolescent years. Perception and interpretation of social cues as well as subtleties in meaning communicated through vocal intonation play an important role in conversation among adolescents. Students with ALLD may find themselves socially removed from the peer groups from which they gain and establish their identity.

Auditory language learning deficits continue to present many unanswered questions. Increased knowledge in areas related to sensory, cognitive, and linguistic processing and the physiology of the neurological system will contribute to and expand our current understanding. In the meantime, remediation perspectives that emphasize auditory function as a basis for cognitive performance and spoken language are necessary. Auditory capabilities entail a complex continuum of analyses, decisions, and processes in conjunction with cognition and language that make auditory experiences useful.

Case Study 16-3. JQ is a 19-year-old high school student whose auditory learning difficulties had been identified when he entered first grade. The impact of ALLD during his primary and elementary school years was reflected in reading and writing problems and frustration in auditory tasks. He received learning disabilities resource services from second through ninth grades, but opted to complete high school without resource assistance. He passed all of his required academic subjects except Spanish which he had taken during his junior year. Repeated attempts to pass the class, even with generous amounts of tutoring, were unsuccessful.

In addition to the frequently cited ALLD characteristics attributed to him by his teachers, assessment data documented the impact of ALLD on JQ's retention of information learned over time and his immediate recall of unrelated information, such as names or individual words. He presented slightly better recall of related information, such as sentences. His aptitude for learning a second language was nearly non-existent. His coping strategies included his interest and involvement in weight lifting and athletics, his interactive personality, and his disciplined practice of reading all academic materials a minimum of three times to understand and gain information. He was successful socially and academically, except for Spanish. Both teachers and peers were positive toward him.

REFERENCES

1. Cawley JF, Miller JH: Cross sectional comparisons of the mathematical performance of children with learning disabilities: are we on the right track? *J Learn Disabil*, 23 (1989), 250–254, 259.
2. Linville WJ: The effects of syntax and vocabulary upon the difficulty of verbal arithmetic problems with fourth grade students. Unpublished doctoral dissertation (State University of Iowa, Ames 1970).
3. Wiig E, Semel E: *Language Assessment and Intervention for the Learning Disabled.* (Columbus, OH: Charles E. Merrill, 1984).
4. Rosenthal D, Resnick D: *Children's Solution Processes in Arithmetic Word Problems. J Educa Psychol,* 66 (1974), 817–825.
5. Hasenstab MS, Laughton J: *Reading, Writing and Exceptional Children.* (Rockville, MD: Aspen Publications, 1982).
6. Laughton J, Hasenstab MS: *The Language Learning Process.* (Rockville, MD: Aspen Publications, 1986).
7. Sariff LS: An innovative use of free field amplification in regular classrooms, in Roeser R, Downs M, eds, *Auditory Disorders in Children.* (New York: Theime-Stratton, 1981).

CLASSROOM INTERVENTION STRATEGIES AND RESOURCE MATERIALS FOR CHILDREN WITH HEARING IMPAIRMENT

Virginia S. Berry, M.S.

17

The eye is the mirror to the soul;
The ear is its gates.

—Helen Keller, 1880–1968

The child with hearing impairment in the mainstream is often manipulated by the well-meaning educator falling prey to the self-fulfilling prophecy.[1] Public Law 94-142 and all other education of the handicapped laws are often a double-edged sword. Certainly, one of the most positive outcomes has been an increased sensitivity to identifying children with handicaps and improved awareness of the importance of meeting their educational needs. The result has been the rapid development of services within the local education agency, the home school district.

In turn, an outgrowth of these positive trends has been the surfacing of increased labeling of children. Granted, a necessary evil, categorizing a child is a prerequisite to providing service. However, it is, in fact, this process that is the catalyst for the educator's submission to the self-fulfilling prophecy.[1]

Teachers react, although often indirectly, to labels assigned to children. When told a child is "gifted," expectations are set. This child is often given increased attention and special privileges. If you expect creativity, a child frequently responds accordingly. After reading a previous teacher's notes on the discipline difficulties associated with a child, there is often a tendency to misjudge those small misbehaviors frequently overlooked or excused in other children as outrageous disruptive acts.

Teachers who have had a child with hearing impairment in their class, particularly if the child comes with the label of deaf, may also create some inappropriate assumptions. Well-trained and experienced educators are outstanding professionals in many areas. However, with limited exposure to children with hearing impairments,

(or adults), they are likely to be holding on to many misconceptions.[1] Thus, the self-fulfilling prophecy begins.

The intent of this chapter is to provide the tools an educator needs to manage successfully the child with hearing impairment in the classroom. Also, it is hoped, this chapter will illustrate that the strategies needed for the child with hearing impairment are no more overwhelming than those basic strategies that make for a good educational setting in general.

Certainly, if an educator was modifying or redirecting all teaching to serve the child with hearing loss, then placement staff should ask the question, "Was mainstreaming premature?" Successful mainstreaming should include only a few overt classroom changes, with most techniques being subtle differences in style. One of the most important keys to the process will be a teacher with a positive attitude and confidence, who is not being transformed into an educator of the deaf. This chapter will discuss the skills necessary to eliminate forever the fear of deafness and, therefore, bury for good the self-fulfilling prophecy.

WHO ARE THE KIDS?

So often as professionals, we are plagued with the attitude that the only children who have special needs are those with the most obvious, most visible, and, therefore, the most severe problems. It is ironic to think that the child who is hearing impaired and who often has the least difficulty "making it" in the regular classroom is the child with the more severe hearing loss.

The reason for this is likely attributed to the direct relationship between severity of handicap and level of intensity of staff involvement. The child who is mainstreamed with a severe hearing impairment is often older than the child with a mild hearing impairment, received years of previous direct intervention, utilizes in class interpreters/ tutors, has use of special assistive devices, etc. In addition, teachers selected to serve this child are chosen after careful consideration of knowledge and experience.[2]

On the other hand, children with lesser degrees of hearing loss of varying natures are often not afforded such advantages. Are their special needs any less important? In fact, these children are often more difficult to serve in the regular classroom. Children with mild hearing losses, fluctuating losses, unilateral deficits, or high-frequency disorders are often overlooked when needs are outlined or programs are planned. For many years, these children were thought to be unaffected educationally by their hearing loss (Table 17–1).

Table 17–1. Teacher Tips for Identifying a Possible Child with Hearing Impairment

1. Inattention
2. Frequently requests to have a statement or word repeated
3. Frowning or straining forward when addressed
4. Easily fatigued
5. Failure to participate in class discussions
6. Inability to localize sound
7. Gives inappropriate answers to simple questions
8. May isolate himself or be isolated by his peer group
9. Is overly dependent on visual clues
10. Low tolerance for frustration
11. Often speaks too loudly
12. Has poor reading skills
13. Tends to do better in mathematics than reading
14. Poorly spoken or written language
15. Sounds distorted or omitted from words
16. Voice quality harsh, breathy, nasal, or monotone
17. Pitch, rhythm, stress, and inflection inappropriate
18. History of frequent earaches or ear discharge
19. Mouth breathing or other nasal symptoms
20. Complaints of ringing, buzzing, or other noises in the head

Certain techniques specific to all populations of student with hearing impairment are essential to incorporate in the classroom. As professionals, we must recognize the unique differences among children with hearing loss. In many states for a number of years, the guidelines that qualify and quantify special education funding have considered hearing impairment a low incidence handicap. Such a distinction often translates into less

monies applied to public education needs and services for students with hearing impairment. If considering only severe to profound, bilateral hearing losses, then perhaps such an equation is justified because only 1 child in 1000 births exhibits such deficits. However, if other types and degrees of hearing loss are factored into the formula, a drastic increase in numbers occurs. Six children in in every 1000 births reveal mild to moderate losses; 2 in 1000 exhibit minimal and unilateral losses. Examining those figures and including fluctuating, conductive, and numerous acquired losses, some studies have noted in excess of 3 million schoolchildren who reveal educationally significant hearing disorders.[3] These figures should certainly reinforce the critical need to reexamine how education of the hearing impaired is prioritized and funded.

WHERE ARE THE KIDS?

In addition to often overlooking certain populations of children who are hearing impaired, educators and other professionals often neglect the issue of what placement is chosen for the child. Currently, 79% of children with hearing impairment are served in some form of mainstreamed setting.[3] However, mainstreaming can be a fairly generic term, sometimes simply meaning the child attends lunch or recess with regular classes. The remainder of the day, it may be that his educational needs are best met in a non-categorial, self-contained special education classroom. In many districts there are not enough children with hearing impairment to justify a teacher of the deaf. Children with hearing loss are often served successfully by special education teachers holding certification in another area and in classrooms housing a variety of children with disabilities and with differing needs. The intent of this chapter is not to debate the validity or appropriateness of such placement.

The point to be made, rather, is that professionals serving the hearing impaired often assume that information on hearing loss and intervention goals does not need to be provided to any special educator.[4] Our goal should be to direct the strategies of the regular classroom teacher who has no experience with children with special needs. After all, special educators received all the training they needed in every exceptionality, including deafness. If professionals are operating under this philosophy, they are missing an area of great need. My experience has proven that, with the exception of certified teachers of the deaf, special education classroom teachers need suggested techniques and guidance in working with the hearing impaired, and are anxious and receptive to receiving such.

We cannot neglect the environment in which the child is placed. Regardless of whether the child with hearing impairment is in a regualr classroom full time, or a resource room for a portion of the day for isolated tutoring in selected areas, or in a self-contained room for the entire day, neither his special needs nor the intervention plan to meet these needs change. Equal time and energy should be placed on informing all varieties of educators of these needs.

GETTING READY

Teacher Motivation

The successful implementation of any educational program is only as strong as the professional responsible for it. All the training and experience in the world does not guarantee the will to succeed. Success hinges on the motivational level and attitude of those involved with the program.

Hearing professionals convince themselves that simply supplying school staff with pertinent case hisotry information on the child, a previous services summary and tips for teaching will provide into the classroom that will be trouble free.

We forget one all important variable—motivation. Regardless of what role particular school staff plays in the program of a child with hearing impairment, that person must have a receptive attitude toward serving the child. The responsibility of working with this child means extra work for everyone, including the child himself.[5]

The first important step in establishing the necessary receptive climate is to ensure the classroom teacher feels a part of the child's total program. Too often, hearing professionals enter a school situation bringing in their "better mouse trap." We fail to keep in mind that educators are too have some critical insight to add as to what makes for good teaching practices. We often forget to listen to their suggestions or their concerns.[5]

In addition, hearing professionals typically have one goal when approaching school staff— meeting the needs of the child with hearing impairment. Although commendable, we often overlook the needs of the educator.

In many situations, individuals are significally more receptive to hard work or change if they feel they were allowed input into the direction of the change. Therefore, temper our enthusiam for our "better mouse trap" and allow school staff to describe their needs and take an active part in the planning of any special training they are to receive. Specific teaching strategies are much more likely to be incorporated in the classroom if the manager of that room has assisted in their design.

Administrative Preparation

An individual who is often overlooked as a critical element in the success of a mainstreamed child who is hearing impaired is the school administrator. Familiarization of these persons to the design of the program will have lasting effects on the outcome.

Administrators can assist in the commitment to the child and supply confidence to the staff. They can foster the positive attitude of "We can make a difference for this child." They can arrange for the redistribution of duties for teachers serving children who have special needs. Administrators can support the funding of equipment and materials essential to school staff implementing teaching strategies necessary for success.[6]

Therefore, professionals working with schools must include administrators in all activities, particularly during the initial stages of program development. They have needs that should be addressed ,just as classroom staff do. Provide information relevant to their role; utilize strategies directed to meeting their needs; provide answers geared to eliminating their fears. The end result will be a cohesive program with a long-term emotional, professional and financial commitment.

Team Management

If a child with hearing impairment is expected truly to succeed in a mainstreamed educational environment, it is naive to consider this a "one-man show." It is certainly a team effort. Members of the team are all individuals concerned with this child's progress. Each member has specific responsibilities and goals and, therefore, requires specific intervention practices and strategies.[7]

The recognition of the importance of team management is a prerequisite to getting ready for any program. Identifying the team members and providing them useful and relevant management information is essential. One individual should be designated team manager. Too often, hearing professionals who are not school staff and are brought in only on a random consultant basis feel they are this designee. However, the role of the team manager is to provide consistency and continuity among members in the implementation of classroom strategies. Is it possible for an individual who visits a school only a few times to serve in this capacity?

Granted, although the hearing consultant is likely the individual with extensive knowledge and expertise in the area of the needs of the hearing impaired, this is not the individual who can guarantee daily application of good educational principles. The primary teacher, for example, might be the more appropriate choice for team manager. This individual can assist the school counselor, the speech-language pathologist, the music teacher, the school secretary, and others in carrying over successful management strategies from the classroom.

The underlying assumption here, however, is that this primary teacher has been given the necessary tools for effective management to pass on. Here enters the hearing professional. Although these consultants cannot guarantee continuity of daily programming, they can take responsibility for intensive training and education of school staff, particularly the team manager.

If adequate staff preparation occurs, the team manager and, subsequently, each team member can take charge of consistent implementation.

Team professionals often ignore the parents. So often, we consider parents a nuisance, a threat, an intimidation. Certainly, there are parents who make it difficult to enjoy working with the child because of their pushy "You work for me" attitude. However, if this aggression was traced back through the child's special service career, we may find it stems from parent needs that were ignored, questions that were unanswered, or concerns that were pushed aside and not addressed.

Most parents want to have an active role in their child's programming, but not to the point of domination, as many professionals often think. Parent's can be important assistants in the process of identifying strategies that work. Who better to explain some techniques in successful communication practices than the individual who uses them 24 hours a day?

Professionals need to listen carefully and attentively to parents. Information they supply will give insight into the child that educators often miss. Communicate to parents that their input is important and that their suggestions will be incorporated into the child's program.

Finally, one essential member of the team is the child. For those children who are old enough to provide meaningful input, use it. The child is the only true expert on what facilitates learning. Allow him or her to set the example for strategies that are useful. If the child is of an age that cannot describe these strategies specifically, then observation and manipulation of various procedures will provide the answer.

In-Service-Training

No matter what specific information is included in in-service training sessions or what style or form these sessions take, the intent should be on developing a knowledgeable and accepting attitude toward hearing loss and students with hearing loss. The outcome of such training should be the establishment of a realistic educational environment in which children with hearing impairment can function and progress.[4]

As hearing professionals who may likely be responsible for conducting in-service training, we must not be dogmatic. Remembering the principles of teacher motivation and team management, it is critical that participants do just that—participate.[8] They must feel that the information presented gives them options for intervention.[4] Preparing staff for working with children with hearing impairment should not take away from their flexibility or creativity.

When establishing an in-service training program for a school, it is helpful if the information presented can be specific to the child with hearing loss *in the school*. It is the responsibility of the professional conducting the in-service to know the child in question. Rather than general information on hearing loss, hearing aids, or teaching practices, present the topics chosen for discussion as they relate to the specific child with hearing impairment Discuss the child's loss and its educational implications. Discuss classroom activities as you understand them. It is helpful to have observed this child in some sort of teaching environment so that specific examples can be given. Know the specific curriculum and textbooks used in the child's class so you can explain modifications necessary to them in terms of vocabulary, content, etc.[9] Many sources are available that can provide specific information to be gathered during the observation. There are several observation protocols that are commercially available or each professional can create their own. Data should be collected that describes the participation of the child in classroom activities, such as interactions among child, teacher, and classmates; communication style, level, and modality; physical environment; teaching style; and curriculum structure. If possible, it is certainly meaningful to have the child present during a portion of the in-service so that demonstrations of certain teaching strategies can be given.

There is a wealth of information that hearing professionals feel obliged to convey to school staff during in-service preparation. We must keep in mind that a goal of such training is to instill the attitude that students with hearing impairments are a challenge not a burden and they can be an asset to the school. Often we are overambitious and attempt too much during the preparation stage of programming. Certainly, our ambition is well meaning in that we recognize several areas of need that warrant discussion. Staff preparation should include information on language, communication, reading, behavior management, peer orientation, speech, hearing aids, and classroom techniques[4] (Table 17-2).

Table 17-2 In-Service Training Topics: Teacher, Other School Staff, and Classmates

Definition of hearing loss and nature of the problem
Specific assessment information as it relates to each child who is hearing impaired (audiological data, previous academic history, speech/language abilities, etc.)
Orientation to hearing aids and FM systems, including operation, placement, and maintenance
Auditory training
Speech and language activities
Behavior management
Individual educational planning and implementation
Teaching strategies
Materials and resources
Use of an interpreter, tutor, notetaker, or other supportive staff
Acceptance in the classroom
Communication needs
Sign language classes

The timing and scheduling of in-service training can be the variables that dictate the success of the program in general. School staff are already burdened with many extracurricular assignments, so we must guard against lengthy, after-school meetings. Also, brief, frequent meetings are often better received than 2- to 3-hour workshops. Each session could focus on one particular issue.

Although some initial in-service preparation is certainly necessary prior to a teacher assuming responsibility for a child with hearing impairment, educators will have a much better understanding of this child's needs following time in direct classroom contact. Therefore, it is critical that in-service training be an ongoing, continuous process. Staff preparation sessions preceding direct child contact do just that—prepare staff. They do not and certainly cannot acquaint staff with all situations that may arise. Individuals responsible for staff education should be willing to schedule several meetings throughout the school year.[9]

In addition, professionals should keep in mind that in-service training cannot meet its goals if it does not keep the interest of its audience. Therefore,a straight lecture format is typically not effective. Demonstrations, visual aids, and open discussion forums are generally excellent techniques to maintain interest level. Also, although there are, as previously mentioned, many areas that need discussion, some areas are more relevant to certain school staff than others. It is helpful, therefore, to conduct in-service training on specific topics with specific types of staff. Specialized sessions can be scheduled for speech-language pathologists, school nurses, and others.

INTERVENTION STRATEGIES

General Considerations

Previous educational structures met the needs of children with exceptional needs by removing them from the mainstream of regular classrooms, serving them in self-contained classes or separate schools. With the shift in emphasis toward the least restrictive environment of the regualr classroom, all teachers are now expected to meet the needs of the exceptional child, with little preparation.[7] During a school day, children are expected to listen and respond, integrate information, and generalize. They must interact with spoken language, written language, peers, and adults. They must apply thinking skills to learning and problem solving.

When a regular educator is asked to enroll a child with a hearing impairment in a school program, it is likely their first contact with such a youngster. For this reason, it is critical that some basic elements of the mainstreamed program be analyzed before specific educational strategies can be addressed. These elements are child, family, class, and teacher centered.

Child

1. The student should be able to participate at or near grade level of the regular class in both academic and communicative areas (regardless of communication type).
2. The child's social and emotional maturity should be at least equal to that of his or her classmates.
3. The student should be able to function somewhat independently and exhibit self-confidence.
4. The child's ability to learn, as measured from standardized testing, should be at least average.
5. The child should be comfortable with his or her peers who are hearing and should be willing to communicate openly regarding his or her hearing loss and not be embarrassed by the handicaps. It is often helpful for the child with hearing loss to teach the class about the hearing aid or about sign language.
6. The student's chronological age should be within 2 years of his or her classmates.
7. The child should have a realistic view of mainstreaming and be prepared to receive extra help and program modifications.[2]

Family

1. The family of the student with a hearing loss should show interest in his or her mainstreamed enrollment, such as helping with assignments or participating in regular school activities.
2. The family should consistently attend conferences so as to provide needed input into educational planning.
3. The family should be aware of the difficulties to be expected in regular class placement and, therefore, should not be critical of school staff or place unrealistic demands on the teacher.
4. The family should be prepared for both success and failure and not become discouraged prematurely.[2]

Class

1. The other students in the class should be prepared and ready to accept the child with hearing impairment as a member of the class and treat him or her with consideration.
2. The enrollment of the class should be somewhat smaller than traditional classes, particularly during initial mainstreaming.
3. It is critical that the class be informed through an in-service process, just as teachers are, about the nature of a hearing loss, communication techniques, etc. Classmates and their awareness of the needs of a child with hearing impairment are as closely linked to the success of mainstreaming as are the specific teaching styles of the teacher.
4. Classmates should incorporate many of the same techniques necessary for improved comprehension for the child with hearing impairment as school staff must use.[3]

Teacher

1. Teachers must disregard any misconceptions they possibly held previously regarding the intelligence, communication, or behavior of a child with hearing impairment.
2. Teachers should expect basically the same kind of behavior, responsibility and dependability from the student with a hearing loss as they expect from the rest of the class. A child with a hearing loss is first of all *a child*. What is good for any child is good for the child with heari ng impairment. Teachers should treat him or her as they do a child with normal hearing.[5]
3. Teachers should create a climate in which experiences of success are frequent, thus assisting the adjustment to the regular class and developing a positive attitude for the child.
4. Teachers should not overemphasize the hearing loss but be considerate of the child's special needs.
5. Teachers should not sympathize but give assistance.
6. Teachers should give those privileges that are only absolutely necessary. The child with a hearing loss should not be allowed to take advantage of his or her handicap. The child should not be pampered or overprotected.
7. Teachers should ensure that the child with a hearing impairment shares in all class experiences and extracurricular activities.
8. Teachers should try to accept the child with a hearing impairment positively no matter how impaired his comprehension, speech, or vocabulary. Teachers are the role models for the class and set the example. Their reactions or attitudes will generate similar ones from the other children.[5]
9. Teachers must remember that no two children with normal hearing are alike so they should not expect every child with a

hearing loss to be the same. Even those children with identical hearing losses will function very differently. Teaching practices that are successful vary among children.

10. Teachers should make a consistent effort to communicate frequently with all individuals involved in the program of a child with hearing impairment (special educator, speech-language pathologist, etc.).[6]

Classroom Arrangement and Environment

Any educator would agree that the noise level in every classroom should be kept as low as practical. There is certainly no elementary school class whose noise level is 0 dB. As normal hearers, we often take for granted sources of classroom noises, such as papers rustling, pages turning, hallway traffic, pencil sharpeners, playground activity, student chatter, and classroom animals. With normal hearers, adequate comprehension of orally presented information is found to occur in the presence of a +20 dB sound pressure level (SPL) signal-to-noise ratio.[3] Considering an average vocal volume of 60 dB SPL, combined with often present classroom noise of 73 dB SPL, the chances of such a listening condition occuring are obvious.[10] For the child with hearing impairment, even with the utilization of personal amplification, the effects of these conditions are even more devastating. It is important to remember the limitations of personal hearing aids. All sounds are amplified, thus prohibiting the child with hearing impairment from sorting out the important from the unimportant. Teachers should be aware that hearing aids do not correct a hearing loss but only assist in improving awareness or discrimination. The presence of excessive noise often counteracts the benefits of these improvements. As discussed in Chapter 12, the use of frequency modulation (FM) systems can eliminate many of the adverse effects of classroom noise.

In addition, the teacher should be aware of classroom acoustics. Although there is usually little a teacher can do to alter the construction of the room, she can control some of the adverse effects. Hard surfaces, such as glass, wood floors, and blackboards reflect sound and can add to extraneous noise. Reverberation results as speech is repeatedly reflected back and forth from each surface with a time differential. This will cause the child with a hearing impairment to pick up echoes of several different words at the same time.

There are some materials in the room that can absorb sounds and, therefore, assist in decreasing noise. Soft porous materials such as fabrics, paper, carpet, window shades, and cork can be used strategically throughout the room. The rear wall of the classroom is often the starting point for reverberation. Posters or cork bulletin boards arranged in this area as well as on the blackboard and shades or curtains on windows are certainly helpful. Carpet squares can be placed under each desk to help with sound absorption. The human body also provides effective dampening of sound. If the teacher can stagger the student's desks instead of arranging them in straight rows, less sound will travel to hard surfaces. The physical size of the classroom and the number of students will also be contributing variables to room acoustics.

Teachers should take care not to schedule a verbal presentation or lecture during periods of high activity or noise, either in other parts of the classroom or directly outside.

Lighting is a variable that can significantly affect the comprehension of a child with a hearing impairment. There is an obvious correlation between lighting and speechreading ability, which will be discussed in more detail in another section. The best situation is the use of overhead lights and natural lighting. They should supply sufficient light but not be so bright as to cause shadows or a glare. If lights come primarily from one wall, the teacher should arrange it so that this is the back wall of the class. It is best if the light comes from behind the child and falls on the teacher's face. This illuminates the teacher's face and the child is not blinded by the glare. The teacher should be careful not to stand near a window in bright sunlight, as it often casts a shadow on the face. The teacher should also be aware of the effects of time of day changes on lighting and make appropriate adjustments.[11]

The importance of preferential seating cannot be underestimated. The seating placement of a child with a hearing impairment certainly depends in part on the type of hearing loss, but it also is important to look at classroom format and activity.

If a bilateral loss is present, placement should be in a central location approximately 3 to 5 feet from the teacher. This allows for optimum use of the hearing aids. The teacher needs to take care not to be too close so that voice is not directed above the child with a hearing loss. Therefore, second row seating, near the center is typically most effective. This also can help eliminate back and neck strain from looking up at the teacher. If a significant asymmetry exists between the ears or a unilateral loss is present, a similar placement in the second row is recommended but with the child seated off-center so that the better ear is angled toward the teacher.

Special seating should not necessarily isolate, separate, or further identify the student with a hearing loss as "special." The front row is not only a disadvaantage for optimum hearing aid use, but also, at times, puts the child on the periphery of the class and causes him or her to "stand out."

Preferential seating by itself is not the complete answer to the problems of a child with a hearing loss. The teacher does not do all the talking or teaching in a classroom. Much information comes from class participation. Incidental or third-party learning is critical to every child's progress. A child should be allowed some flexibility in seating or orientation. This might mean different seats for different class activities. Or, if such movement is too attention-getting, the student should be placed where turning the body will assist in monitoring other student's questions or discussions, thus improving overall comprehension. The teacher may need to cue those students with hearing impairment who are unaware of other classmates' participation. Whenever possible, a circular class arrangement could be utilized which allows for better peer monitoring.[12] See Case study 17–1 for an example of improvements that can be made in the classroom setting.

Communication

Speechreading is a skill on which all children with hearing impairment exhibit heavy reliance. The success of speechreading is based on the principle of redundancy (the ability to predict the total message after receiving only a part of that message). Speechreading is not absolute. There are many more speech movements per second than the eye is capable of perceiving. In addition, many speech movements are not visible, whereas at the same time many sounds and words look identical. Such homophenous elements can confuse a child and certainly affect the accuracy of comprhension. Imagine a child's fustration if he thought the teacher said to "sit by Pat," when the actual instruction was to "sit on your mat."

The following are some guidelines to assist in optimum speechreading abilities and to guarantee improved comprehension:

1. It is critical to make certain that the child with a hearing impairment is attending, not just listening. However, it is unrealistic to expect continuous attention of a child with hearing impairment. Afterall, we do not expect such a level of attention from childen with normal hearing. Some inattention should be tolerated if we are not to wear the child out. Speechreading can be exhausting. Therefore, presenting as many important lessons as possible in the morning hours can help avoid fatigue.[11]

2. Teachers should speak clearly with moderate speed. Voice should be pleasant and unstrained. Lip movements should be natural and not exaggerated. Raising the voice or overarticulating will make understanding more difficult for the child.

3. Teachers should try to speak to the class from a position in the room that allows adequate light to fall on the face. It is nearly impossible to speechread in a glare; therefore, abundant light should be avoided. Also, teachers should not stand with their back to the window for this places their face in a shadow.

4. Teachers should avoid excess movements during critical speechreading times. They should try to stand as still as practical for their teaching style.

5. Teachers should try to face the class as much as possible. Writing on the blackboard and talking at the same time should be avoided. In addition, teachers should keep books and papers down from their faces when speaking.

6. Teachers should expect adequate speechreading behaviors from other students as well. They should be instructed to speak normally. The child with hearing impairment should be encouraged to turn and face other children while they are speaking.

7. Teachers should be aware that many words look alike on the lips. They should, therefore, always put single words into a sentence so that the child with a hearing impairment can take advantage of the principle of redundancy. The more contextual clues a child obtains, the better their comprehension. Also, teachers should be patient and understanding with any confusions that occur in comprehension.

Case study 17–1.   Adam, age 11, exhibits a moderately severe sensorineural hearing loss in his right ear and a profound, fragmentary loss in his left. Adam utilizes an ear-level hearing aid on his right ear and no amplification on his left due to its minimal hearing. Adam receives excellent benefit from his monaural aid, responding within normal limits.

Adam entered the fifth grade this school year. He has consistently been placed in regular classrooms throughout his school experience, receiving resource room instruction and speech/ language services. Adam functions near grade level in all academic areas and has good communication skills.

Adam's fifth grade teacher has complained that he often has difficulty following directions and understanding orally presented class material. She finds him a bright student who is capable of all work, with minimal resource assistance. However, she is concerned about Adam's auditory comprehension skills and questioned his ability to maintain adequate progress because of this deficit.

Examination of the class by the area's consultant for the hearing impaired found a large room with wooden floors. One wall was all windows with no shades. Two walls were long blackboards. The back wall of the class was plaster. In addition, the class often divided into groups to complete different activities or projects. Significant background noise is often present caused by the hum of the heating or cooling unit in the rear of the class, pupils' conversations during small group work, and street noise from the unshaded windows.

Several recommendations were made to improve the class signal-to-noise ratio. Window shades were added. Also, corkboard was placed on the rear plaster wall, which was also used as a class bulletin board. Inexpensive room dividers were used to section off small group work. Also, such a divider was placed around the heating or cooling unit. Portions of each long blackboard were used to display class projects, assisting with decreasing the amount of hard surface. Student desks were staggered so as to create a body-baffle effect for noise and reverberation.

Further examination also revealed inappropriate seating for Adam. He was seated in the front desk on the far right-hand side of the class. Such a seat places Adam's unaided, poorer left ear nearer the teacher. It was recommended that he be moved to the second row, off-center to the left. Such placement would provide Adam improved auditory clues, placing his better, aided right ear toward the teacher. Also, such seating would provide Adam better visual access to both blackboards. The teacher was also encouraged to allow Adam flexible seating so as to be better able to follow orally presented materials from all points in the room.

To monitor Adam's comprehension, his teacher had been asking questions such as "Did you understand what to do?" Adam's response was typically a head nod for yes. It was recommended that the teacher begin asking open-ended questions such as "Which pages in your science book are you to read?"

These simple recommendations were well implemented. A 9-week review conference was held to examine Adam's progress. His teacher was surprised at the changes in Adam's abilities. She particularly commented on the effectiveness of flexible seating and the use of open-ended questions. In addition, some of her other children with normal hearing had mentioned how much easier it was to concentrate with the decreased noise.

8. Teachers should be aware that it is difficult for the student with a hearing impairment to speechread a new person who might come into the classroom. Also, although lipstick often assists speechreading abilities, fancy hairstyles, some clothes, moustaches, and beards will detract from speechreading.

9. It can be helpful to have one location in the classroom that is routinely used for oral presentations by both the teacher and other classmates.

Although part of the communication success that takes place in a classroom is dependent on visual clues, many students with hearing impairment can also rely on audition. Therefore, the teacher must use strategies that ensure adequate comprehension through listening. Auditory and visual clues should be used together to ensure that the child is obtaining as much information as possible. As with speechreading, however, for many students with hearing impairments, auditory clues will not be absolute. As normal hearers, we often forget the subtle language/ meaning changes that occur simply with inflectional or intonational differences. Emphasizing one word over another in a sentence can change its meaning. A statement can be turned into a question simply by altering our inflection. Also, the phonemes of /s/ and /z/ are responsible for a significant amount of linguistic information. Plurals, possessives, or some verb tenses, are conveyed by these speech sounds. These high frequency sibilants are difficult to discriminate through audition alone. Even with the ambiguity of much of the auditory information received, a child with a hearing loss should be encouraged to use their listening skills to the fullest extent possible. From responding correctly to roll call to following a story read aloud, any traditional auditory activity successfully completed will allow the child with a hearing impairment to feel like a part of the class.

As mentioned previously, it is important that the teacher makes sure the child is attending. Asking an open-ended question requiring a specific response can often determine if he is alert to the content. Teachers cannot assume that the child with a hearing impairment understands information presented one time. These children are "famous" for the neutral response technique. Teachers should learn to never trust a nod.[5] However, it must be emphasized that simply repeating what was said a second time does not guarantee comprehension. Rephrasing information is helpful, using different vocabulary, less complex sentence structure, and shorter sentences. Such practices are even more improtant when dealing with new or complex information or when listening conditions are poor. Here again, asking a question can check the child's ability to use or apply what was presented. Children with hearing impairments hear in a distorted manner and encounter unfamiliar vocabulary and language structures daily.[13] Teachers will find it necessary to go over any verbal instructions or directions given to the child.

In addition, classmates' presentations will require similar strategies. It is difficult for the child to follow discussion when speech is coming from several different directions. Teachers will often need to repeat or rephrase the main points stated by other students during such discussion. The consistent use of repetition with rephrasing provides the child with a hearing impairment increased input and the advantage of redundancy, thereby aiding comprehension.[9]

Often, hearing professionals place so much emphasis on the communication skills of teachers that they forget there are strategies the child should practice as well. Teachers must remember that children with hearing impairments have special vocabulary limits. Many words that children with normal hearing use may not be common to the student with a hearing impairment. Teachers should encourage activities that strengthen vocabulary and enrich communication. Dictionary assignments are helpful. In addition, professionals should develop in the child an interest in reading. Teachers should reinforce and reward attempts to learn or use new vocabulary, and, professionals must remember that the use of slang is important to communication.[5] Children with hearing impairments should have the benefit of this exposure as well.

Teachers need to make the child with a hearing loss speech conscious.[9] Goals should be developed that address his communication skills, posture, attitude, and fluency. Classromm staff can work closely with speech-language pathologists so they can be aware of specific speech goals and targets. Encourage the child to "practice" his or her speech goals in class and modify speech as appropriate. Naturally, this is not to mean the use of constant interruption or speech nagging. Sometimes rather than correcting poor speech the teacher should simply model appropriate production.

Teachers should compliment correct speech, as well. Reinforcement and reward are important keys to carry over. Often, the child with hearing impairment cannot hear improvements but must depend on the listener to judge his accuracy. Educators should not protect children with hearing impairments from speaking assignments. They should be provided the same opportunities as other children.[7] Depending on the degree of the hearing loss, the speech of the child with a hearing impairment may be difficult to understand at times. As the teacher becomes more familiar with the child's pattern of speech production, intelligibility will improve. Teachers should not be overly hesitant to ask the child to repeat what he said if he or she is unsure. When requesting information or a response, it is helpful to give the child time to "attack" and organize the communication attempts. Also, providing the child with a limited number of choices to use in selecting responses will assist the teacher in interpreting the answer.

Many children with hearing impairments may exhibit inappropriate volume by either talking too loudly or too softly. Teachers should assist children to work out their own "measuring stick" for monitoring the loudness of their voice.[11] Teachers can help the child recognize the loudness level that he should maintain. Also, at times, children with hearing impairments vocalize to themselves or make unnecessary noises. This can be disturbing to the class so the child should be taught to identify these times through cuing or other means.

It is important that educators instill in children with hearing impairments feelings of speech competency. Also, they must learn not to be ashamed or embarrassed if they do not understand. Children should express their confusion immediately. Teachers should watch for signs of poor understanding and not be impatient if the child with a hearing impairment asks for clarification.[8] The art of asking questions is a critical skill for all children to master.

Teaching Methodology— Hints and Recommendations

No amount of in-service training or chapters in books can prepare classroom teachers for all situations they will encounter with children with hearing impairments or develop in them all skills necessary for successful management of these children. Each classroom is different, as is each teacher and each child. However, there are many areas of common ground and, therefore, many universal methods that should be incorporated in classrooms housing children with hearing impairments.

Teachers must be realistic. No teacher is expected to be all things to all students, particularly those with handicaps. Often texts overemphasize how professionals should not frustrate children with hearing impairments, but they forget to stress the frustration of the teacher and its negative effects. Educators cannot reinvent the wheel with every lesson. Rather, they should be expected to simply be aware of this population's special needs, be eager to meet them, and do their best. A failure to grasp the concept of multiplication in a student with hearing impairment is not necessarily a reflection of poor teaching or an absence of teacher enthusiasm (Table 17–3).

Teachers of students with hearing impairments must be aware that the active listening and concentration required of these children will cause them to fatigue more easily than others. Greater effort is necessary of these students, and as a result, they will tire.[2] At the end of a school day, they may appear not to be paying attention or to be daydreaming. In actuality, they may be exhausted. It is helpful to alternate class activities that require close attention or precise comprehension. Listening breaks are useful. Give the class

Table 17–3. Ways to Impact Positively on Learning of Students Who Are Hearing Impaired

1. Be careful about the assumptions made about the child
2. Be word and vocabulary conscious. The child encounters new words daily with which other children may already have familiarity
3. Be conscious of students' questioning abilities
4. Be aware of opportunities to develop word attack abilities, including both phonetic and contextual analysis
5. Keep up with all available resources and materials useful to the hearing impaired
6. Be aware of the importance of figurative language, syntax, memory, sequencing, inferencing, and comprehension, not only to reading but to all learning areas
7. Be alert to students' attitude and motivational level
8. Develop test-taking abilities of students
9. Recognize importance of expanding students' general world knowledge
10. Expose students to a variety of printed materials
11. Read to children daily and provide time daily for children to read silently

seat work to complete.[4] This is not to mean, however, that teachers should not expect the student with a hearing loss to pay as close attention as others.

Teachers should organize their schedule so that children with hearing impairments can anticipate subjects and thereby predict vocabulary, etc. It is helpful to provide the student with a hearing impairment with a preview of topics or subjects to come. They could be given assignments to read ahead so that they are familiar with new concepts and vocabulary. Vocabulary lists could be sent home. Early exposure to subjects to come can prepare the child for the visual properties of the new vocabulary and acquaint them with contextual clues.

Teachers should reduce as much to writing as practical to their classroom style. New vocabulary words should be written on the board, as well as said. Blackboard outlines of topics being discussed assist in orienting students to the subject matter and allow them to keep up with the sequence. Homework assignments should also be written on the board as they are given. It is helpful if the same portion of the blackboard is consistently used to note assignments.

Teachers should use natural gestures just as they would during informal conversation. Gestures and cuing assist children with hearing impairments with comprehension. When talking about a specific child or object, point to, walk over to, or touch the child or it.[7]

Visual aids are very helpful to comprehension. Diagrams, graphs, pictures, maps, etc, are excellent supplements to lecture materials. They assist in reinforcing verbally presented material and increase visual input. Such aids give context and clarify the message. Overhead projectors are particularly helpful. Information may be written on a transparency as the lecture progresses, cuing students with hearing impairments to new vocabulary, subject changes, etc. Visual aids increase the number of sensory associations.

The use of slides, movies, and tapes is often not as helpful, however. Their sound tracts are frequently poor and the pictures are too small and far away for adequate speechreading. If these are used, it is often beneficial to provide the student with hearing impairment with a script or summary before the film or slides are shown, it they are not captioned.[5]

Instituting a buddy system for the child with a hearing impairment can be of great benefit to both the teacher and the child. One or two students in the class can be named as the assistant to the child with a hearing loss. Such "buddies," if chosen appropriately, can take some of the demands off the teacher. Buddies can alert the child with a hearing impairment to critical listening times. The buddy can repeat directions or instructions to ensure comprehension. In addition, note takers can be assigned to help the student with a hearing impairment. Not that the child with a hearing loss should be excused form note taking, but teachers must remember that it is difficult to write and speechread at the same time. Notes supplied by another student can supplement any information missed. Carbonless paper copies are excellent tools for note takers. When choosing a buddy for the child with a hearing impairment, it should be a classmate who is reliable, willing, and an above average student.[8]

With the implementation of cooperative learning centers in many classrooms, the child with a hearing loss will face some new, yet needed, challenges in education. The purpose of cooperative learning is to provide students the opportunity to work together in small groups and to target a specific task, such as reviewing for a test, solving mathematical problems, or writing a book report. The advantages to this practice are obvious. Students learn how to share ideas, encourage participation from others, become responsible for their own learning, and increase their attention to tasks.[4] For the child with a hearing impairment, these are also important byproducts of cooperative learning. In addition, however, the child will develop improved social skills and acquire necessary exposure to pragmatic skills, such as turn-taking and interactive communication. It will also provide increased opportunity to utilize targeted auditory, speechreading, and speech production skills. It is critical that teachers not eliminate children with hearing impairments from cooperative learning experiences.[8]

Teachers should recognize that subjects that involve manipulative activity or experimentation such as home economics, mathematics, or science are more readily understood than those subjects with high language content, such as reading or creative writing.[4] Experimental activities assist in comprehension, as well. After discussing farm animals, a trip to a farm should be scheduled. Pictures can be taken by the students to bring back to class. This helps with carryover and provides consistent exposure to new concepts. Also the use of role-playing or dramatic play assists concept development. All children learn best by doing (Table 17–4).

Table 17–4.   School and Learning Can Be Fun

IF YOU. . .
1. Provide for individual differences
2. Avoid overarousal
3. Work to strong areas
4. Allow time for response
AND. . .
5. Work sequentially
6. Watch vocabulary
7. Increase redundancy

Teachers should avoid yes or no questions. This type of response provides no guarantee that the child with hearing impairment grasped the material. Teachers can have the child repeat what was said or summarize in his own words. This reveals if the student with hearing impairment did understand the message.

Teachers should avoid introducing new topics without preparing or cuing the child with a hearing impairment. Verbal and visual connectives and transitions should be used between subjects. Situational clues can be provided, which can clue children to what is to come.[5] In lower grades where vocabulary enrichment is a daily event, teachers can label items in the room so that the child is exposed to the vocabulary in printed form.

Obviously associated with impaired hearing is a poor auditory memory. Teachers should break verbal directions down into a step by step explanation so that the child is not required to process multiple components. For complex written directions, it might be helpful for either the teacher or the student to highlight each stage or component with a different color marker. Again, although it is critical for children with hearing impairments to be held accountable for similar levels of responsibility as other students, at times it may be necessary to provide them additional time to complete some assignments. Based on the complexity of the language used or reading requirement, some extra time will allow the child to sort through the information presented, process the task, and, therefore, provide a more accurate picture of his true abilities on that activity. Also, there may be times due to difficulties in timely task completion that some assignments need to be decreased in length to safeguard self-esteem. Perhaps the child with hearing loss could complete 15 of the 25 mathematical problems. It is also helpful to increase the spacing between questions or problems on a page, decrease the number on a page, enlarge the print, and put all information on one page to avoid page turning as the child with a hearing impairment is often distracted by too much material.[4] Also, teachers must remember that word order is not always the same as meaning order. The direction "Before you do your spelling assignment, complete your math worksheet," can be confusing to a child with a hearing impairment. Again, when possible, teachers should be concrete and specific in their language, rephrase the information if confusion appears or check the child's comprehension by asking him to repeat what was said.

Oral tests place the child with a hearing impairment at an obvious disadvantage. Although written tests are recommended, they cannot always be used. When oral testing is used, an overhead projector could be utilized to reveal one question at a time after it is presented orally. This does preserve some of the elements of oral testing. Teachers should be confident that they are testing the knowledge of the student who is hearing impaired rather than his listening skills or language.[12] Also, children with hearing loss often perform better on closed-set tests where choices are provided rather than in an open-set format.

Teachers can provide the resource room teacher or the speech-language pathologist with special vocabulary or topics that will be covered in class. These individuals can reinforce classroom instruction or work ahead on certain subjects, providing these students the edge they often require.

In addition, it is helpful if the resource room teacher or speech-language pathologist can go into the child's class during key times to assist with instruction. This will also provide them an awareness of the child's group learning style.

Teachers need to encourage students with hearing impairments to participate in extracurricular activities. Such involvement fosters acceptance and truly makes them a part of school. Activities such as scouts, school sports, and school clubs, are critical to a successful school experience. Music is an area often thought inappropriate for children with hearing impairments. After all, how could someone with impaired or distorted hearing succeed in such an auditory area. Most children with a hearing impairment enjoy music-related activies and gain significantly from them. Music improves listening skills and rhythm. Children should not be deprived of this school experience.[7]

Teachers of younger children often speak negatively of comic books. These books can be excellent learning tools, paricularly for the child with a hearing impairment.[5] They use short, simple sentences, always paired with pictures. This assists the child in language development and reading acquisition. Comic books can assist the child in understanding idioms, one of the most difficult language structures they will encounter. During the language learning process, children with hearing loss are very literal and concrete. The teacher must keep in mind that idiomatic expressions such as "Don't knock yourself out over the assignment" will be confusing; or "You're pulling my leg" will mean just that to children with hearing impairments. Comic books can help eliminate the confusion prompted by idioms through their use of pictures.

Teachers should be aware that school announcements over a public address system are difficult listening situations for the hearing impaired. Nor only are they typically distorted and of poor quality, they provide no visual clues. Teachers should either repeat such announcements or have the buddy explain them to the child with a hearing impairment.

Teachers need to be aware of the safety hazzards in the classroom that may not be as obvious to the child who is hearing impaired. Precautions need to be taken against such hazards. School crossings and bus loading zones are hazzard areas for all children. Teachers need to be aware of areas of hazard where hearing acts as signal or warning (fire alarm, cooking timer, traffic, etc).[8]

Teachers need to recognize that the hearing of all children can fluctuate during the presence of colds or allergies and that children with documented hearing losses are not immune to the temporary acquisition of additional loss because of these illnesses.[3] Inattentiveness or decreased performance may not be due to conscious behavior on the part of the child, but rather temporary conductive involvement. Teachers should be alert to such problems and refer the child for needed evaluation.

To assist in making the child feel a part of the class and if he is not bothered by the attention it may draw, teachers can incorporate the child with a hearing imapriment into an instructional activity. A unit on hearing loss or hearing aids can be taught during science. A speechreading lesson can be taught to the entire class. The child with a hearing impairment could instruct the class about his hearing aid and its use (see Case study 17–2).

Teachers need to communicate frequently with parents. They are, after all, the "at home" teacher. Teachers need to be willing to discuss both the strengths and weaknesses of the child with a hearing impairment. They should be

---

Case study 17–2. Emily, age 15, exhibits a bilaterally symmetrical, severe sensorineural hearing loss. She utilizes binaural ear-level hearing aids that provide her adequate benefit, improving her acuity to within the borderline mild to moderate hearing loss range. For the last 3 years, Emily has become somewhat more self-conscious about her loss and hearing aids. Emily often leaves her aids at home or fails to have spare batteries.

Emily is currently enrolled in the 10th grade. Until this school year, she received the majority of her academic instruction in a resource room. Emily was mainstreamed into regular classes for mathematics, physical education, and extracurricular activities only.

School staff involved with Emily had observed her motivation to be very high to return to regular classes for additional periods. Assessments had shown her abilities to be in the average range. Although Emily was not on grade level for high language content courses, such as civics, history, and English, staff agreed to attempt increased mainstreaming, with resource/tutoring services cut to 1 hour a day.

Initial observation of Emily in many of her classes revealed a high level of motivation to succeed. Teachers believed that she was capable of keeping up with the work as long as the resource teacher could review content with her on a one to one basis. Teachers were concerned, however, about Emily's reluctance to discuss her handicap with her peers and her inconsistent use of hearing aids. In addition, Emily's regular teachers had been relying on Emily communicating to the resource teacher what class material with which she need assistance. A 9-week conference revealed that Emily was often confused about assignments and had a significant amount of missing information in her class notes.

In attempts to decrease Emily's self-conscious feelings about her handicap, her science and history teachers approached her with some ideas to introduce her classmates to hearing loss. Although reluctantly, Emily did agree to the teachers' ideas.

An entire unit in Emily's science class was devoted to anatomy of the ear and hearing disorders. Although Emily initially was bothered by the increased attention drawn to her loss, she quickly was pleased to see her classmates were nothing but positive and supportive. Their curiosity and frequent questions about her loss and her hearing aids seemed to improve Emily's self-concept and acceptance of her handicap. Following encouragment to bring her aids to school by her peers so that they could listen to them, Emily exhibited more consistent use of amplification.

In addition to the science unit, Emily's history teacher prepared lectures on Alexander Graham Bell and his interest in deafness following his marriage to a deaf woman. This reinforced Emily's improved relationship and openness with her classmates.

Once Emily's confidence was enhanced and she appeared more comfortable in her classes, her communication skills improved and her eagerness to participate in class discussion was obvious.

To ensure that Emily was obtaining all material presented in her classes and comprehending all assignments, a buddy system was implemented. A good student in each class was assigned to make carbon copies of all notes for Emily and to repeat to her essential verbal instruction.

Other strategies to assist Emily with keeping up with new material presented in class included each teacher supplying the resource teacher a weekly preview of new topics and vocabulary.

Pre-teaching of material, the buddy system, improved self-concept, and consistent use of amplification all contributed to a successful year for Emily. She maintained a B or C average in all classes.

encouraged to keep a management diary for the child to take home daily. It could include vocabulary lists, a preview of subjects to come, or teaching strategies that work. Using parents to work on topics at home can only improve carry-over. Parents can use certain vocabulary introduced at school in different contexts, which certainly facilitates comprehension of multiple meanings.

Special Adaptations

Although many of the teaching strategies previously described are applicable to all children exhibiting impaired hearing, regardless of type or degree, they are often associated only with those children with identified losses in the severe to profound range. Children "classified" as hearing impaired by most educational standards are those requiring special services, those children with academic deficits and more significant impairments.

However, there are many children attending school who exhibit hearing losses of varying types and degrees who may be functioning with no difficulty in academic or other school-related areas. They may not require the extent of intervention that the more severely impaired do, but they do require some amount of special classroom adaptation for their needs to be met.

Children exhibiting fluctuating, conductive hearing losses can cause a dilemma for the teacher. On many occasions, the child responds with no difficulty and without problems in comprehension. At other times, the child seems to be "in a dream world" and follows very little of what goes on in the class. These children may be exhibiting fluctuating degrees of hearing loss due to temporary episodes of upper respiratory involvement, middle ear disease, etc.

At these times, they may perform and function just as the severely hearing impaired child does who reveals a permanent sensorineural loss. Teachers should be alert to changes in responsiveness and understanding. If a history of fluctuating hearing loss is documented in the child's records, then the teacher might assume such a loss is the cause of the changes and begin incorporating those necessary teaching practices already described. If this is the first indication of poor awareness, the teacher should refer the child for testing and consult with the district's specialists on hearing impairment.

For many years, the presence of a unilateral hearing loss was thought to have no effect on the educational achievement of children. As professionals, we now know that is certainly not the case. Unilateral losses (in the presence of one normal ear) have been found to play a significant role in the abilities of the child exhibiting such disorders.

The intent of this chapter is not to debate the controversies that surround the skills of the child with a unilateral hearing loss. Rather, it is only important that teachers be aware that such a loss exists and, if so, program for it appropriately. After reading in the child's records that a unilateral loss is present, teachers should not assume that the one normal ear will compensate for that disorder. Obviously, special consideration must be given to seating the child with the better ear directed toward the speaker. Also, as appropriate to the unilateral nature of the loss, modifications should be made to teaching styles, as previously described.

Children with high-frequency losses pose an even greater challenge for the classroom teacher. Similar to those children with fluctuating losses, these children exhibit inconsistent abilities in awareness and comprehension. Special consideration is necessary for children with high-frequency hearing loss, as well. These students will often respond normally and comprehend with little difficulty. However, the presence of such a loss will certainly prompt more evident problems when noise occurs, when visual clues are absent, when speech is complex, etc. These children will have greater difficulty processing plurals or other morphological elements that are high frequency in nature.

Educational Interpreters

Many students with hearing impairments in the mainstreamed environment take advantage of a communication interpreter. School districts employing such a professional utilize varying titles for this position. These individuals are often classified as tutors, aides, or communication facilitators. Regardless of their "official" title, if these individuals are held responsible for communicating classroom information to the student with a hearing impairment, certain guidelines are critical.

Guidelines for interpreters for persons with hearing impairments are clearly outlined in the Code of Ethics of the National Registry of Interpreters for the Deaf.[1,4] These guidelines serve the purpose of assuring high-quality interpreting services for individuals with hearing impairments. However, as increasing numbers of young students with hearing impairments are mainstreamed into public schools, schools are experiencing unique interpreting situations that are not addressed in these guidelines.

Special situations develop for several reasons. One is related to the fact that the very young child with a hearing loss does not yet understand how to use an interpreter. In addition, typical early childhood behaviors call for a great deal of flexibility by all people involved, including an interpreter. A further explanation is the lack of trained interpreters. The response to this in many schools has been to use an employee who, in addition to other duties, also facilitates communication with the child with a hearing impairment by using existing sign language skills.

Guidelines have been developed that are designed to assist with the unique interpreting problems school staff they may face. Although most of these guidelines are addressed to the interpreter, the responsibility of the regular classroom teacher and the school administrators should not be overlooked. The use of an interpreter in educational programs truly calls for a team approach by all professionals involved.

Supportive Services

Many states have developed a network of consultants to assist public school staff with their management of the student who is hearing impaired. In addition to the traditional support personnel housed within each specific school district (speech-language pathologist, certified teacher of the deaf, counselor, etc.), many districts or educational regions also have the service of a consultant management of the hearing impaired available to them. Although these individuals are not in schools on a daily basis to teach reading or facilitate communication, they can provide an essential services: in-service training necessary before embarking on a mainstreamed program; educate school staff in successful teaching strategies; acquaint personnel on the significance of consistency of amplification; assist in due process completion; assist in the guarantee of a least restrictive and successful education.

RESOURCE MATERIALS

Many discussions of resource materials useful with the hearing impaired might like readers to believe that there are not many materials available that are appropriate for use with this population.[15] Regular teachers, as well as special educators, then feel abandoned, at times. Their responsibility is to "teach" these children, but yet there are no "tools of the trade" useful to them.

I would like to reject the theory that curricula materials or resources appropriate to education of the hearing impaired are limited. Rather, I contend that not only are there published sources for this population, but most materials designed for *all* students are more than adequate for the hearing impaired, with some modification. Too often, professionals fall prey to the philosophy that teaching methods and materials must be "laboratory tested" on the designated population before its usefulness can be proven. With the implementation of the strategies previously described in this chapter, many of the traditional or established materials used in the classroom will teach all students, including the child with hearing impairment.

In surveying professionals involved with the education of the hearing impaired, many themes emerge in the description of their approaches for organizing activities and content. Emphasis is placed on a natural language/whole language approach and strategies that are based on normal developmental information. There should be reliance on teacher judgment and experience to organize content areas and individualized instruction that best meets the child's needs.[16] I find little difference between these emphasized priorities for programming for the hearing impaired and those that would be beneficial to *any* student.

Although I am not a teacher by profession, years of experience have provided exposure to many "tried and tested" curricula and programs. Each of the materials described in the Appendix are useful tools in the areas they are listed. It must be emphasized, however, that these listings are not intended to represent all materials or products beneficial to persons who are hearing impaired. Although this listing only begins to identify helpful materials, readers might recognize a trend in publishers or distributors. Many of the other products available through these groups are also helpful.

SUMMARY

I hope that the information contained in this chapter eliminates the need for educators to live under the influence of the self-fulfilling prophecy. Students with hearing impairment deserve the chance to prove that they can be a successful member of any class. The inclusion of these children can have many positive effects on the teacher and all the children.

The teacher and class work together to make the student with a hearing impairment feel accepted. This cooperative effort results in a class enthusiastic and eager to learn.[12] Also, the experience of getting to know a disabled child can emphasize the fact they are *a child first*, a child with similar needs, likes, and dislikes. Being hearing impaired certainly requires specific teaching strategies, but it also requires being allowed to be a child.

As detailed in this chapter, teachers need to be more precise and graphic in their teaching style for the child with a hearing loss to have a clear understanding of the information presented. Such precision and clarity can only benefit the entire class. Also, because the teacher serves as an example, the class will make an effort to be clear and specific in their communicative endeavors.[11]

Educating a child with a hearing impairment can certainly be both frightening and overwhelming, but it can also be exciting and rewarding. Is not that the case with educating any child?

APPENDIX

Resource Materials and Curricula

Reading
AG Bell Association for the Deaf
3417 Volta Place NW
Washington DC 20007
  Reading and the Hearing Impaired Individual
  Teaching Reading to Deaf Children
  Guide to the Selection and Use of Reading Instructional Materials
  Sentences and Other Systems
  World Traveler Magazine
  The Raindrop
Edmark
P.O. Box 3218
Redmond, WA 98073
  Simple Language Fairy Tales
  Reading Milestones
  My Words
  Simple English Classic Series
  Fables/Myths
  Building Stories with Julie and Jack

Garrard Publishing Company
Champaign, IL 61820
  Dolch Basic Vocabulary Books
  Dolch First Reading Books
Harper and Row Publishers
10 East 53rd Street
New York, NY 10022
  Design for Reading
Lingui Systems
3100 4th Ave.
East Moline, IL 61244
  Access to Reading
McGraw-Hill Book Company
1221 Avenue of the Americas
New York, NY 10020
  Lessons for Self-Instruction in Basic Skills
  New Practice Readers
  Reading for Concepts
  Step Up Your Reading Power
St. John's School for the Deaf
3680 South Kinnickinnic Avenue
Milwaukee, WI 53207
  Basic Vocabulary Worksheets
Continental Press, Inc.
Elizabethtown, PA 17022
  Reading Skills Spirits Masters
Allied Educational Council
P.O. Box 78
Galien, MI 49113
  Mott Basic Language Skills Programs
Scott Foresman & Company
1900 East Lake Avenue
Glenview, IL 60025
  Activity Concept English
  Easy Reading Books
National Association for the Deaf
814 Thayer Avenue
Silver Springs, MD 20910
  Library Classics
Communication Skill Builders
P.O. Box 42050-NC
Tuscon, AZ 85733
  Speech, Language and Reading Workbooks
CC Publications
P.O. Box 23699
Tigard, OR 97223-0108
  Before Reading: A Language Comprehension Program

Language
AG Bell Association for the Deaf
3417 Volta Place NW
Washington, DC 20007
  Basic Vocabulary and Language Thesaurus for Hearing Impaired Children

Blueprints for Conversational Competence
Curriculum Guide: Hearing Impaired
  Children 0-3 and Their Parents
Dictionary of Idioms for the Deaf
Language and Literary Guide
The Language of Directions
The Language of Toys
Listening and Talking
Parents and Teachers: Partners in Language
  Development
Schedules of Development in Audition,
  Speech, Language and Communication
Communication Skill Builders
P.O. Box 42050-NC
Tucson, AZ 85733
  Communication Competence: A Functional-
    Pragmatic Language Program
  TOTAL: Teacher Organized Training for
    the Acquisition of Language
  Teaching Morphology Developmentally
  Pictures, Please
  Developing Expressive Language: A Func-
    tional Approach for Children 3–8
  Language Remediation and Expansion Series
  Shape Up Your Language
  Natural Language
  Emerging Language 3
  UniSet Kits
  Communicards
  A Sourcebook of Pragmatic Activities
  Concept Formation
  A Guidebook for Instructional Materials for
    Speech and Language Development
CC Publications
P.O. Box 23699
Tigard, OR 97223-0108
  PALS: Developing Social Skills Through
    Language
  Steps Toward Basic Concept Development
  PLUSS—Putting Language to Use in Social
    Situations
  Language Rehabilitation
Reed Education
182 Wakefield Street
Wellington, Australia
  Tate Language Program
Edmark
P.O. Box 3218
Redmond, WA 98073
  Apple Tree Language Program
  Pronoun Pages
  Lessons in Syntax
  TSA Syntax Program

Imaginative Adjectives/Prepositions
Vocabulary Building Exercises for the
  Young Adult
Vocabulary in Context
Basic Vocabualry Study Cards
Newby Visual Language Series
Building Sentences Step by Step
Building Blocks for Developing Basic
  Language
The Potomac Program
American Guidance Service, Inc.
P.O. Box 99
Circle Pines, MN 55014
  Peabody Language Development Kits
Continental Press
Elizabethtown, PA 17022
  Spirit Masters Series
Educational Services, Inc.
Box 219
Stevensville, MI 49127
  The Spice Series
Academic Therapy Publications
1539 4th Street
San Raphael, CA 94901
  Helping Your Child at Home
Teaching Resources Corp.
100 Boylston
Boston, MA 02116
  Fokes Sentence Builder
Children's Hospital
Washington, DC 20001
  Structured Language for Children with
    Special Learning Problems
Learning Concepts
2501 North Lamar
Austin, TX 78745
  Developmental Concepts
Lingui Systems, Inc.
3100 4th Ave.
East Moline, IL 61244
  HELP—Handbook of Excercises for
    Language Processing
  Workbook of Activiţies for Language and
    Cognition
  Language Processing Remediation
  Follow Me
  Question the Direction
  ACHIEV Series
Rhythm Productions
Los Angeles, CA 90034
  Steps Up to Language
  In, Out and Round About
  Mix and Match

Council for Exceptional Children
1920 Association Drive
Reston, VA 22091
  Helping Young Children Develop Language
    Skills
Instructional Industries
Executive Park
Ballston Lake, NY 12019
  Project Life Program
Milton Bradley Company
Springfield, MA 01101
  GOAL Language Program
General Printing Services
1910 N. Providence Rd.
Columbia, MO 65202
  A Process Approach to Developing
    Language with Hearing Impaired
    Children
Wadsworth Publishing Co.
Belmont, CA 94002
  The Sourcebook
Gallaudet University Press
500 Florida Avenue NE
Washington, DC 20002
  Structured Tasks for English Practice (STEP)
  Communicate With Me
Sheffield Publishing Company
P.O. Box 359
Salem, WI 53168
  An Anthology of Figurative Language Stories
Pro-Ed
8700 Shoal Creek Blvd.
Austin, TX 78757
  Idiom Workbook Series
  Multiple Meanings
  Communication Training for Hearing
    Impaired Children and Teenagers

Speech
AG Bell Association for the Deaf
3417 Volta Place NW
Washington, DC 20007
  Speech Assessment and Speech Improve-
    ment for the Hearing Impaired
  Teacher/Clinician Planbook and Guide to
    the Development of Speech Skills
  Cumulative Record of Speech Skill
    Acquisition
  Speech and the Hearing Impaired Child:
    Theory and Practice
CC Publications
P.O. Box 23699
Tigard, OR 97223-0108
  Articulation Modification Program
  Phonemic Context Articulation Program

Communication Skill Builders
P.O. Box 42050-NC
Tucson, AZ 85733
  Articutales
  Articulation Worksheets
  Carry-Over Stories for Articulation
    Therapy
  All the Games Kids Like
  Articulation in Sentences
  Forming Sounds
  Speech and Auditory Training: A Program
    for Adolescents with Hearing Impairments
    & Language Disorders
American Guidance Service
P.O. Box 99
Circle Pines, MN 55014
  Peabody Articulation Cards
Interstate Printers and Publishers
19–27 North Jackson
Danville, IL 61832
  The Big Book of Sounds
  Speech Activity Card File
St. John's School for the Deaf
3680 South Kinnickinnic Ave.
Milwaukee, WI 53207
  Speech Books for the Deaf

Auditory Training
AG Bell Association for the Deaf
3417 Volta Place NW
Washington, DC 20007
  The Joy of Listening: An Auditory Training
    Program
  Auditory Training
  I Heard That!
  Auditory Learning
  Auditory Enhancement Guide
Foreworks
Box 9747
North Hollywood, CA 91609
  Auditory Skills Curriculum
Houston School for Deaf Children
726 Diamond Leaf
Houston, TX 77079
  Developmental Approach to Successful
    Listening
Communication Skill Builders
P.O. Box 42050-NC
Tuscon, AZ 85733
  What's That I Hear?
  Sound Investments: Carry-Over Activities
    for Listening Skills
  CLAS: Classroom Listening and Speaking
  Learn to Listen
  Attending

Educators Publishing Service
75 Moulton St.
Cambridge, MA 02138
   Learning to Listen
St. Joseph Institute for the Deaf
1483 82nd Boulevard
St. Louis, MO 63132
   ABC of Auditory Training
Interstate Printers and Publishers
19–27 North Jackson
Danville, IL 61832
   The Auditory Training Handbook for Good
      Listeners
CC Publications
P.O. Box 23699
Tigard, OR 97223-0108
   Auditory Rehabilitation
   Auditory Memory for Language
   Auditory Discrimination Training Program
Gallaudet University Press
800 Florida Avenue NE
Washington, DC 20002
   Developing Auditory Skills

Speechreading
AG Bell Association for the Deaf
3417 Volta Place NW
Washington, DC 20007
   Lipreading Made Easy
   Stories and Games for Easy Lipreading
      Practice
   Lively Lipreading Lessons
   Lipreading for Children
   Messy Monsters, Jungle Joggers and
      Bubble Baths
Rochester Institute of Technology
NTID
1 Lomb Memorial Drive
P.O. Box 9887
Rochester, NY 14623-0887
   Association Cues
   Speechreading Strategies
Interstate Printers and Publishers
19–27 N. Jackson
Davville, IL 61832
   Speech and Lipreading Instructional
      Program
Charles C. Thomas Publishers
301–327 East Lawrence Avenue
Springfield, IL
   Total Communication Used in Experience
      Based Speechreading and Auditory
      Training Lesson Plans

Gallaudet University Press
500 Florida Ave. NE
Washington, DC 20002
   Speechreading: A Way to Improve
      Understanding
   Speechreading in Context

Other Academic Related Subjects
Edmark
P.O. Box 3218
Redmond, WA 98073
   I Can Write
   HEP—History, Economics, Political Science
   Time Concept Series
   Green Mountain Math
   Joy of Learning
   Controlled Language Science Series
AG Bell Association for the Deaf
3417 Volta Place NW
Washington, DC 20007
   Learning to Write and Writing to Learn
   Science for Deaf Children
   The Tutor/Notetaker: Providing Academic
      Support to Mainstreamed Deaf Students
   Manager's Guide for the Tutor/Notetaker
   Teaching Geography to Sensory Impaired
      Children
   Teaching Social Skills to Hearing Impaired
      Students
Rochester Institute of Technology
NTID
1 Lomb Memorial Drive
P.O. Box 9887
Rochester, NY 14623-0887
   The Tutor/Notetaker Comic Book
   Tutor/Notetaker Pads
Fearson/Pitman Publishers, Inc.
6 Davis Drive
Belmont, CA 94002
   The Pacemaker Arithmetic Program
Continental Press, Inc.
Elizabethtown, PA 17022
   Arithmetic Step by Step
Frank E. Richards Publishing Co., Inc.
P.O. Box 66
Phoenix, NY 13125
   Useful Arithmetic
   Using Money Series
   Science Series
McGraw-Hill Book Company
1221 Avenue of the Americas
New York, NY 10020
   Foundations in Mathematics

David C. Cook Publishing Company
850 North Grove Avenue
Elgin, IL 60120
  Science Themes
  Social Studies Picture Sets
Follett Publishing Company
1010 West Washington Boulevard
Chicago, IL 60607
  Beginning Science Books
  Beginning Social Studies Books
Milliken Publishing Company
1100 Research Boulevard
St. Louis, MO 63132
  General Science Series
  Geography Through Maps
  Map Reading Series
Benefic Press
10300 West Roosevelt Road
Westchester, IL 60153
  Basic Concept Series
  Basic Understanding Series
Lingui Systems
3100 4th Avenue
East Moline, IL 61244
  Crash Course for Study Skills
Harris Communications
6541 City West Parkway
Eden Prarie, MN 55344
  *Beginning Reading and Sign
    Language*
Gallaudet University Press
500 Florida Avenue NE
Washington, DC 20002
  Pre-Reading Strategies
  The Deaf Student's Curriculum Guide
  *Kendall Demonstration Elementary School
    Curriculum Guides*
TJ Publishers
817 Silver Spring Avenue
Suite 206
Silver Spring, MD 20910
  Tomorrow We're Taking a Test

Computer Software
AG Bell Association for the Deaf
3417 Volta Place NW
Washington, DC 20007
  *Natural Processing Program with Com-
    puterized Language Lessons*
Edmark
P.O. Box 3218
Redmond, WA 98073
  Lessons in Syntax
  Write this Way

Communication Skill Builders
P.O. Box 42050-NC
Tucson, AZ 85733
  Computer Managed Articulation Treatment
  Computer Managed Language Treatment
  Idioms in America
  *Computer Courseware for the Exceptional
    Student*
  Wizard of Words
  First Words I and II
  Twenty Categories
  First Verbs
  *Micro—LADS—Microcomputer Language
    Assessment and Development System*
  Stickybear Reading
  Juggles Rainbow Story Machine
  Ship Ahoy Word Scramble
  Gertrude's Secrets
  Tuk Goes to Town
  *Planning Individualized Speech and
    Language*
  Intervention Programs
Gallaudet University Press
500 Florida Avenue NE
Washington, DC 20002
  Computer Assisted Notetaking
  Software to Go

Audio-Visual Materials
Captioned Films for the Deaf
5034 Wisconsin Avenue NW
Washington, DC 20016

Associated Films, Inc.
866 Third Avenue
New York, NY 10022

Modern Talking Picture Series
5000 Park St. North
St. Petersburg, FL 33709

National Catalog of Films in Special
  Education
Ohio State University Press
Columbia, OH 43210

AG Bell Association for the Deaf
3417 Volta Place NW
Washington, DC 20007

National Association of the Deaf
814 Thayer Avenue
Silver Springs, MD 20910

Modern Signs Press
P.O. Box 1181
Los Alamitos, CA 90720
  Signing Exact English Video Tape Series

Harris Communications
6541 City West Parkway
Eden Prarie, MN 55344
  Beginning Reading and Sign Language
    (video tape)
Health Services Consortium
103 Laurel Avenue
Carrboro, NC 27510
  Language and Hearing Impaired Children
    (video tape)
See Sign Productions
116 Volusia Avenue
Dayton, OH 45409
  See Sign Videos
See-A-Sign Videotapes
2 Connell Drive
Little Rock, AR 72205
  See-A-Song (videotape)
  See-A-Story (videotape)

In-Service Training

Bono Film Service, Inc.
1042 Wisconsin Avenue NW
Washington, DC 20007
  Lisa, Pay Attention! (film)
AV Resources
319 15th Avenue SE
Minneapolis, MN 55455
  Hearing Aid Demonstration (audio tape)
AG Bell Association for the Deaf
3417 Volta Place NW
Washington, DC 20007
  Show and Tell: Explaining Hearing Loss to
    Teachers (video tape)
  A Child with a Hearing Loss in your
    Classroom (book)
  Mainstreaming: Practical Ideas for Educating
    Hearing Impaired Students (book)
Gorden Stowe Assts
Custom Records Dept.
RCA Victor
Northbrook, IL 60062
  How They Hear (record)
Anne Seltz
Title III Interdistrict Project for Hearing
  Impaired Children
807 N.E. Broadway
Minneapolis, MN 55413
  Team Approach (slide tape program)
  PACT—Procedural Adaptations for
    Classroom Teachers, Tutors and
    Therapists (slide tape program)
  Guidelines for Preparing Case Manage-
    ment Conference (handout material)

  Questions to Promote Discussion (handout
    material)
  Teacher-Tutor Communication Forum
    (handout material)
Instructor Publications, Inc.
Dansville, NY 04437
  Hints and Activities for Mainstreaming
    (book)
Harris Communication
6541 City West Parkway
Eden Prarie, MN 55344
  Special Needs in Ordinary Schools
Gallaudet University Press
800 Florida Ave. NE
Washington, DC 20002
The Science of Sound
  Say That Again Please
  There's a Hearing Impaired Child in My
    Class
  A Very Special Friend
  Chris Gets Ear Tubes
  The Day We Met Cindy
  What is an Audiogram
  Ear Gear and Wired for Sound
  Deaf Like Me
  Mandy
  Now I Understand
  Belonging
  Let's Learn About Deafness
  Growing Up Without Hearing

Sign Language Materials

Gallaudet University Press
800 Florida Avenue NE
Washington, DC 20002
  Come Sign With Us
  Sign Word Flash Cards
  The Signed English Schoolbook
  Signing for Reading Success
  Word Signs—A First Book of Sign
    Language
  Discovering Sign Language
  Sesame Street Sign Language Fun
  Signing for Kids
  My First Book of Sign
  ASL in Schools: Policies and Curriculum
  Signing at School
  Learning to Sign in My Neighborhood
Dawn Sign Press
9080 Activity Road
Suite A
San Diego, CA 92126
  Signs for Me
  Sign Language Coloring Book Series

Modern Signs Press
P.O. Box 1181
Los Alamitos, CA 90720
*Signing Exact English Vocabulary
Development*
Harris Communications
6541 City West Parkway
Eden Prarie, MN 55344
Signing for Kids
Academic Communication Associates
4149 Avenida de la Plata
Oceanside, CA 92058
Sign Language Classroom Resource
Pro-Ed
8700 Shoal Creek Blvd
Austin, TX 78757
Teaching Sign Language

***Additional Companies Representing
Educational Materials***
Hear You Are
4 Musconetcong Ave.
Stanhope, NJ 07874

Laureate Learning Systems
110 E. Spring St.
Winooski, VT 05404

The Speech Bin
1766 20th Ave.
Vero Beach, FL 32960

Parrot Software
P.O. Box 1139
State College, PA 16804

United Educational services
P.O. Box 1099
Buffalo, NY 14224

DLM
P.O. Box 543
Blacklick, OH 43004

The Psychological Corporation
555 Academic Ct.
San Antonio, TX 78204

REFERENCES

1. Ross M, Calvert DR: The semantics of deafness, in Northcott WH: *The Hearing Impaired Child in the Regular Classroom* (Washington DC: AG Bell Association, 1973).

2. Davis JM: Management of the school age child: a psychosocial perspective, in Bess FH: *Hearing Impairment in Children* (Parkton MD: York Press, 1988).

3. Watkins S, Schow R: Aural rehabilitation for children, in Schow R: *Introduction to Aural Rehabilitation*, 2nd ed (Boston: Allyn and Bacon, 1989).

4. Ross M, Brackett D, Maxon AB: *Assessment and Management of Mainstreamed Hearing Impaired Children* (Austin TX: Pro-Ed, 1991).

5. Gildston P: The Hearing Impaired Child in the Classroom, in Northcott WH: *The Hearing Impaired Child in the Regular Classroom* (Washington DC: AG Bell Association, 1973).

6. Brackett D, Maxon AB: Service delivery alternatives for the mainstreamed hearing impaired child. *Lang Speech Hear Serv Sch*, 17 (1986), 115–125.

7. Conway L: Issues relating to classroom management, in Ross M: *Hearing Impaired Children in the Mainstream* (Parkton MD: York Press, 1990).

8. Maxon AB, Brackett D: *The Hearing Impaired Child Infancy Through High School Years* (Boston: Andover Medical Publishers, 1992).

9. Brooks N: Educational support services, in Froehlinger V: *Today's Hearing Impaired Child: Into the Mainstream of Education* (Washington DC: AG Bell Association, 1981).

10. Olsen W: The effects of noise and reverberation on speech intelligibility, in Bess FH, Freeman B, Sinclair JS: *Amplification in Education* (Washington DC: AG Bell Association, 1981).

11. Brackett D: Communication management of the mainstreamed hearing impaired student, in Ross M: *Hearing Impaired Children in the Mainstream* (Parkton MD: York Press, 1990).

12. Flexer C, Wray D, Ireland J: Preferential seating in the classroom. *Lang Speech Hear Serv Sch*, 20 (1989), 11–21.

13. Olsen WO: Classroom acoustics for hearing impaired children, in Bess FH: *Hearing Impairment in Children* (Parkton MD: York Press, 1988).

14. Caccamise F: *Introduction to Interpreting* (Silver Spring MD: Registry of Interpreters for the Deaf, 1980).

15. McCarr D, Wisser MW: Curriculum materials useful with the hearing impaired (Beaverton OR: Dormac, 1979).

16. Fristoe M: Language intervention systems: programs pubilshed in kit form, in Lloyd L: *Communication Assessment and Intervention Strategies* (Baltimore: University Park Press, 1979).

COUNSELING FOR PARENTS OF CHILDREN WITH AUDITORY DISORDERS

18

David M. Luterman

I'm not a teacher: only a fellow-traveler of whom you asked the way. I pointed ahead—ahead of myself as well as you.

—George Bernard Shaw, 1856–1950

Education of individuals with deafness in the United States began essentially as a school-based program within a residential setting. Since deafness is a low incidence disorder, prospective students were scattered throughout the countryside. Each state would set up one school supported with tax dollars, generally in a rural area. The prevailing belief was that children who are disabled should be educated in a setting that was structured for them and was not visible to the rest of society; consequently, parents often had to travel enormous distances to reach the school. Since travel was so difficult and communication between home and school minimal, the school personnel assumed the total responsibility for educating the child; in fact, it was common for parents to be required to sign release forms granting custody of their child to the school.[1] Parents were seen as peripheral to the education of the child. There might be an end of the year conference with the teacher and occasional visits but very little detailed involvement of the parents was expected in the educational program. When parents did try to be involved, it was often seen as a threat by the school personnel. The principal of the Ohio School for the Deaf in 1917 admonished parents "to accept the recommendations of the school authorities. They know. It is their business to know."[1]

With the urbanization of the United States and the technological improvements in transportation and communication, which occurred in the early to mid 20th century, the schools for the deaf became more accessible to families, but attitudes did not change appreciably. School personnel (and parents themselves) still saw parents as peripheral to the educational process. Now that the school was more accessible, however, parents were more available to the professionals; thus

began the Parent-Teacher Association (now known as the PTO). In this model, parents were viewed as "resources" to the schools; often, they were enlisted as fund raisers and school volunteers to fill in for office personnel. Occasionally, they were enlisted as classroom aides. Education of the parents consisted of lectures and hurried conferences with teachers in which parents were expected to be passive recipients of the professional expertise. There was no emphasis or even feeling that educating the child who was deaf was in any way a collaborative effort between parents and the educators. Parents were seen at best as helpers and at worst as potential adversaries. This attitude was reflected in the training of teachers in which there was no mention of parent involvement and no training facilities that would demonstrate to the neophyte teacher an attitude toward parents other than the restrictive, patronizing one that was then considered good, standard operating policy for the school.

It was not until 1940, with the establishment of the Tracy Clinic in Los Angeles,[2] that parent education and active participation in the educational process was demonstrated. With this pioneering effort, which was confined to preschool children, the Tracy Clinic established the notion that parents can be and should be participants in the education of their children. It has taken us quite a while to make that cultural shift, and now almost all training programs in the United States and almost all schools for the deaf, at least, pay lip service to the notion of a parent-school partnership. This attitude also reflects the greater cultural shift that has taken place in the United States in which "consumers" are afforded a great deal of influence on the final "product." It remains to be seen, however, whether active parent participation has truly filtered up from the preschool program to invade all aspects of academics. Most schools seem to involve parents heavily in the pre-school years and then revert to the PTO model in the school years.

A computer search of the literature reveals almost no articles and very few chapters about parents of school age children with auditory disorders. Although there is material on the parents of preschool children; it is as though parents of school age children had fallen off the face of the educational map. This chapter, then, was written mainly from an experiential and anecdotal framework. To aid me in preparation of this chapter, I solicited information from parents of children with hearing impairments who were associated with Emerson College's family-centered program when their children were young (0 to 3 years old). This program has been described elsewhere.[3] Parents were asked to comment in an open-ended way on three questions: (1) What are or were your specific needs as the parents of a school-age hearing-impaired child? (2) What programs do (or did) you wish the school had or did provide for you? (3) Aside from the academic considerations, what were your child's needs and were they met by the school? Thirty-four parents responded of 121 solicited with children ranging in age from 5 to 30 years. Many of the parents wrote lengthy responses going much beyond the scope of the questions posed. This chapter then is written mainly from my own 30 years of clinical ex-perience of working with families of children who are hearing impaired and data gleaned from the questionnaires.

To understand parent's behavior, we need first to understand parental feelings. In the early stages of the diagnostic process the feelings are usually very apparent and felt acutely. For the parents of the school-age child, the feelings are present but may not be readily apparent. The parents live a life of deafness that seems normal to them until their adjustment is challenged; the feeling then emerges acutely whenever, for example, there is a change in the educational plan or the parents are reminded again of the loss that they have sus-tained (with congenital deafness the loss is always felt by the parents; in acquired deafness it is a shared loss). One father of a 17-year-old child commented: "When you first find out your child is deaf it hurts like hell. Then it becomes a dull ache that doesn't go away."

GRIEF

The loss for which parents grieve is of the dream that they had of how their life was going to be and how their child would turn out. This dream or expectation is very real, and when that dream must be abandoned, it is experienced as a fundamental loss much akin to the death of a loved one. This loss is not to be minimized, as it determines much of the subsequent behavior of the parent. As with the death of a loved one, it is the little incidents in subsequent years that remind parents again of their loss and throw them back into acute grief. One frequently hears pro-fessionals commenting in amazement on how a parent of an older child with deafness broke down in tears when they put a frequency modulation (FM) system on the child "And I thought," com-mented the teacher, "she has accepted it so well." In actuality this mother was accepting the deaf-ness quite well, but seeing her child so wired for sound brought the abnormality and loss to light again, and she needed some space and time to grieve anew. It often does not take much to re-mind the parents of their loss. Birthday parties and family gatherings are particularly hard be-cause they force a comparison of the skills of the child with deafness with the skills of the child who hears normally. Invariably, the child with deafness is found to be deficient and the parent's tenuous adjustment is shattered: at least for the moment. For hearing parents of children who are deaf, the deafness is a wound that when assaulted by reality bleeds a bit. Acceptance is not without pain and I do not know of any hearing parents of a child with hearing impairment who does not at some time break down and grieve the loss. These breakdowns in subsequent years usually are short-lived and are part of the normal adjust-ment process.

INADEQUACY

To understand parenting is to understand that all parents are scared. Any parent, who is the least bit introspective, recognizes the awesome responsibility that being a parent entails. Some-how, parents have to find the resources and wis-dom to raise their child to responsible adulthood. Usually these feelings of inadequacy are sub-merged into the everydayness of raising a child.

The feelings emerge acutely whenever there is a crisis to be confronted. Deafness in a child is a matter of confronting a series of crises for parents, beginning with the diagnosis and, for many parents, never ending, as they remain very much involved in the adult life of their child with deafness. When life-changing decisions need to be made, parents often feel overwhelmed and scared because they do not want to make a bad decision and, in their eyes, "ruin their child's life."

The feelings of inadequacy often lead to trying to find someone else to make the decisions and at least share the responsibility if not take it. In short, the parents want to be rescued from their feelings of inadequacy. Often this felt inadequacy corresponds to the helping professionals strong need to be needed, and an unholy alliance is formed in which the professional does a great deal of dysfunctional rescuing. When we rescue persons from their felt inadequacy, we reinforce their low self-esteem and lack of confidence in their own ability to cope. The more parents are rescued from taking responsibility, the more we contribute to their feelings of inadequacy. In previous writing, I have called this phenomenon "the Annie Sullivan effect,"[4] whereby over-helping of parents by professionals leads to the ceding of responsibility for their child to the professional. The "Annie Sullivan relationship" leads to a disempowered, impotent parent—the obverse of what we want to accomplish. Schlessinger's[5] research shows that the best predictor of literacy in a deaf third grader is the degree to which the mother is empowered, and the quality of the parent-child interaction.

Empowerment of parents is best accomplished by not rescuing; by assuming that the parents are capable of making good decisions for themselves and their family when *they have all the facts*. The professional's responsibility is *to* the parents not *for* the parents and is to provide the facts as needed and trust the parents eventually to make good decisions for themselves. This is often a difficult thing for most professionals to do as they see foundering parents and children not being immediately helped. To rescue only leads to more rescuing and it becomes difficult, if not impossible, to break the dependency cycle once initiated. To be sure, professionals need to help, but the helping should be covert and not so obvious that it diminishes the self-confidence of the parents. At all stages, we need to be empowering the parents and all clinical and educational interactions need to be examined in light of whether they lead to parental empowerment.

There is no more potent educational intervention than enhancing parental self-confidence.

ANGER

At some fundamental level, all hearing parents of children with deafness are angry. Anger occurs in our life whenever there is a violation of an expectation. For parents of school-age children, their expectation was around being the parent of a "normal" child: whenever the disability of hearing loss asserts itself, the parent gets angry because it reminds them of their failed expectations. The parents who go to school and see their child wired for sound and socially isolated will get angry. Anger is usually one of the first emotions to emerge, and it often masks other emotions, frequently becoming a cover for the chronic grief that the parent feels.

Anger also stems from a loss of control. We all like to think of ourselves as having unlimited degrees of freedom to control our own fate. When we cannot do what we want to do, we feel thwarted and angry. One of the angriest men I ever encountered was the father of a 10-year-old child with deafness. He had been working for a number of years in his business trying to get a promotion to regional sales manager. When he finally got the position, he found out he was required to move to a small town in the midwest that had no services for children who are deaf. His child would have to be sent to the regional school for the deaf on a residential basis: this was an anathema to both him and his wife. If he took the job, then he would injure his child, and if he failed to take the job, he would hurt his own chances for promotion. He was furious.

Another source of anger stems from the feelings of impotency. It is a fury stemming from the feelings of powerlessness that parents experience when they cannot "fix" their child's deafness. All parents are pledged to make things better for a hurting child and when they find they cannot— that this child will always have to wear hearing aids and probably be subject to the taunts of children who are hearing—the parents get furious. It is the kind of anger that makes us want to kick the cat, put a fist through the door, and anyone or anything that gets in the way better watch out.

The anger is sometimes at the child for being deaf and is masking the parents' guilt that they might have done something to cause the deafness: this is very difficult to acknowledge. Parents will often dream or fantasize that their child is dead, and in one sense their expected child has died.

Anger is something most people have trouble dealing with because it is equated with a loss of love. In actuality there is a great deal of caring in anger—the opposite of love is not hate but indifference. It is difficult for parents to see this, and the anger is often suppressed or displaced. These are the most common means we have to deal with anger; unfortunately, neither is psychologically healthy. Suppressed anger often leads to depression, and displacing the anger onto professionals who are trying to help often leads to alienation of the parents and the child from the people who can best ameliorate the situation. What the professional must do is help the parents to acknowledge the anger that they feel toward their child's deafness, by helping the parents to see that they are really upset by the situation rather than the child. This often means confronting a furious parent, something most professionals find difficult to do. Anger is a useful energy that can be harnessed to work in the child's best interest, and it must be harnessed by careful counseling.

GUILT

Almost all mothers of children with hearing impairments feel guilt. It seems women in our society are acculturated to take responsibility for everything bad that happens—one mother said to me once "I even feel guilty when it rains." Guilt at a very fundamental level is really a power statement, it is saying that one has some control over that event (worry does the same thing). Often that power is an illusion but it serves to assuage the feeling of powerlessness that many women feel. In the long run, this is a psychologically expensive way to feel power because the flip side to guilt is always resentment. Guilt is such a corrosive, uncomfortable, and controlling feeling that we resent the person or the event that causes us to feel guilty. Relationships that are built on a foundation of guilt are often unstable because the resentment can bubble up to sabotage them.

The mother's role is usually to protect the health of the family members. When someone is sick, mother has failed in her responsibility. Mother guilt is particularly evident around the cause of the deafness. In most cases of congenital deafness the cause is not known, at least by the professional. The mother then goes over her pregnancy, day by day, looking for something untoward that happened that she can blame on having caused the deafness, and thus is born the guilty secret. Often the mother "knows" that she

did something to cause the child's deafness, this leads her to dedicate her life in an attempt to "fix" it. In effect, she tries to make it up to the child by devoting all her energy and time becoming a super dedicated parent. This often has very serious long term repercussions in the family.

Father guilt stems from his role in the family as protector; when people are hurting father has failed in some way. Fathers tend to play the guilt out by denying it. They try to make other family members feel better and not respond directly to their pain or to even acknowledge it. If they cannot "fix" it, they tend to withdraw. Occasionally, one does get to see a super-dedicated father, but more often as not, the father's solution to guilt is to get very involved with work. The pattern of the dysfunctional family begins to be established early in the educational process as the mother becomes over involved in her child's deafness, the father becomes over involved in work, and there is less and less time and energy devoted to maintaining the marriage. When this happens, the relationship spirals down into increasing levels of marital dissatisfaction. I have found over the years that the most successful children with deafness are the products of a happy marriage, and children from the dysfunctional families are often limited severely in their abilities to have satisfactory interpersonal relationships.

In the preschool years the super dedicated parent looks very good to the professionals who are working with the family. These are the parents who are in two or three different programs and who never fail to attend a PTO meeting or a conference. The negative consequences of super dedication begin to emerge later. For the school-age child the dedication is apt to become suffocating. The superdedicated, guilt-driven parent finds it very difficult to let go—trust of professionals is usually minimal ("If I let something bad happen how can I trust these less invested professionals with my child?") and the child is overprotected ("I let something bad happen (to my child) once; I am not going to let it happen again.") Because so much energy has gone into the parenting of this one child, there is little left for the marriage or for the other siblings. When one examines families of the superdedicated parent of a school-age child, one often finds a marriage that is not functional and siblings who are at risk. It is not a happy or supportive environment to raise a deaf child.

Ultimately, all parents must give up their children. This is a painful process, and the super-dedicated, guilt-driven parent finds this almost impossible to do. So much of the parent's time and energy has revolved around the child's deafness that to let go of the child leaves a huge void; parents are often horrified at the prospect of losing their child and a large chunk of their lives. The tight bonding that is created by the guilt-driven parent often creates a very dependent child who has not been allowed to have sufficient life experiences to enable him or her to develop the skills necessary for becoming a responsible adult. Counseling parents around their guilt feelings is essential if we hope to create independent, responsible adults who happen to be hearing impaired.

VULNERABILITY

The existential truth of life is that it is hard and there is no way that we can encounter life without, at some point, suffering pain. At some fundamental psychological level, we are aware of this truth, and it causes us anguish. In the desire to assuage that pain we pretend that we are invulnerable; "bad things only happen to other people" becomes our mantra and we proceed to live life as though we are indeed invulnerable. When a bad thing does happen to us, we realize anew at some fundamental level what we have always been most fearful of; we are naked and alone in the face of what seems to be an indifferent universe. Childhood deafness is just such a defense-piercing event and often leads parents to overprotective behaviors.

By counseling parents and having them recognize that the overprotection stemming from these feelings of vulnerability are leading to destructive behavior, the parents can begin the process of transforming these feelings into self-enhancing acts. The recognition and acknowledgment of vulnerability can lead to a restructuring of life's priorities, parents can now live more authentically because they know what is truly important in life. Knowing that our loved ones are fragile (they are just on loan to us) can lead us to appreciate them more.

The parent of a 16-year-old said:
Deafness in my child has been the best thing that ever happened to me. My life now has a focus and meaning that it never had before. I was fated to become a suburban housewife whose main concern was whether or not the neighbor thought my house was clean. I now see how shallow that life was.

There is a potential for much good in deafness—the deafness can become a powerful teacher. David Wright,[6] an adult who is deaf had this to say about his deafness:
The handicapped are less at the mercy of vague unhappiness that afflicts so many, especially those without an aim in life, whose consequent boredom promotes what used to be called spleen. The disabled have been given a built-in ready-packed objective which is always present: a definite impediment to get the better of. Like the prospect of hanging, it concentrates the faculties wonderfully. (p. 111)

Counseling can help unlock and unleash the potential good that is in deafness.

Unfortunately for most professionals working with parents of school-age children, they often must undo the mistakes and insensitivities of professionals who encountered the families in the preschool years. These parents are often locked into the unproductive behavior stemming from their unacknowledged feelings of inadequacy, guilt, anger, and vulnerability leading them to dependency, overdedication, overprotection, and the displaced anger that alienates them from professionals seeking to help. With proper help, the anger can become a positive energy to make things happen, the guilt becomes commitment, and the acknowledged vulnerability become an opportunity to restructure lives and values. The grief becomes a sadness that will always be there and serves to intensify all other feelings.

There is also much joy in deafness. I often tell parents that this child has come bearing a gift; albeit the gift is buried under much pain and sheer hard work, but it is a gift nonetheless. Their task is to find this gift because with it there is much joy. It is the joy of having a purpose and direction in life, it is the joy of hearing that first word and knowing who put it there.

COUNSELING

It is beyond the scope of this chapter to go into detailed descriptions about the counseling process in communication disorders. The interested reader can pursue this subject further in other volumes.[7-9]

I think the notions of the discipline of Humanistic Counseling have great implications for the field of communication disorders. According to Carl Rogers, the founder of Humanistic Counseling, there are three prerequisites to encouraging client growth: counselor congruence, unconditional regard, and reflective listening. It is the relationship that is established between the counselor and the client that promotes growth. In this relationship the counselor needs to provide unconditional regard that releases the client from feelings of being judged that might inhibit risk. With openness and acceptance in the relationship growth can take place. There also needs to be an authenticity (congruence) in the counselor and all counselor communication that enables trust to be established in the relationship. The key to growth is the nonjudgmental reflective listening that the counselor does. This listening and valuing of the client within an atmosphere of acceptance allows clients to work through their own problems. Information is provided as needed, and the counselor trusts the clients ultimately to make good decisions for themselves. We diminish a parent's self esteem when we advise and try to "fix" things for them.

Here are some notions about working with parental feelings:

1. Listening is the single most powerful skill for a professional to have—listening enables the parent to work things out.

2. People can take care of themselves: the corollary of this notion is that people are not fragile. Sensitive and reflective listening elicits feelings that need only to be acknowledged and validated. When that happens, the feelings no longer control the person's behavior.

3. Feelings are neither good nor bad, they just *are*. Parents do not have to be responsible for how they feel; they must always be held responsible for how they behave. Behavior can be judged as to whether it is productive for both the parents and the child.

4. We all have a need to control events in our lives. After feelings have been elicited and validated, the professional and the parents need to embark on a journey examining what can be done now. Mental health lies in doing what is doable, and accepting what is not subject to change, and wisdom, as the old saying goes, is knowing the difference between the two. Counseling should encourage that wisdom.

Counseling is often approached fearfully, if at all, by professionals working with the families of children who have auditory disorders. In part this stems from a lack of course work at the training program level[10] and a mistaken notion that parents are extremely fragile and somehow we can harm them irreparably if we say or do the wrong thing. I think as a profession we need to

address the lack of training but also we need to recognize that we really cannot hurt anyone by using the reflective listening, valuing model proposed here. How can someone be hurt if we just listen to them and believe in their competency? We can be destructive when we prescribe and overhelp and ignore the important role that feelings play in determining behavior. It must always be borne in mind that we are dealing with people who are normally upset, not emotionally disturbed. Listening in a nonjudgmental manner and valuing other people's competency so as to build self esteem are not skills that are or should be exotic. These skills are within the scope of all caring professionals and need to be a part of every professional encountering individuals who are hearing impaired.

PARENTAL ISSUES

The major parental issue of the school-age child is the "success" of the child (and really the success of the parents) in accordance with the parental dream established in the preschool years.

In examining the questionnaires that were sent to the parents, it became clear that many of the parents could not distinguish between their needs and their child's needs, even though the question was clearly worded as "What were *your* needs?" Here are some typical responses (it must be borne in mind that these are all rather sophisticated parents who have participated in a family-centered program):

"That he didn't lose out on his scholastic social classes that fit him in with his peers."

"We want our child to live as normal a life as possible."

"We want him to always be challenged further in his development mentally and physically."

"Teaching faculty willing and able to adapt classroom activities and learning environment to the needs of a hearing impaired child."

"To receive a good education."

"Teachers able to sign well."

When they did get around to talking about their needs it became readily apparent that no school program offered anything to the parents other than the rather haphazard catch-as-catch-can programs of the traditional PTO model. Many of the parents were turned off and angered by the insensitivities of school personnel to parents' needs. For example, parents of a 19-year-old needed:

To have educators who themselves were the parents of school-age hearing impaired children. We found that the educators, while with good intentions, seldom showed that they truly understood how it was to not only be involved with the education of these children but how it was to deal with the daily parent-child problems which all parents deal with when working with hearing children but which are multiplied over and over when dealing with hearing impaired children.

A single parent mother of 5- and 7-year-old children who are deaf needed:

A support group consisting of parents that have (had) their hearing impaired children mainstreamed. I still have trouble separating which problems are connected to their hearing loss and normal 'growing pains.' Now that the kids are becoming aware of their difference they are having all kinds of emotions—anger, pain, why me? Blame. I need advice on how to deal with their feelings as well as my own.

A parent of a 24-year-old child which deafness listed the following needs:

1. Knowledge of programs available and quality.
2. Other parents with similar experiences.
3. Relationships with parents of hearing peers so that my child had experience and relationships with other kids in her class.
4. Knowledge of how to make the public school system work for her and skills for me to provide inservice for working with the classroom teacher.

From the mother of a mainstreamed 16-year-old boy:

"Program" has become a dirty word. The term has come to symbolize a complex, generalized set of obstacles organized within a rigid academic institution which guarantees that no one child's needs be evaluated correctly, acknowledged, or met. Having witnessed (and suffered along with) my son's program of the absurd, I can only be thankful there were none for me.

The parent of a 20-year-old mainstreamed child:

Would have liked to have been more involved in decision making as far as what the parents felt was 'in their child's best interests.' So often the 'professionals' made decisions about the child's placement in programs that were not the choices of the child or parents. When parents raised questions about the choice, there was always a 'sterile' explanation by the educator which the less informed could not challenge or succeed in changing any minds. Over a period of time it would often show that the child would suffer the consequences of a bad decision and would lose years of his education as a result of the changes necessary to correct the errors. Listen to the child and the parents more often.

The school-age years are when the methodological decisions made in the preschool years come home to roost. Often the results leave the parents subject to profound feelings of disappointment. The school age years are those times when the parent begins to compare their dream of what their child with deafness was going to turn out to be with the actual emerging reality. A common strategy for a hearing parent in dealing with the initial pain of having a child with hearing impairments is to adopt the notion that the child will be a special case; that he or she will become a super adult with deafness in which there is at worst a very minimal handicap associated with the deafness. The reality for almost all parents is that the deafness has loomed large in their child's life and, although they still love the child very much, they are also experiencing disappointment at the result of the educational choices made. For many parents, this is still a child who is not "normal" and they are disappointed and must somehow come to grips with the child who is there as opposed to the child they wished they had. This is a painful, delicate time for all parents and professionals need to be sensitive to the parents renewed pain. It seems that parents who opted for an oral/aural, mainstreaming route for their child were generally happy with their child's academic skills and communication abilities, but very concerned about the social isolation that a mainstreamed situation entailed. Parents who chose a school for the deaf were generally happy about their child's social abilities but not pleased with their academic accomplishments.

One parent of a 13-year-old currently mainstreamed child who is deaf summed it well when she wrote:

A socially/culturally enriched deaf curriculum with *high academics* . . . . He is grade appropriate in his hearing school—has been on the honor role (sic) every semester. My dream would be for 2 or 3 deaf 13-year-olds to move to our town and mainstream with Todd. I am now in favor of mainstreaming only because of my disappointment in deaf education: the low expectations—the limited offerings—the narrow curriculum. I wish it could all come together and we have tried by trying to split Todd (1/2 day hearing/1/2 day deaf).

The concern about the social isolation of their children and of themselves worries all parents of mainstreamed children. Although many of these children (and parents) would be considered successful by most educators, it is apparent that there are many problems that are not being addressed by the school systems. I think confining our definition of success mainly to speech, language, and academics competency is too narrow. Somehow we must also look at the social and emotional consequences of our educational methodologies as well. The message of the deaf community must be heeded—we all hunger for community and many children who are hearing impaired who are oral successes are severely lacking in community, and although they seem to be educationally successful, they are lonely, isolated, and not very happy. The schools for the deaf, on the other hand, must look at their academic standards and low expectations for youngsters with hearing impairments which severely limit the children's ability to compete vocationally in a very complex world.

The route through this educational morass is, in part, an educated, empowered parent who can keep the educators aware of the broader picture that education of students with hearing impairments should entail. As educators, we must look at the consequences of our educational choices; it is the parent who must live with them. It is only through a true parent/educator partnership that the child benefits. Empowered parents seem to work out their own solutions, often quite creatively. The following letter was received from the mother of a 5-year-old child who is empowered and is fashioning her own program (note how she is not afraid to move her child in and out of programs as needed):

Tyler was enrolled in a School for the Deaf for two years after he left Emerson. The first year he was in a total communication program. In January of his first year, he received a cochlea implant at the MEEI in Boston. He began to hear sounds and speech all around him and began to develop some oral skills. His second year at the School for the Deaf he was enrolled into an oral program that was just developed that year.

Tyler did good both years, but I felt there was a lack of communication between the school, teachers and parents. I think the parents need to be more informed and have an open line of communications with all of the teachers, speech therapist and others that are all working with your child. I think everyone working together and keeping in communication on a regular basis would be very beneficial to everyone involved and you would see faster and more productive progress with your child.

Tyler at age five, has now had the cochlea implant for almost two years. He is now mainstreamed into a special needs pre-kindergarten program with his peers, but they have normal hearing. He is doing fine! I find the teachers to be open and cooperative with me and we all work as a team. We have a common journal that we all write in to keep everyone informed of Tyler's areas of need and progress. The team consists of a head teacher, asst. teacher, speech therapist, and a special aide. He also still sees an outside speech therapist once a week. I think I am fortunate to work with a team of professionals that don't feel intimidated by other professional's opinions and most of all I get to share my opinions!

Tyler's program is a language-based program, which is wonderful. Academically, Tyler needs to work hard in all areas, but math seems to be his best subject. Socially, he is so happy. He is making friends and talks about them all the time. They tell me he loves to sing and recite poems. I have not had the pleasure to see that yet!

I would like to see more programs that offer an aggressive language-based program, teacher-parent teamwork with open lines of communication and a challenging environment that would give them the maximum opportunity to succeed.

For anyone who takes a dispassionate view of the learning/education process, it is quite obvious that parents do play a key and perhaps primary, role in their child's education. At one level, it is a matter of sheer arithmetic. Few children with hearing impairments educated in residential schools[11] (8.6%) and most programs for children with deafness are either day schools or mainstreamed situations, which means that, on a weekly basis, the child has far more contact with the family than with the school. It seems logical, then, that a much more efficient use of school personnel would be to work with the families to ensure that the home environment is conducive to ameliorating the effects of childhood deafness. In short, if we can make the home educationally responsive to the child's needs, we should be able to succeed mightily. To give a single example, we have been teaching deaf children the pragmatics of language skills through conversation.[12] It is obvious that the child would have the most opportunity to converse with the family and, in particular, the parents. Would we not do well to teach the parents how to converse with their child? This means that we must direct our energy at the parents and give them a much more central role in professional thinking than they currently seem to have.

Occasionally, one hears criticism of parent involvement with the statement that "parents should not be teachers." I think this begs the question because all parents, by virtue of their central role in their child's life, are teachers. The goal of parent education should be to enhance the natural teaching that all parents do so as to create a home environment in which the child who is deaf can learn best. To accomplish this goal, we will need parents who are educated and empowered. The recent very cogent studies of Schlessinger[5] demonstrate the value of an empowered parent; she studied 40 families over a 20-year span and found that literacy in the child was most related to empowerment of the mother. An empowered mother was more important to the child learning to read than socioeconomic status, methodology, or hearing loss. This is an incredible finding, and it substantiates what most educators know intuitively: that they need to direct energy and time to incorporating the parents into their educational planning although this seldom seems to happen at the school-age level. Parent education and involvement pays huge dividends. An empowered parent is the greatest asset a child or the school has; it is clear that we need to cultivate and use that asset fully, if we are to succeed in educating children with hearing impairments. Beyond the preschool years, there is no evidence that schools are doing anything actively to educate and involve parents in the educational process so that there is truly a parent-school partnership. There is never any need for an adversarial relationship between the parents and the school because both want the same thing—good things for the child. Yet it seems so difficult to achieve a true working partnership.

Here are some suggestions for school personnel to consider in thinking about parents and perhaps going beyond the limited PTO model that seems to be currently in vogue:

1. Before the school year begins, all parents should be visited at home by the teacher. The purpose of this visit is in part to draw up a contract of parent participation in their child's education for the year. This is beyond the individual educational planning meeting, which is a group meeting. The purpose of this meeting, on the parent's turf, is to discuss the nature of the parent's participation in the child's schooling. This can be minimal if it is arrived at by parent-teacher decision. These contracts need to be flexible in nature and renegotiated over the school year. I think there always needs to be some element of parent involvement in every contract.

2. Schools should try to establish support groups for parents. These groups need to deal with affect issues as well as content discussions; the content should emerge from the needs of the group. For parents of mainstreamed children, the groups will probably have to be established on a regional basis and may take the format of an intensive day-long workshop where by the parents receive information and also have an opportunity to network. School personnel need to look at the learning vacation model sponsored so enthusiastically by Gallaudet University, where parents and children are enrolled in a camp-like environment to actively learn together and recreate together.

3. Attitudes of school personnel need to change. Parents must be seen as central to the educational process. Educators will need increased skills in dealing with parental needs, which they probably did not receive in their training programs. Schools, therefore, will have to provide ongoing in-service experience for their personnel. All educators must understand fully the notion that if you take good care of the parents, the children will turn out well.

REFERENCES

1. Bodner-Johnson B. The family in perspective, in Luterman D, ed: *Deafness in Perspective* (San Diego, CA: College Hill Press, 1986).
2. Lowell EL: Parent infant programs for preschool deaf children. The example of the John Tracy Clinic. *Volta Rev*, 81 (1979), 323–329.
3. Luterman D. A family centered program for hearing impaired children, in Roush J, ed: *Infants and Toddlers with Hearing Loss: Family-Centered Assessment and Intervention*, (Parkton, MD: York Press, in press).

4. Luterman D: *Counseling the Communicatively Disordered and Their Families.* (Austin TX, Pro-Ed, 1991).

5. Schlesinger H: The elusive X factor: parental contributions to literacy, Edited by Walworth M, Modres D, O'Rourke T, eds: *A Free Hand* (Silver Springs, MD: TS Publishers, 1992).

6. Wright D: *Deafness.* New York: Stein & Day, (1969).

7. Shipley K: *Interviewing and Counseling in Communication Disorders.* (New York: Macmillan Publishing, 1992).

8. Clark C, Martin, F: *Effective Counseling in Audiology* (Englewood Cliffs, NJ: Prentice Hall 1994).

9. Rogers C: *Client Centered Therapy* (Boston: Houghton, Mifflin, 1951).

10. McCarthy P, Culpepper N, Lucks L: Variability in counseling Experience and Training Among ESB Accredited Programs. *ASHA* 28 (1986), 49–53.

11. U.S. Department of Education. Twelfth Annual Report to Congress on the Implementation of the Handicapped Act (Washington DC: U.S. Government Printing Office, 1990).

12. Kretchmer R, Kretchmer L: Language in perspective, in Luterman D, ed: *Deafness In Perspective.* (San Diego, CA: College Hill Press 1986).

ENHANCING THE SELF-IMAGE OF THE MAINSTREAM CHILD WITH AUDITORY DISORDERS

Susan P. Russell

The greatest magnifying glasses in the world are a man's own eyes when they look upon his own person.

—Alexander Pope, 1688–1744

Self-image is most often defined as the manner in which a person describes the way he perceives himself. There are different domains of self-image. For a child, some of the most important domains include the *academic*, how a child defines himself or herself as a student and how the child perceives his or her own achievement in a classroom setting; *the social/emotional or personal*, which includes relationships within the family, as well as other interpersonal exchanges; and *the physical*, how a child perceives his outward physical appearance and related physical or athletic abilities. Each domain develops and changes as a child grows and matures and is by the impact of the experiences encountered throughout the years. Within these domains, a child's self-image is going to be influenced by the people and experiences in two important environments: home and school.

Parents have the earliest and perhaps the major role in influencing the development of a positive self-image in their children. Parents have the opportunity, right from the start, to establish an atmosphere of acceptance, and to plant the seeds of confidence and competence in their children. As the child grows older, teachers join parents in this endeavor and play an important supporting role. There are many books and articles for parents and professionals on enhancing children's self-concept. "Seven Secrets for Building Kids' Self-Esteem"[1] is described in Table 19–1. These guidelines help the adults create an *environment* at home and at school conducive to and supportive of building a strong and positive self-image. Marshall's ways to influence self-concept in children[2] addresses more the *skills* on which to focus when a good self-concept is the goal (Table 19–2). We can see that both the climate that is created for the child and the direct teaching of

skills impact significantly on the development of self-image.

Development of self-image for children who are deaf or hard of hearing will also be influenced by all of these factors and strategies, and each one can make a positive difference. However, there is much more to the picture. Each of the three domains mentioned, academic, social/emotional, and physical, is likely to be impacted on by hearing loss.

There is no dispute that having a hearing loss has consequences within the parameters of a hearing world. Maxon et al[3] delineate the potential separateness that a student who is deaf may experience in a mainstream setting: communication difficulties in both academic and social situations; the visibility of necessary amplification; difficulty in listening situations; and the need to leave the classroom for support services. Additionally, the following factors also impact on the self-concept of a student who is deaf: the global impact of language and communication skill development, the role of these skills in developing age-appropriate social interactions, and the often resulting isolation, exclusion, or rejection;[4] the different settings or programs in which a student's self-image might be high or low (ie, mainstream vs residential); the role that degree of hearing loss, age of onset, or gender plays;[3] the significance of having deaf or hearing parents.[5,6]

The measures used for evaluating self-concept in students who are deaf have proved problematical in their own right. Oblowitz et al[4] have examined the linguistic-related issues and problems for students who are deaf, using a variety of standard measures of evaluating self-concept. Suggestions that have come out of these studies include controlling the linguistic content of the test items and modifying the presentation to be more

Table 19-1   Seven Secrets for Building Kids' Self-Esteem[1]

Build in success	Success builds self-esteem, especially when the chain of successes remains continuous and unbroken
State the positive	Acknowledging the positive in a nonevaluative but validating way nurtures success
Capitalize on successes	Children will feel success is possible if you can help them build a history of similar successes
Watch for growth sparks	Children with low self-esteem tend to believe they cannot grow, learn, or successfully relate to other people. Often they do not until a spark of interest is ignited
Value and acknowledge	Evidence of success that is visible and tangible has a strong positive effect on a child's self-esteem
Keep expectations realistic	Clearly stating reasonable expectations will help children with low self-esteem feel less anxious about pleasing others
Do not be boring	Boredom depresses self-esteem; interest and excitement increase a sense of self. Active involvement in life nourishes self-esteem

Table 19-2   Ways to Influence Self-Concept[2]

Help children feel they are of value	Listen attentively to what they say; ask for their suggestions
	Help them identify their own positive and prosocial behavior
Help children feel they are competent	Provide experiences for children where they can succeed
	Provide new challenges and comment on positive attempts
	Teach strategies to accomplish tasks
	Allow them to carry out and complete tasks themselves
Help children feel they have some control	Provide opportunities for choice, initiative, and autonomy
	Avoid comparison between children; avoid competition
	Help children learn to evaluate their own accomplishments
Help children learn interpersonal skills	Help children learn skills to enter interactions with others
Become aware of your own expectations for children	Be open to perceiving new information about children and looking at them in new ways
	Be aware of whether your expectations differ for boys and girls

pictorial/conceptual. New items need to be added to current evaluation tools, including items related to communication, acceptance of disability, feelings of being different and excluded, perceptions of positive regard, and perceptions of academic competence in a context beyond the world of individuals who are hearing impaired. It will be beneficial to have further research in these areas, as they are all issues that are important to examine when looking at the self-image of a student who is deaf.

When a child who is deaf has deaf parents, the overall process of development is more parallel to that of hearing children of hearing parents. Language growth goes through comparable stages of development, and the child is likely to see himself like his parents. However, when the parents are hearing, as is the case in 90% of the families, the child who is deaf may have a more difficult time sorting out how he sees and defines himself and how he fits in as a member of the family. This often results in significant issues of acceptance that can adversely affect the development of self-image.

That same dynamic can occur with a child who is deaf in a mainstream setting. The mainstream program in a public school system mirrors that scenario of a child who is deaf in a hearing family—and brings the same potential for feelings of isolation and rejection. Just as family dynamics differ, so do mainstream programs; like families, some are more successful at meeting these challenges.

When examining the concept of mainstreaming for students who are hard of hearing or deaf, and the qualities and destinies that these students may possess, the literature often begins with a look back at the period since the passage of Public Law 94-142 in 1975, and the successes and failures of the almost 20 years since that law was enacted. The field of education of children who are deaf or hard of hearing has been greatly impacted on by this legislation. However, this field of education has never been free of controversy and debate, and the law did not change this fact.

Today, as we learn and experience more about deaf culture, the concept of "least restrictive environment" and indeed, mainstream programs themselves are under greater scrutiny. Regardless, in 1994, mainstreaming is a reality. So is the likelihood that the parents of children who are deaf or hard of hearing will be hearing people. These are facts that are not going to disappear in the very near future. In light of these realities, the purpose of this discussion is not to look at what is good or bad about the law, and not to debate the merits of a residential school versus a mainstream experience. Rather, this discussion seeks to identify specific ways to enhance a deaf student's self-image in a mainstream setting. This is really the crux of the matter: maximizing a student's potential by making the mainstream setting as productive as possible within the parameters that exist.

Unfortunately, there has not been much written specifically for students with deafness in the mainstream for enhancing self-image. *Skillstreaming* techniques,[7] although not specifically developed for deaf students, deal with special education students in general, and the increasing need for teaching prosocial skills. This is a tremendously important area for students in a mainstream setting, where social skills may lag behind other skills. In this book there are a total of 60 skills covered in five basic areas: classroom survival skills; friendship-making skills; skills for dealing with feelings; skill alternatives to aggression; and skills for dealing with stress. It is well laid out for parents and professionals, and is an excellent resource for building students' confidence in social and mainstream settings.

Schwartz[8] delineates four critical areas that impact on the psychosocial development of children who are in a mainstream setting: clear communication; parental support; extracurricular activities; and social skills. These issues are key in the development of children who are deaf, and are interwoven in many of the strategies related to strengthening self-image. Grimes and Prickett[9] give an overview of the issues involved in self-concept of children who are deaf, and do provide ideas for enhancing its positive development, although not specifically from a mainstream perspective. They describe a positive self-concept as comprised of many wonderful components—including pride, acceptance, responsibility, and independence. These are indeed the positive qualities for which to strive.

The ideas presented in this chapter reflect my experiences working with the staff, families, and students in the Montgomery County Public Schools, Programs for Students Who Are Deaf and Hard of Hearing (formerly the Auditory Program). This is a day program for children who are deaf and hard of hearing within the public school system in Montgomery County, Maryland, a suburb of Washington, DC. This program has a total population of approximately 320 students, from birth through age 21 years. The students have a range of degree of hearing loss, receive a broad continuum of services, and use different communication approaches (sign language, cued speech, oral/aural). Reflecting the accepted statistics, hearing parents outnumber deaf parents. Although the focus here is on the mainstream environment, many of the following ideas are appropriate for public school programs where there are special classes for children who are deaf. Regardless of the placement, the more focused the attitudes are of the families and staff working with the students, and the more effectively home and school can work together, the stronger the self-image will be for these students who are deaf.

The mainstream life of a student with deafness, and the strategies to achieve success will be divided into two environments: at home and at school. These two environments are both important when developing and enhancing self-image. Each of these environments will be examined from two perspectives: strategies that impact on the overall climate, making it more accepting and positive for the students with deafness; and those skills that the student needs to develop to strengthen and enhance his or her self-image.

AT HOME

Climate

Parents are the first and most important people who affect the development of a child's self-image. The single best predictor of self-concept among children with deafness is related to parental child-rearing attitudes.[10] The attitude that a parent projects of acceptance of deafness, commitment to clear and consistent communication at home, and involvement in school with the related guidance and support all play an important role for building a positive self-image. Home should be a place of unconditional love and unconditional acceptance.

Acceptance of Deafness. When hearing parents have a child who is deaf, there is often a sense that the child is different from themselves.

There is an emotional process of understanding and acceptance parents go through, each at their own rate. Professionals need to work with parents to help them arrive at the conclusion that their child, while unique in his or her deafness, is also special simply as their child. This relates to the social/emotional domain of self-image. What parents then do for their relationship with their child with deafness affects the way this child looks at himself as a member of the family, and as a potential member of both a hearing society and a deaf culture.

Support for Parents. Parents need support, in different ways, at every level of their child's development. A parent who feels confident and secure is more likely to be successful at developing a good self-concept in their child. A *parent group* can provide a venue for gaining information, validating practices, and sharing concerns. At the parent-infant or preschool level, this group addresses the parents' more basic and immediate needs about deafness, interacting and communicating with their young children, issues of amplification, and support from other parents.

For a parent with an older child, there is an additional need of being able to support and cope with a child who may be experiencing feelings of isolation or rejection. Although evidence shows that attendance at parent groups declines as the child progresses through school, the need for information and support continues. Talking with other parents continues to help put feelings and anxieties in perspective, to enable a parent better to deal more effectively with the child.

In conjunction with, or as an alternative to parent groups, a trained *parent educator* or *counselor* for parents of children who are deaf can be a tremendous resource for parents. This professional can help parents deal with all aspects of child-rearing, as well as with issues specifically related to deafness. Such a person should be available to parents in groups or individually to link up parents who may have similar needs or suggest a "veteran" parent for one facing a new experience. Knowing what is part of "normal" development (which many of us tend to lose sight of) is often helpful, as is having someone with whom to share thoughts, who can offer ideas and solutions. In our program there is a teacher who recruits the parent counselor for monthly discussion groups, where parents can come together and share ideas and concerns in conjunction with a planned topic presentation. Being able to deal with your child as an individual with deafness, and being able to say that deafness is fine, has

an incredible effect on how the child sees himself and how his self-image develops. This is one of the basic tenets of self-concept.

Access to Deaf Individuals. Having access to individuals with deafness can be beneficial for hearing parents to get a different perspective on what it is like to be deaf and perhaps to understand better life from their child's viewpoint. One approach is to present a "panel" of teens who are deaf or adults from different backgrounds and experiences, perhaps as part of a parent meeting series, or the previously mentioned parent group. This kind of presentation provides an opportunity for sharing valuable information and feelings that books cannot adequately communicate. The Washington, DC, area is fortunate to have a large population of individuals with deafness, and the opportunities that go with this community. There are social events, dramatic performances, and sporting events through Gallaudet University and local organizations that are available for families. All of these can provide parents with an inside view of deaf culture.

A school program or parent organization can call on their resources to sponsor informational meetings and workshops. One well-received workshop is a Deaf Awareness Day for parents and the community. A variety of presentations on cultural topics, opportunities for questions and answers, as well as time for more informal social interactions can be scheduled. It can be a positive experience for the parents and can lead to a greater overall understanding of deaf culture.

In a different type of outreach, the Deaf and Hard of Hearing Program has developed an educational videotape series, through the Montgomery County Public Schools educational cable television channel. The series, "Stop, Look and Listen," is designed to inform and educate parents of young children with deafness. Each show, as part of the format, spotlights teens and adults from the community who are deaf. These segments, which have received positive feedback from parents, help present a view of what their child can grow up to be, supporting a positive sense of potential and possibility. This "can do" attitude is showcased on "About Me," which examines ways to build self-esteem in children who are deaf. The series is open captioned, which in itself alerts parents of the technology available to serve individuals with deafness. Having a technological resource like television, and the ability to reach out to parents in their own homes through cable and videocassette, has proved to be very valuable.

Communication. Part of accepting a child's deafness is understanding the kind of communication challenges that deafness can bring, and the commitment that parents and the family must make to be part of that communication system. It is widely accepted that one of the most powerful factors influencing a student's development and achievement is appropriate, clear and consistent communication at home. For a child with deafness with parents with deafness, this communication happens automatically and naturally, from birth. No time is lost; the diagnosis of the child's hearing loss is secondary.

In contrast, with hearing parents, effective communication does not happen from the start. The hearing loss may not even be diagnosed for 2 or 3 valuable language-learning years. This starts the deaf child of hearing parents off at a disadvantage. If parents do not make the commitment to effective communication, the child can be more vulnerable to developing a negative self-image. A child who feels included as part of the family dynamic will feel positively about himself and his role in the family. Parents need to take the responsibility to develop their child's communication skills, while building their own, as well.

As a child goes through the normal stages of development, during childhood and adolescence, parents will have to deal with the range of feelings that will inevitably occur. Being a child who is deaf in a mainstream setting can magnify feelings of isolation and rejection, real or perceived; these same feelings should not have to be experienced at home, or, for that matter, away from home, at a store or restaurant. For example, the child needs to know that this commitment to communication is full-time, and neither child nor parent should feel any embarrassment about using their hands in public to communicate. A parent needs to develop the communication skills and competence to discuss any thoughts, ideas, and issues on a level appropriate for their child. Parents and adolescents with deafness also need to be able to discuss honestly the differences between the deaf and hearing worlds, an openness that ultimately leads to a feeling of parental acceptance.[11] Communication at home addresses the social/emotional domain of self-image, the necessary ability to have meaningful relationships among family members. Parents who make that commitment to clear and consistent communication have a greater ability to give the kind of support, and show the kind of acceptance, that a child needs to feel part of the family.

Instructional Classes and Materials. Parents often need encouragement and assistance in finding appropriate instructional classes and materials to help them meet the communication needs of their child with deafness. Contacting a local college or the adult education office in their area about classes is a good place to start. Organizations for individuals who are deaf and their families have resources and materials available for parents.

Instructional classes for parents and family members may be offered through the local parent organization or the school program. Instructional classes such as these are welcomed by parents, and not only do the parents who attend feel good about themselves and their efforts, but teachers also report a positive impact on the children, which is ultimately the goal.

Building on the known accessibility of videotape technology, there are instructional videotape series for both sign language and cued speech, which the staff may provide to parents. Montgomery County Department of Public Libraries has a Special Needs Library devoted to materials and resources for people with disabilities. There is a wide range of videotape and print materials not only on developing communication skills, but on deafness in general. When a parent takes advantage of these classes and resources, it sends positive messages of support and value to the child, translating to a positive feeling of self-worth.

School Involvement. Parent involvement at school is important for all children, and this may be even more true for deaf children in a mainstream setting, where the school attended may not be their neighborhood school. Sometimes, as a result of not living in proximity to the school and not being part of that community, parents may have the feeling of needing to prove that they, and their child, "belong" to the school. Some parents view themselves in a "public relations" role in the school, feeling that a constructive level of visibility and contribution is necessary. Being involved in school activities and projects provides a way for parents not only positively to impact on their child, but also the whole school program with regard to having students with deafness as part of that program. In Montgomery County, schools have a "special needs chairperson" for the PTA. This role may be filled by a parent of a child with deafness, and can help ensure that programs and extracurricular events take into account the needs of deaf children (eg, interpreting services for school programs).

Supporting the School Team.   Children need to feel that all the adults in their environment are working together for their benefit and that all fronts are united. Krupp[12] supports the concept that parents and teachers who are willing to work together have the best chance of helping students develop a sense of higher self-esteem. When parents openly work against the school team, it can confuse a child and make him question his support system, as well as his place in it.

This does not mean that parents should be spectators, simply sitting back and agreeing with the professionals. There should be an appropriate process in place for disagreement, discussion, and resolution. When a child sees that there is open communication between school and home, that everyone knows the same information, his confusion is lessened. Establishing appropriate channels of communication helps give parents feelings of comfort and control. For a child to feel comfortable and secure in a classroom setting, it is necessary to have teamwork among all the adults.

Student Skills

Parents have a critical role in the development of skills that will enable their children to feel positive and successful in life, and to develop a strong self-image. For a child with deafness in a mainstream setting, parent involvement is just as important, if not more so. Parents of children who are deaf have expressed that, although they practice their own child-rearing philosophies, nothing magical or different, they do so more consciously and purposefully for their child. A resource such as *MegaSkills*[13] can provide parents with useful and practical information on the kinds of skills that all students, including students who are deaf, need to develop to be confident and successful students. It may take more effort for students who are deaf, but the payoff is well worth it. The two major areas in which parents can play a direct role are language skills and social skills, addressing both the academic and social/emotional domains of self-image.

Language Skills.   The most pervasive problem that a student with deafness can experience is one of a language delay. As discussed previously, when a child who is deaf is born to hearing parents, the hearing loss may not be detected for several years. In the meantime, valuable language-learning time is lost. If the child is to be successful in school and in life and reach her

potential, there must be a strong language base on which to build. Therefore, language learning must take place at *all* times, not just at school. Home is a place for language input as well, and parents must be prepared to take on this task.

The parent first and foremost needs to develop the communication skills discussed before. There is so much communication and language that happens (or should happen) on a day to day basis. Experiences at the supermarket, at the dinner table, or at the gas station all contribute to a child's comprehension of the world around him. Clear communication impacts on overall language development, which correlates to how the student who is deaf is going to function in a mainstream class.

Academic Support.   For a child in a mainstream setting, supporting academic goals at home is an area where parents can and should play an important role. Having the communication skills and understanding enables the parent to go over a spelling list, drill and practice mathematical facts, and review for a social studies or science test. These kinds of activities are important, and contribute to increased confidence in the classroom. A child who is well-prepared for school each day, ready with homework, and familiar with the vocabulary used and the concepts being taught, will feel better about himself, and more willingly participate in the teacher's questions and classroom discussions. That feeling of success will build on itself.

There are other areas of language that a parent can and should continue to support, which may not seem at first glance directly related to school, but are relevant to supporting a stronger self-image in a mainstream setting. An understanding of the language of the world around them is critical. This effortlessly "happens" for hearing students, but needs to be consciously presented to students with deafness. Knowledge of current local and world events can put a student who is deaf in a better position to participate in class discussions and understand references and comparisons presented in their subject areas. Just as important if not more so is the awareness of the current pop culture. When children are concerned about "fitting in," there are few things that have the potential to impact on them like the social concerns of television, movies, radio, fashion, and, of course, the latest social slang. These are media to which a child with deafness may not have access. Decoders are helpful, as are other printed materials, such as books, newspapers, and magazines. However parents can play a major role in presenting and discussing these concepts, and supporting this aspect of language development.

Students may get academic support from in-school personnel, but the home support provided from parents can make a critical contribution to the way the child perceives himself as a student in a competitive classroom as shown in Case study 19–1.

Case study 19–1.   David is in the fourth grade and has been in mainstream classes since kindergarten. His parents demonstrate the kind of commitment to consistent communication that results in a child who feels part of his family and part of his class.

Starting with an oral education, investigating cued speech, and currently using sign language primarily, these parents saw the value in assessing what would work best for their son, and then how they worked to support it. Between them, they have taken many instructional classes to develop and refine their skills. To make communication as clear as possible for David, they use a combination of these communication approaches as appropriate.

Always thinking about ways to expand David's language and cognitive development, these parents make the effort to include him fully in all communication that takes place at home. For them, this ranges from explaining the humor of a popular television show to discussing the latest United States involvement overseas.

At home, David knows that his parents are a dependable source of information, support, and guidance, and he takes this knowledge and support to school with him. Although the specific topics may not directly relate to the curriculum units, he is developing an understanding of the world around him. This knowledge is powerful. David feels more confident in classroom discussions and peer interactions.

Social Skills.   A child with deafness needs to have appropriate social behaviors and manners, as does any child. Children with appropriate manners and positive interpersonal skills are more attractive to other children, and for a child in a mainstream setting, these behaviors and skills help increase the likelihood of acceptance.

Responsibility and Independence.   Building qualities such as responsibility and independence can contribute to school success and a positive sense of self for a child in a mainstream setting. There are many ways to build these qualities at home that carry over to school. It can be as simple as a child dressing himself, doing household chores and duties, getting his own things ready for school, or getting out and completing his homework. All of these things can develop pride in a job well-done and done on his own. This pride in accomplishment and of doing things himself makes a more confident student. Parents may be too overprotective, trying to compensate for a perceived deficiency they think comes with deafness. However, fostering independence gives the child a chance to do for himself, perhaps to try and fail, but to learn from mistakes and then try again. These skills, when supported by parents, help develop confidence along with the risk-taking skills so critical for success.

Social Opportunities.   Having the opportunity to be in a variety of social situations helps to develop the familiarity and confidence that will be important for working in a mainstream setting as well as in society later in life. Parents should try to seek out a variety of playmates for their child, both deaf and hearing, to give the child the chance to learn how to deal with different people and personalities, experiment with different social strategies, and practice the interpersonal skills that they may be learning in school or at home. Also helpful is providing opportunities out in the community, perhaps at a restaurant, where the child has the chance to build appropriate manners and etiquette and parents can be there as a support. These are opportunities and strategies built and supported by parents that will positively effect the child's behavior and comfort level in the mainstream and enhance her self-image.

AT SCHOOL

Climate

The school environment encompasses a large number of people who can have an impact on the self-image of the student with deafness. The climate of a school sends a message to the child: one of acceptance or rejection. School climate encompasses all three of the domains of self-image: academic, social/emotional, and physical. Our goal here is to examine strategies that help support a more positive and accepting environment, one where deafness is respected and celebrated.

There are successful practices that positively influence a school's climate, which in turn affects the student's perception of herself as a member of that school. History, or how long students have been part of the overall school population, influences this climate. The longer the history, the more there is a sense among staff and students of ownership and permanence, rather than a situation that will go away. In our Program for Deaf and Hard of Hearing Students, schools are not dispersed throughout the county, as is often the case in public school programs. Instead, schools were selected that were in the same "cluster," so that the school population, deaf and hearing, stays constant as the students move through the grades from preschool through 12th grade. The goal is for familiarity with deafness to foster understanding, sensitivity, and acceptance among students, staff, and principals who are hearing.

Deaf Awareness. In developing a positive climate in a school it is important to educate the staff, students, and community about deafness and the population of students with deafness. There are many practical and effective ways of providing this kind of information on an ongoing basis to the school community.

Staff and Student In-Service Programs. Providing information and ideas to the staff and hearing students in the school is one effective way of demystifying deafness. Included in a presentation would be the "physical" attributes of deafness: anatomical and audiological information, and explanations of equipment and assistive technology used (decoders, teletypwriters (TTYs), hearing aids, frequency modulation (FM) trainers). Also important is the discussion of the communication systems used by people who are deaf (and by the students in that school, if different) and effective communication strategies that can be utilized.

Individuals who are deaf (students, staff, and community) can and should play an integral role in an in-service program. Consulting ahead of time with the student with deafness who may be in the mainstream class, explaining the presentation, and soliciting feedback, are all important steps to take before going into a classroom. Feedback shows that when done respectfully, the student who is deaf feels proud to be able to share something very unique to him.

Bulletin Boards and Classroom Displays. Displays of information in and around the school can provide ongoing reinforcement of a variety of topics, from use of the national relay system and TTY etiquette, to audiological equipment, to people in history who were deaf. Bookcovers or clippings from recent newspaper articles can also be posted. Included should be whatever is most relevant not only to the population of students who are deaf in that particular school, but also items of interest and relevance to deaf culture and the larger circle of people with deafness.

School-Wide Assemblies and Programs. School-wide functions can provide a way to present people who are deaf in a variety of roles. In our program, a visiting production by a deaf/hearing drama troupe from the National Technical Institute for the Deaf performed at several schools where students with deafness attend. The performances provided insight into the deaf perspective. In addition to theatrical presentations of fairy tales and stories, there were skits dealing with deaf culture as well.

A local performing arts academy has also incorporated students who are deaf into its productions, forming a deaf access company which performs publicly, including performances at school functions, for school staff and students during the school day, and in evening school programs for parents and the community.

Participation of students with deafness in school productions also sends a positive message to the students who are deaf and to the school as a whole. Students with deafness in Montgomery County schools have had leading and backstage roles in several productions at both the elementary and secondary levels. Some of the schools have taken a slightly different direction and have put on all-deaf student productions. These have been presented to the entire student body with voice interpretation, and in some cases to other school programs where there are students who are deaf. These types of productions put students who are deaf in a positive spotlight for the whole school to see, and it is an inspiring sight to see the hearing student audience wave their hands in applause.

One school program currently has a music teacher who cultivated an interest in sign language, developed her skills through classes, and then made sign language an integral part of her music program.[14] She formed a unique choral group, "The Fabulous Flying Fingers," made up of 5th graders who are hearing and deaf, which performs all of their numbers in song and sign. It has developed a special reputation for all students in the school. The group travels and performs around the Washington, DC, area, and showcases the recognition and respect in the school for students with deafness and sign language.

Presence of Interpreters.   Working with interpreters for students with deafness and staff is new for many school staff members, but it should be an important part of the school program. Educating the school staff that interpreter coverage needs to be arranged not only for classroom instruction, but assemblies and programs, lunchtime, "special subjects" like art, music, and physical education, as well as visits to the school nurse or principal, is important. The high visibility of interpreters can become a good source of public relations. Having staff who are deaf in the school provides an ongoing awareness of the need for including interpreters, for they will be seen at faculty meetings and conferences. Understanding this need for interpreters, and the role they play in and out of the classroom, contributes to the climate for students with deafness in the school.

Role of Deaf Students, Teens, and Adults.
Recruiting a variety of persons who are deaf in different roles in a school is very important. Role models are invaluable in developing a greater understanding about deafness, as well as creating a positive school climate. Adults who are deaf not only provide a perspective of "what it's like to be deaf," they also show that children with deafness grow up and can aspire to the same goals as other children. This can be accomplished by hiring staff who are deaf at the school, by inviting adults with deafness from the community as guest speakers or mentors, welcoming parents who are deaf as volunteers in the classroom, or inviting teens with deafness from the secondary program to the preschool or elementary level as interns or aides.

Staff with deafness at school gives the rest of the school staff an ongoing learning opportunity, while providing them with a unique view of the needs of students with deafness as well. Such staff will require interpreters (as mentioned) or note-takers at staff and team meetings and can share first-hand experiences with other staff members.

Montgomery County currently runs a program, "Montgomery Exceptional Leaders (MEL)" which was developed by the Superintendent's Advisory Committee on the Rights of Disabled Individuals. This group consists of teams of high school students with disabilities who travel across the county to different elementary schools, presenting first-hand accounts of their own disabilities, and more importantly, their own abilities. These presentations give young children not only the exposure to deafness, but the opportunity to ask questions and get to know a person who is deaf as an individual.

This program also plays an important role in the development of self-image for the high school students with deafness who participate. The student with deafness gets a positive sense of contributing to a better acceptance and understanding of deafness. This leads not only to the development of poise and confidence in public presentations, but also to a different understanding about being a deaf person and more positive feelings about themselves as shown in Case study 19–2.

> **Case study 19–2.** Matthew is a 22-year-old college senior and a graduate of our program. In mainstream classes from the upper elementary years through high school, he was academically successful. During his high school years, he was a member of the Montgomery Exceptional Leaders (MEL) program. Looking back at the experience, Matthew was able to see how much his involvement in this program affected the way he saw himself as an individual, and as a deaf person.
>
> As a child, Matthew was very shy and reserved. When he got to high school and joined the MEL program, he saw he had the chance to influence how young children developed an understanding and acceptance of deaf people. In preparing for this endeavor, he had to look closely at himself, at his strengths and at his limitations.
>
> The actual presentations gave Matthew the confidence and poise that would carry over to his mainstream classes and his interpersonal relationships, both in high school and college. He was able to compile a definition of himself that *he* liked and felt comfortable with. It helped *him* feel good not only as a person, but as a deaf person.

Having people with deafness in the environment is positive for the hearing students, but students who are deaf need appropriate role models who are deaf, and this is particularly significant for those students in a mainstream setting. While getting an academically challenging program, these students also need opportunities to connect with other individuals with deafness. In Montgomery County, our program is fortunate to be large in comparison to other public school systems. There may be more than one student in a mainstream class, if not for the full day, for at least part of the day. This allows for some creative rolemodeling within the program.

There are effective strategies for widening the circle of peers who are deaf. Telephone numbers for a student TTY directory can be collected and distributed to students who are deaf and their families, to put them in touch with other students at different schools within the county. Pen pal letters or electronic bulletin boards on the computer can supplement these opportunities. Newspapers done by students at the elementary and secondary levels can be shared among deaf students at other schools. A newspaper of this sort is particularly beneficial for the itinerant population, where a student may indeed be the only student who is deaf or hard of hearing in the school. The "Montgomery Messenger" brings stories and experiences to the hundred or so students who are deaf and hard of hearing across the county who contribute to this newspaper. The students report positive feelings of knowing there are other students out there like themselves. Teachers and parents can use these connections to develop relationships further between students, who may be in different schools but share common experiences.

Young students always look up to the older students in their school or program. Older students with deafness can fill a variety of roles for the younger ones. Within a school, pairings of older and younger students who are deaf, perhaps for a story time, can give both parties a sense of connection and belonging. Teens who are deaf doing their community service requirement or child development practicum in the preschool or elementary program, or volunteering in the summer school program, contribute to positive feelings among the younger students. Older students are uniquely able to support and advise younger students in a mainstream setting, as those who have "been there." Sharing feelings between those who share a special bond is invaluable for helping students feel comfortable with who they are.

Communication Skill Development. The nature of deafness means unique communication needs. How these needs are met is often the center of controversy. Our main concern here is how to ensure that a mainstream setting will effectively meet the communication needs of students with deafness so that isolation can be minimized as much as possible. Obviously, a mainstream program has to be creative in its approach to achieving the goal of complete communication access for students who are deaf. Working successfully with interpreters, as already mentioned, certainly plays a critical role in the communication between both populations. However, there is value in developing the communication skills of the hearing staff and students, trying to build a bridge of acceptance for all.

Instructional Classes.   Achieving a level of effective communication for both staff and students is critical to any successful school climate. It is made more challenging when students with deafness are part of that environment. Offering instructional classes and opportunities for learning sign language or cued speech, perhaps as a lunchtime or after-school activity, is one way to encourage direct interaction and communication between students and staff who are deaf and hearing. Where sign language and cued speech classes or clubs are offered, students who are hearing often develop excellent communication skills which fosters positive relationships with students who are deaf. Staff members, from teachers to secretaries to cafeteria workers should have the opportunity to develop these skills as well.

In-School Opportunities.   Developing creative in-school activities for students who are hearing to build communication skills addresses students who may not be able to participate in after-school classes. By offering specific activities during the school day, an attitude of acceptance is reinforced.

One creative and effective approach involves the music teacher previously mentioned. In this case, sign language is integrated into the students' music program from kindergarten through grade 5. This is done regardless of whether there is a student with deafness in that class. This provides a uniquely comfortable atmosphere for the students, with deafness, particularly considering that music is not often thought of as a positive activity for them. For the students who hear, the result is not only a greater familiarity, but often fluency in sign language. Students who are deaf are likely to feel more included in classroom activities if those around them have some comfort level with their communication method.

To encourage communication between classmates who are deaf and hearing outside of school, a TTY loaner program has been developed. Hearing students have a training session on using a TTY and then borrow one to take home to call deaf classmates. This gives students who are deaf a chance to develop relationships with classmates outside of school, and provides a social link important to the development of a strong self-image (see Case study 19–3).

Extracurricular Activities.   Extracurricular activities are of great value, and must be available to all students, including the students in the school who are deaf. Transportation may be an impeding factor, but it is well worth the effort on the part of parents to try to make necessary arrangements. In extracurricular activities students are often put

Case study 19–3. Brian is in the seventh grade in mainstream classes, but the work does not come easily to him and he has to put forth a lot of effort. "Fitting in" and having friends are important to him, as they are to any child.

When in elementary school, Brian's class was involved in a TTY loaner program. The communication specialist in the school implemented the TTY loaner program, which was successful in his class. Many students were anxious to participate.

The result? Brian was able to call his classmates. He was able to initiate communication comfortably. This provided the vehicle for sharing homework assignments and sports statistics. He had the opportunity to feel special in his experience and expertise, and the TTY activity helped him to see himself more as a member of the class. In fact, the program was so successful that Brian and other members of the school's student council raised money for a TTY for the school.

on a more equal plane, quite different from the competition in the academic arena. Students have the opportunity to show different sides of their personalities, skills, and talents that may not be recognized in the classroom.

Athletic activities are an example of this. A student who has physical and athletic talents becomes a sought out classmate, as the respect and admiration from the playing field carries over to the classroom. A recognized school-wide honor like patrols also relates directly to a student's self-concept. This special position, like participation in student government, is one that is highly regarded throughout the school. These activities provide the student who is deaf with a chance to develop not only a sense of responsibility and teamwork, but also confidence and positive feelings about herself.

Deaf culture clubs, deaf awareness activities, "Deaf and Hearing Power," and the Junior National Association of the Deaf (NAD) are extracurricular types of activities that can be implemented at both the elementary and secondary levels. These groups may be made up of only students who are deaf, or mixed deaf and hearing. Planned events can include guest speakers and field trips in addition to the use of videotaped materials. These activities provide ongoing opportunities for all to learn more about Deaf Culture and American Sign Language through drama,

literature, and informal interactions with other people who are deaf, as shown in Case study 19–4. Exposure and acceptance from this perspective cannot come too early.

Case study 19–4. Amy is in the fifth grade and is fully mainstreamed. She had been struggling with her identity and self-esteem as a deaf person. The factors she perceived that made her feel "different," including hearing aids and an interpreter, are magnified in a mainstream setting.

Amy's school has started a Deaf Awareness Club. As part of this program, a graduate of our program, a young man who is now a professional athlete, was invited to be a guest speaker. He presented to the entire student body. Everyone was excited and enthusiastic.

Amy was positively impressed by the presentation on several accounts. She saw a popular and successful adult with deafness wearing hearing aids, using his audition and speechreading skills to the maximum, without hesitation. She saw him use an interpreter in front of this large audience without embarrassment, and she saw that all of these "differences" had not made a difference in his aspirations and achievements. For Amy, having this experience helped her look at herself in a more positive light.

Teacher Attitudes.   Attitude can be one of the most subtle, yet one of the most critical factors in how a student perceives his place and success in the classroom. Difficult to measure objectively, the presence or absence of the "right" attitude can definitely be felt by students and staff alike. Does the teacher view the student with deafness as an individual, as her own person, or are all of the students with deafness lumped together, as one mass composite? Teachers and other staff have the tendency to have one particular student in mind, and then define all students with deafness that way. Or, when there is more than one student who is deaf in the mainstream class at a given grade level, those students are often so closely identified together that it is easy for their individual identities to be lost. Teacher recognition of individual characteristics, preferences, skills, and needs is important to each student. And the teacher's attitude influences the other students' attitudes as well. Students with deafness want to be valued for who they are.

How the classroom teacher uses the interpreter in the classroom also sends a message. Teachers should talk to and face the student who is deaf, and not face the interpreter or say to the interpreter, "Tell him. . . ." Even if the teacher does not know sign language or cued speech (whichever the student uses), communication should still be face to face. Direct communication reflects an attitude of respect.

Consistent Expectations and Equitable Treatment. It is important that accepted school rules and behavior exist. A student who is deaf needs to know that he is responsible for his own actions, and the consequences are the same for him as for any student in the school. This not only influences the way the student who is deaf feels about herself as part of the school, but also how the hearing students perceive the situation: what exceptions are necessary because a student is deaf, by nature of the deafness, and what exceptions are not made, in terms of academic and social behavior.

There are, of course, accepted classroom accommodations that a student who is deaf will require. It is important for teachers to understand what these accommodations are and their importance. Teachers then need to transmit this understanding to the other students. Interpreters and notetakers are but two examples of these accommodations; they are services that may be vital to the student who is deaf in the mainstream and should be used appropriately.

For example, the interpreter should not be used as a disciplinarian for the student who is deaf alone or for the class as a whole. When the interpreter disciplines the student with deafness, he feels judged by the person who should be there to facilitate communication objectively. No one should feel they have their own personal "watchdog." When the interpreter is put in the position of responsibility for the whole class and disciplinary action results, the entire class resents the student who is deaf for needing to have that person in the class. The interpreter as a professional understands the role, but the teacher must understand it, too, for inappropriate use of the interpreter can greatly affect the way the student with deafness perceives his place in that classroom.

It is equally important not to be overly accommodating. Special treatment, while at some level may seem enticing, in fact works against what deaf students are looking for in the classroom, which is acceptance and appreciation. When a student who is deaf gets undue preferential treatment it can build resentment among the hearing

students in the classroom. For example, a student with deafness should not be exempt from staying after school as punishment because he may live a great distance from school and needs to catch the bus to get home. Academic and behavioral standards should be the same for the entire class, and the student who is deaf needs to know that he must follow the same rules.

It is also helpful for a student who is deaf to know that he is not the only student who may get "pulled out" of class to work with a resource teacher or other specialist. It is often a revelation for a student who is deaf to realize that hearing students may also be pulled out of class for a different kind of resource or speech support. It may be psychologically beneficial in the design of a school to have these support personnel, for both students who are deaf and hearing, located in proximity to one another. These attitudes of respect and equality contribute to a student's feelings of acceptance and belonging.

Student Skills

There are strategies and activities that may be used directly through teaching techniques or indirectly through attitudes that can make a difference in not only academic performance in the classroom, but also how a student with deafness perceives himself in a mainstream setting. The focus here is on the instructional program, and the roles of the speech or communication specialist, and the resource (or itinerant) teacher. We often see what Reich et al[15] found: the more available and the better quality of the support services, the better the self-concept of the student. Through this instructional support, the academic, social-emotional, and physical components of a student's self-image are addressed.

Speech and Communication Skills. The words and the body language (including facial expression) that teachers choose are often a reflection of their attitude toward the student who is deaf with whom they work. This may be especially true for the person responsible for speech teaching, because how she deals with the child who is deaf, and the messages, direct or indirect, sent to the child are delicate yet very significant. In fact, in Montgomery County, we prefer the term "communication specialist," a departure from "speech teacher," putting more emphasis on overall communication skill development and not only on speech.

Development of oral and auditory skills present potentially the most difficult skill areas for a child with deafness. Although not a criterion for placement in a regular education classroom (in Montgomery County), it is often the one by which a child is judged by those unfamiliar with deaf people. The balance between communicating encouragement, praise, and realistic feedback can impact on the willingness of the child to continue to develop her skills, as well as the perception she has of herself. The idea of "making mistakes" or "not achieving a goal" puts the student's work in a negative light, one that may build a barrier to further work and successes. Honesty and realism are critical in this area, but they need to be put in a constructive light: you are deaf, and this may mean limits, but it does not mean you make mistakes or fail. One communication specialist puts it very simply: " 'Limit' is a place to go, not a place to stop."[16]

The communication specialist may focus on reviewing current vocabulary and content with respect to pronunciation (or speech approximation), speechreading, or audition, whichever skills are appropriate for the particular student. Related to less academic activities, the communication specialist may review the rhythm, lyrics, or signs for a musical performance, or go over the Boy Scout oath or the Pledge of Allegiance. This kind of reinforcement gives the student more comfort and confidence with the material, and a sense of "owning" the terminology.

Another area of focus is the oral presentations that are required in some classes. The communication specialist works closely with the student, the teacher, and the interpreter to make this a positive and successful activity. It is also relevant to the issue of respect, as the student is not "required" to use his voice or speech. Not every student who is deaf feels comfortable using his voice in everyday classroom situations or formal presentations. The staff works with students to learn how to use visual aids effectively, and how to use the interpreter appropriately and effectively. Of course, for students who do want to speak for themselves, the communication specialist will review the presentation and give feedback regarding the rate, rhythm, etc., that will help that student be more intelligible and successful in this classroom endeavor.

The student who is deaf needs to realize his own areas of strength and areas of need and learn how to accommodate for himself. The goal is to maximize all of the student's communication skills, enabling him to feel more comfortable and confident with his communication in the mainstream classroom.

Audiology. The need for and the use of amplification relates to the physical domain of self-image. Deafness itself is not a visible disability, but hearing aids and the FM auditory trainer make it visible. This is an area that becomes a more sensitive issue as the student who is deaf gets older. With advances in technology, this kind of equipment has become smaller in size, and the hearing aids and auditory trainers of today are much smaller and more "acceptable" than in years past. But that still does not make it easy for a child or adolescent to accept wearing them.

At the elementary level, having an in-service program, as mentioned previously, can be effective for educating the hearing students in the mainstream about audiological equipment, while helping the student who is deaf try to have a more positive and accepting outlook. The in-service teaching should be done with respect for and in cooperation with the deaf student, in the effort to recruit the student and build up his ego in this area. Suggested resources for a student in-service program are listed in Appendix A. Reviewing the equipment is basic, but it is in the explanation of what the equipment can and cannot do that there is an opportunity for the student who is deaf to see a positive response from his classmates, as occurred for Timmy in Case study 19–5. It is one experience that can bring this equipment into a positive light for the student with deafness.

Using the analogy of the hearing aid and a radio is an effective strategy. A radio can be tuned in to a station, and different volumes can make it too hard to hear (too soft) or too distorted (too loud). Then if the tuner is moved in between stations, it is too fuzzy, and turning up the volume does not make it better. It can be very meaningful for a student who is deaf to see looks of frustration and confusion on the faces of his classmates, as they begin to comprehend and empathize. These are feelings that may not have been previously attributed to students who are hearing. It makes a strong connection on a very human level.

As a student who is deaf enters adolescence, "looking like everyone else" becomes so much more important, which is true in the development of self-concept for all children. One thing that has had a somewhat positive effect at the upper elementary and middle school grades is the newer, "behind the ear" FM system. The less visible and noticeable the apparatus is, the more likely a student is to admit that he finds it beneficial and will use it. This can also be

Case study 19–5. Timmy is in the second grade and has been in the mainstream for the past year. He has a difficult time accepting his auditory trainer, and often refuses to wear it. To start off this school year, his communication specialist went into his classroom to explain hearing loss and the audiological equipment that the students wear. She worked with Timmy ahead of time, to let him know what she would discuss, and see if he had any questions or concerns.

Initially, Timmy was not very enthusiastic about this activity. However, as the communication specialist explained that the FM trainer is wireless and can transmit as far as the length of a football field, even through walls (even when the teacher is out in the hall, or in the bathroom), Timmy was surprised to hear the other students exclaim, "That's cool!" and "Can I listen?"

Timmy's feelings changed from embarrassment to pride. He enjoyed "showing off" his equipment and giving other students a chance to listen through his hearing aids. This activity helped him feel more accepting of his need for amplification. He was more willing to wear his equipment and even willing to admit that it helps him.

enhanced by having opportunities to meet older students and adults who are deaf and who may have similarly rejected audiological equipment as a younger student, but perhaps returned to an FM system in college. The goal is to put it in a perspective of usefulness and benefit, with the student being his own advocate for optimum amplification.

Academic Skills. Just as supporting academic skills is important at home, it is even more the business of school. The resource teacher works directly with the student with deafness with the goal of helping him develop the skills to become a stronger student in the mainstream. The stronger and more confident she feels, the more she will perform to his potential and feel good about herself. This may include development or refinement of the following areas that may be challenging for a student with deafness: concept and vocabulary skills, written English skills, higher order thinking skills, organizational and study skills, communication skills, and interpersonal and social skills. These skills impact on learning in all of the content and related areas.

The focus is on building a level of comfort with the information, language, and vocabulary being presented in class for the student. The student needs to feel confident with the work and expectations of the teacher in order to feel more willing to participate appropriately in class. In addition to the internal feelings of success, there will more likely be recognition from classmates of achievement and "sameness," ideally leading to more acceptance of the deaf student.

Social Opportunities. In a mainstream setting, social acceptance can be a challenge to a student with deafness. Providing a variety of social opportunities within the parameters of the school day can be valuable and should include opportunities for interaction with both hearing and deaf classmates.

Within the mainstream class, the way the teacher arranges the seating or the class groupings can impact on the student with deafness. For example, sometimes students are allowed to choose their own seats, but a deaf student may not, and is instead always assigned to the same seat in the front of the room. Although the front of the room is certainly preferable for a student who is deaf, there are choices even within that parameter, and perhaps giving the student some say as to where he sits gives him some control over his environment, and in his social arrangements. For small group work or pairings (as in cooperative learning strategies), not always having the students with deafness together (if there is more than one in a class) can expand the social opportunities within a very structured situation.

Resource teachers or communication specialists may even allow the student who is deaf to choose a classmate who is hearing to join an occasional session. These opportunities provide the student who is deaf a chance to work with other students, to get to know each other as a peer.

Conversely, it is also important for a student with deafness in a mainstream setting to have opportunities to interact with friends who are deaf, whether in the classroom, in the resource room, or during the social times of the day, such as lunch and recess. A student who is deaf expends a lot of energy and effort attending and communicating in the regular education classroom, often through an interpreter. There is an ease of communication that exists between friends who are deaf, and that time and experience allows the student to relax and recharge.

Pragmatic Skills. Students need to develop the necessary and appropriate interpersonal and social skills. These skills can be developed with assistance from either the communication specialist or the resource teacher. One program,

"POWER to Communicate (Practicing Oral and Written Expression Regularly)"[17] is an integrated curriculum developed for the regular education program in Montgomery County, and has been used effectively with students with deafness. It provides a vehicle for working on effective conflict resolution strategies while developing written expression skills, a unique blend of strengthening both the academic and interpersonal. Another resource, a pragmatics checklist,[18] developed by the county's communication specialists specifically for students who are deaf is outlined in Appendix B. This compilation is designed to take a student from preschool through high school and develop the relevant and necessary pragmatic skills at each level. Much attention was given to the skills necessary for working in a mainstream classroom, as well as those for functioning successfully in society. In conjunction with this checklist, at the secondary level, students go out into the community to practice and refine these important skills. The goal is to maximize all of the student's skills, enabling her to feel more comfortable and confident in the classroom, and more prepared to become a positive and productive member of society—pointing to an enhanced self-image.

SUMMARY

The self-image of a student with deafness in a mainstream setting can be positively developed and enhanced by the people and experiences in two important environments: home and school.

At home, parents can positively influence the self-image of their child with deafness by understanding and accepting deafness, by continually developing their own communication skills, and by being a partner in the school team. Parents also play a major role in helping their child develop confidence and competence by building and reinforcing language and social skills.

At school, the overall awareness and understanding by the school administration and personnel, staff and students will greatly impact on how the student perceives himself. A mainstream program that values the students who are deaf in the school as individuals promotes greater understanding of deafness, fosters the development of appropriate communication skills, and works to develop constructive and positive teacher attitudes. Students with deafness will develop healthy, positive self-concepts when they have confidence in their own skills and feel acceptance from others through a variety of social opportunities, effective training in the areas of academics, communication, and pragmatics, and through meaningful interaction with a variety of individuals who are deaf.

Although there is no one answer to the complex issue of enhancing the self-image of students with deafness in a mainstream setting, the ideas presented and discussed here represent an overview of strategies that have proved effective in the Programs for Students Who Are Deaf and Hard of Hearing in Montgomery County, Maryland. The underlying message found in all of the strategies is understanding, acceptance and respect; this is what any program, mainstream or residential, should embrace.

APPENDIX A

In-Service Materials and Resources

Ear Gear—A Student Workbook on Hearing Aids
Carole Bugosh Simko
Gallaudet University Press
Washington, DC

Wired for Sound
Carole Bugosh Simko
Gallaudet University Press
Washington, DC

Hearing Aids for You and the Zoo
Richard Stoker and Janine Gaydos
AG Bell Association for the Deaf
Washington, DC

What Is an Audiogram?
Venita Gragg
Gallaudet University Press
Washington, DC

Let's Learn about Deafness
Rachel Stone
Gallaudet University Pre-College Programs
Washington, DC

How They Hear
RCA Victor
Gordon Stowe Associates
Custon Records Department
Northbrook, IL

Hearing Aid Demonstration
AV Resources
Minneapolis, MN

Using Your TTY/TDD
An Educational Videotape
Telecommunications for Deaf and Sign
  Media
Burtonsville, MD

APPENDIX B

Pragmatics Checklist

I.   Deaf culture
A. Define culture
B. Compare and contrast to other cultures
C. American Sign Language and its history
D. Who is a member of the deaf culture
E. Values and beliefs; experiences and customs
F. Civil rights and political organizations
G. Social organizations for the deaf; clubs
H. Gallaudet University
I. MCPS Deaf Culture Club

II. Deaf awareness
A. Exposure to other deaf children
B. Have pictures of children with hearing aids
C. Exposure to variety of older children and adults
D. Discuss audiology, assistive devices, and interpreting; communication approaches and skills
E. Mainstream in-service: include communication strategies and interpersonal protocols

III. Historical perspectives of deafness
A. History of deaf in ancient civilizations
B. History of the education of the deaf
C. History of the education of the deaf in the United States, including communication controversies
D. Deaf president NOW organization—1988 student protest

IV. Sound and hearing
A. Hearing: anatomy, audiology
B. Hearing aids: types, parts, care, potentials/limitations

V.   Social/interpersonal communication
A. Nonverbal communication: body and facial expression
B. Listening/attending skills
C. Spoken communication
D. Verbal communication
E. Conversational skills
F. Social communication

VI. Communication devices and support services
A. Telephone

B. Conversational skills and etiquette
C. Related skills: operator, information, emergencies
D. TDD calls/assistive devices/services
E. Assistive services, including TEDI (relay)
F. Assistive devices: decoders, flashing lights, alarms

VII. Situational topics
A. Safety
B. Community helpers
C. On the bus
D. Health room
E. Restaurants
F. Medical
G. Mainstream classes
H. Stores/shopping
I. Family meals
J. Celebrations
K. Summertime
L. Law/police
M. Job applications
N. College applications
O. Job applications
P. Job interviewing
Q. Banking
R. Transportation
S. Renting apartments/rooms
T. Budgeting

Adapted from *Pragmatics Checklist*[18]

REFERENCES

1. Berne PH: Seven secrets for building kid's self-esteem. *Instructor*, (1985), 63–65.
2. Marshall HH: The development of self-concept. *Young Children*, 44 (1989), 44–51.
3. Maxon A, Brackett D, van den Berg S: Self-perception of socialization: the effects of hearing status, age, and gender. *Volta Rev*, 93 (1991), 7–18.
4. Oblowitz N, Green L, Heyns I: A self-concept scale for the hearing-impaired. *Volta Rev*, 93 (1991), 19–29.
5. Yachnik M: Self-esteem in adolescents. *Am Ann Deaf*, 131 (1986), 305–310.
6. Meadow K: *Deafness and Child Development.* (Berkeley, CA: University Press, 1969).
7. McGinnis E, Goldstein AP with Sprafkin R, Gershaw NJ: *Skillstreaming the Elementary School Child: A Guide for Teaching Prosocial Skills* (Champaign, IL: Research Press, 1984).
8. Schwartz S: Psycho-Social Aspects of Mainstreaming, in Ross M, ed: *Hearing-Impaired Children in the Mainstream* (Parkton, MD: York Press, 1990).

9. Grimes VK, Prickett HT: Developing and enhancing a positive self-concept in deaf children. *Am Ann Deaf*, 133 (1988), 255–257.

10. Warren C, Hasenstab S: Self-concept of severely to profoundly hearing-impaired children. *Volta Rev*, 88 (1986), 289–295.

11. Leigh I: Parenting and the hearing impaired: attachment and coping. *Volta Rev*, 89 (1987), 11–21.

12. Krupp JA: Self-esteem: how do you feel about yourself? *Teaching PreK-8*, 21 (1991), 63–64.

13. Rich D: *MegaSkills—How Families Can Help Children Succeed in School and Beyond* (Boston: Houghton-Mifflin, 1988).

14. Burdette T: Personal Communication. Montgomery County Public Schools, 1993.

15. Reich C, Hambleton D, Houldin BK: The integration of hearing-impaired children in regular classrooms. *Am Ann Deaf*, 122 (1977), 534–543.

16. Flecker P: Personal communication. Montgomery County Public Schools, 1993.

17. Nordfiord G, Amann R: *POWER to Communicate* (Rockville, MD: Montgomery County Public Schools, 1991).

18. Fernandez JM, Smith J, Flecker P, Broe M, Kittleman R, Munshower C, Michael M, Smith R, Hunt F: *Pragmatics Checklist* (Rockville, MD: Programs for Students Who Are Deaf and Hard of Hearing, 1992).

INDEX